AF479135

CREATIVE BAGS

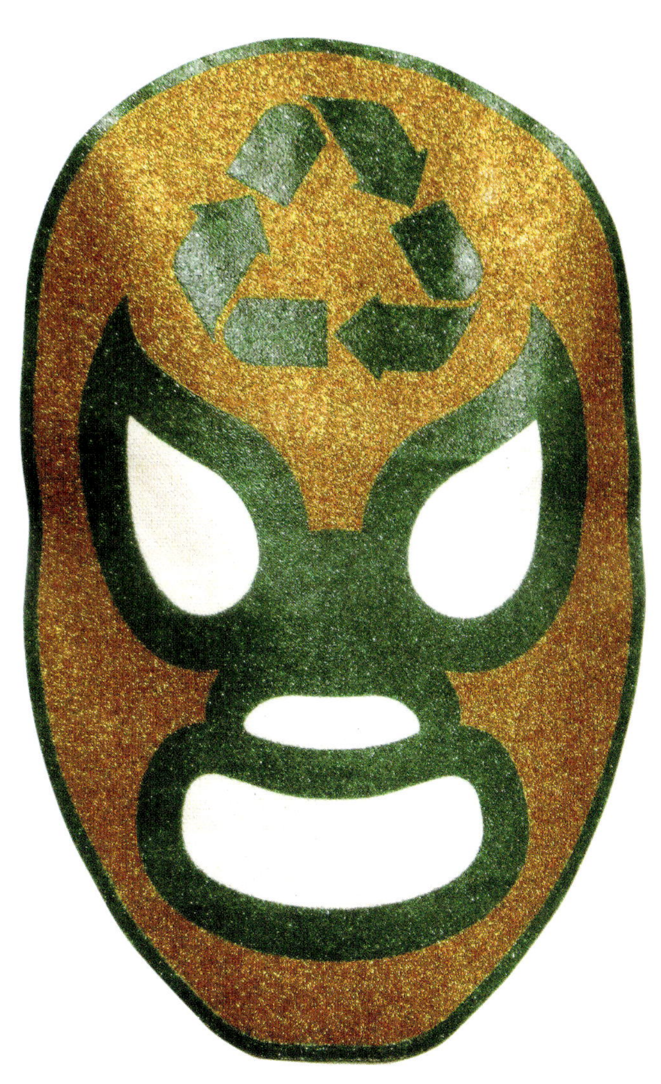

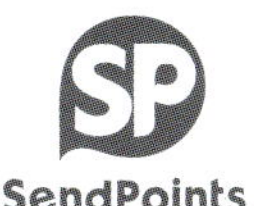

SendPoints

CREATIVE BAGS

© SendPoints Publishing Co., Ltd.

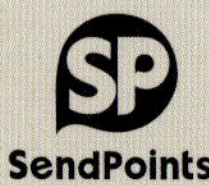

EDITED & PUBLISHED BY SendPoints Publishing Co., Ltd.
PUBLISHER: Lin Gengli
PUBLISHING DIRECTOR: Lin Shijian
EDITORIAL DIRECTOR: Sundae Li
EXECUTIVE EDITOR: Carmen Fong
ART DIRECTOR: Lin Shijian
EXECUTIVE ART EDITOR: Lin Qiumei
PROOFREADING: Sundae Li   Heart Fensch

ADDRESS: Room 15A Block 9 Tsui Chuk Garden, Wong Tai Sin, Kowloon, Hong Kong
TEL: +852-35832323 / **FAX:** +852-35832448
EMAIL: info@sendpoints.cn

DISTRIBUTED BY Guangzhou SendPoints Book Co., Ltd.
SALES MANAGER: Zhang Juan (China), Sissi (International)
GUANGZHOU: +86-20-89095121
BEIJING: +86-10-84139071
SHANGHAI: +86-21-63523469
EMAIL: overseas01@sendpoints.cn
WEBSITE: www.sendpoints.cn

ISBN 978-988-12943-5-7

In the bag design industry these days you will find an
increasing use of natural materials like, paper, wood,
leather and cardboard. The recycling of material is
a topic gaining more and more attention. It is about
reusing materials in an interesting way and telling the
story through the product of bag design. Many designers
are practitioners of these themes of sustainability and
take recycling as a spark for inspiration to develop
their own version of beautiful creative bags. Whether
it is graphic, spatial, multimedia, product design or
architecture, once an idea is physically placed into the
world, each design choice contributes to a sustainable
society. Sustainable design is a broad discipline: there
may be different strategies and there are many aspects in
the design where the focus may lie.

I believe as a designer, you are an important link in
the process of sustainable development. You can make
decisions with major implications for a product: how
it is made and what it does during use. In bag design,
sustainability is now truly happening.

Creative Bags, aims to present works that are as well
inspiring in design, usage of material or printed
patterns. You will find a great variety of beautiful bag
designs: Bags with unusual, bold material combinations,
like leather, wood, paper, textile used in different
ways. Moreover, a lot of shapes handling techniques are
visual in this book, such as braiding and incisions,
to create new 3D shapes, folding, carving, but the
traditional sewing can also see many good examples.

I hope you will enjoy this great book and be inspired.

Ilvy Jacobs
Bag Designer

BAGS

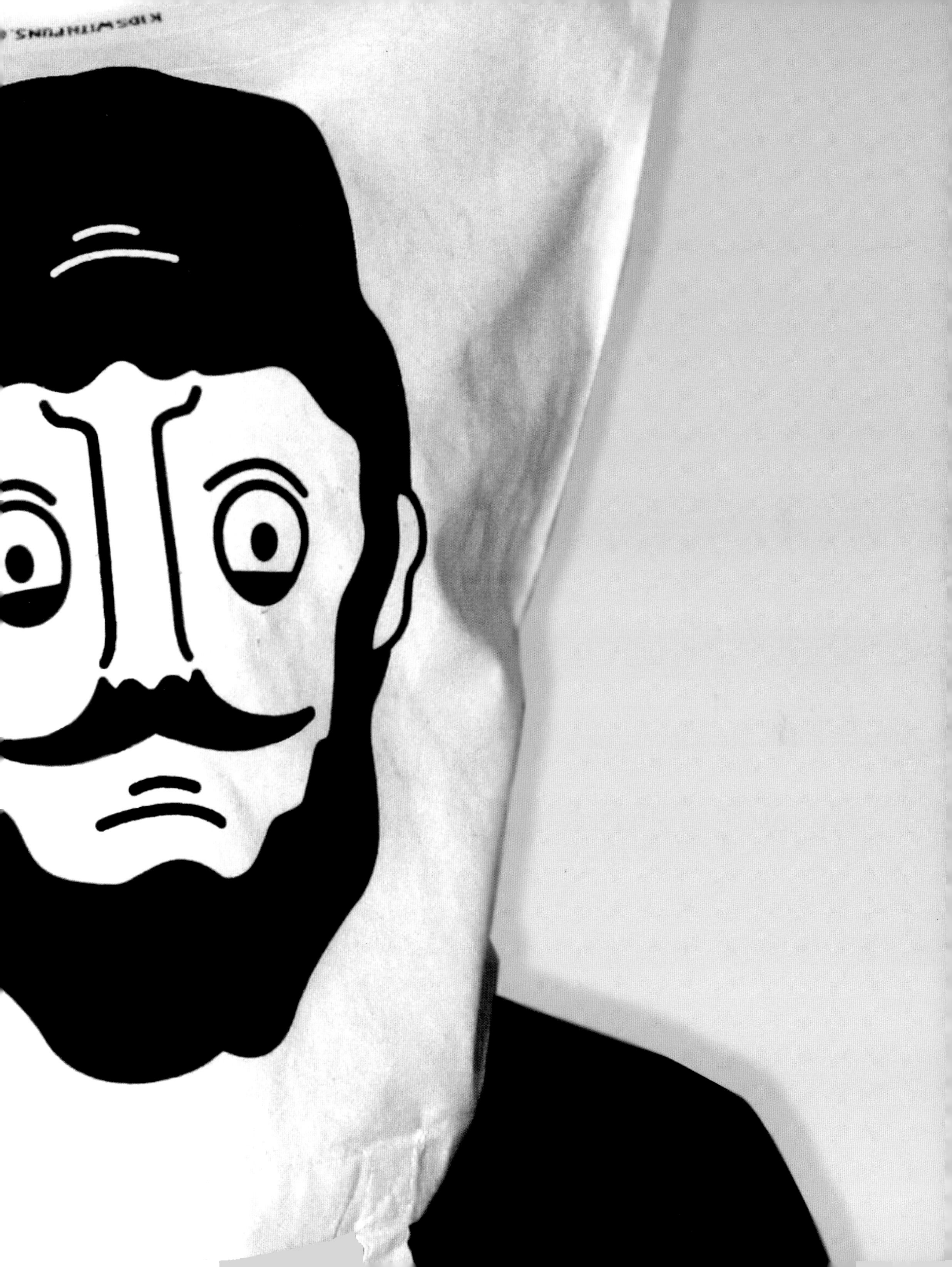

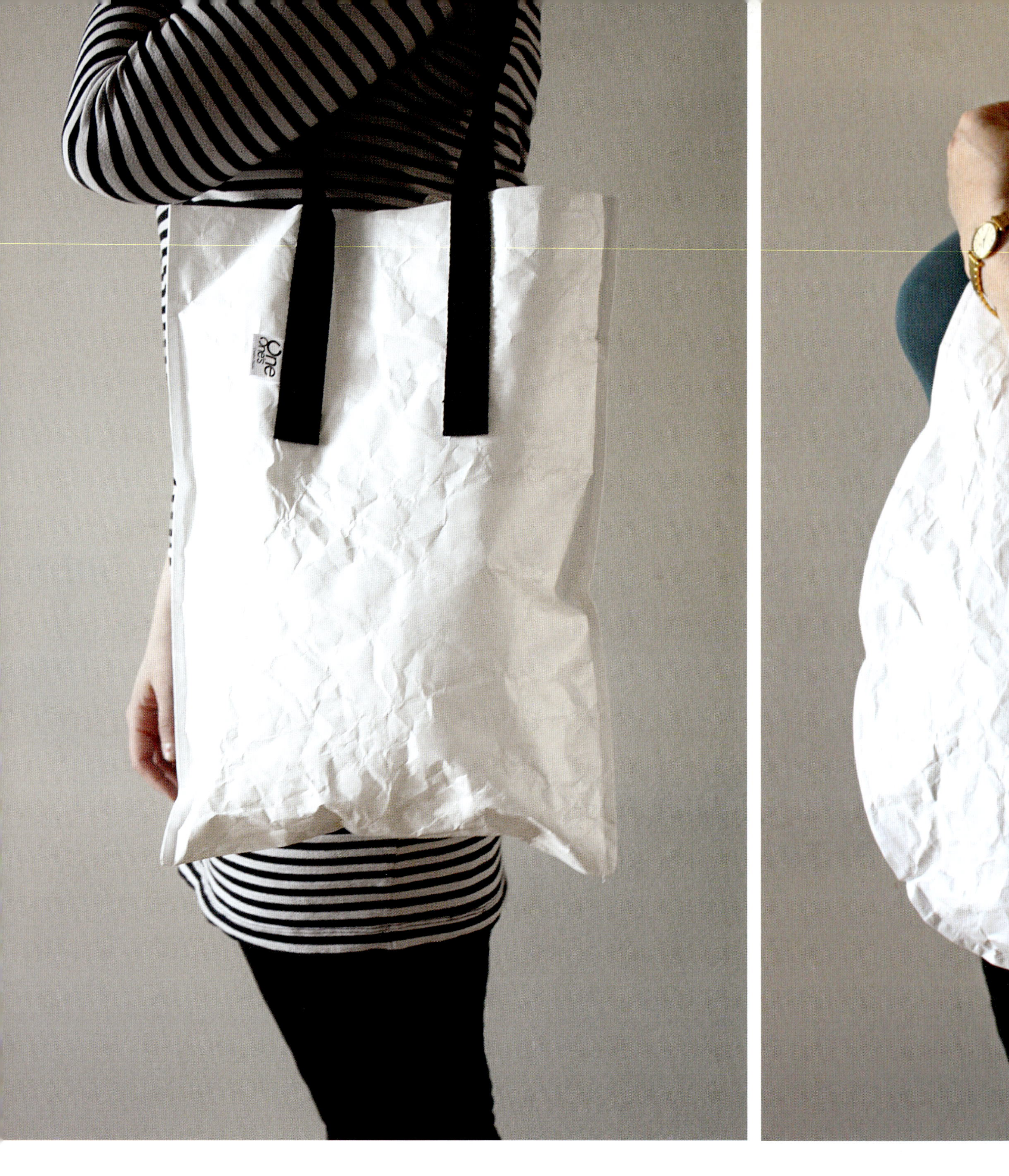

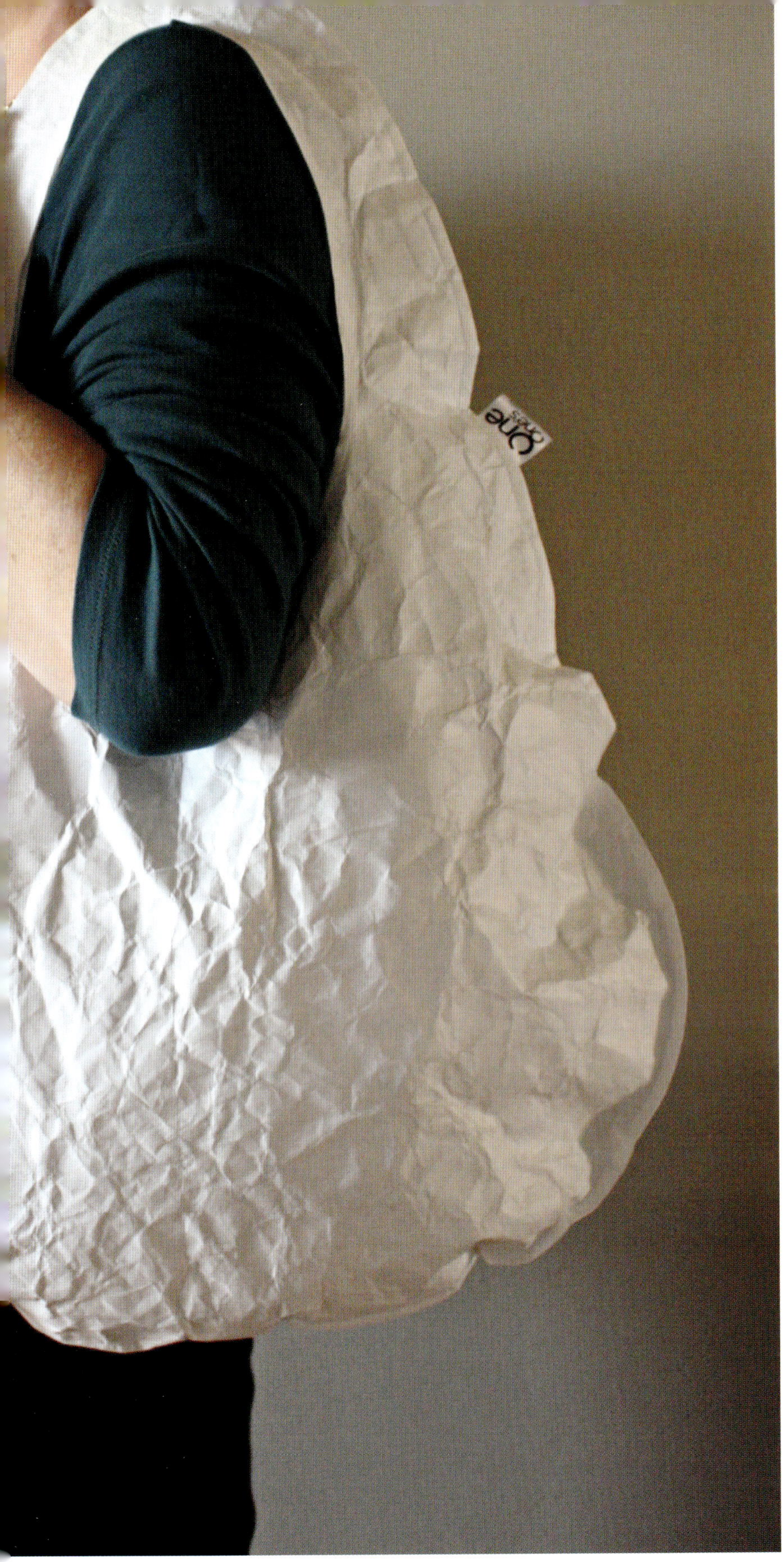

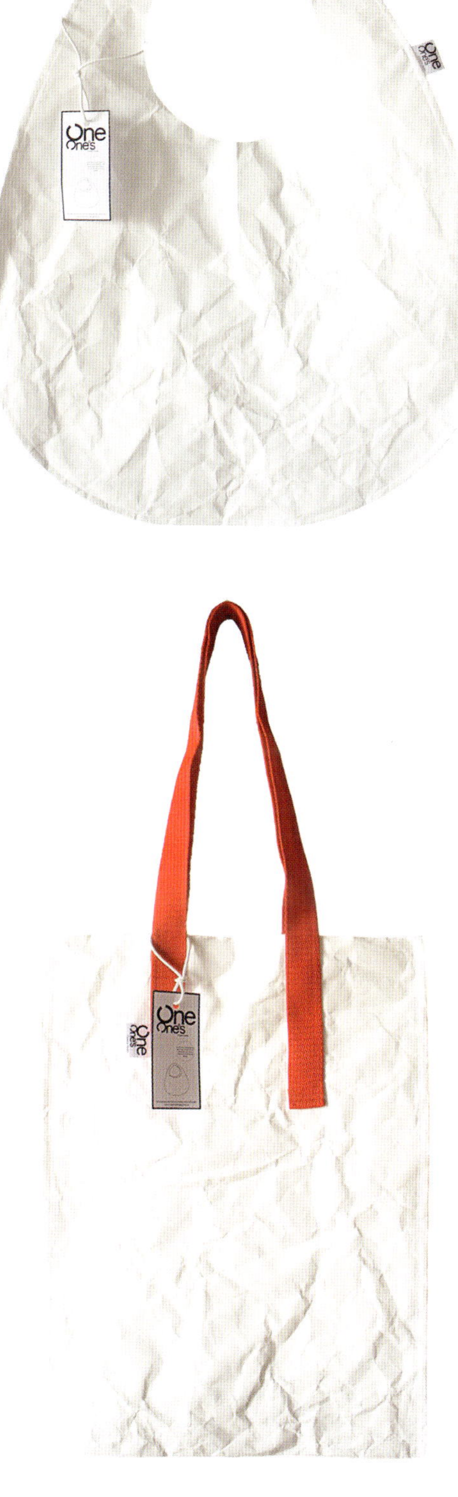

ONE'S BAG SERIES
DE: Dominika Jagiello (OneOnes Creative Studio)

Made of Tyvek, the "One's Bag" series has the look and texture of paper but is waterproof
and washable. The designs were left blank for users to draw on with markers.

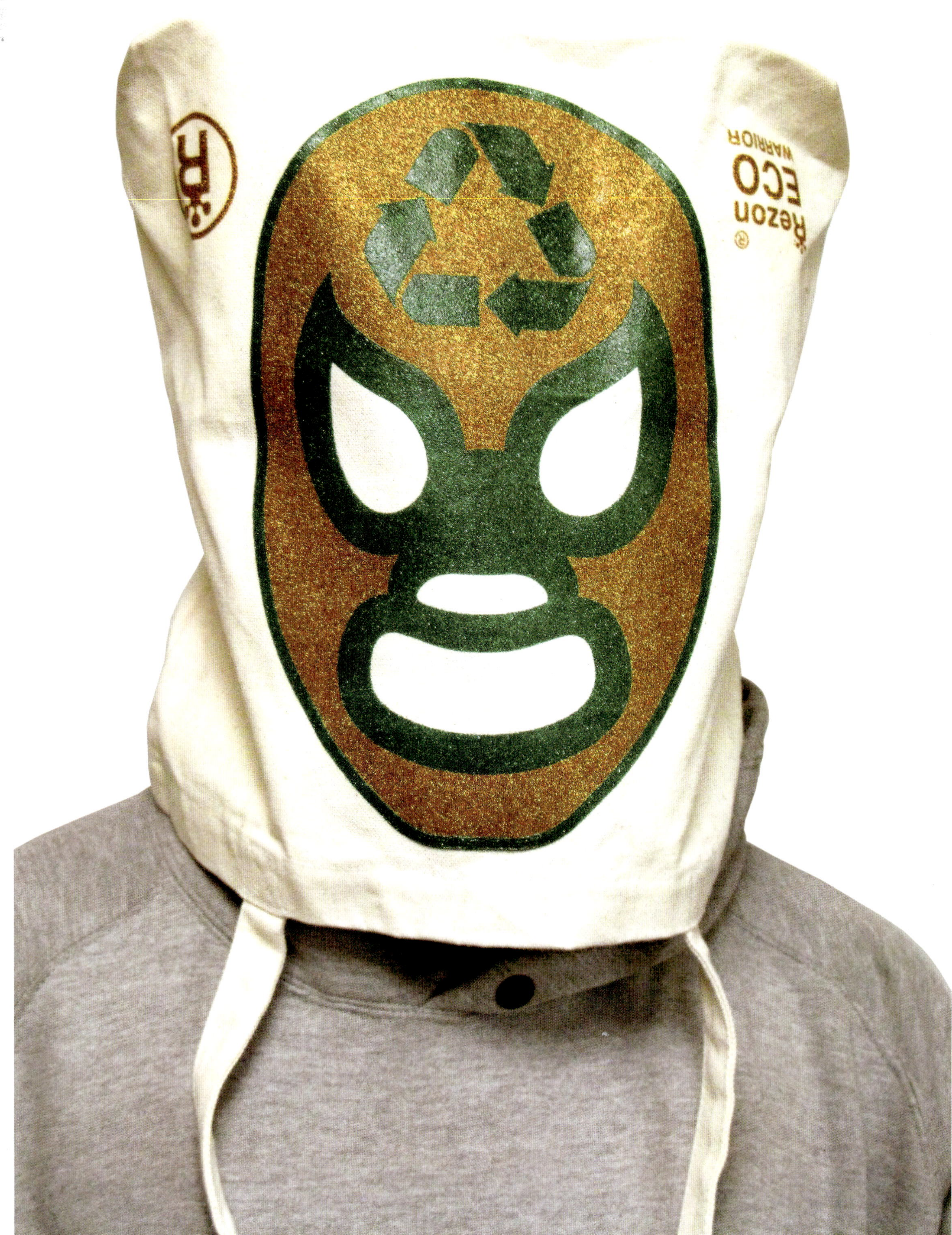

Rezon
ECO
WARRIOR

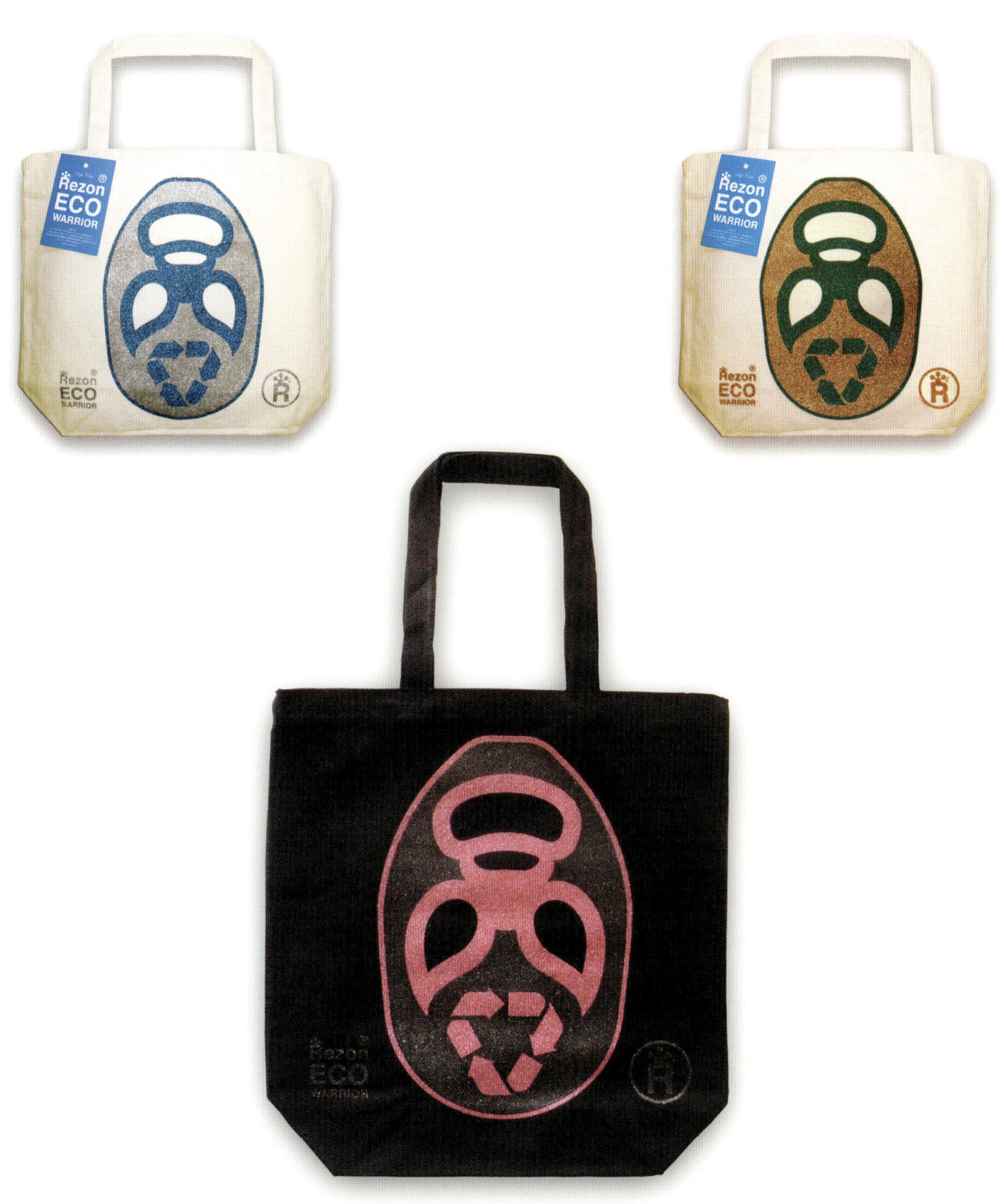

ECO WARRIOR BAG

DE: Hideo Kawamura

Printed with an upside-down mask, the "Eco Warrior" bag encourages people to
act like environment activists. The pattern was printed with metallic ink.

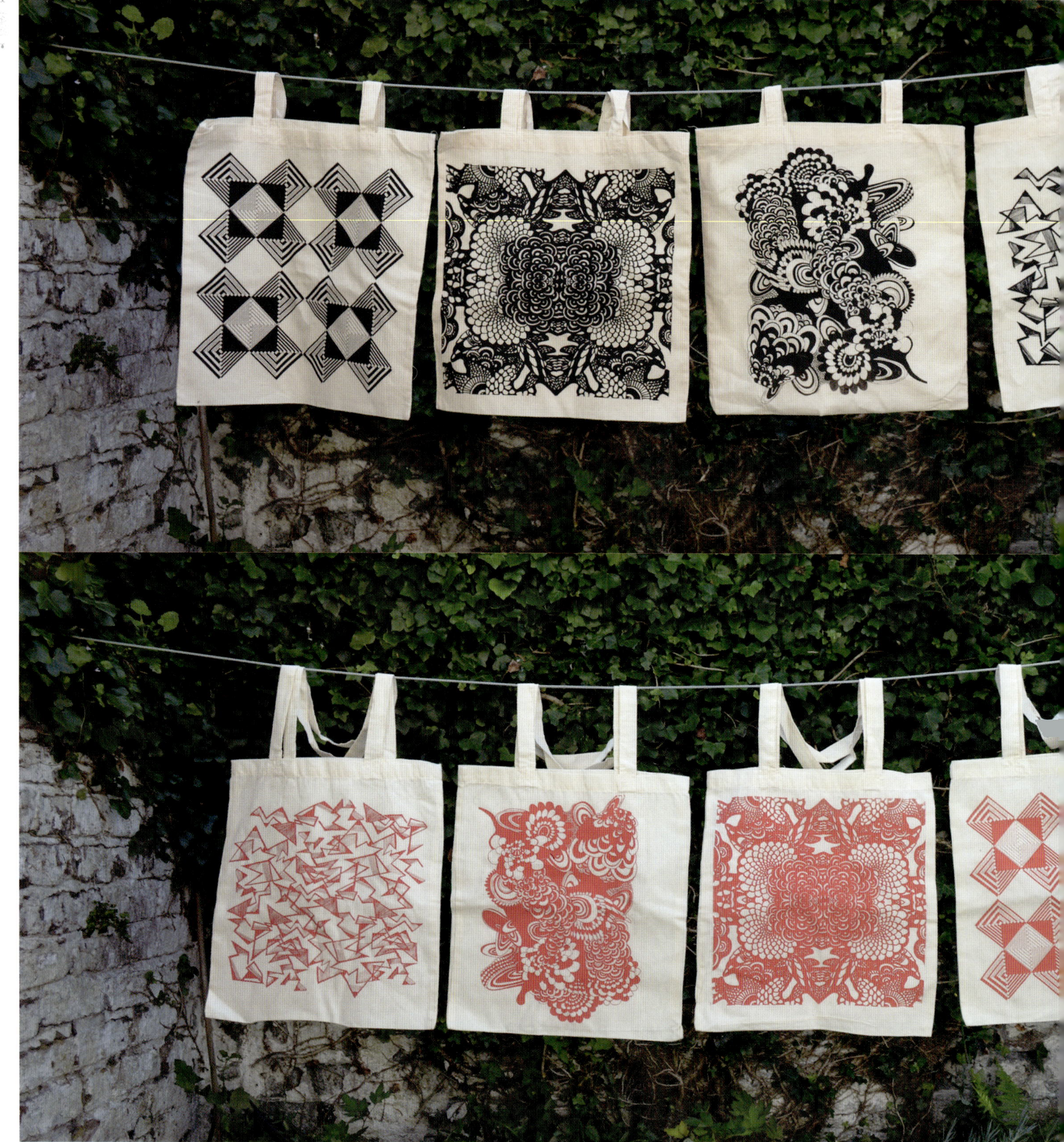

SCREEN-PRINTED CANVAS BAGS
DE: Petra Blahova

The designer printed patterns that were inspired by natural forms to promote
reusable bags and to remind people of the beautiful nature they are damaging
with the use of disposable bags.

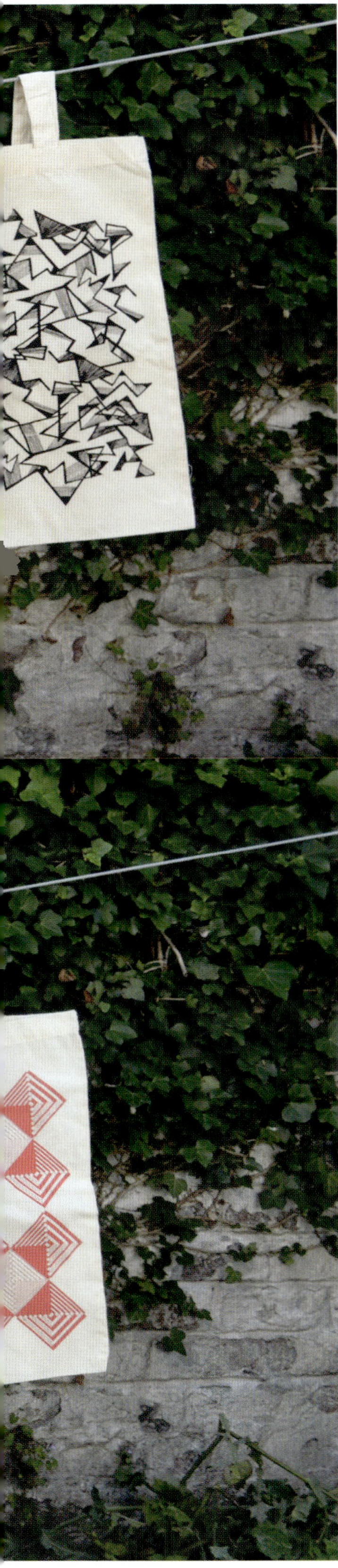

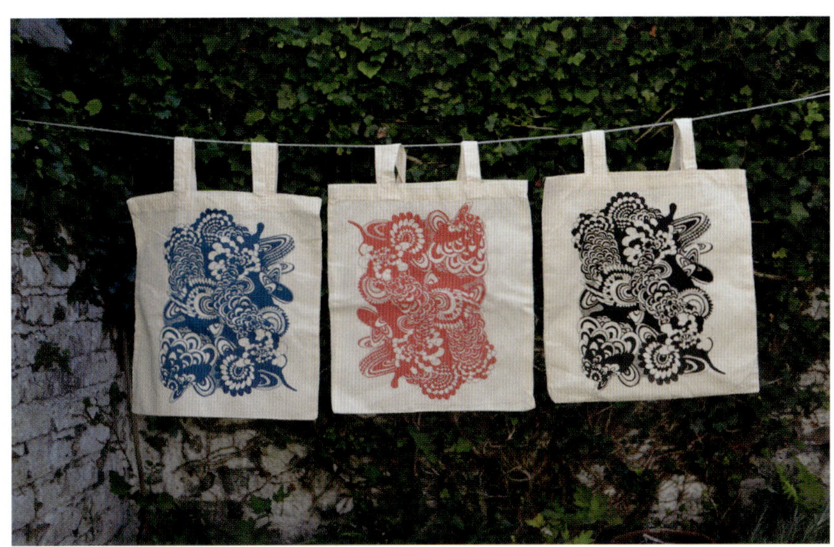

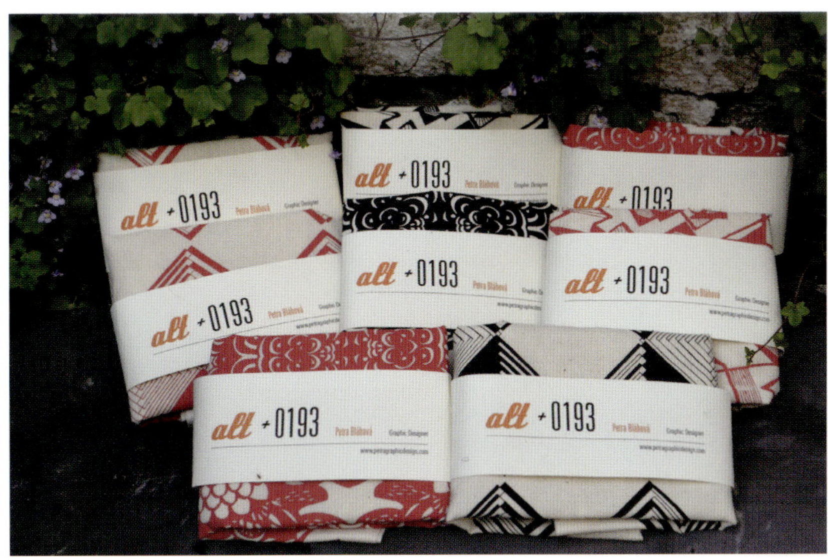

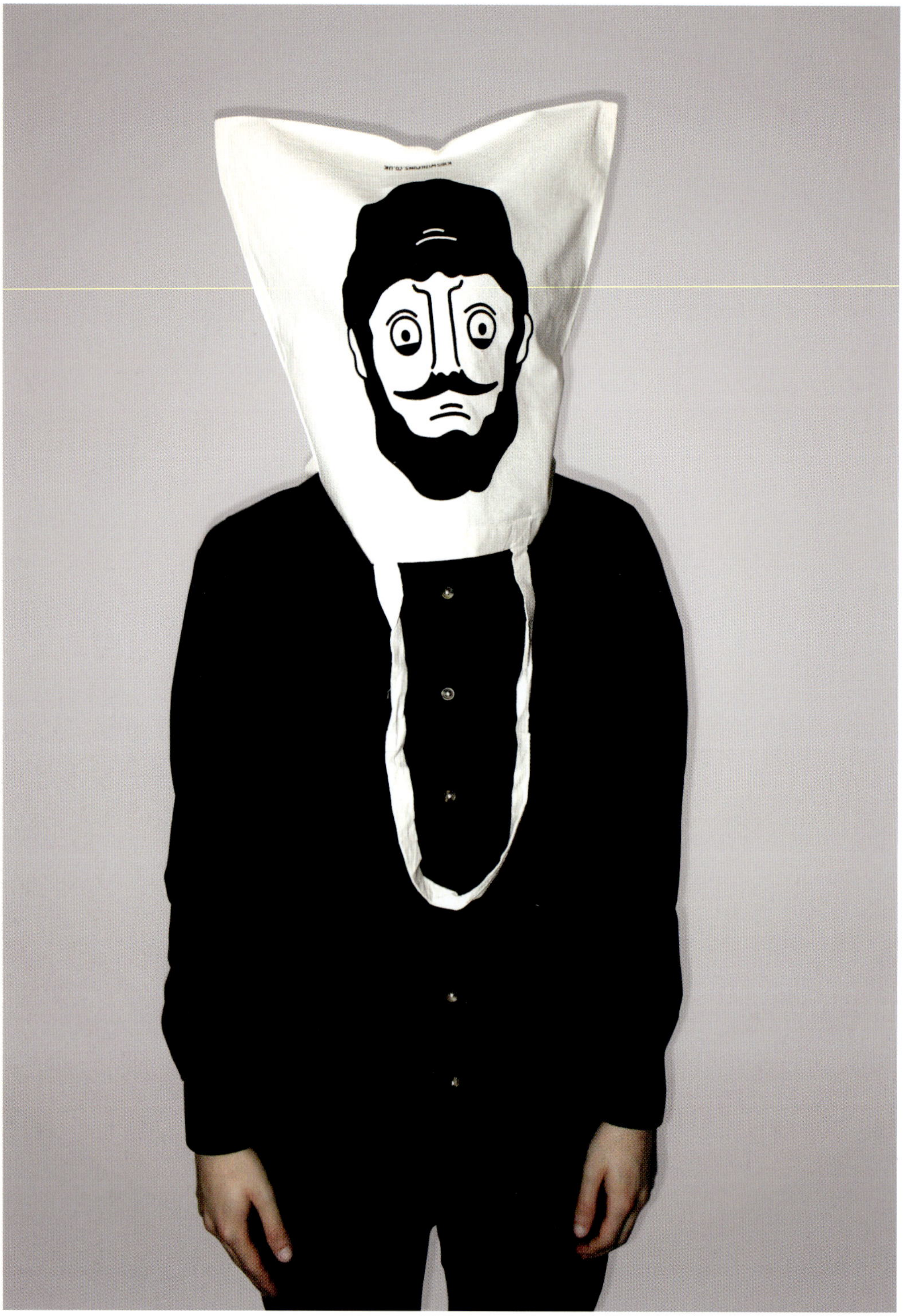

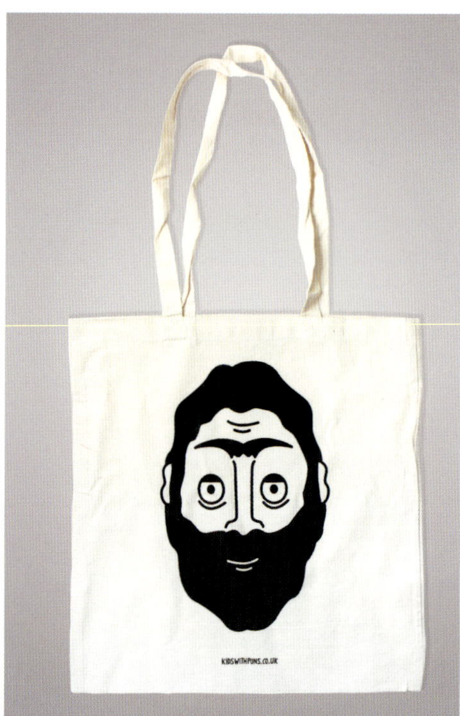

KIDSWITHPUNS.CO.UK

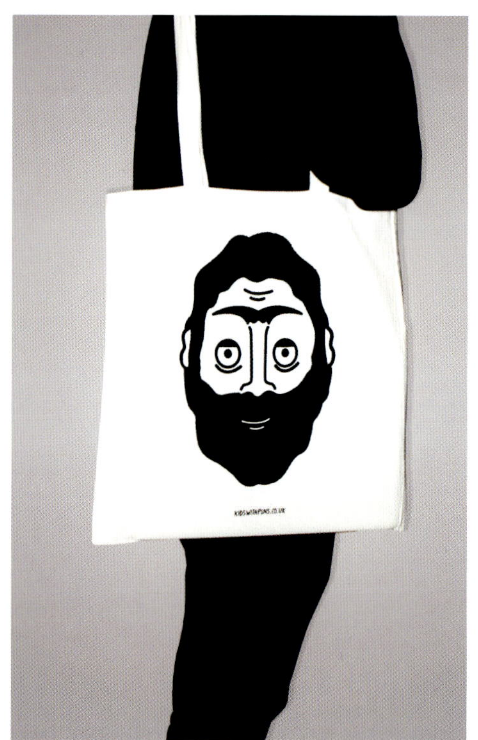

KIDSWITHPUNS.CO.UK

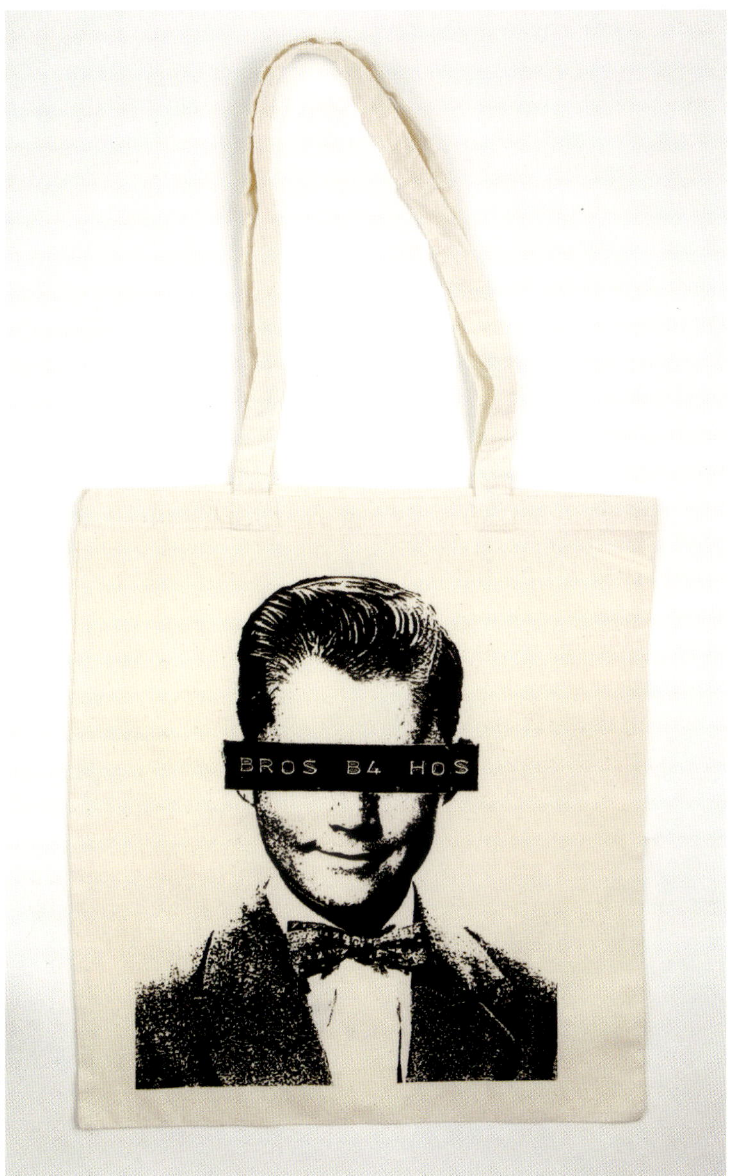

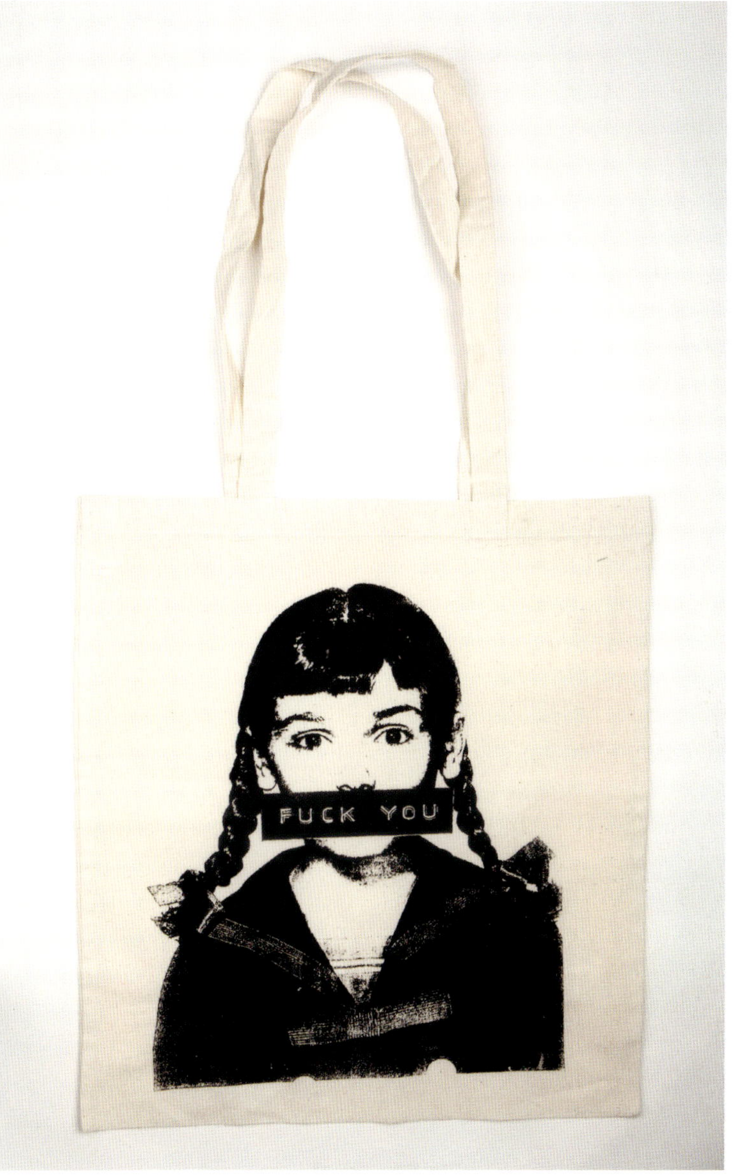

TWO FACED TOTE BAG
DA: Kids With Puns

Used as a promotional item for the Kids With Puns' publication, the bag
itself is a visual pun aiming to bring a smile to the recipient.

SCREEN PRINT TOTE
DE: Rosie Connell

Using screen printing technique, the designer created bags with portraits
using expressions or strong words to create a greater psychological impact.

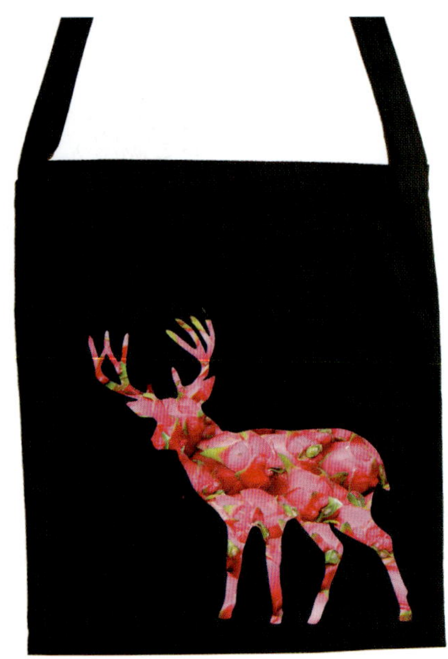
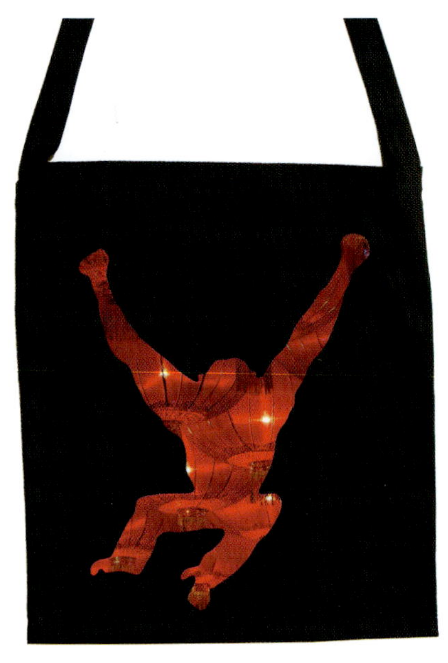
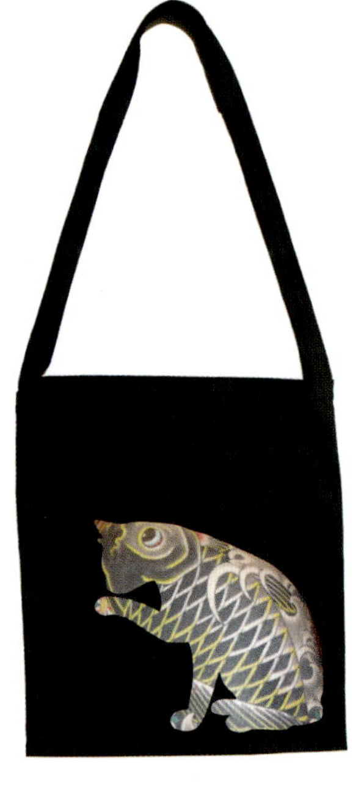
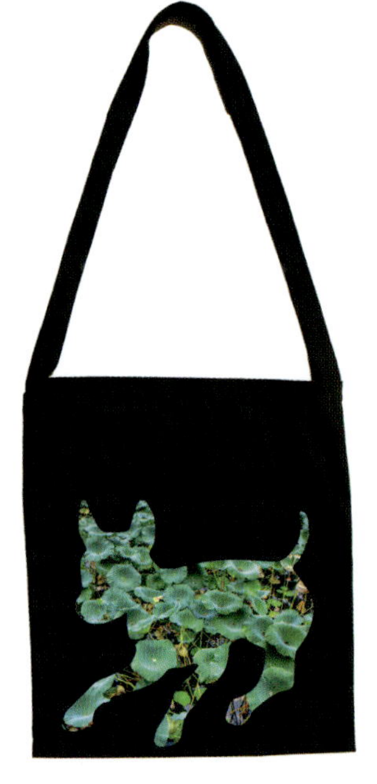
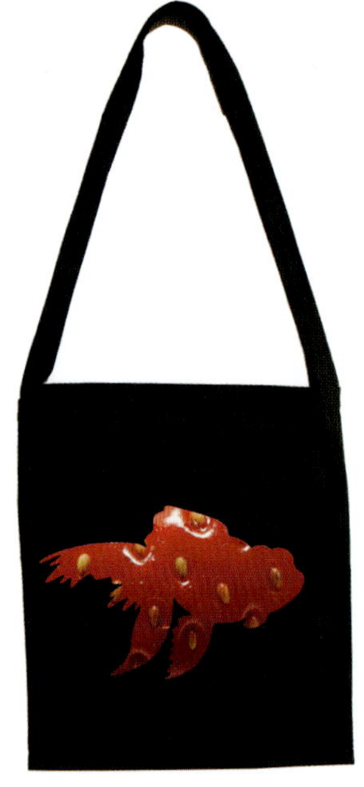
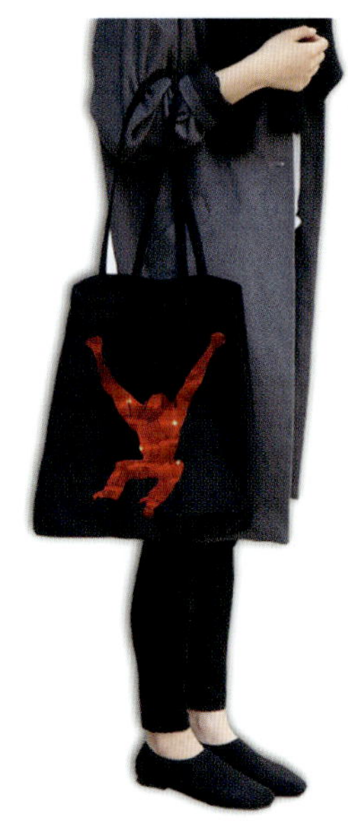

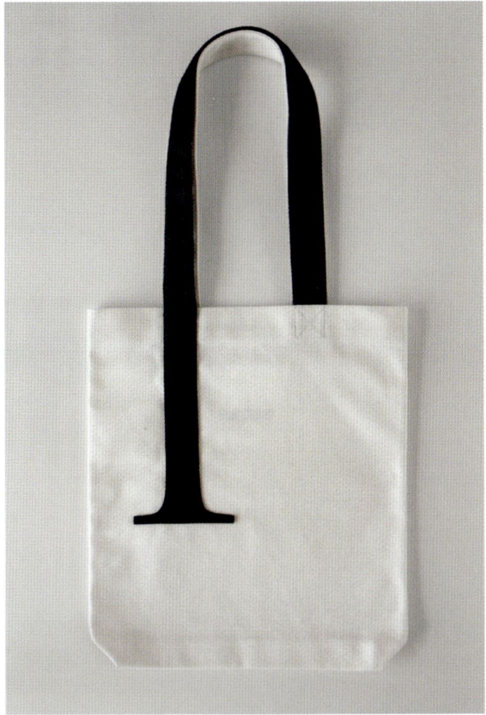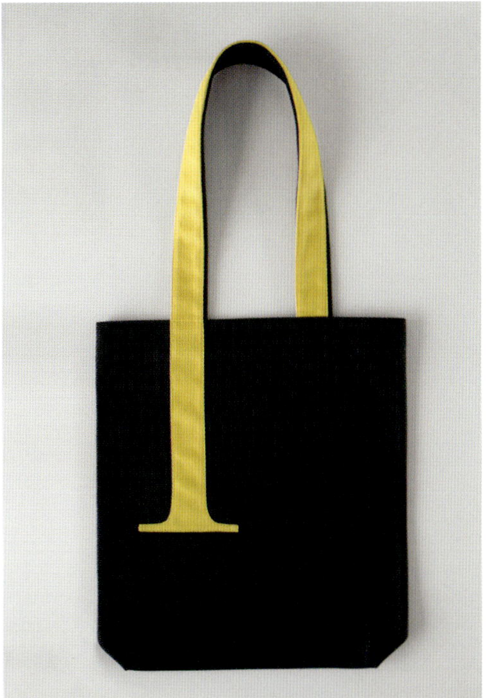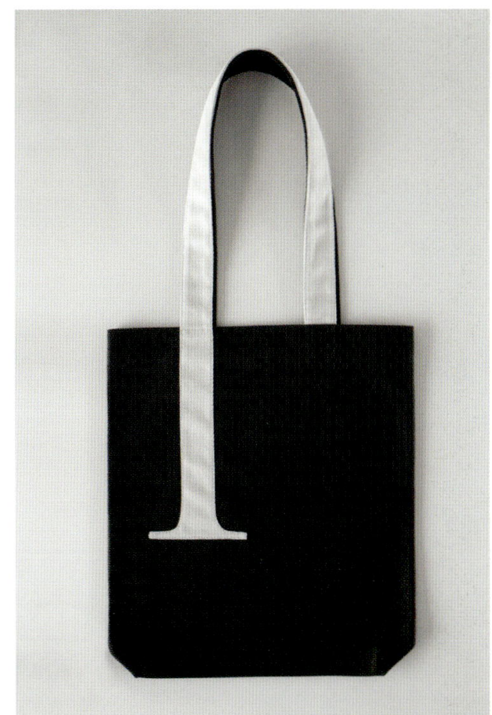
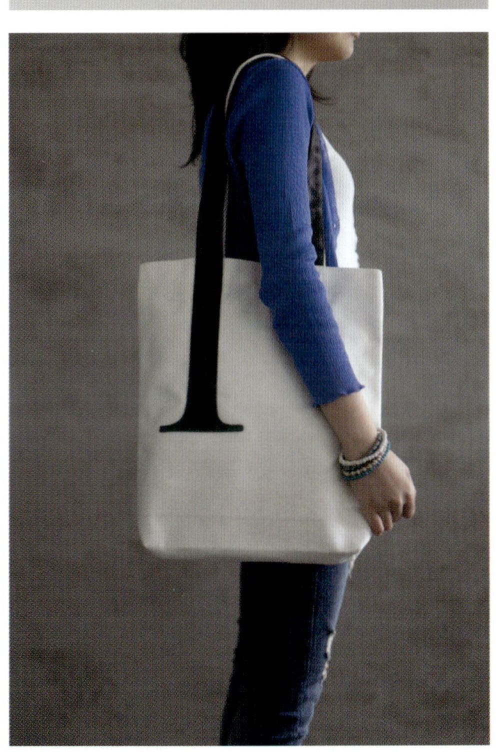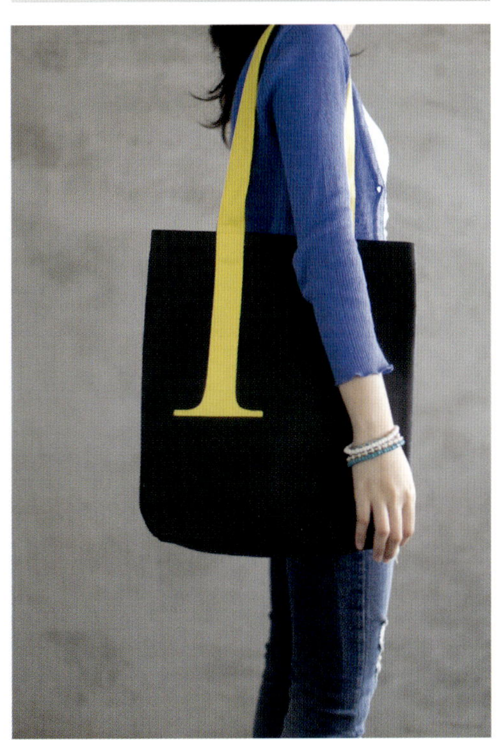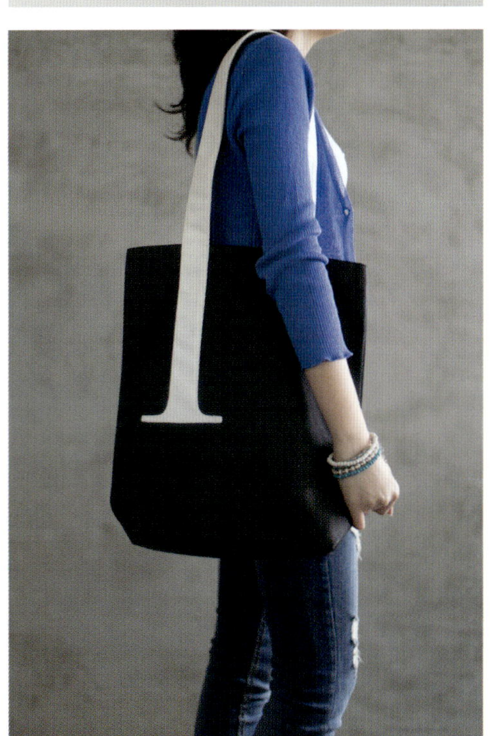

CANVAS BAGS
DA: Nono Muaks

This series was inspired by animal and the patterns of fruits and plants, and it combined the two. They have combinations like: deer-dragon fruit, fish-strawberry, dog-lotus, etc.

SERIF TOTE BAG
DA: Little Factory

Serif typefaces are characterized by the details on the ends of some strokes. The designer tried to apply those details to the tote bag design, with the straps extending to become the serif of the bag.

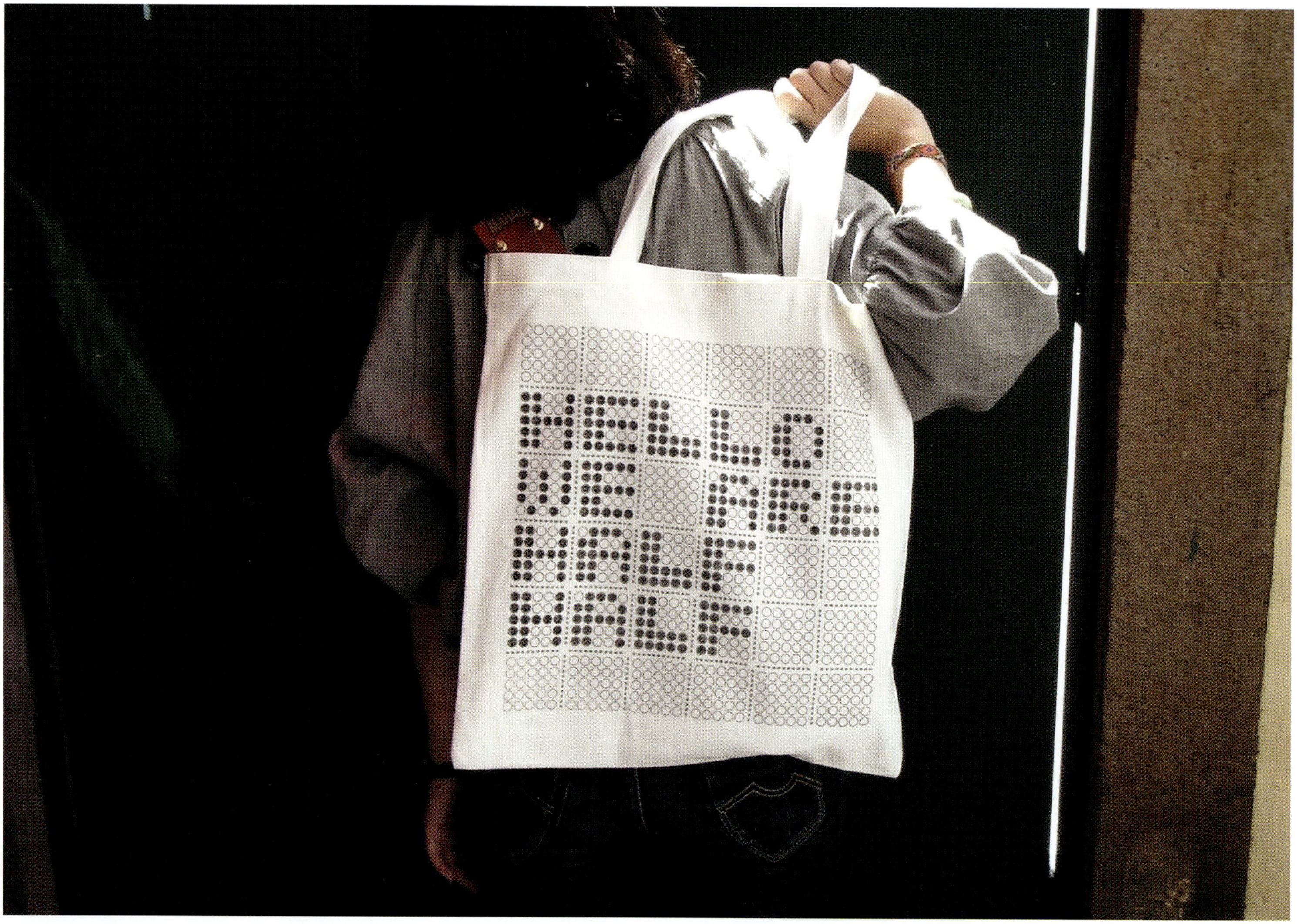

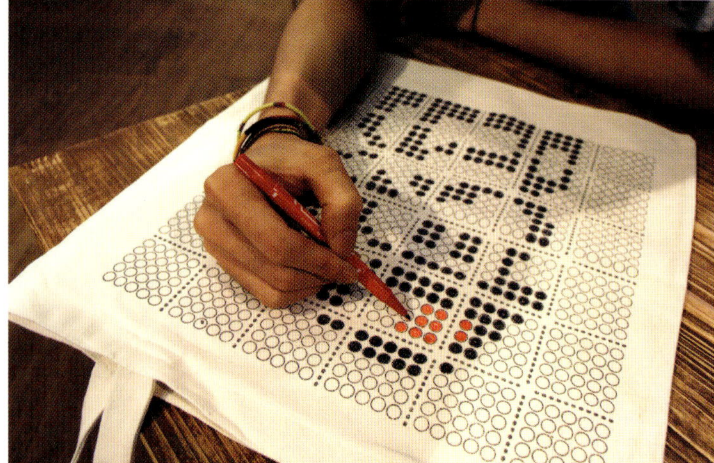 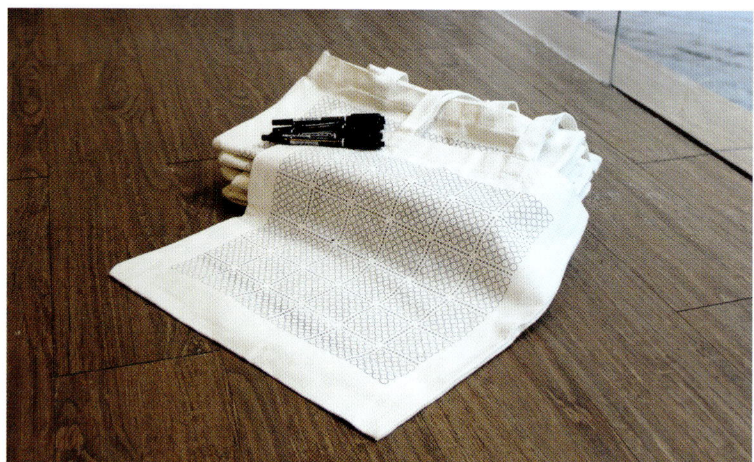

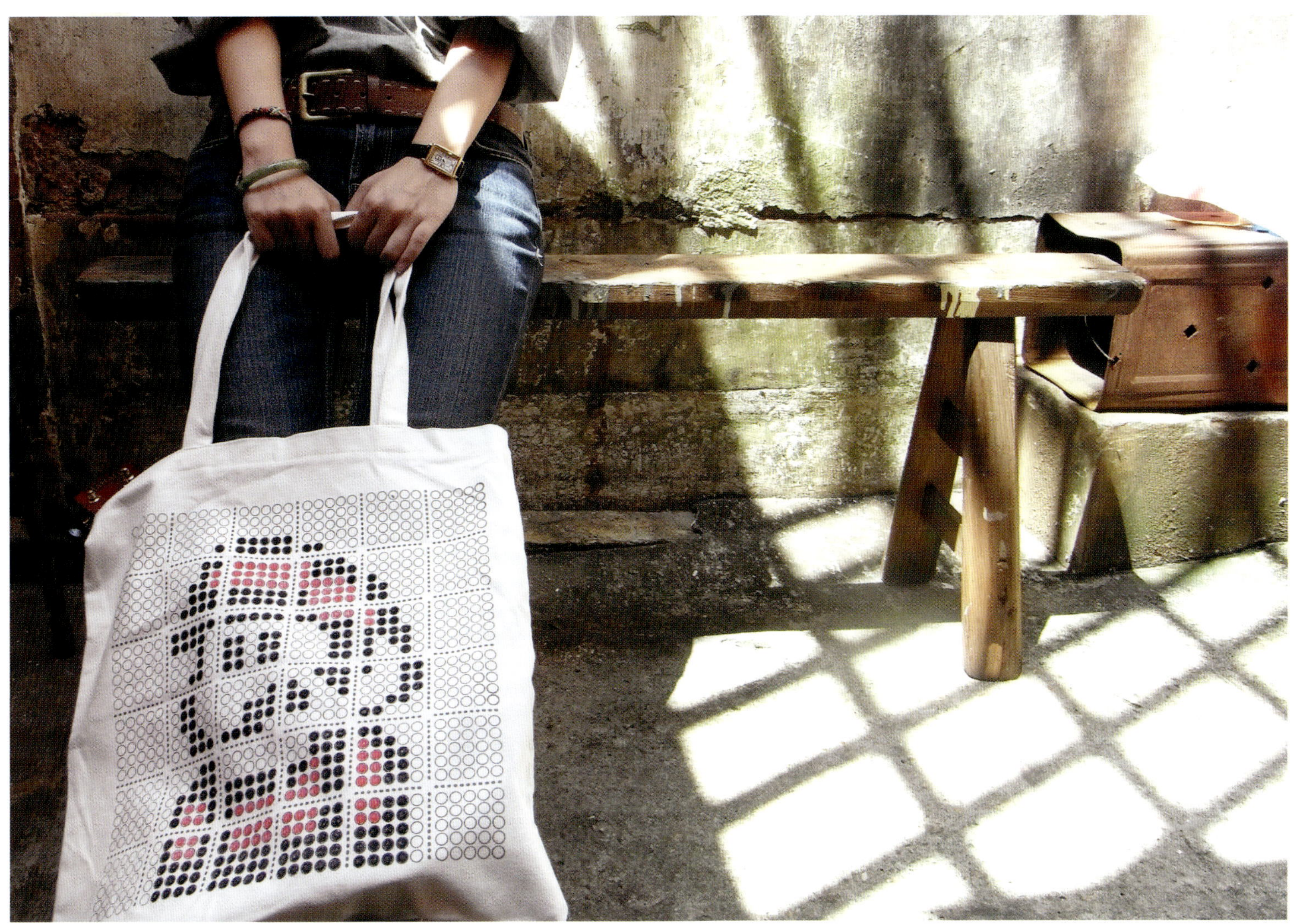

TOLD BAG
DE: Tun Ho

The "Told Bag" is an inviting platform for people to design their very own bag. It has done "half the job" by facilitating the creating process with checks and dots to fill, and leaves the "other half" for users to finalize using their creativity.

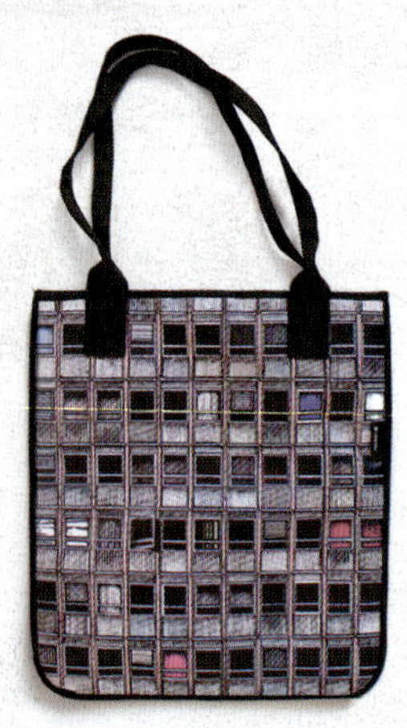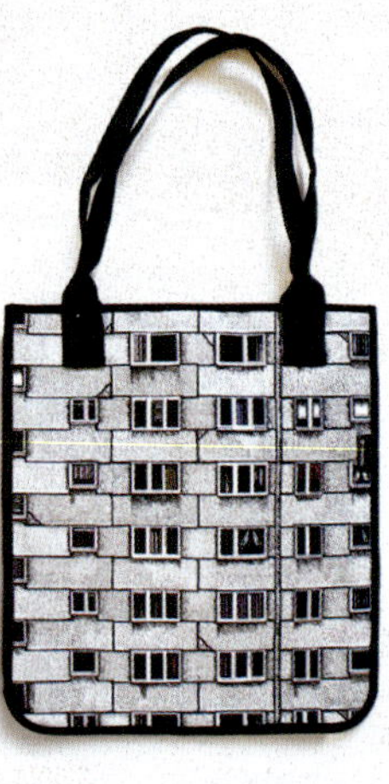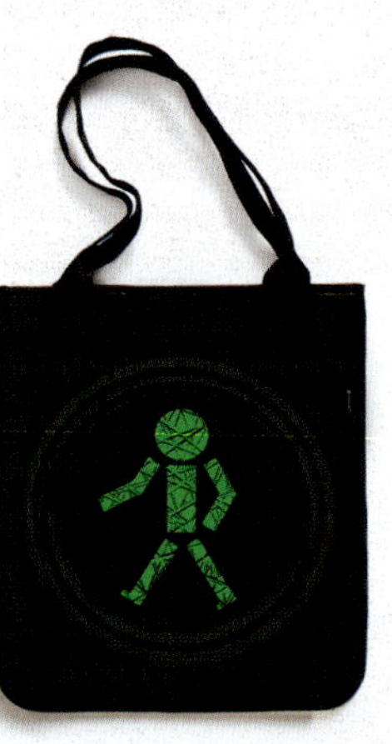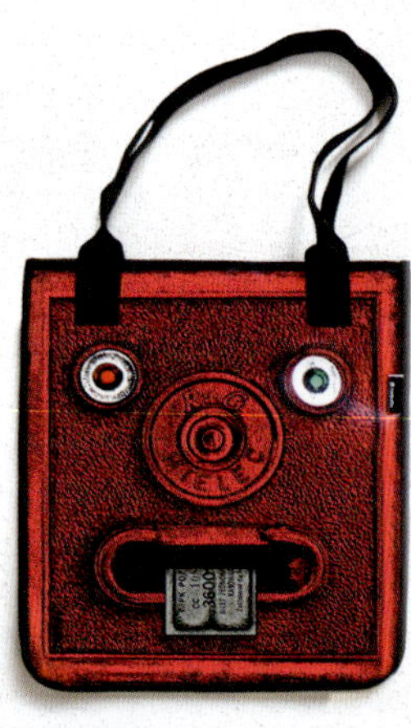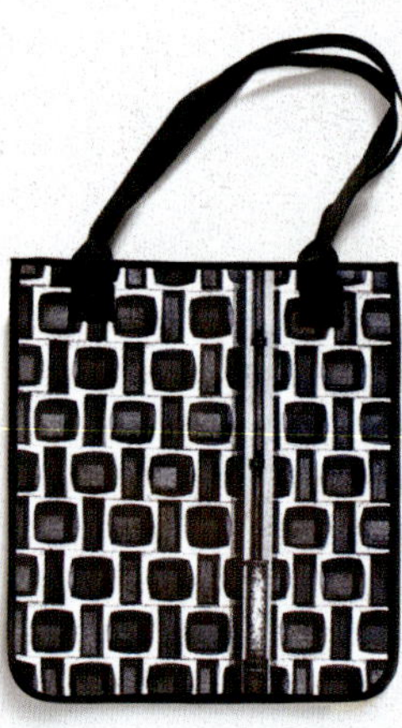

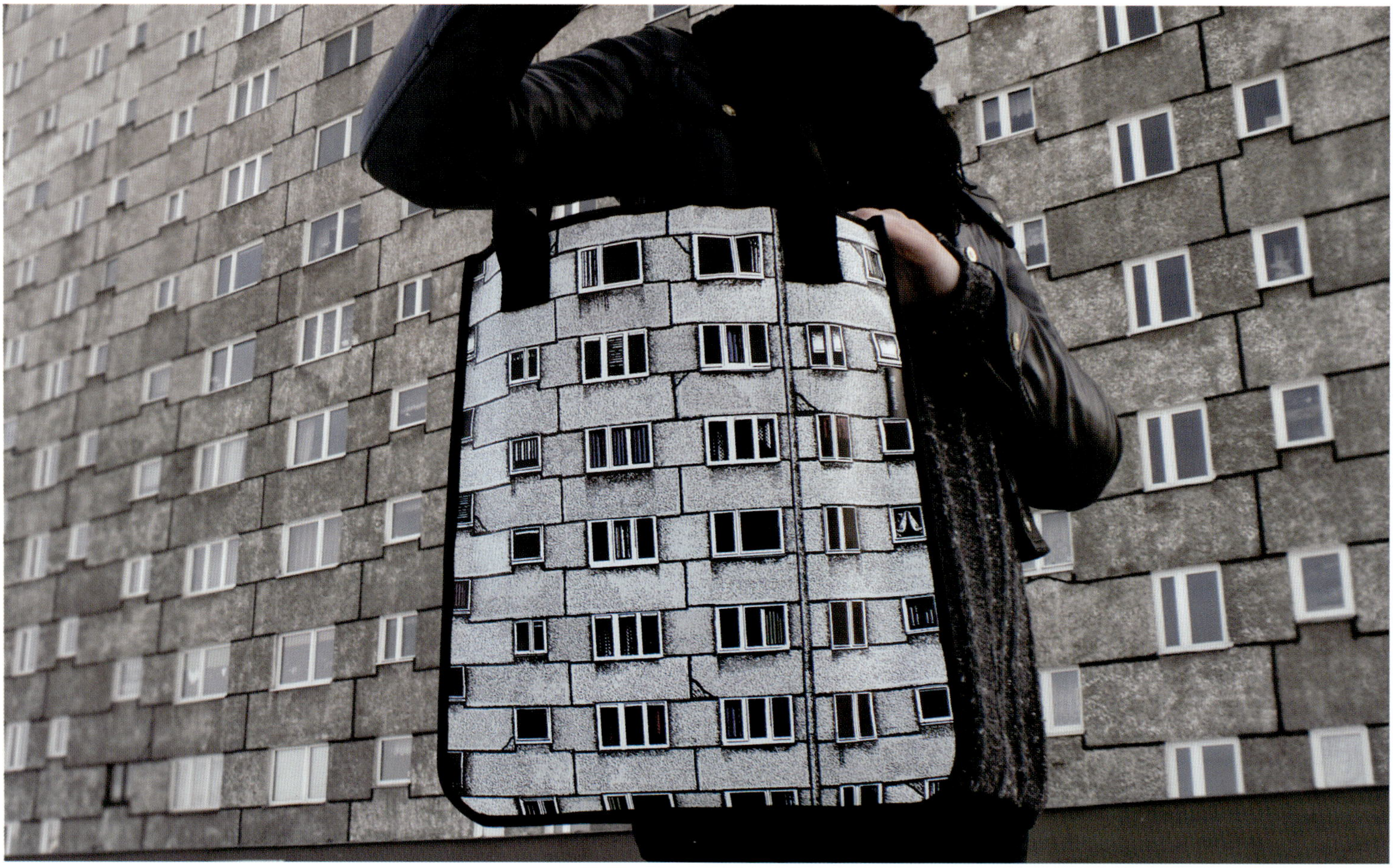

TORBA BLOK
DA: Zupagrafika

Inspired by iconic Polish modernism and industrial designs, the designer
extracted the elements and details of the urban area and reproduced them
with illustration printed on the bags.

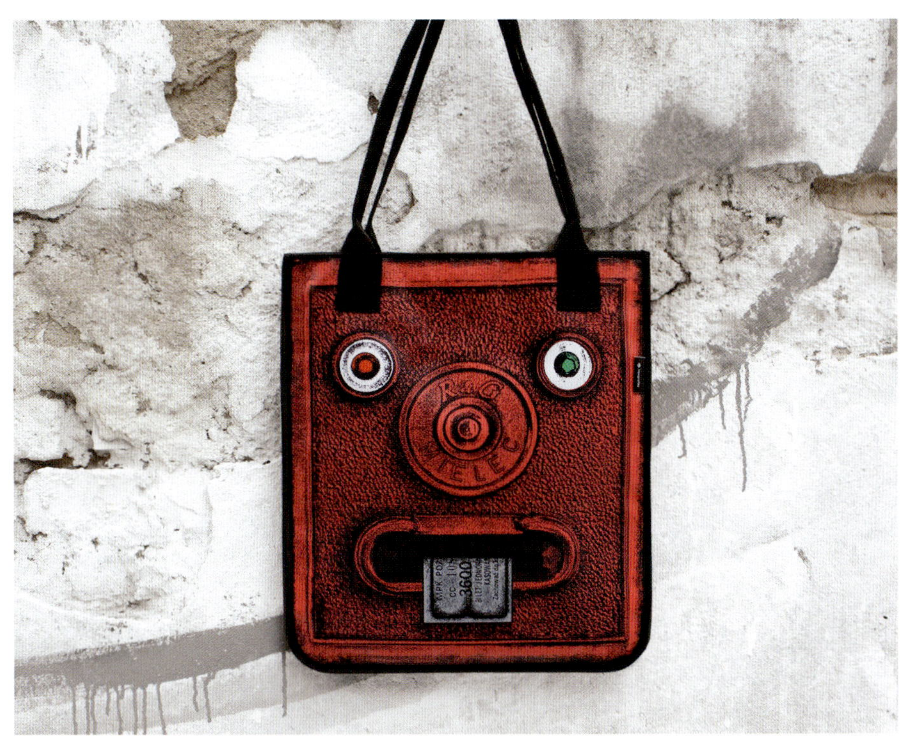

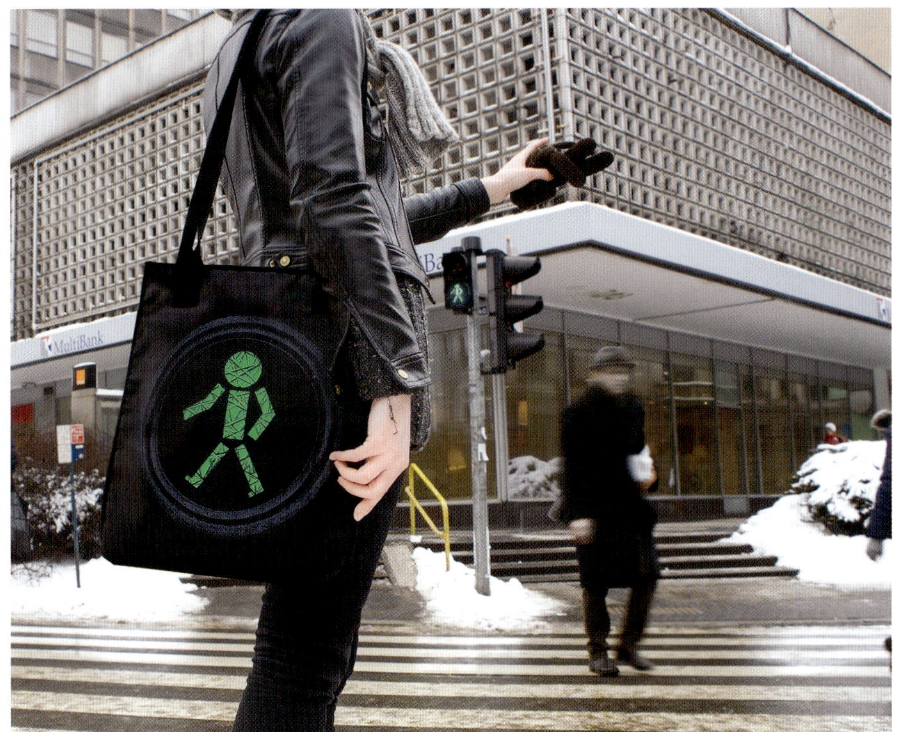

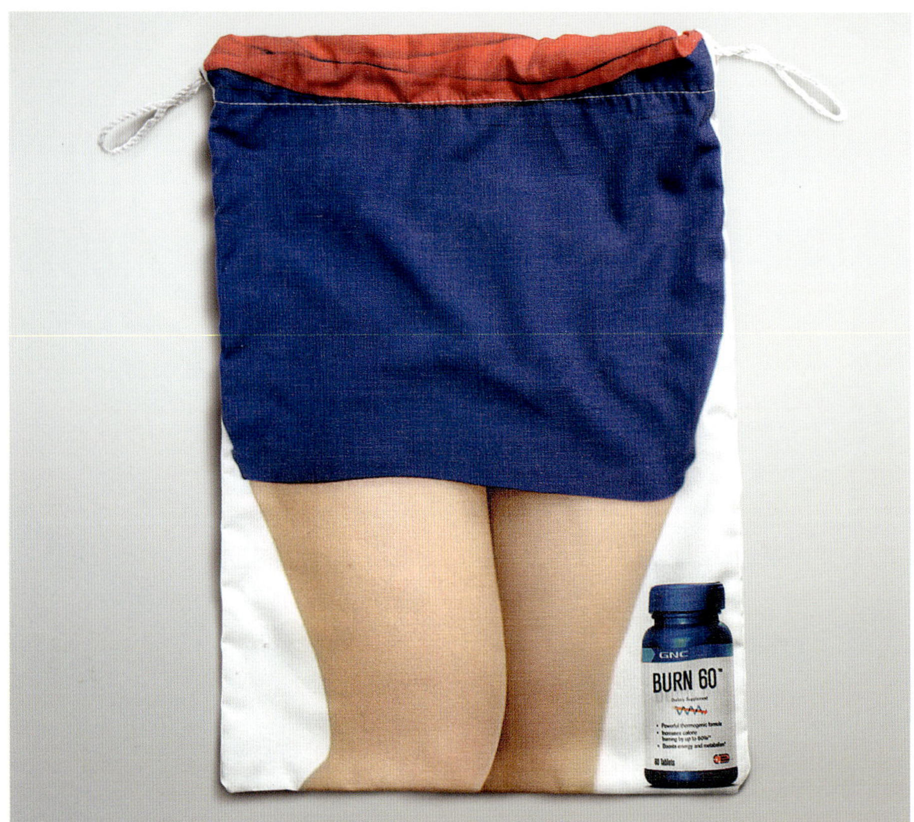

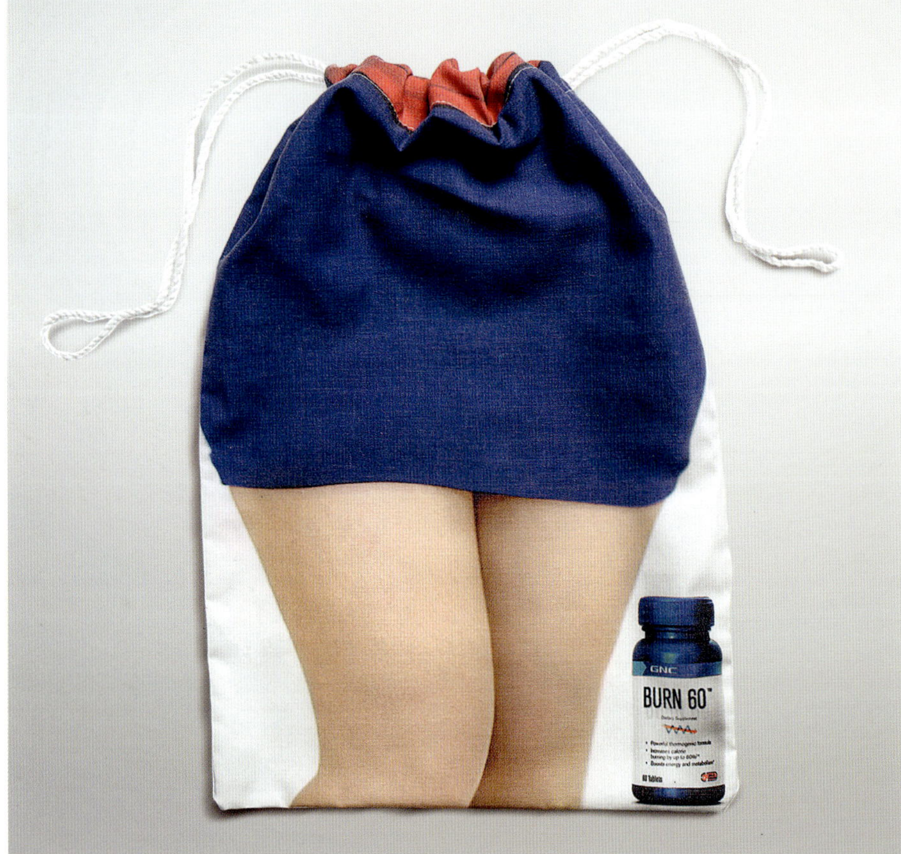

BURN BAG
DA: DM9JaymeSyfu

Designed for a calorie-burning supplement, this bag demonstrates the effect with a simple pull of a drawstring.

SEED ORGANIC
DE: Marcela Cebrowski

To complement the natural and organic food sold in the shop, the bag was made of blurlap and sewed together with yarn.

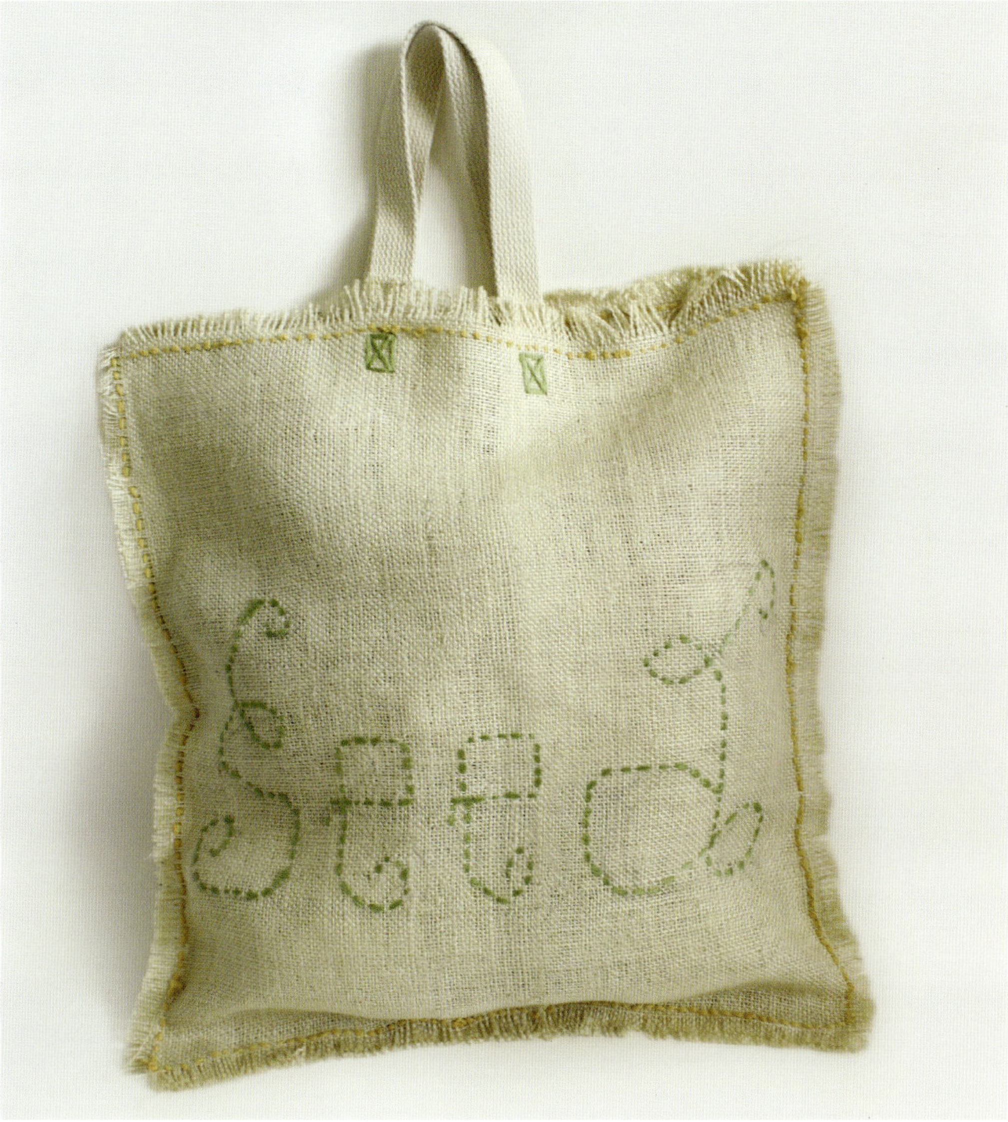

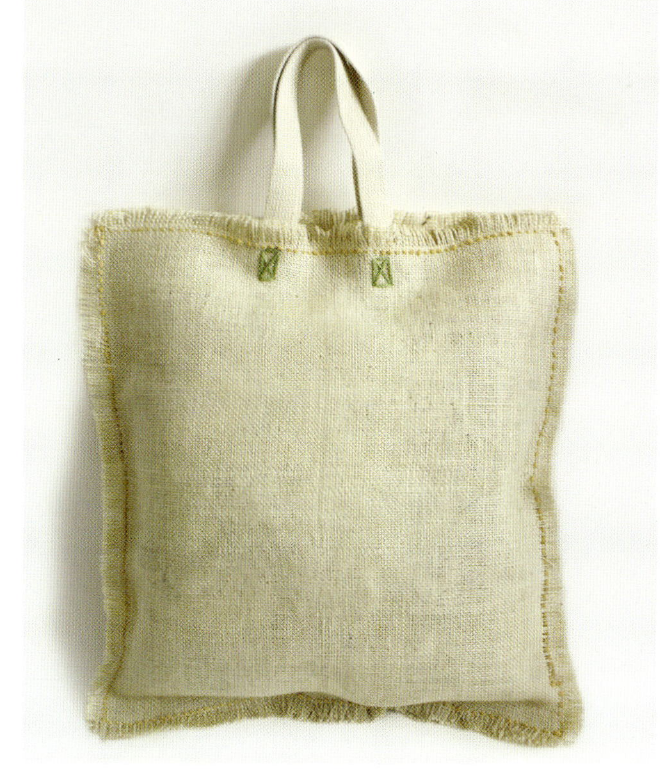

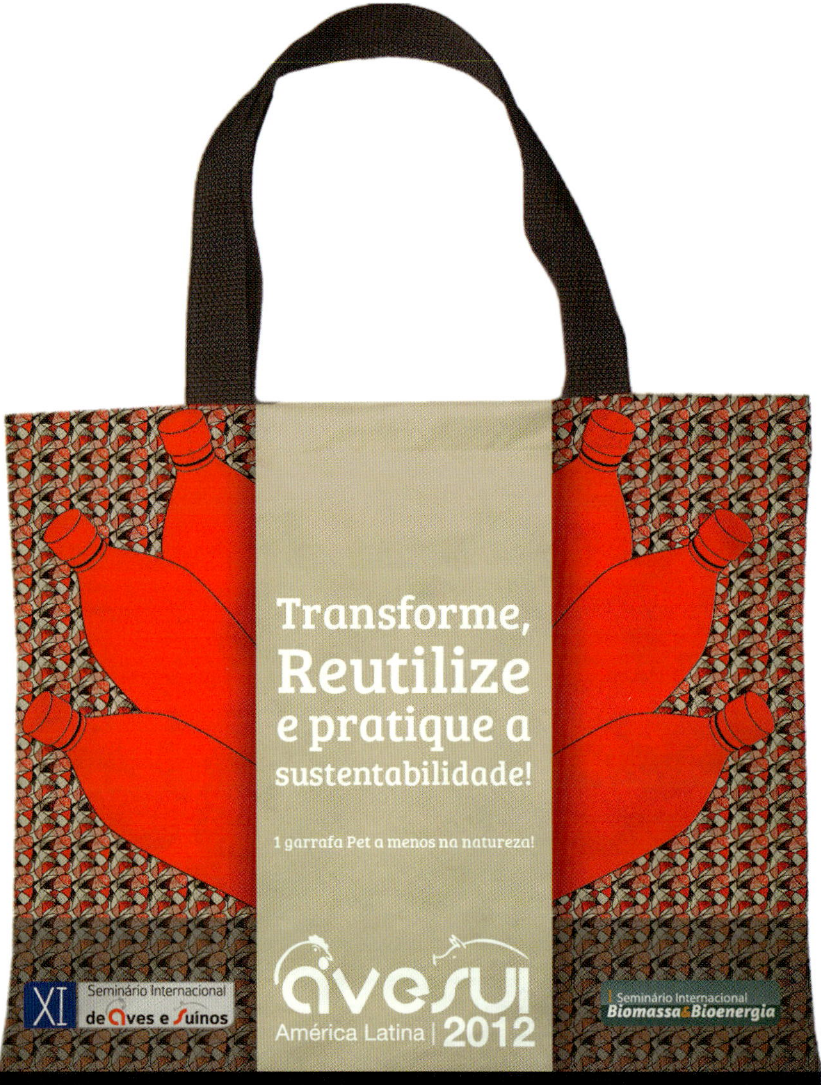

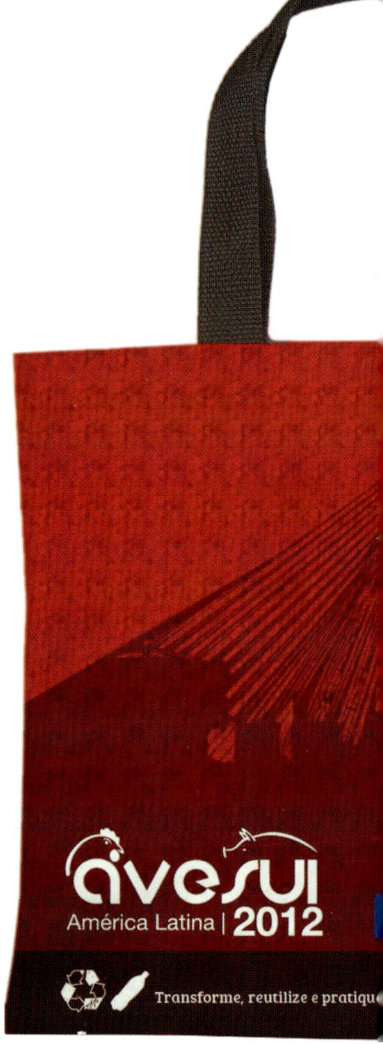

ECOBAG
DE: Thalita Molina

Designed for the Latin American Trade Fair for the Poultry and Swine
Industry, these bags were made from fabric upcycled from PET bottles and
their patterns were inspired by modern art movements reflecting the host
city - São Paulo, Brazil.

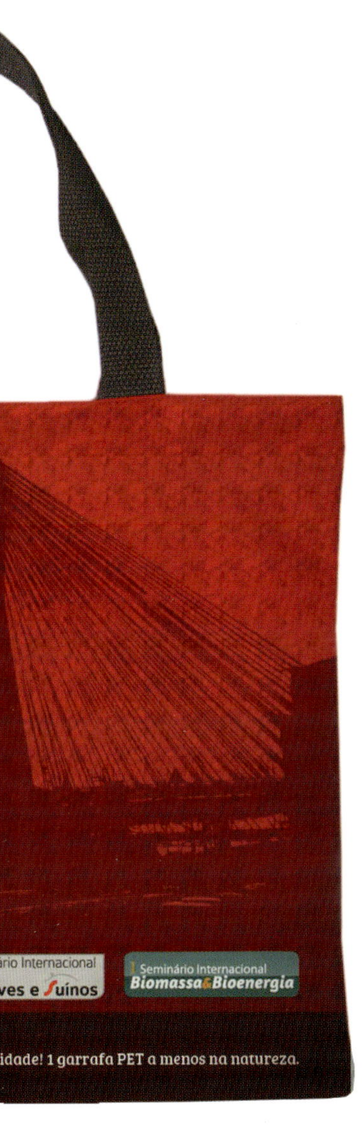
idade! 1 garrafa PET a menos na natureza.
ário Internacional
ves e Suínos
I Seminário Internacional
Biomassa&Bioenergia

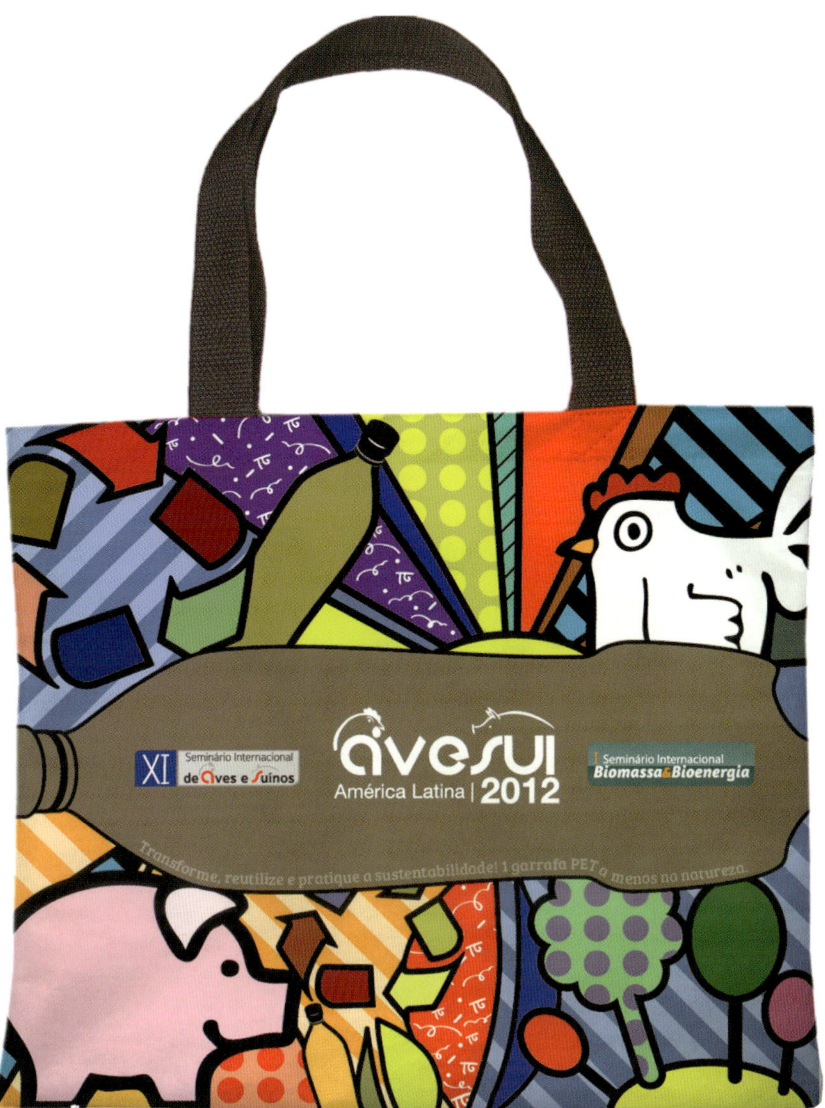
XI Seminário Internacional
de Aves e Suínos
avesui
América Latina | 2012
I Seminário Internacional
Biomassa&Bioenergia
Transforme, reutilize e pratique a sustentabilidade! 1 garrafa PET a menos na natureza.

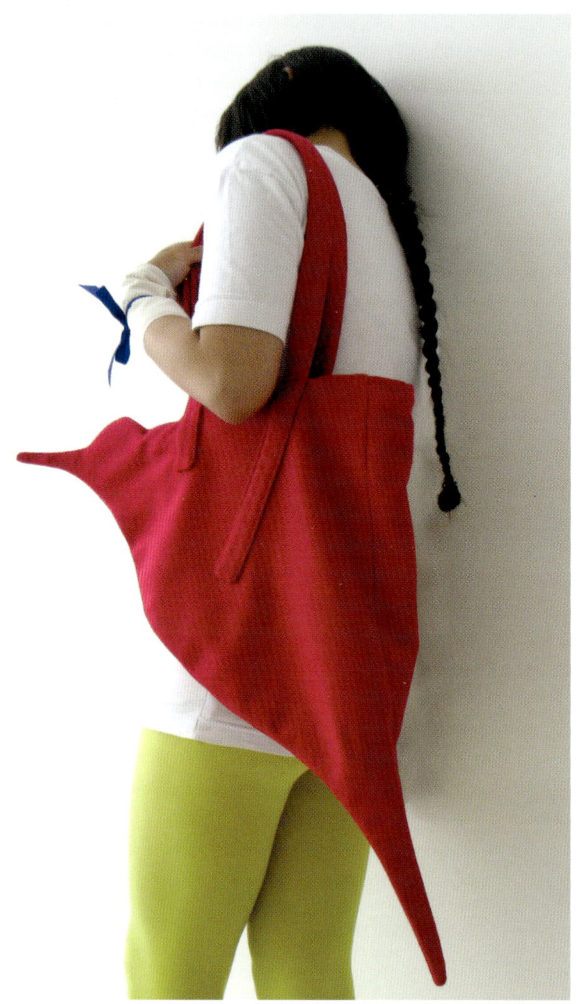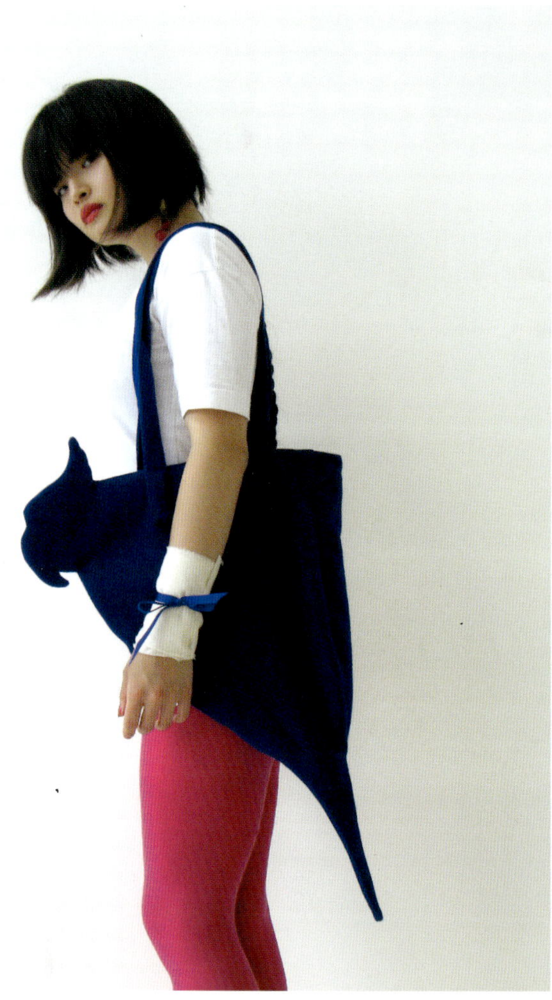

In electric pink or blue, the Birdbag can act as a beach bag, a whimsical
carry-all or a weekend purse. With the joyful design, one can spread wings and
soar through daily tasks and travels.

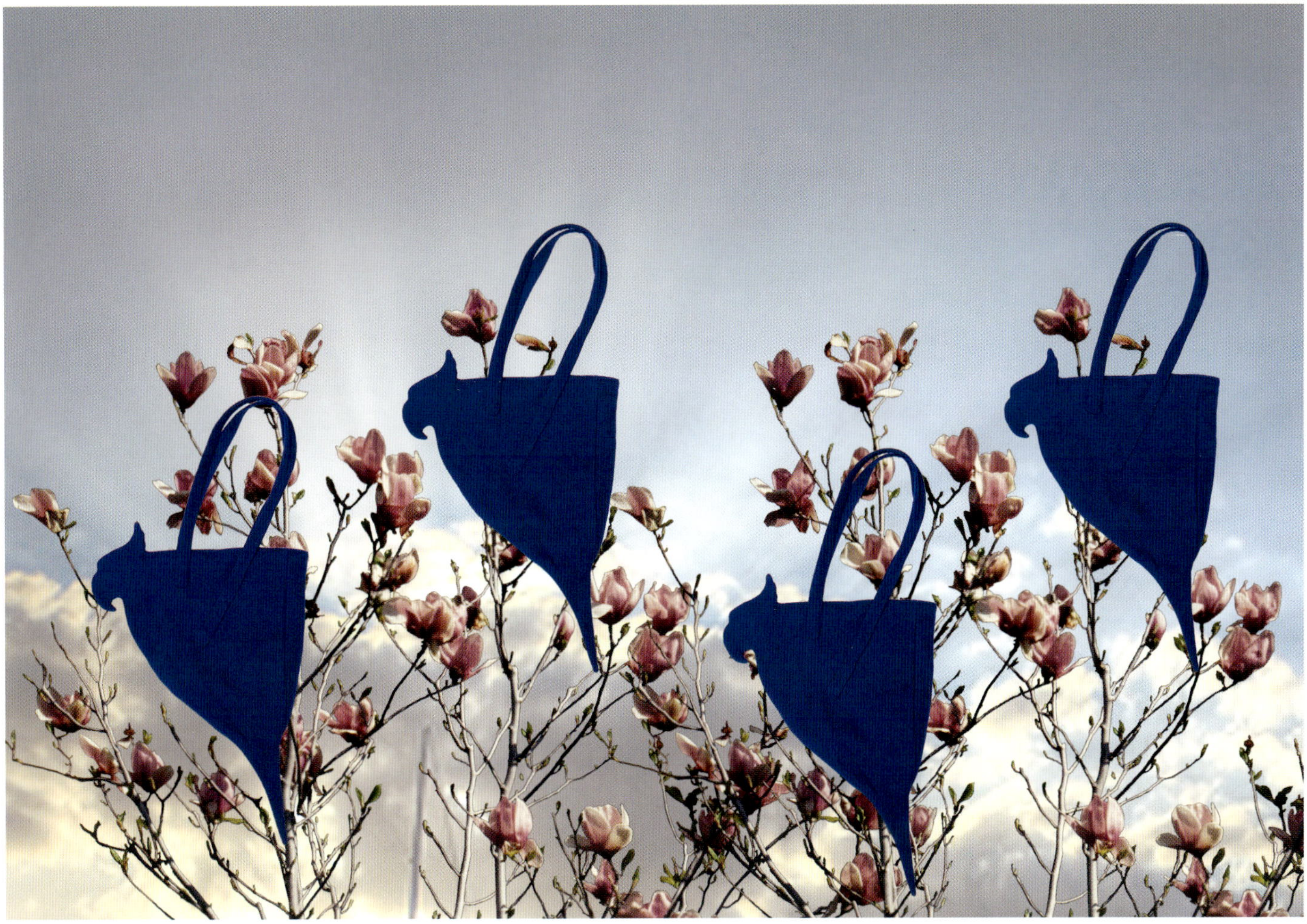

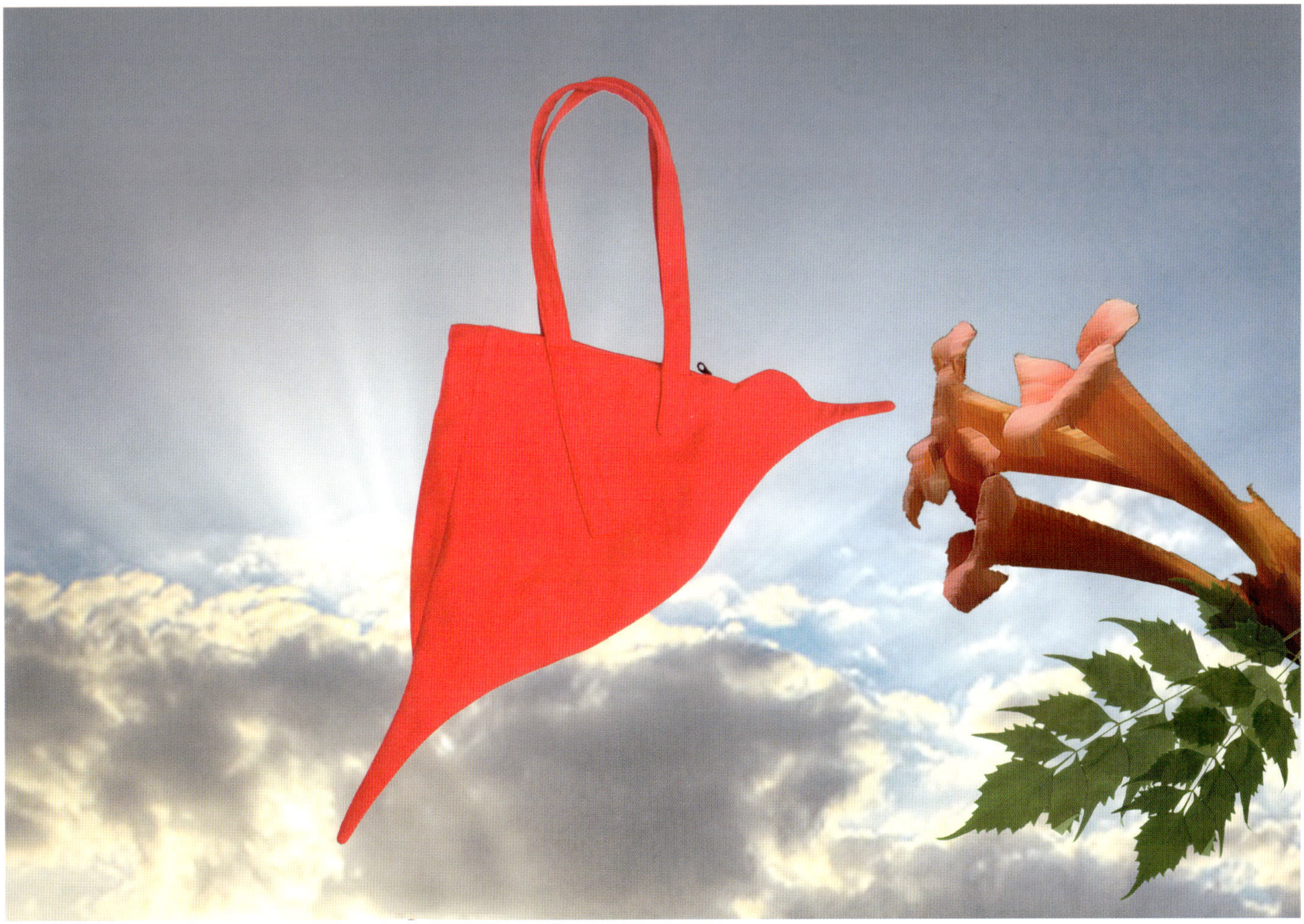

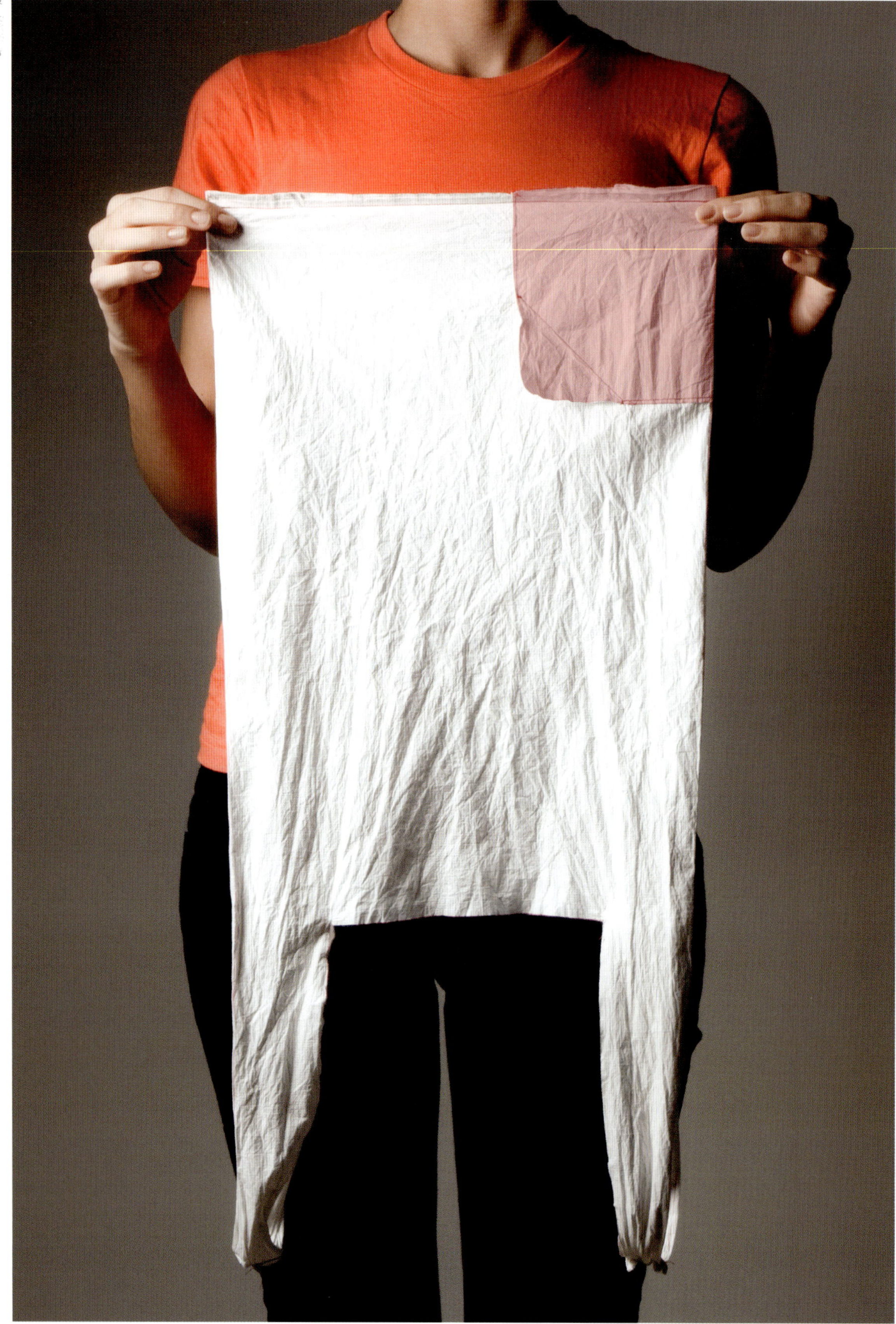

ECCO
DE: Greta D'Angelo

The idea that lies behind the design is: "If it can fit into a man's pocket, then it can fit every woman's bag." Created in Tyvek®, it is recyclable and waterproof on top of being light and sturdy.

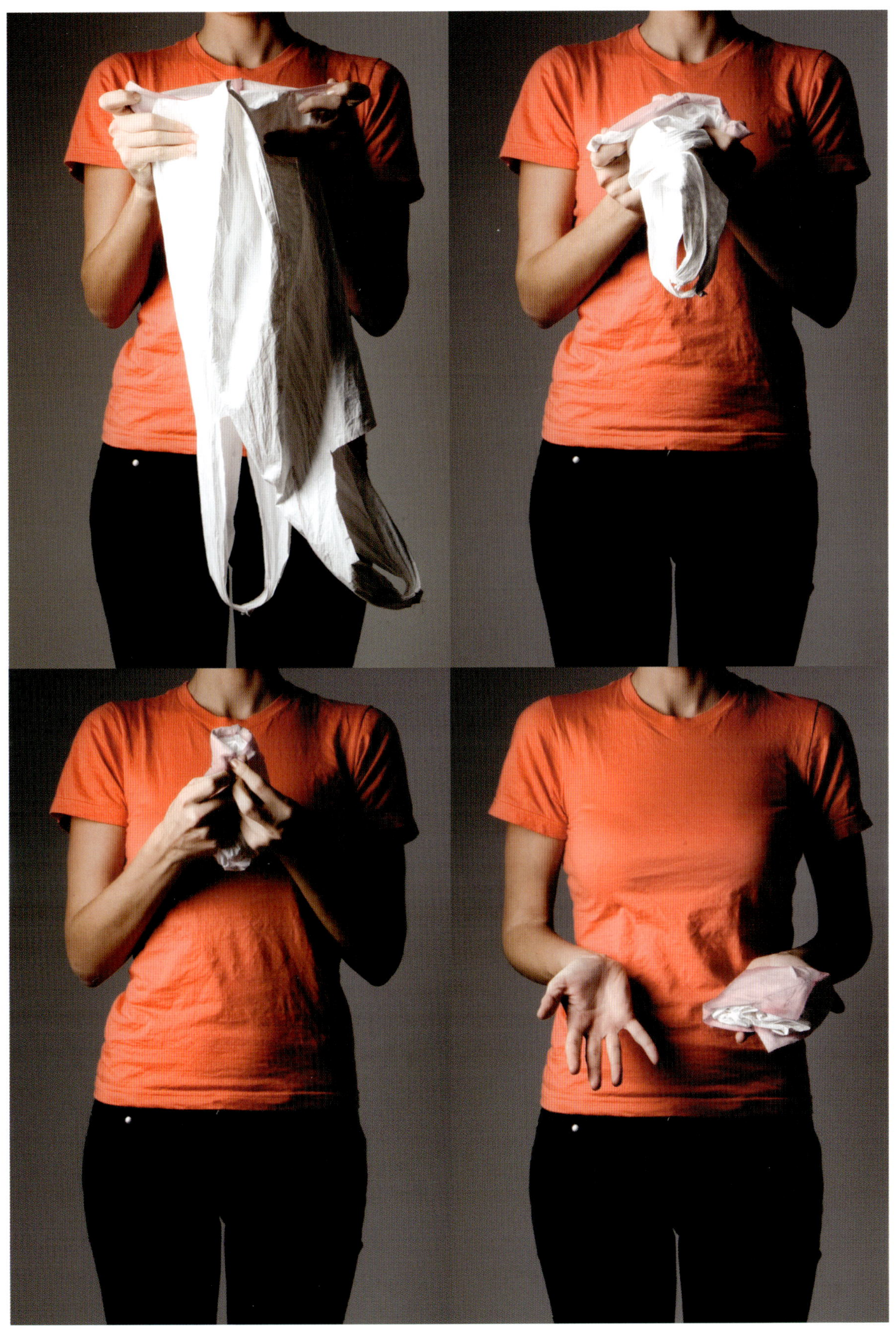

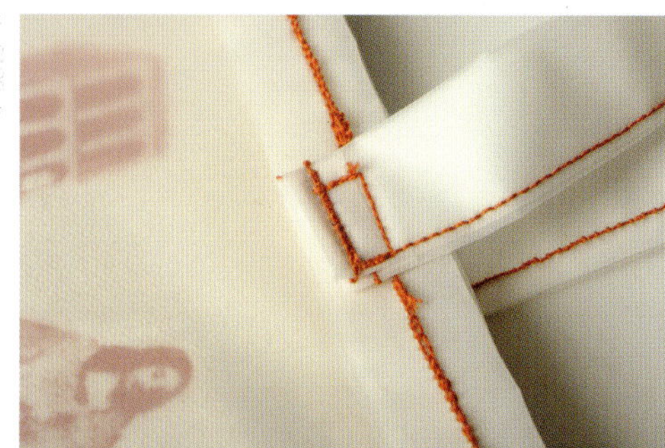
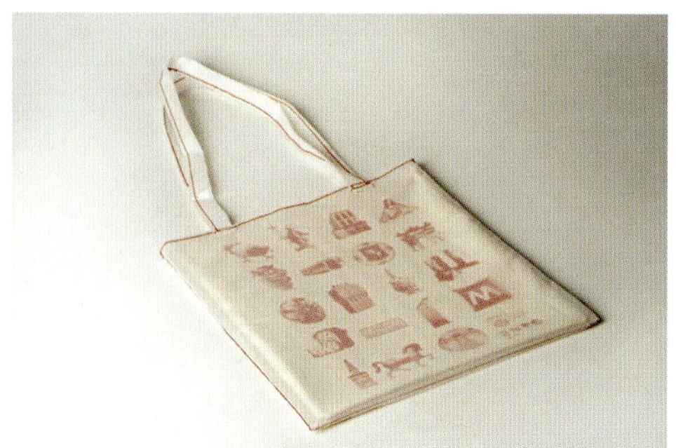
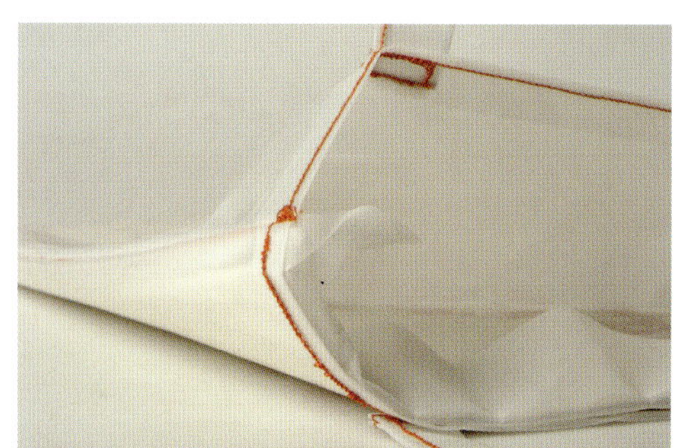
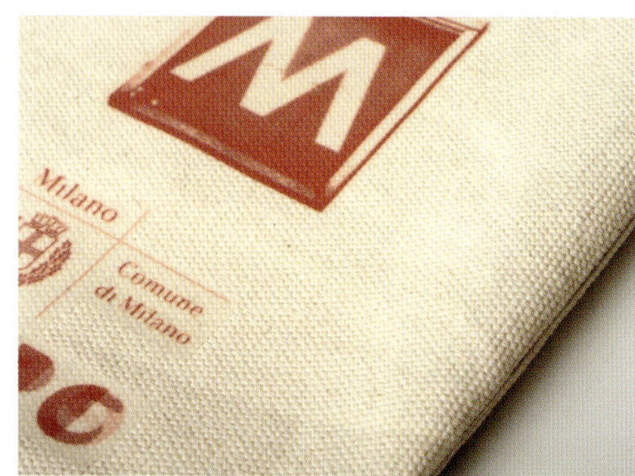

Milano
Comune
di Milano

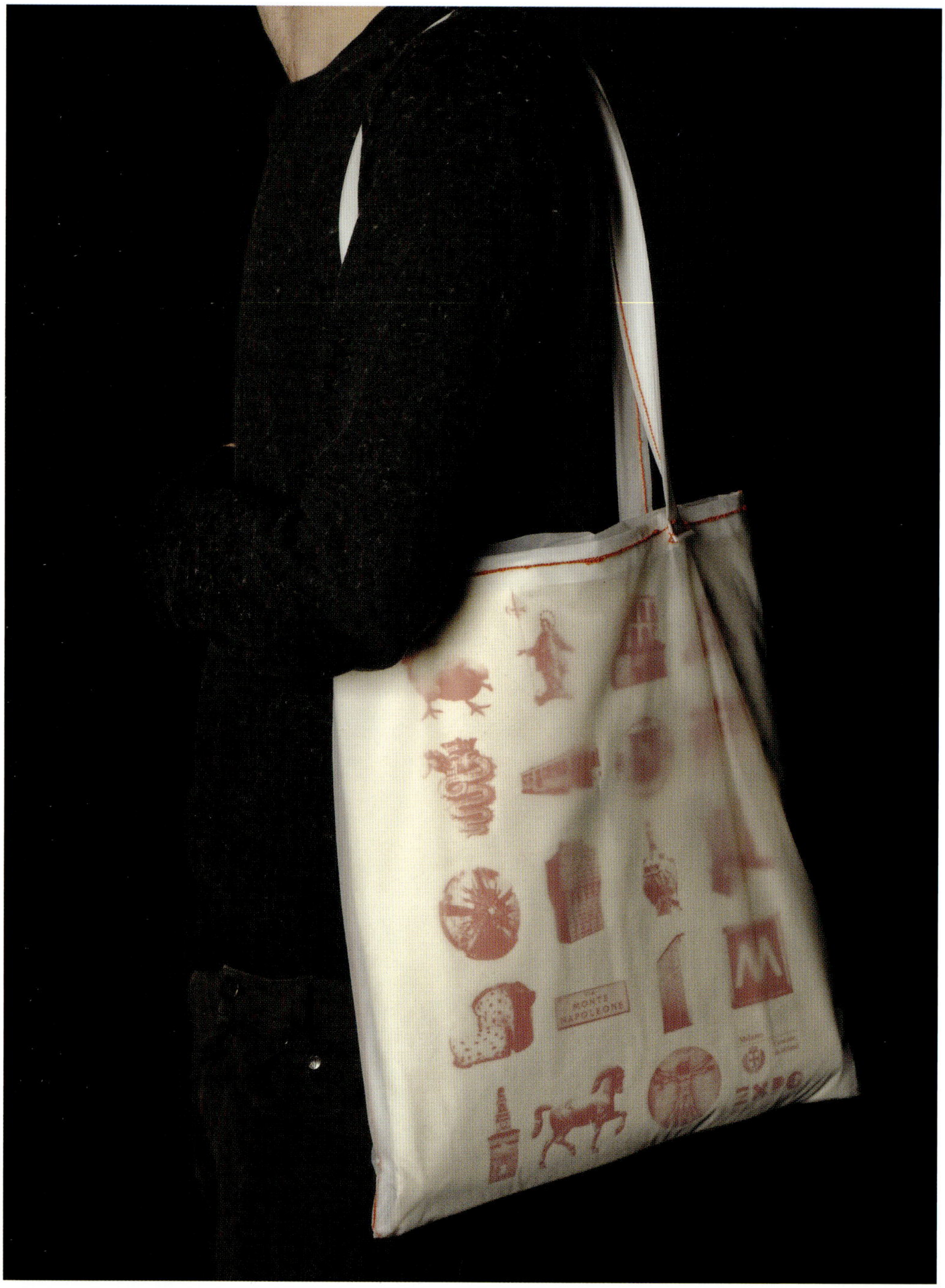

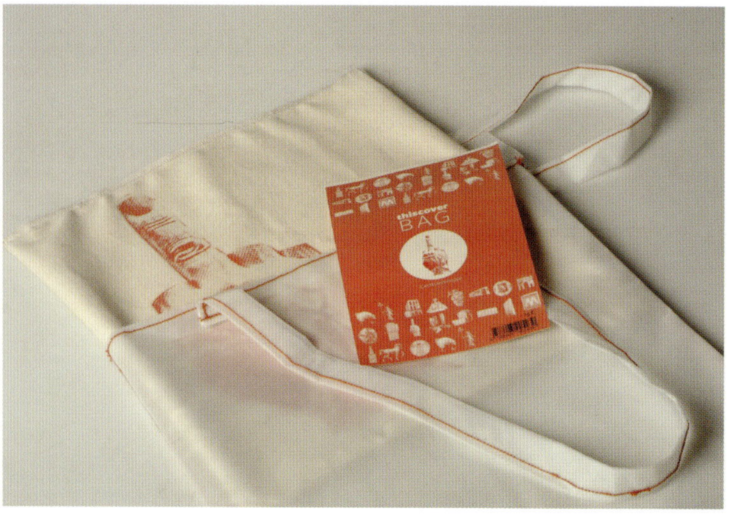

thiscover
BAG

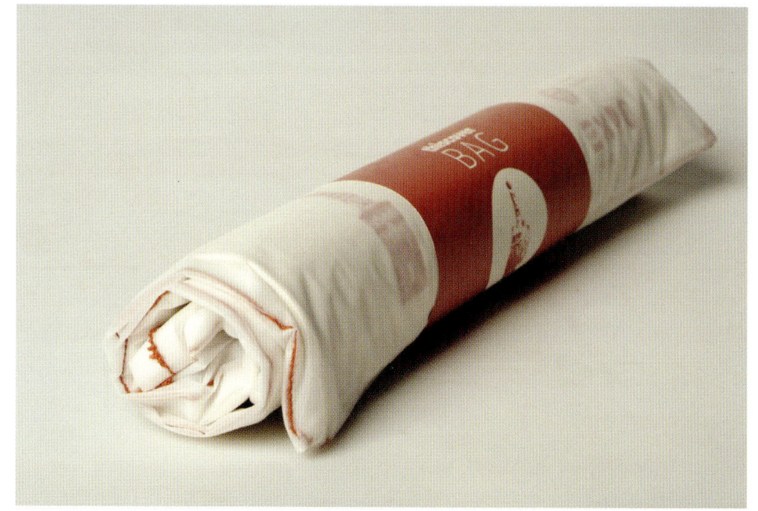

thiscover
BAG

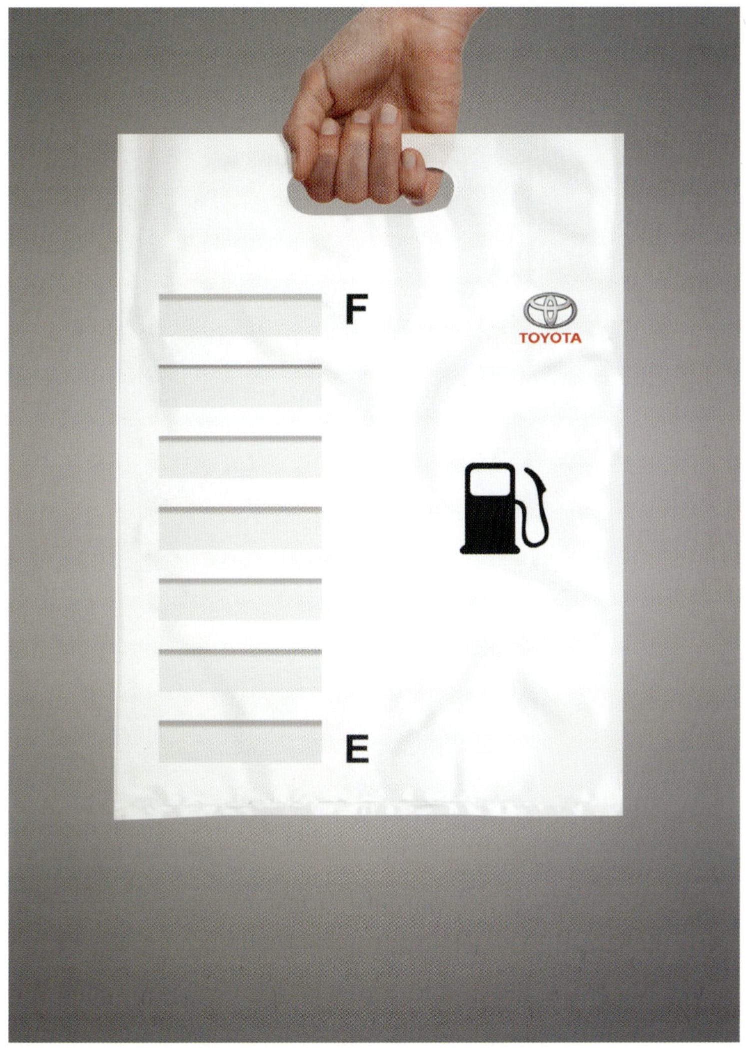

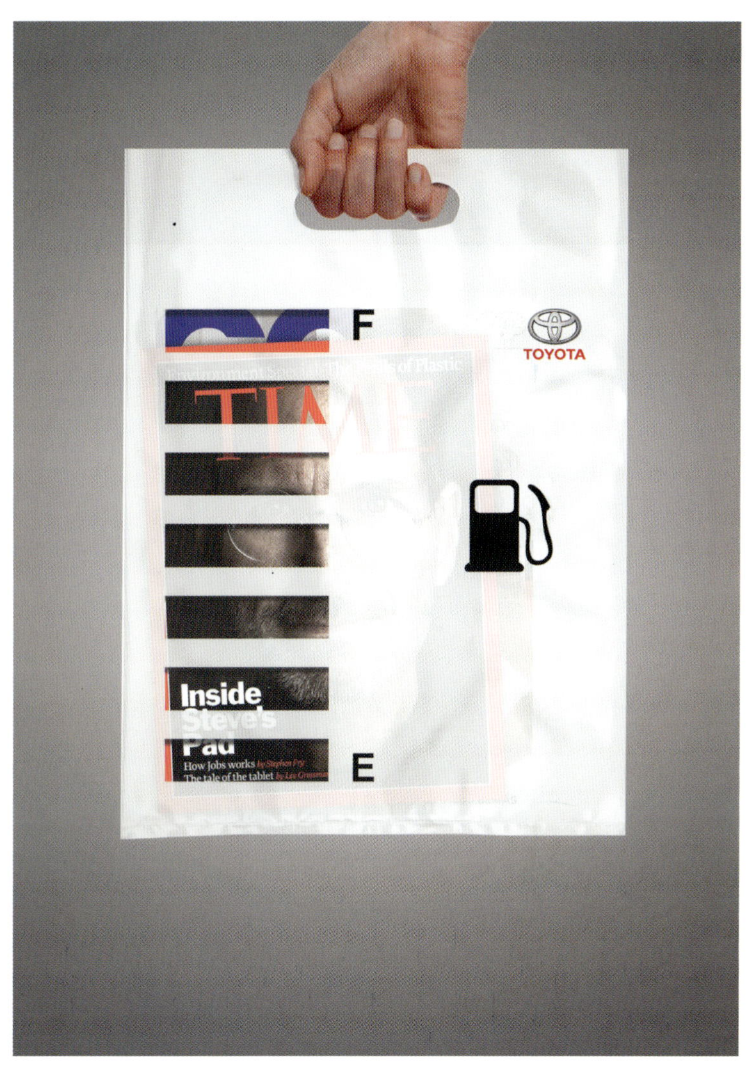

THISCOVER BAG

DE: Rodia Banaei, Hye Wook Chung, Francesca Fornoni, Pietro Lodi, Gabrielle Mathias, Pietro Mazza, Alessio Vanin

The story of Milan is difficult to understand if one does not live there. To tell the intangible story, the bag design employs a "fog" element created using a semi-opaque PVC mask, covering the patterns of the city.

TOYOTA CARRY BAG

DE: Mahir Goktas

As a bag for Toyota, the design leaves a few bars transparent to mimic the gas indicator. When occupied, the contents will appear through the bars.

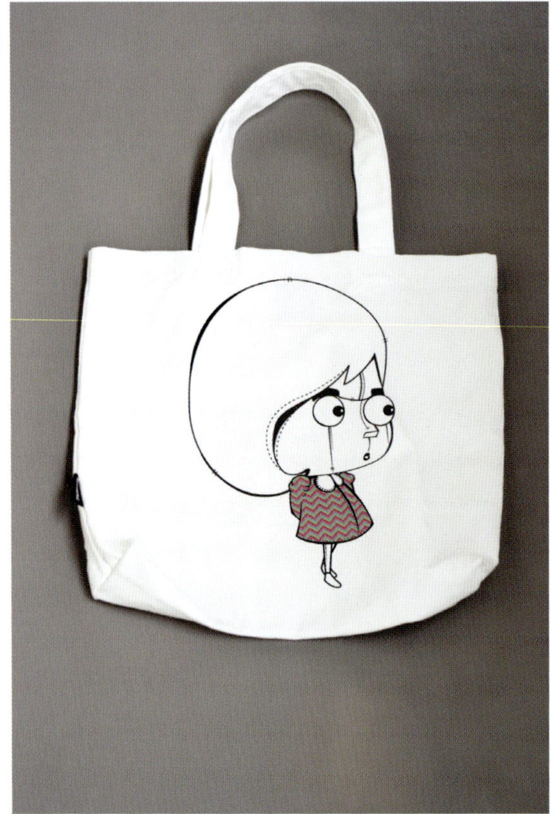

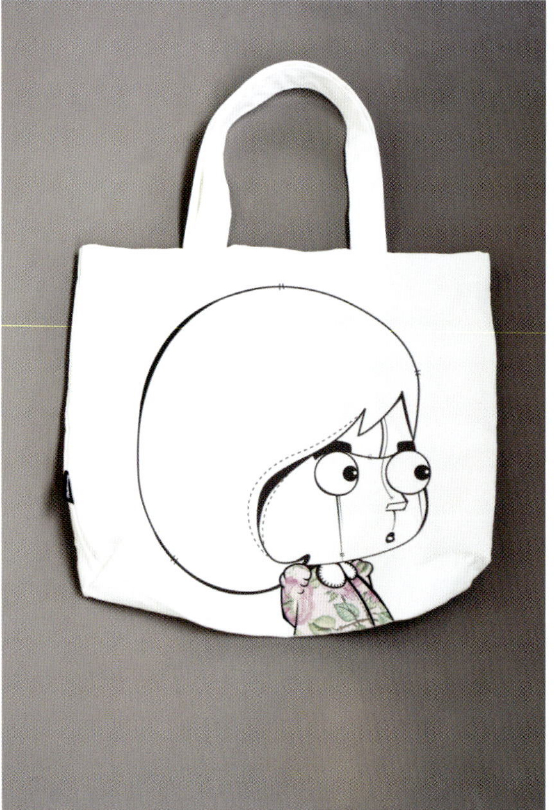

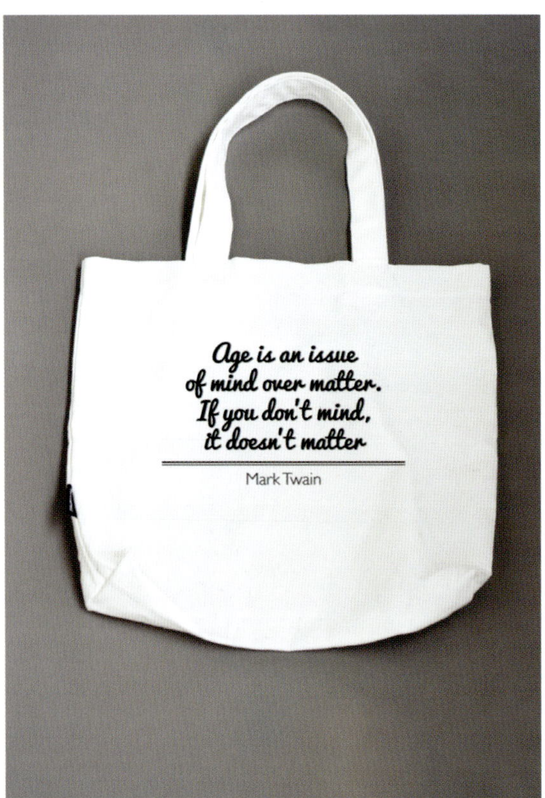

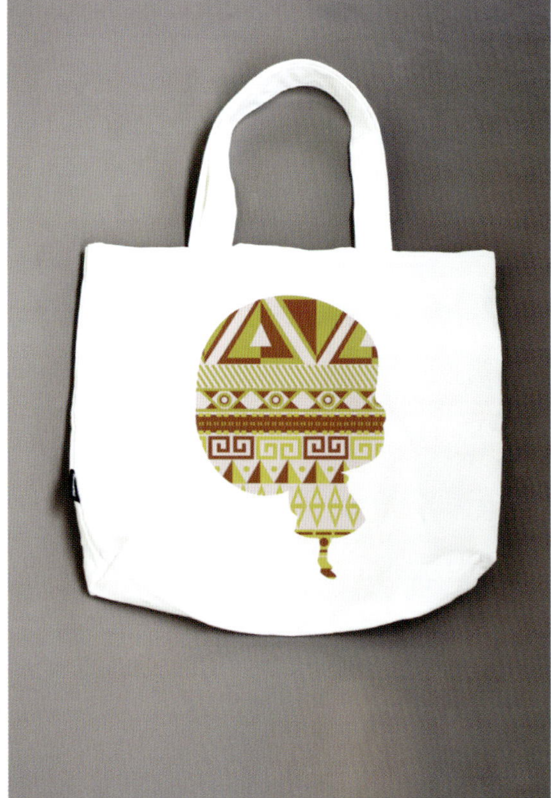

NADIA CHARISSA
DE: Nadia Charissa

As a freelance designer, Nadia Charissa created a set
of tote bags with illustrated self-portraits, which are
professional yet cute and reflective of her artistic
style.

PUF!™ FESTIVAL
CD: Federico Landini(I depend on me),
Jonathan Calugi(Happy lover town)

PUF!™ is a festival about music, art and culture. The
promotional bags feature characters and patterns from
the branding illustration that resonates with the
theme: something new and fresh is growing from the head
of some Pistoia people.

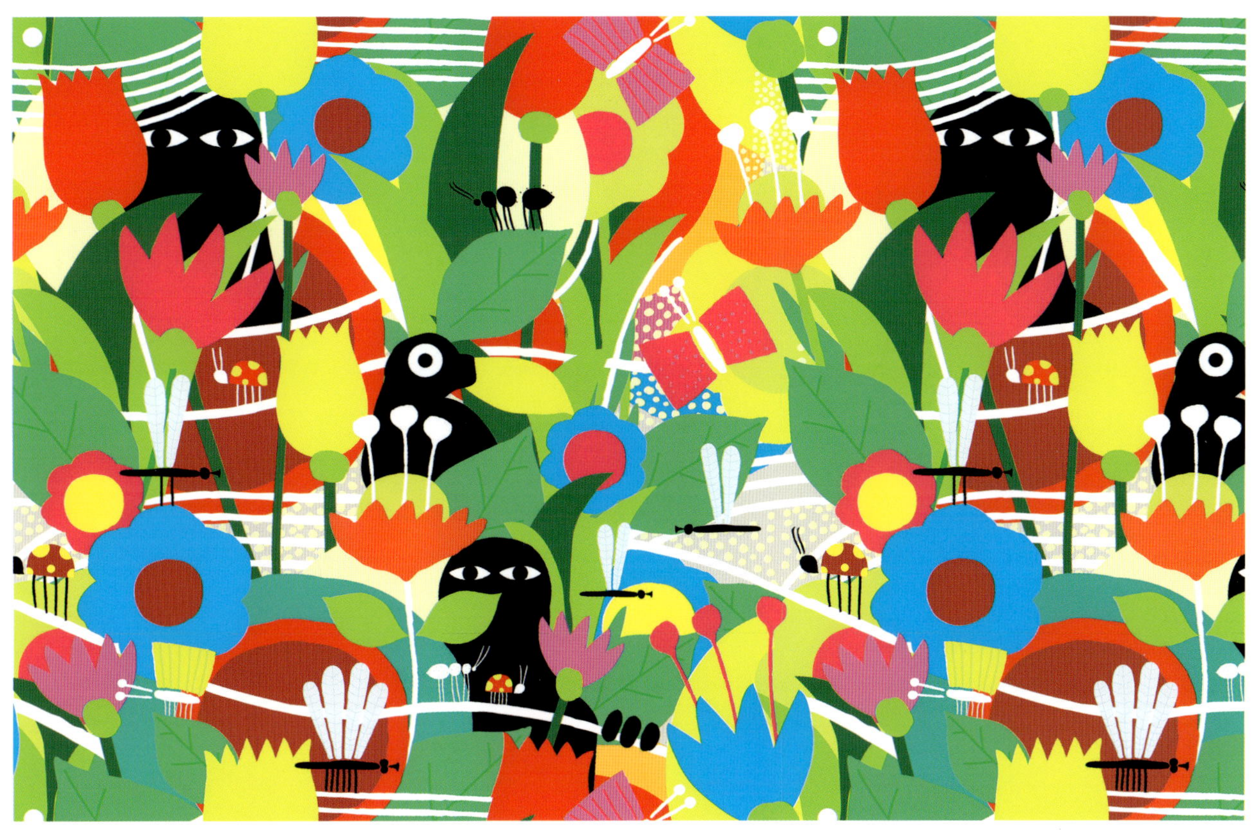

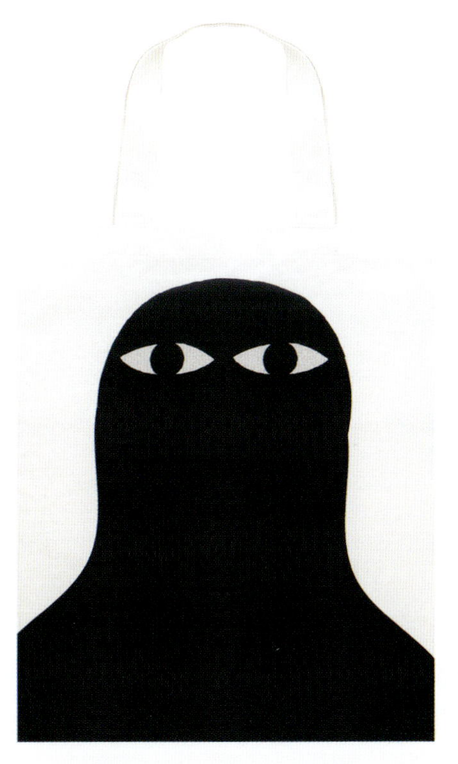

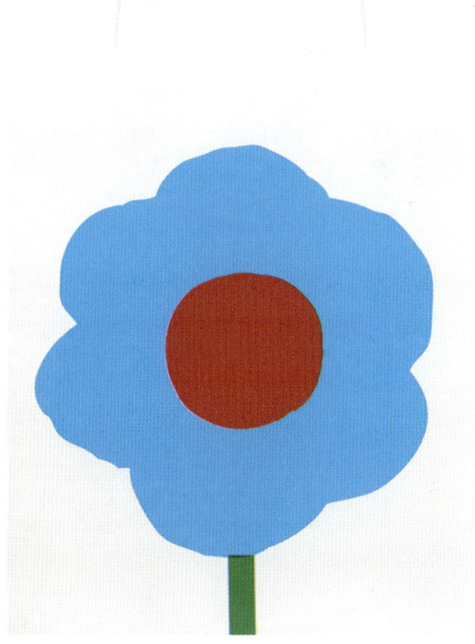

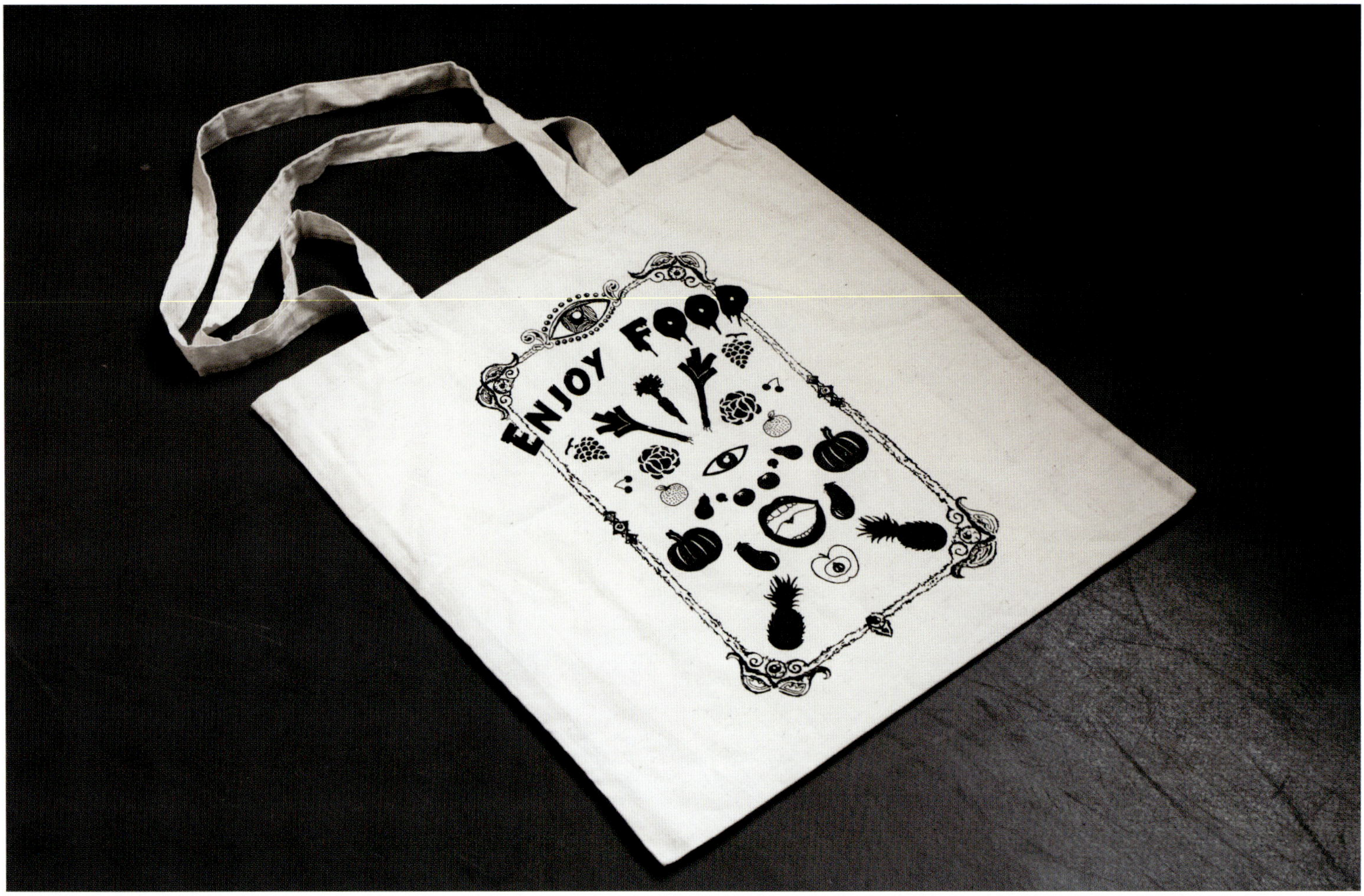

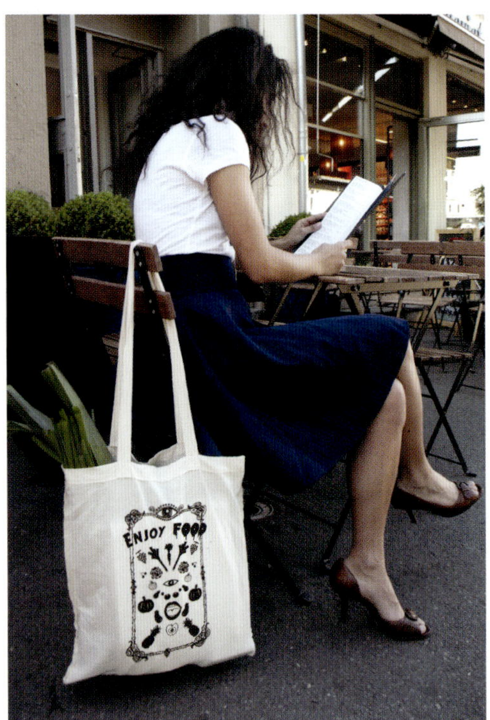
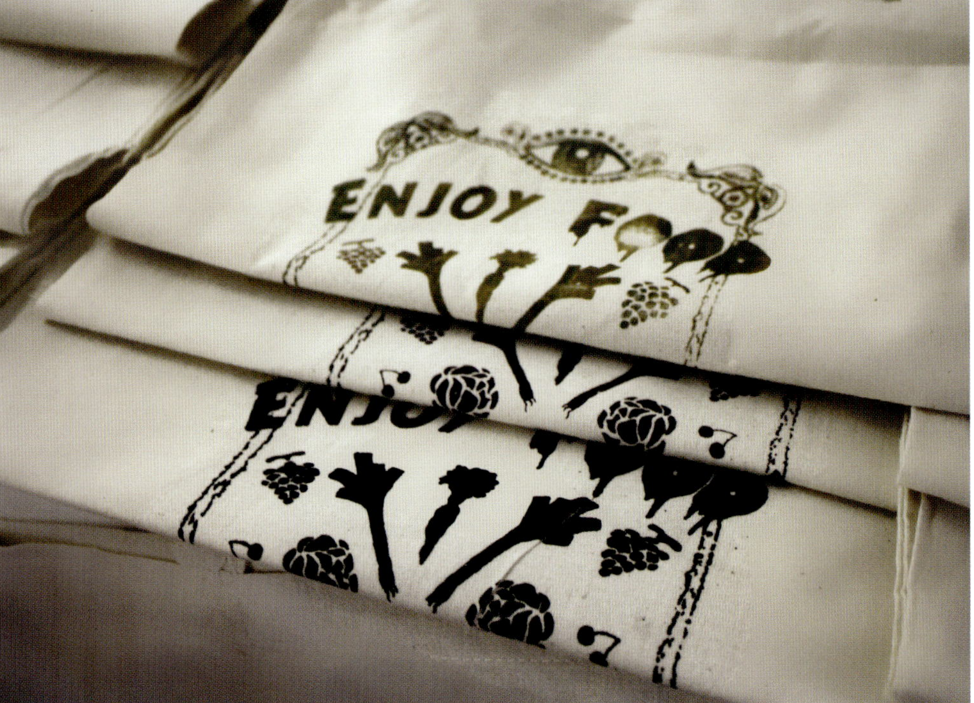

SILKSCREENS FOOD BAG

DE: Julie Chapalain

In exploration of the theme "food," Julie Chapalain created an illustration
playing with patterns of food and facial features.

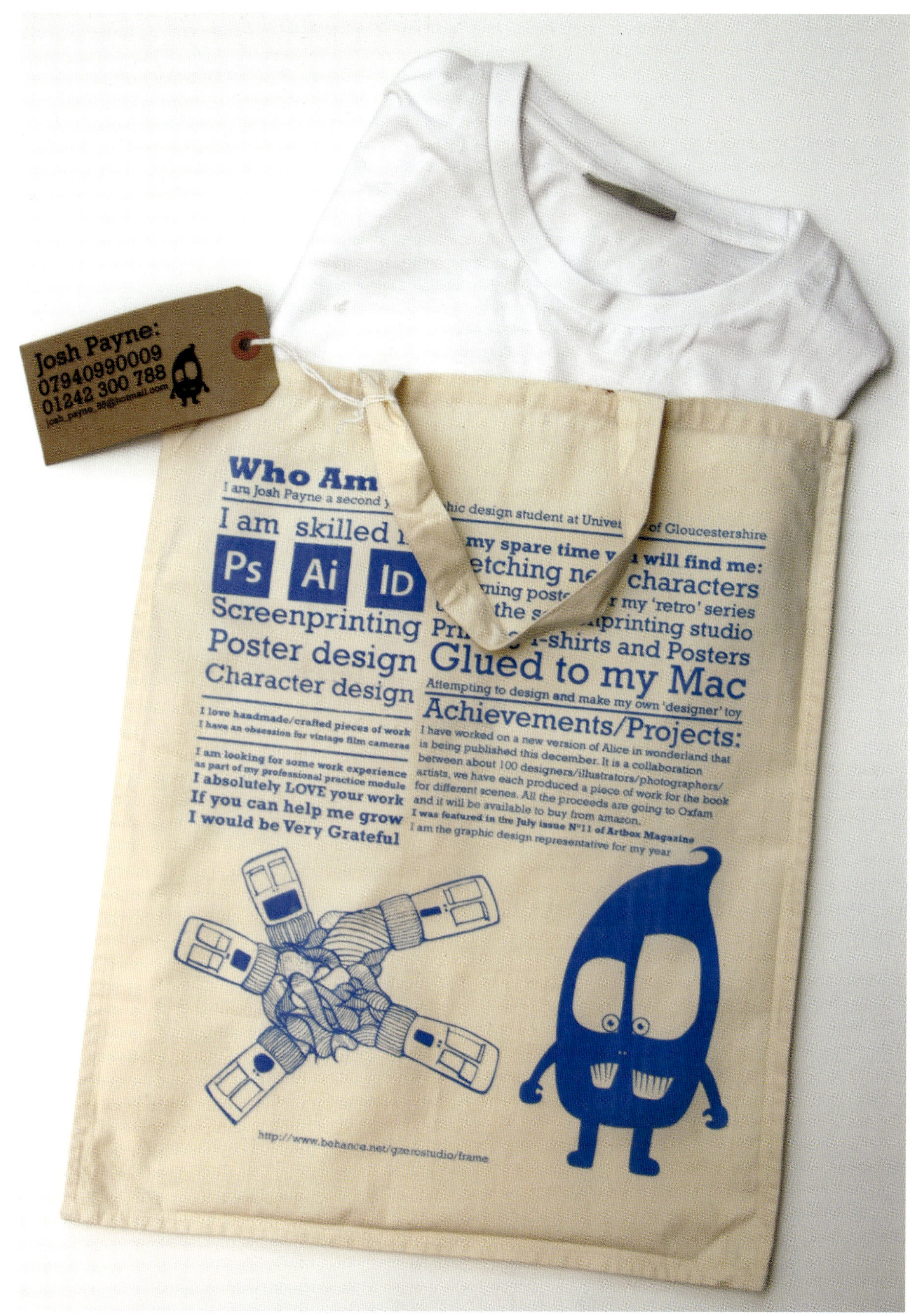

C.V. BAG

DE: Josh Payne

To stand out from the crowd, Josh Payne designed a bag printed with his personal CV to send out in an attempt to secure work. The little card hung on the handle provides his contact information.

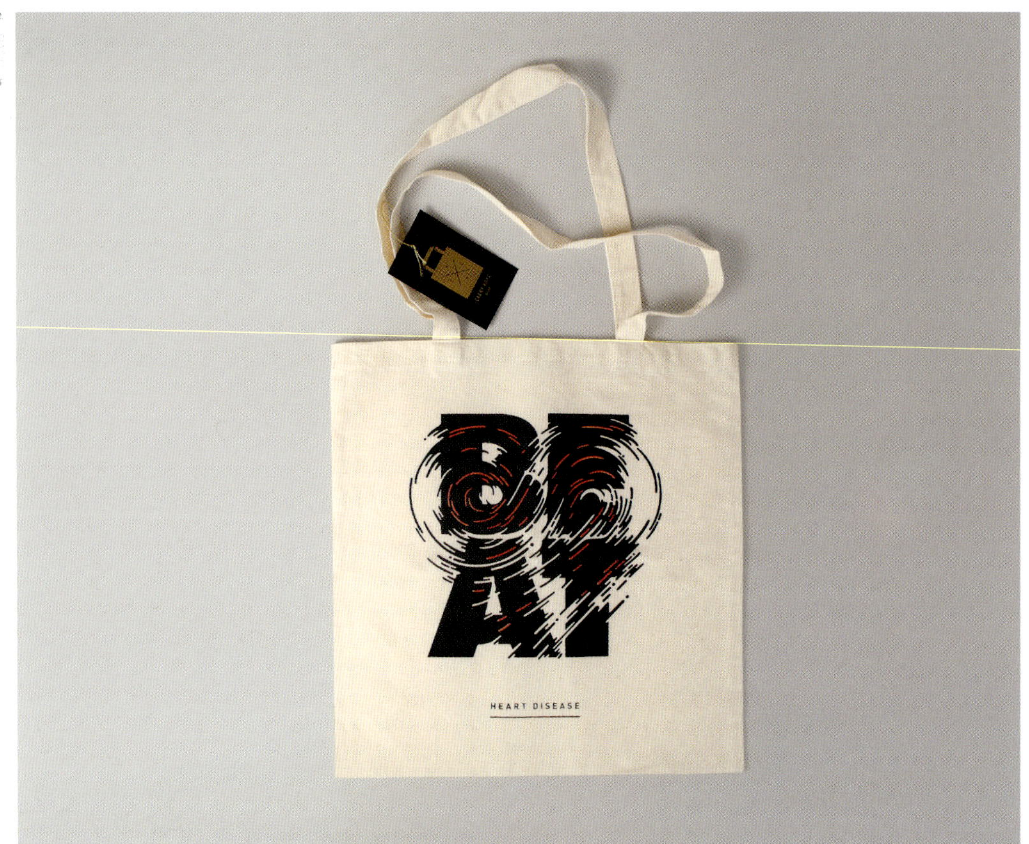
HEART DISEASE

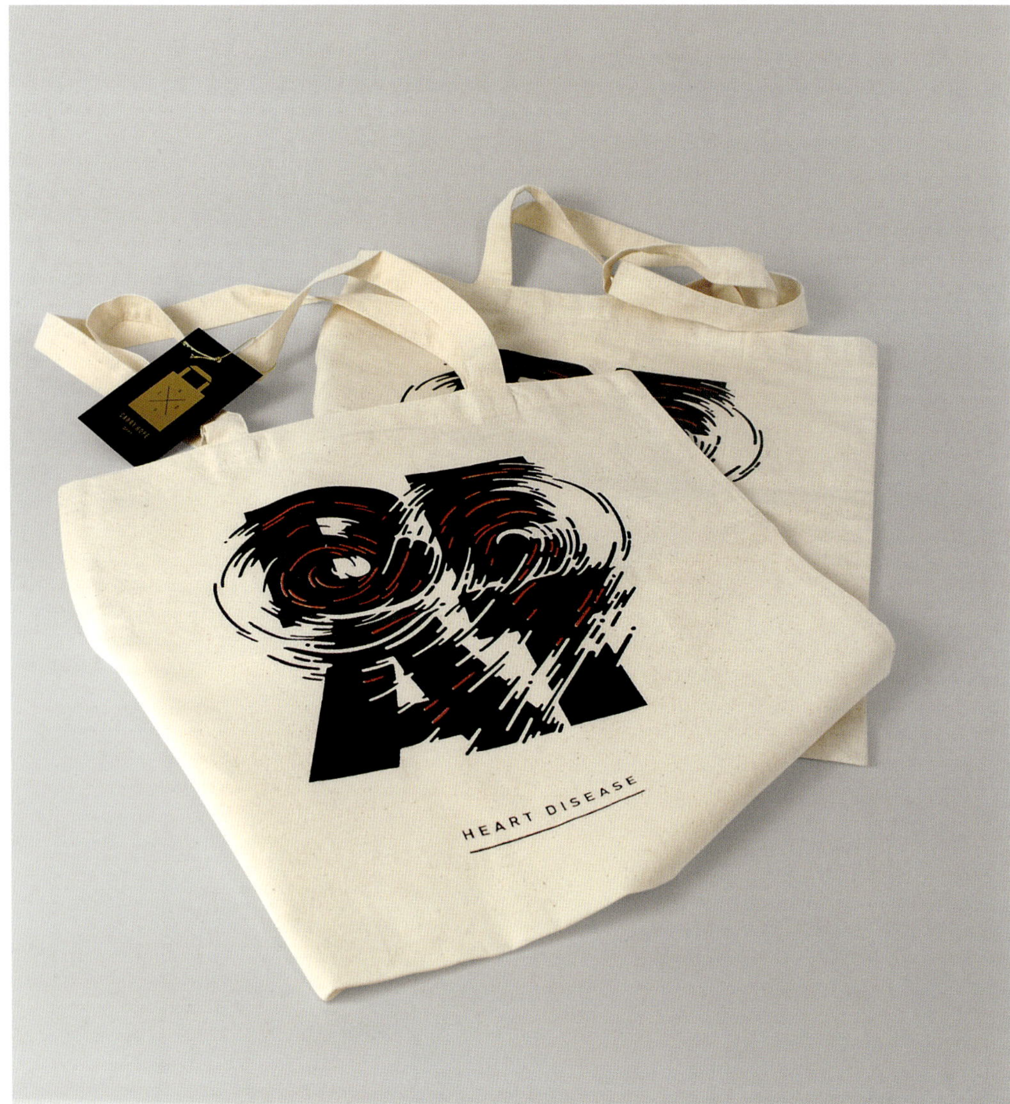
HEART DISEASE

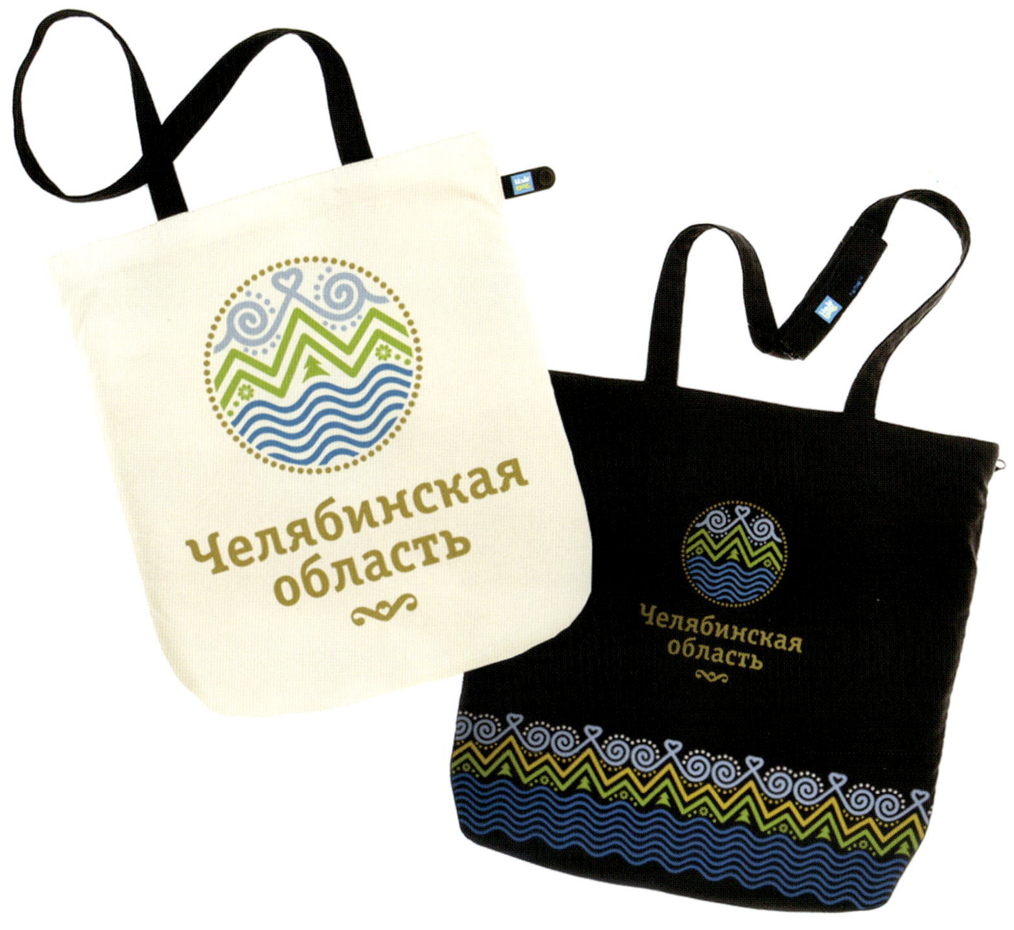

CARRY HOPE
DE: Rob Gonzalez, Jonathan Quainton

Designed for a charity that strives to fight heart disease, the bag uses the word "beat" to demonstrate the resolution to "beat heart disease," while the twirling effect represents the blood flow enabled by the beating of the heart.

CHELYABINSK REGION
DE: Daniil Shumakov

Designed for a tourist brand, this bag was printed with a logo that represents natural elements - the sun, the sky, forest etc.

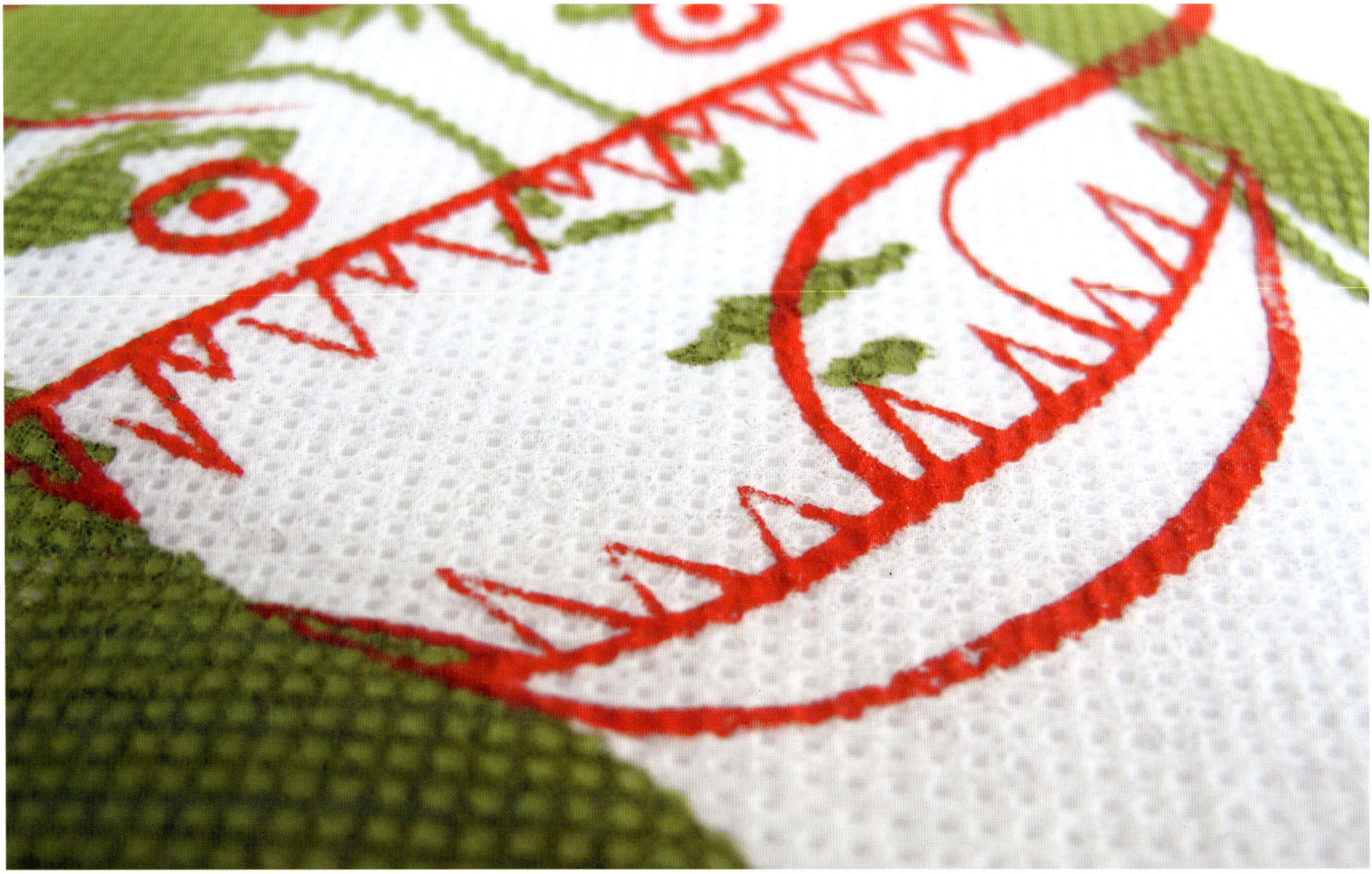

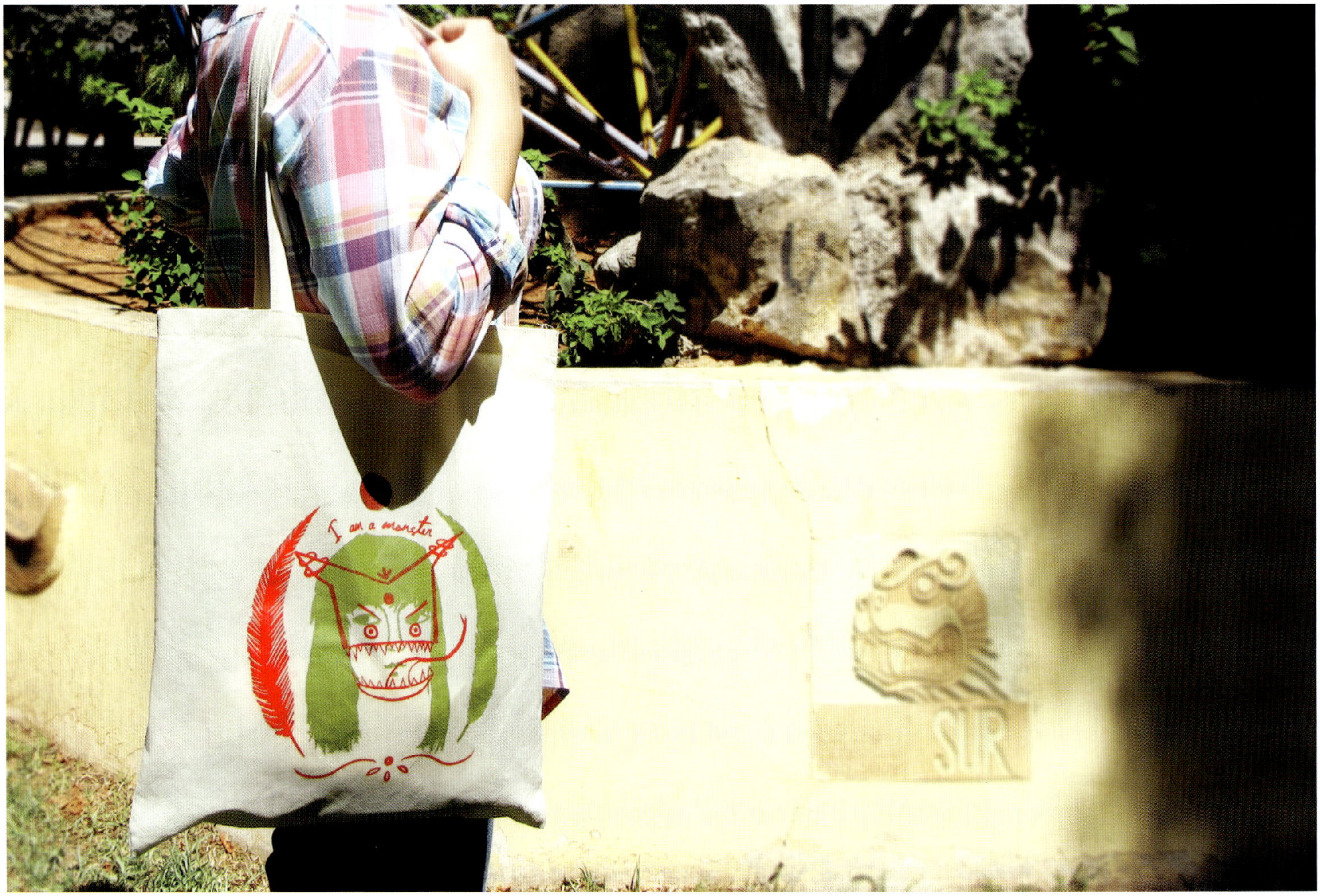

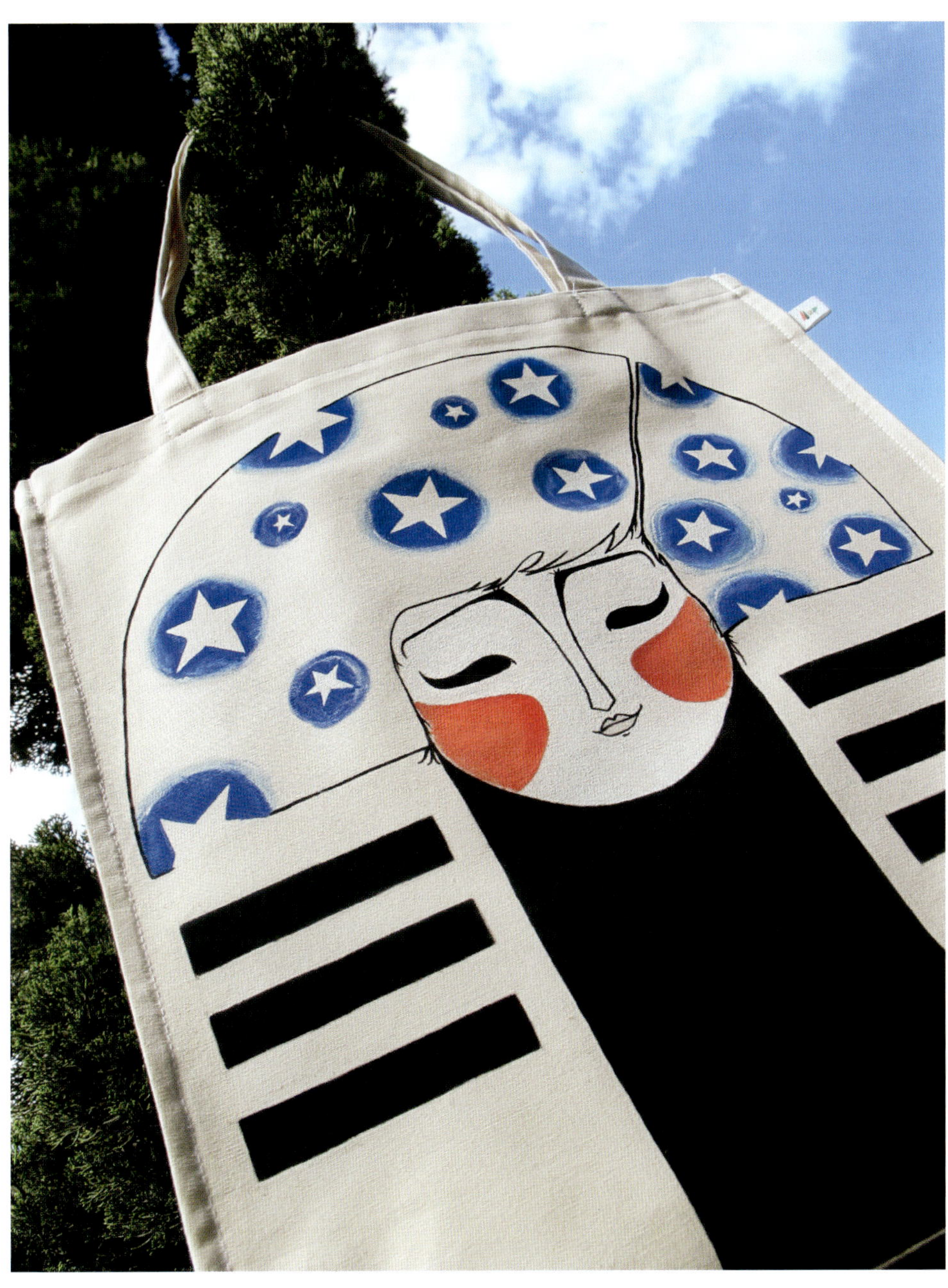

I AM A MONSTER
DE: Llop

Realized in two-ink serigraph, the bag presents an illustration of a girl wearing a monster mask.

STAR GIRL
DE: Llop

This bag was hand-made and illustrated by the artist.

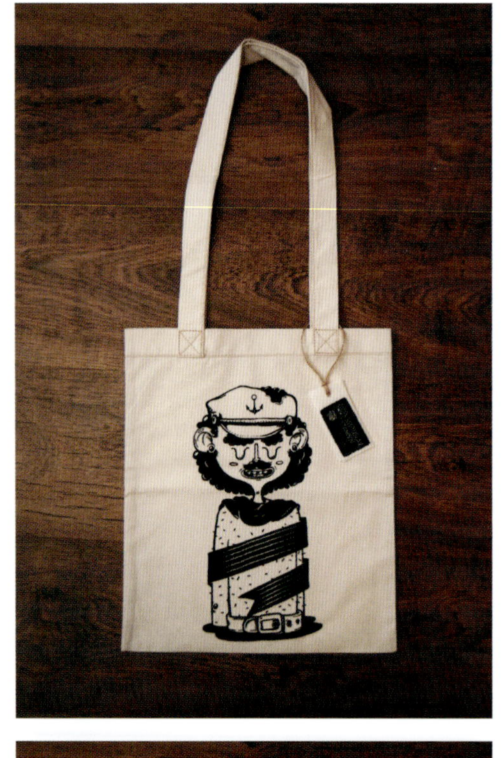
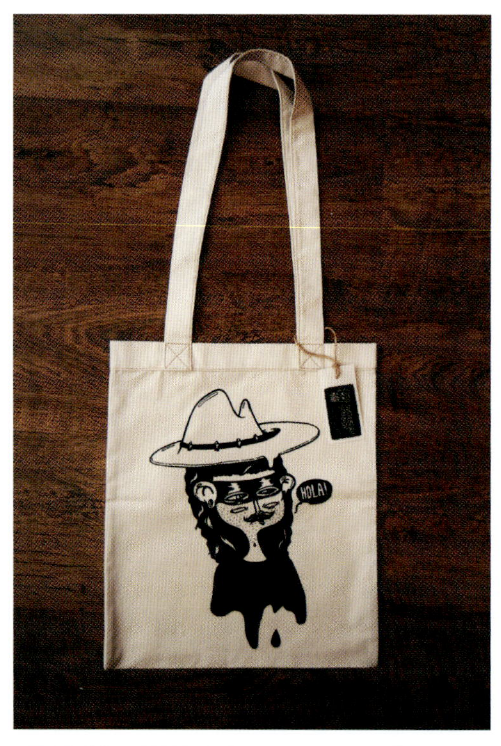
HOLA!
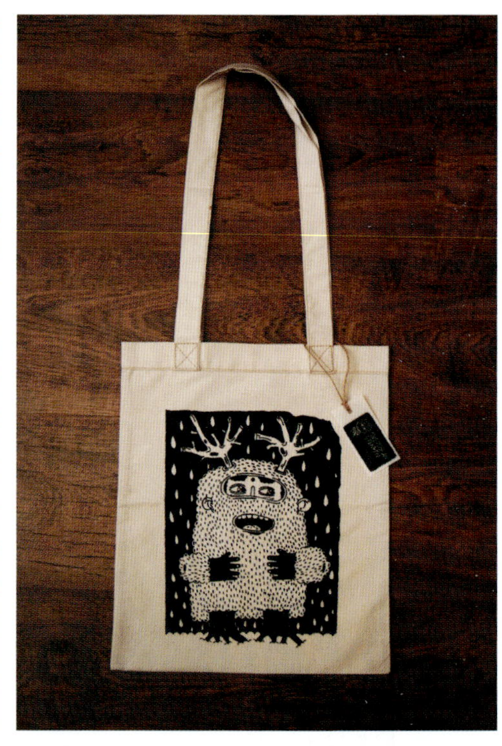
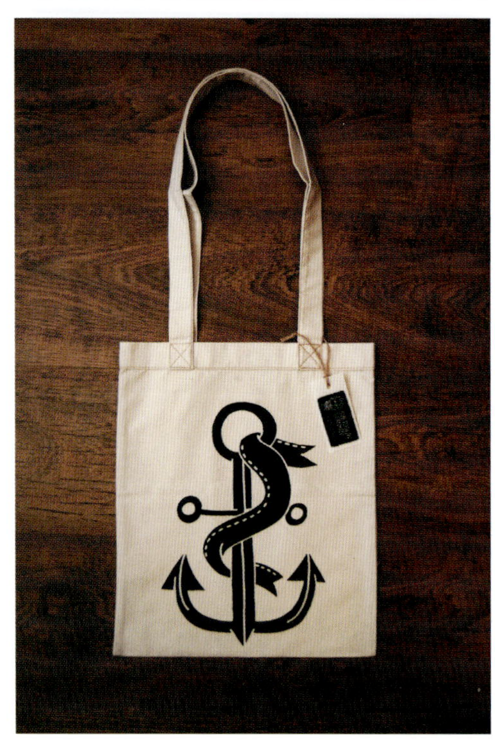
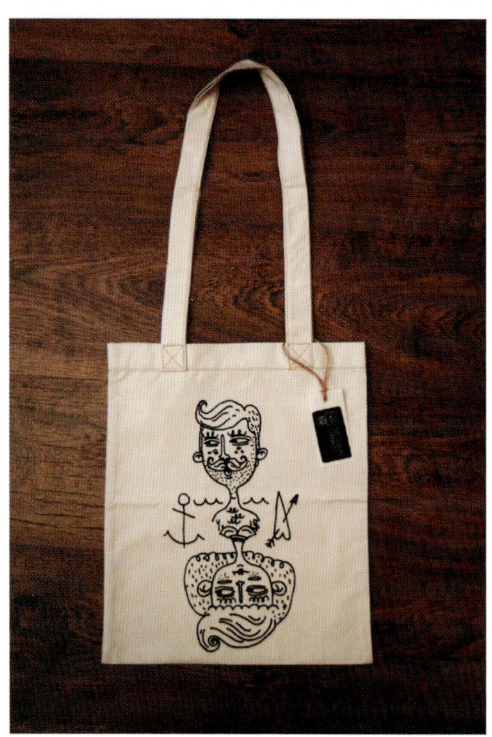
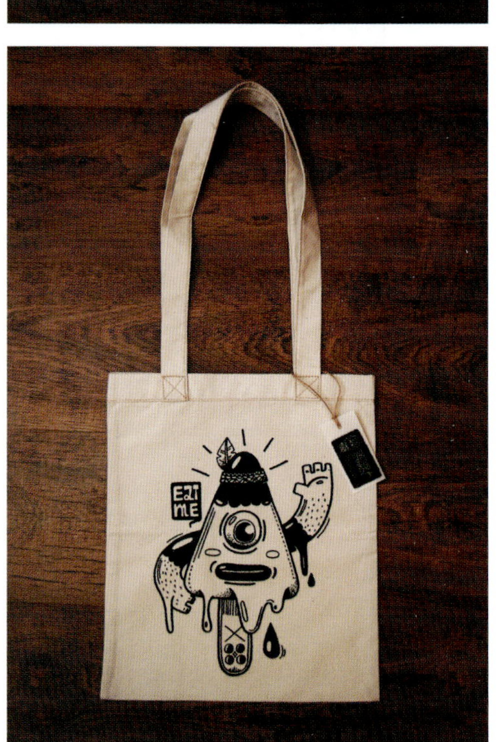
EAT ME

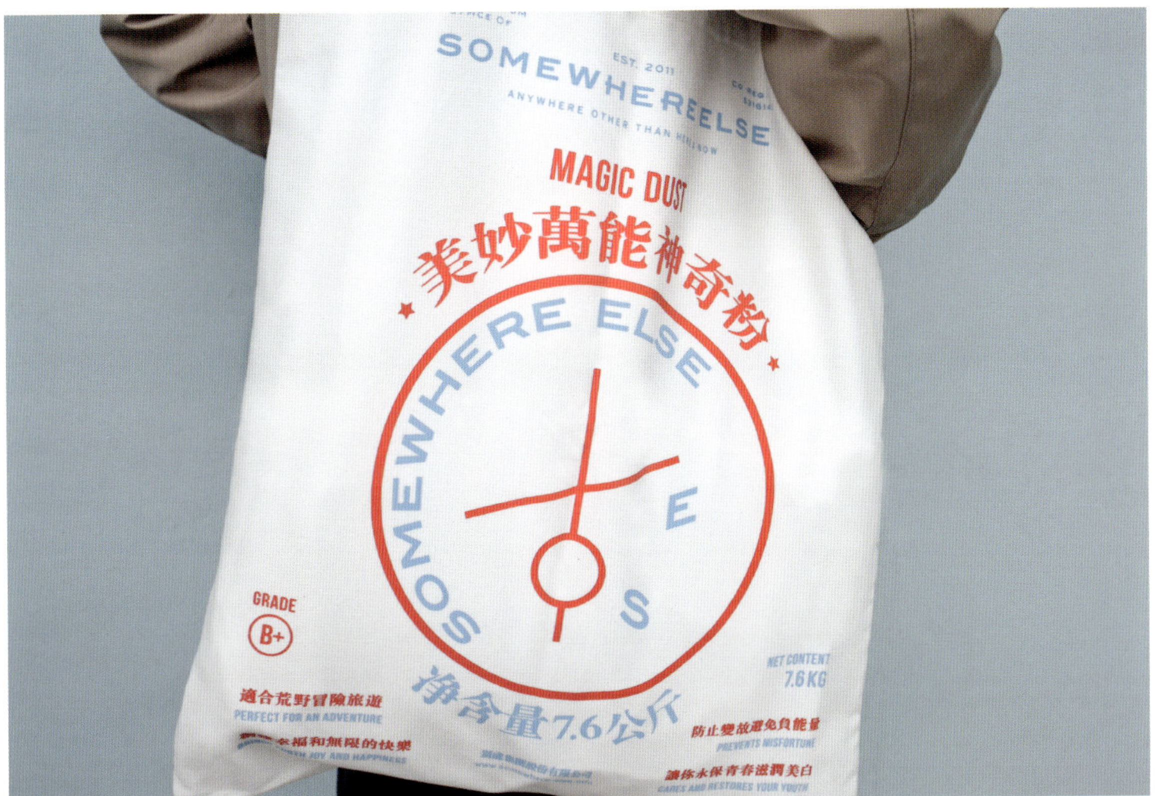

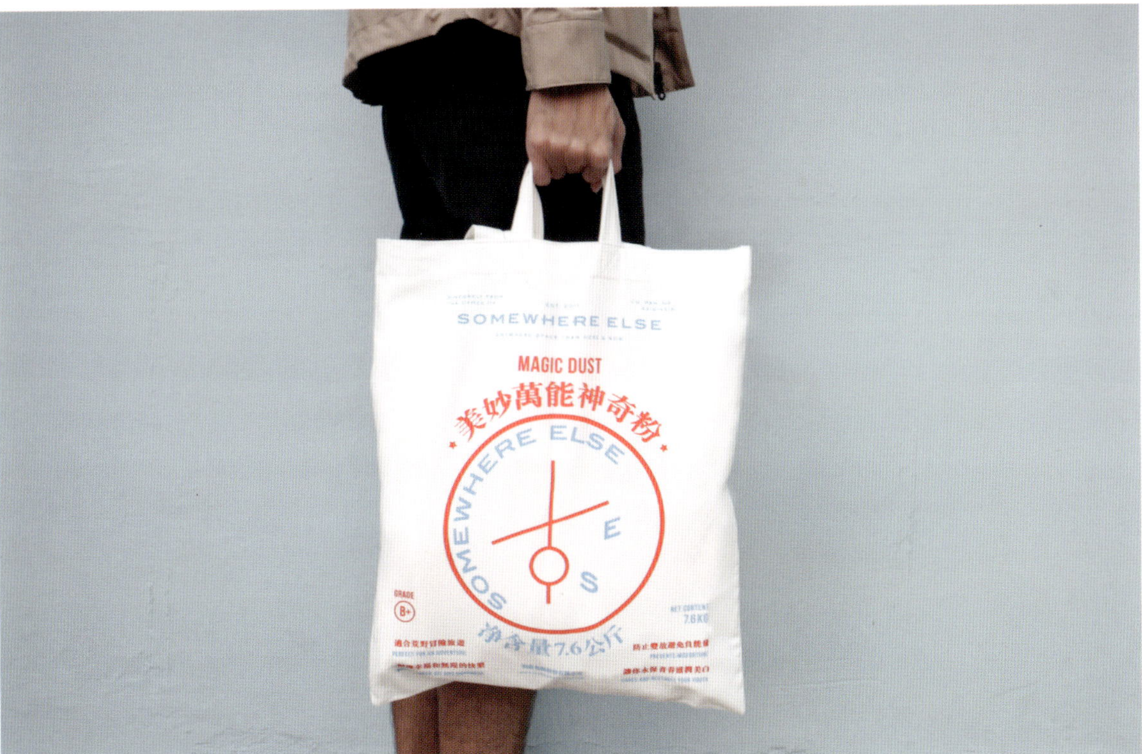

ILLUSTRATED ECO BAG
DE: Svetoslav Stankov

This series features illustrated work that best represents the illustrator, which bring a whimsical feel to the bag.

MAGIC DUST
DA: Somewhere Else

Taking inspiration from rice sacks and herbs used in traditional Chinese medicine, the designer promotes a fictional product: "Magic Dust" with the bag, because everyone needs a little bit of magic every once in a while. The design aims to boost optimism.

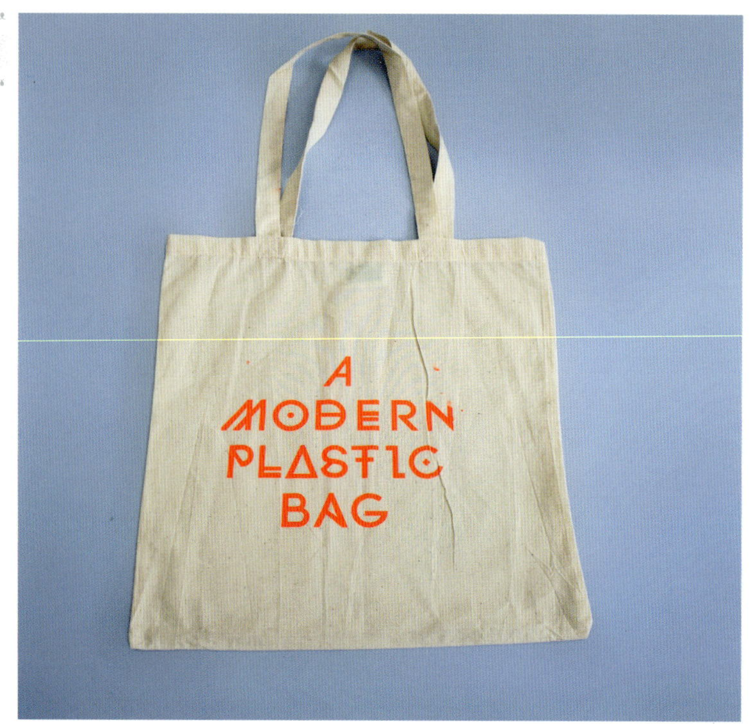
A MODERN PLASTIC BAG

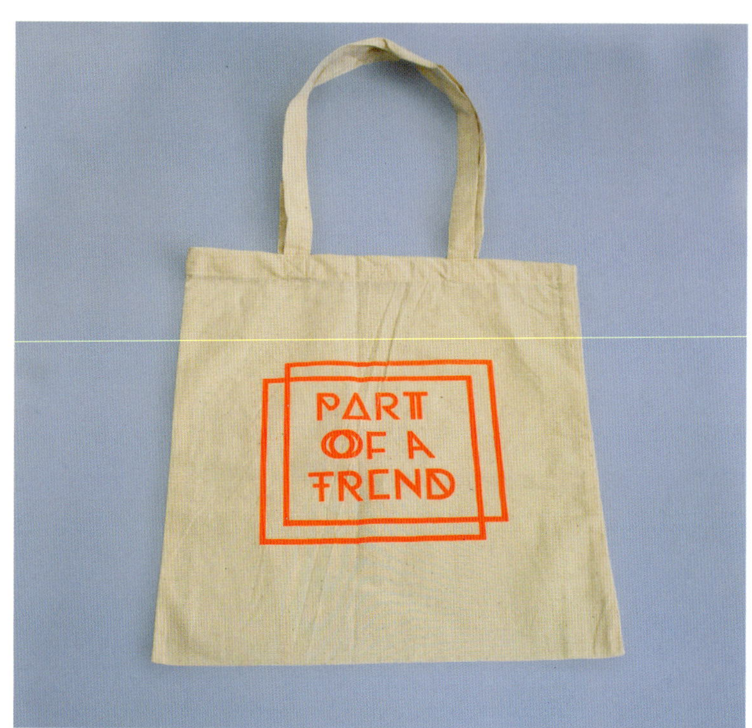
PART OF A TREND

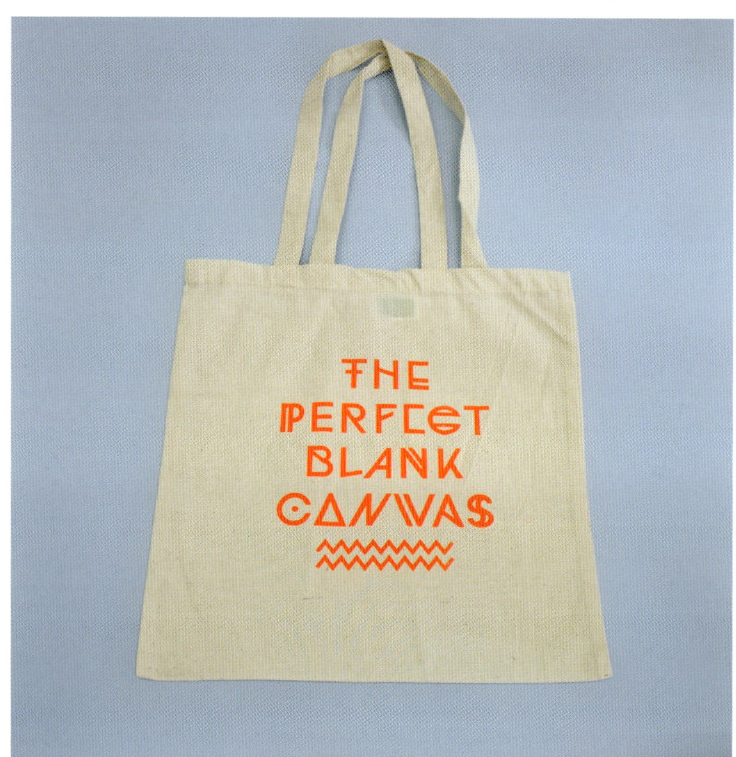
THE PERFECT BLANK CANVAS

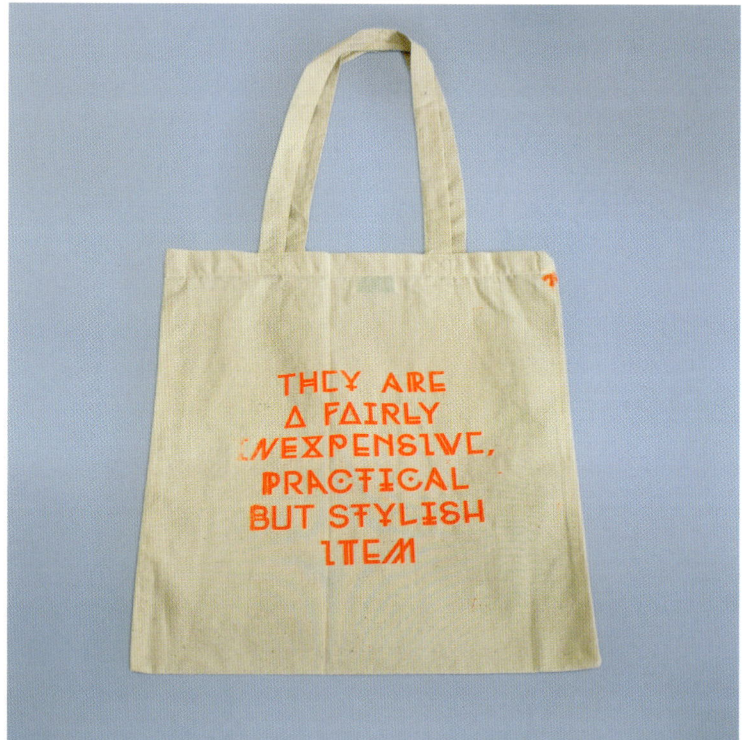
THEY ARE A FAIRLY INEXPENSIVE, PRACTICAL BUT STYLISH ITEM

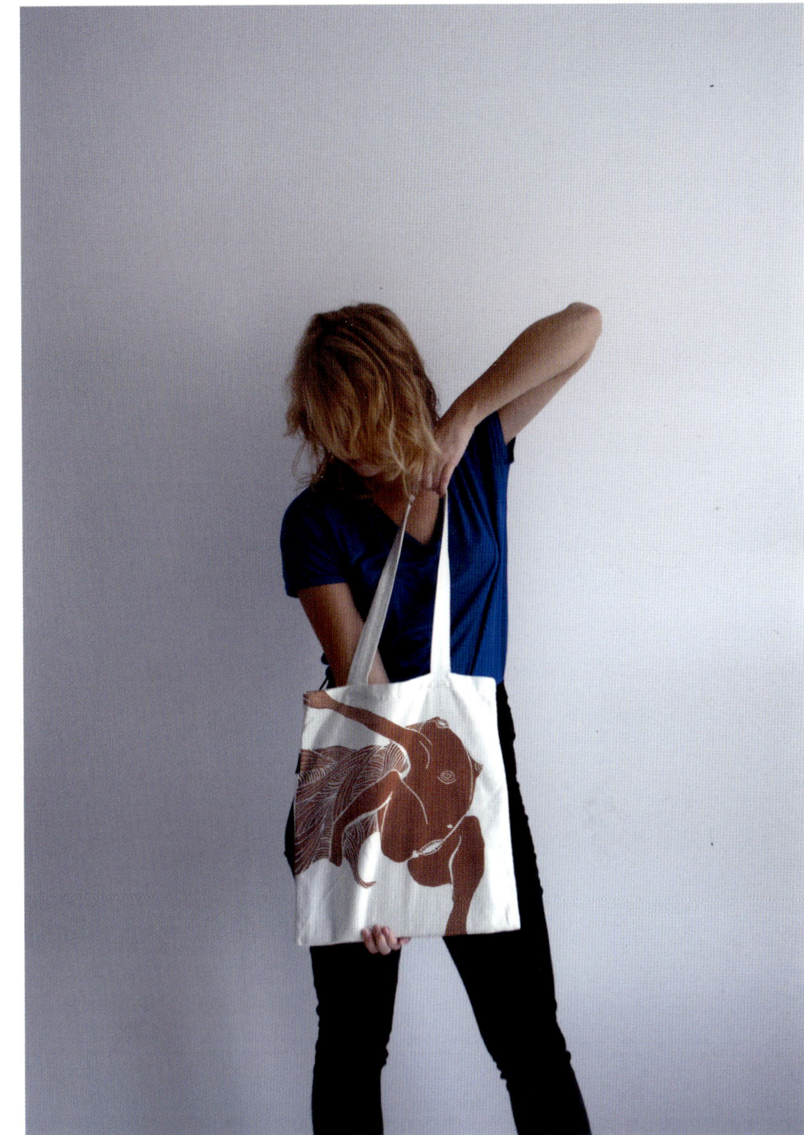

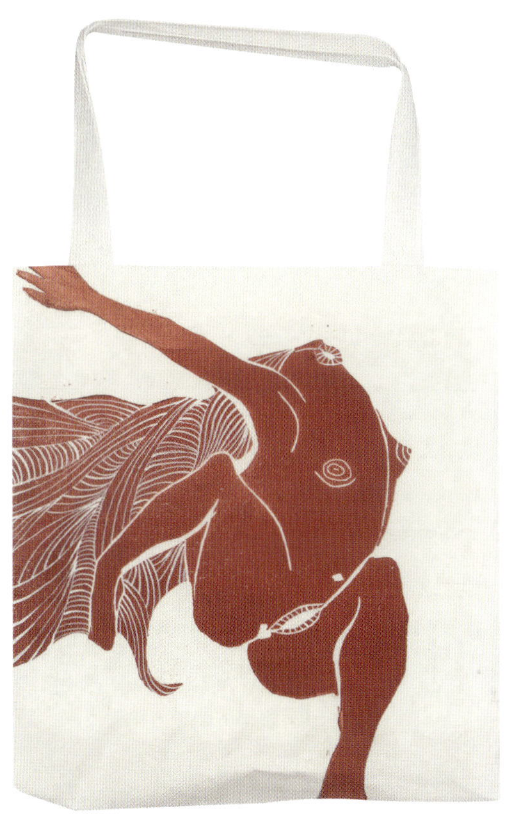

THE TOTE BAG
DE: Helene H. Devold

As a result of a research project, in which Helene interviewed many designers on bag design, the series was printed with quotes from the interviewees in fluoresces ink.

MUJER DESNUDA
DE: Caroline Cracco

This illustration printed on it the bag was conceived during the designer's stay in Barcelona, a place full of passion and zest for life. Inspired, she surrendered herself to her intuition and she created a portrait in such a sensual posture.

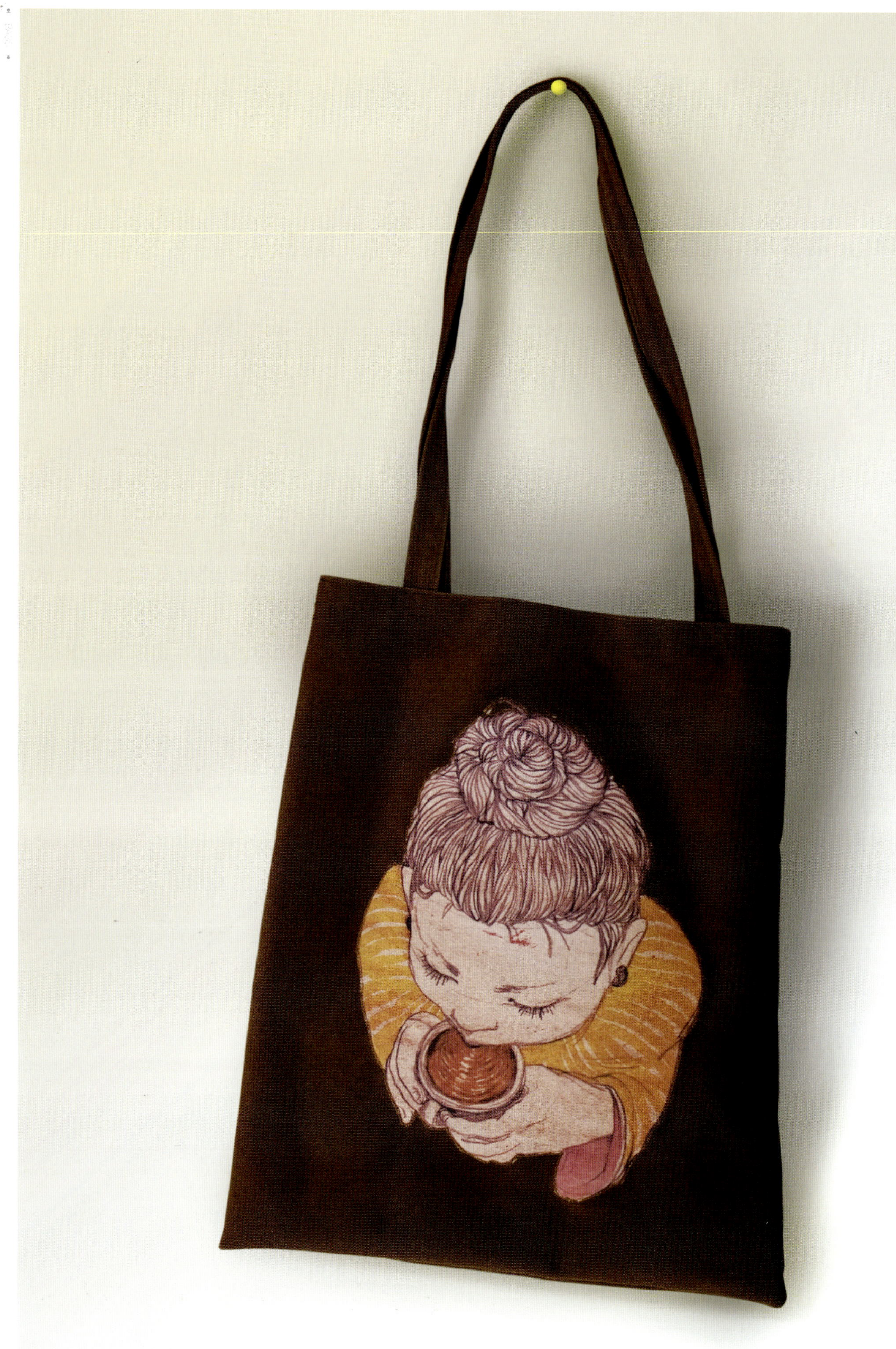

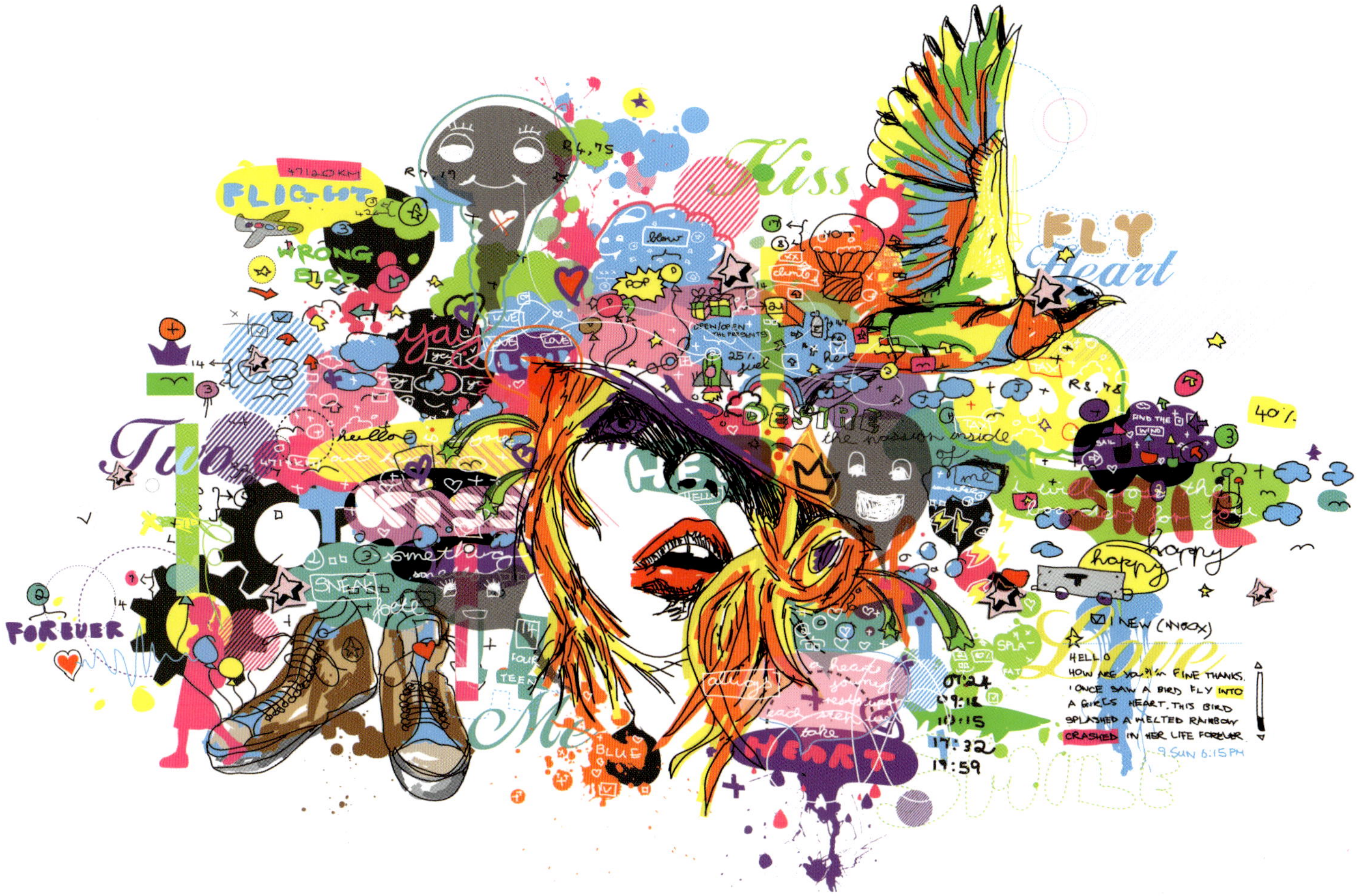

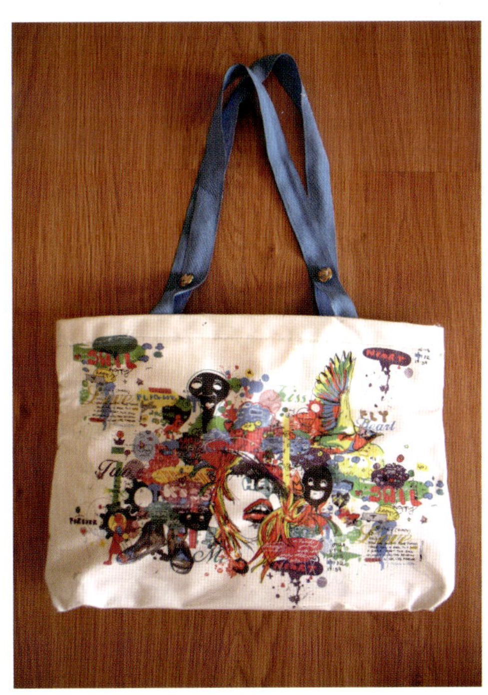

REITERATING THE CONTENT
DE: Daniel Ting Chong

This bag features an image of splashing colors, covering a mixed range of patterns, indicating that the contents inside the bag can be anything that brings excitement to the world.

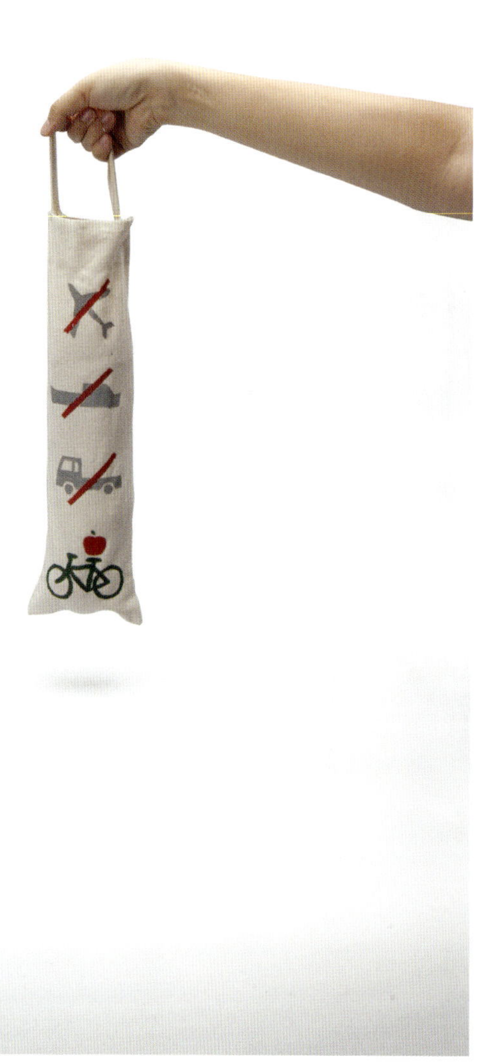

Buy+Cycle
APPLE
EAT Local Food

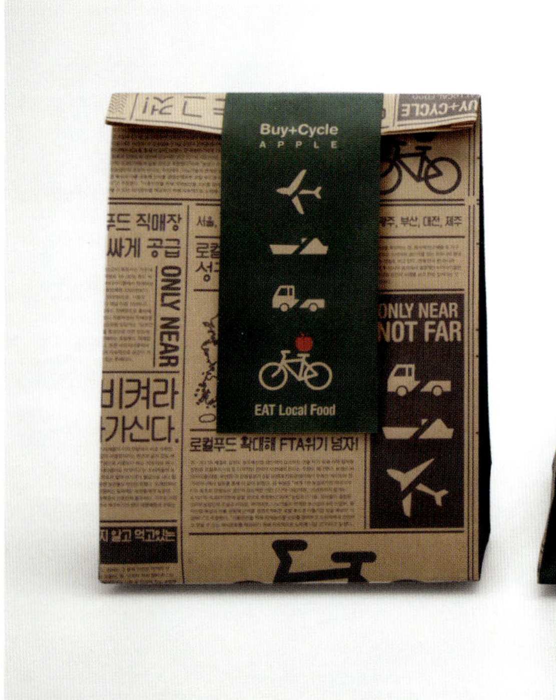

Buy+Cycle
APPLE
ONLY NEAR
NOT FAR
EAT Local Food
ONLY NEAR
비켜라
가신다.
로컬푸드 직매장
싸게 공급
로컬푸드 확대해 FTA위기 넘자!

BUY+CYCLE
EAT LOCAL FOOD

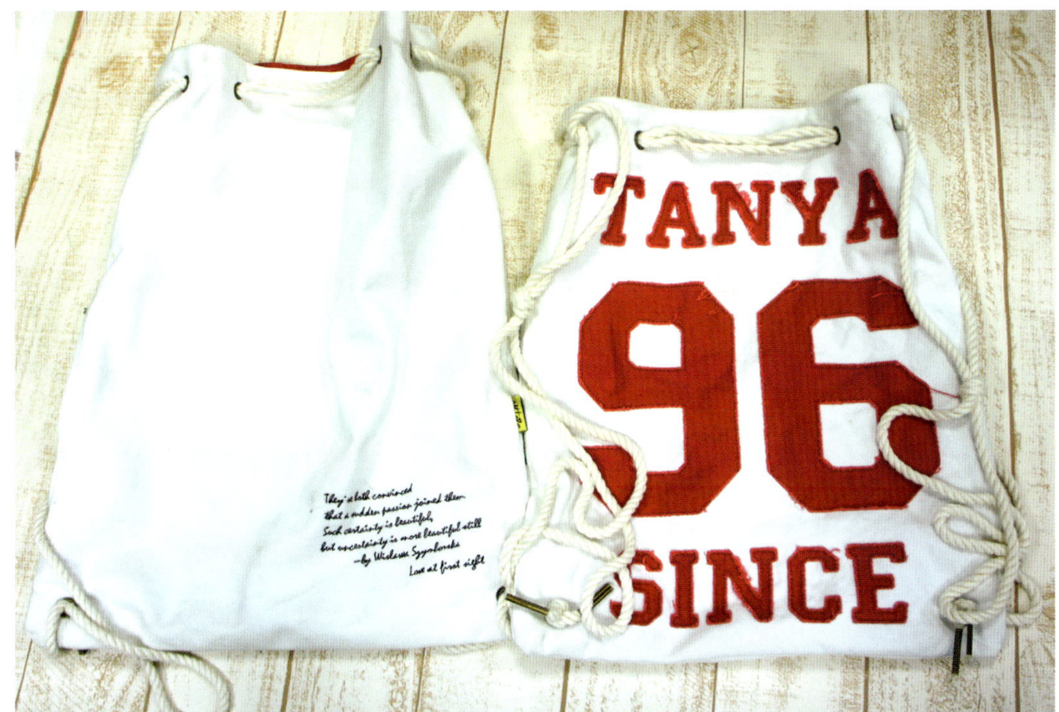

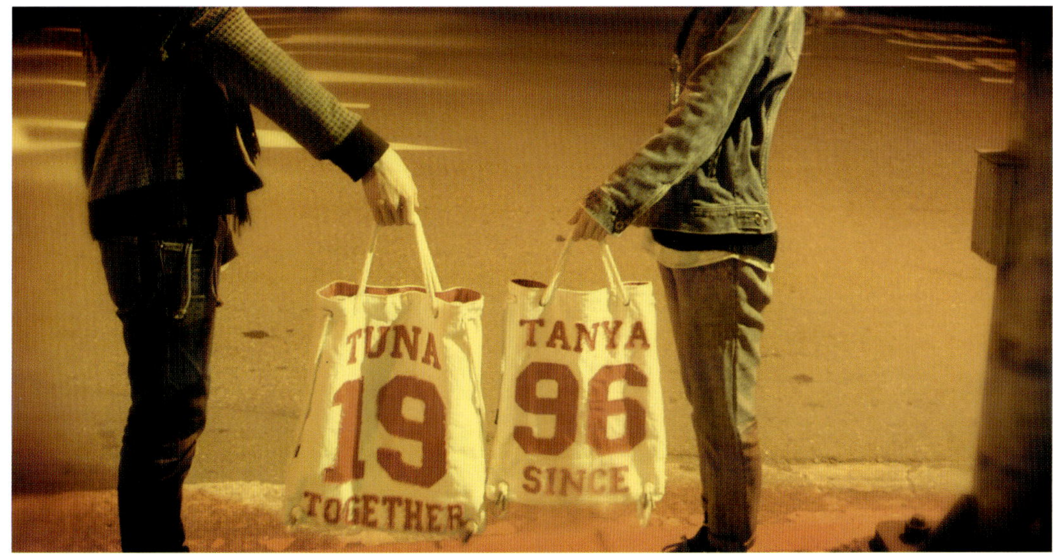

LOCAL FOOD BAG
DE: Kwag Yeon-jung

Intended to encourage the purchase of local food, a cloth bag was designed and printed with patterns that advocate short distance transportation.

LOVE BAG
DE: Ohtoro

The "Love Bag" was designed in pair to commemorate a couple's anniversary, with both people's name and the year they met embroidered on it.

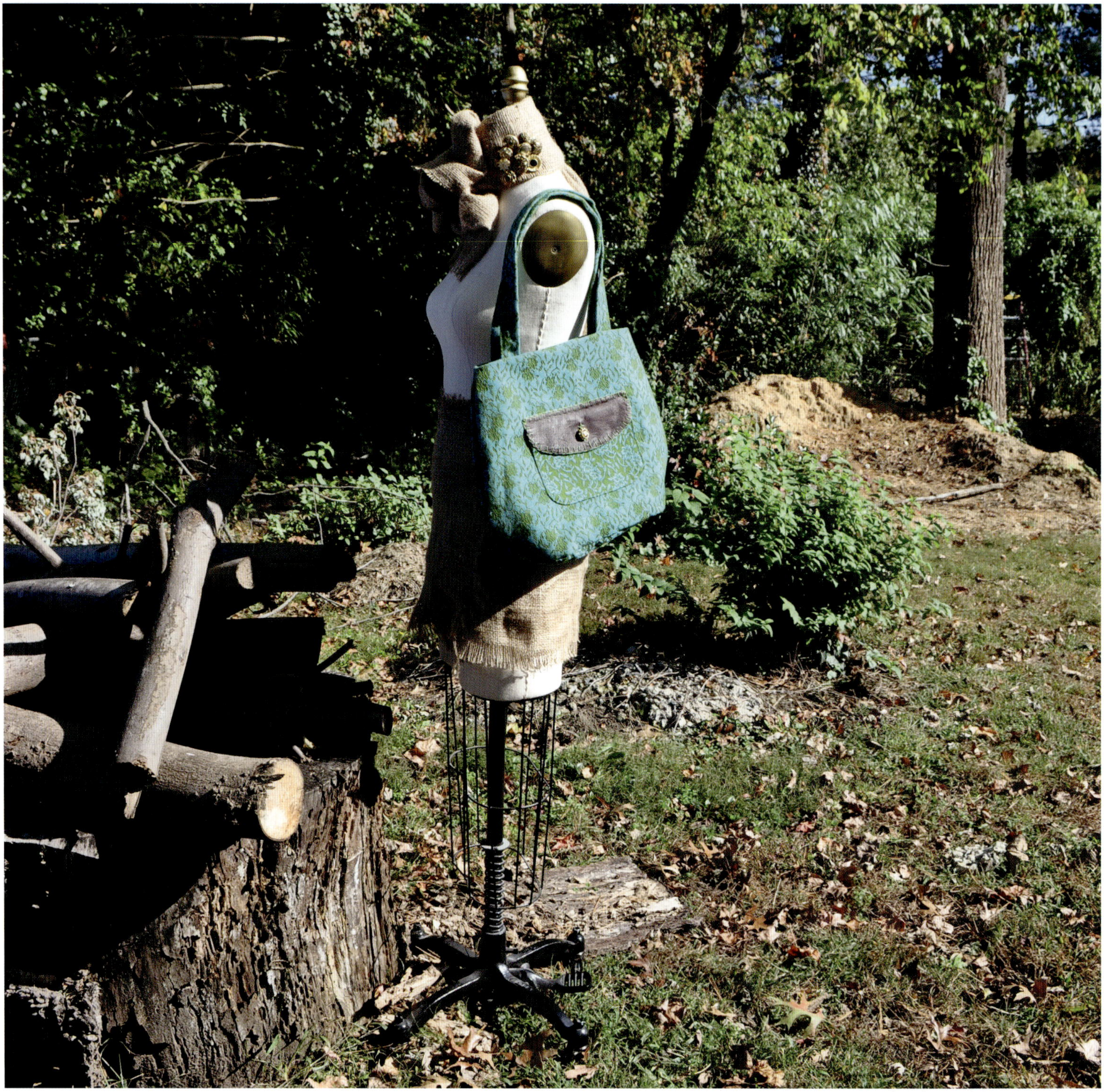

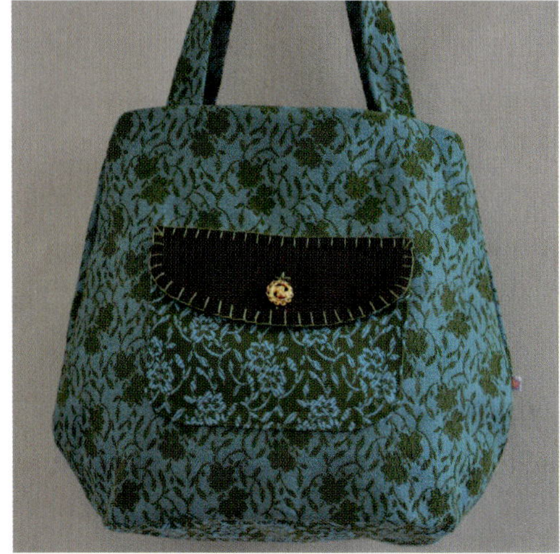
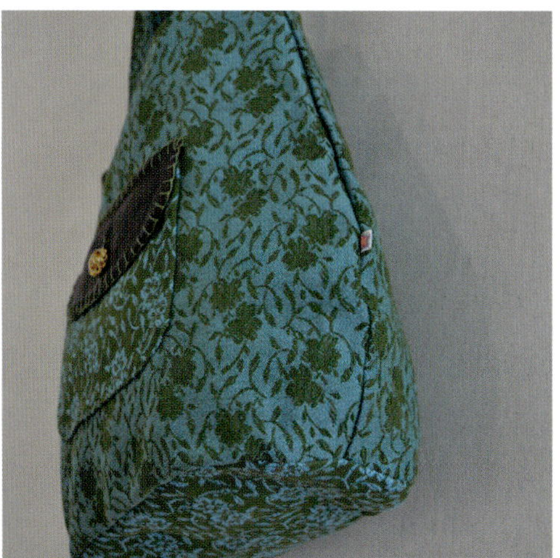
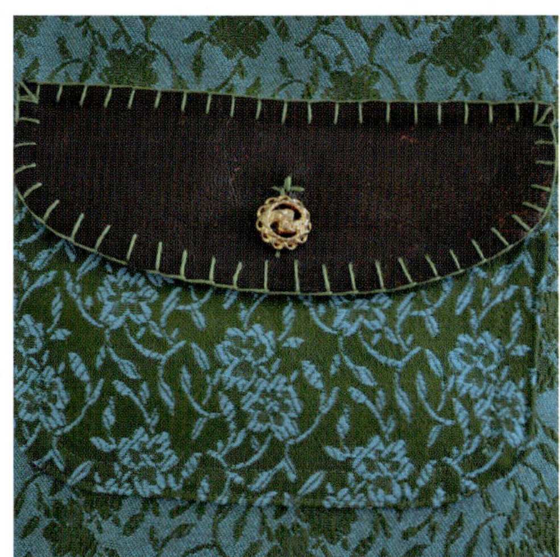

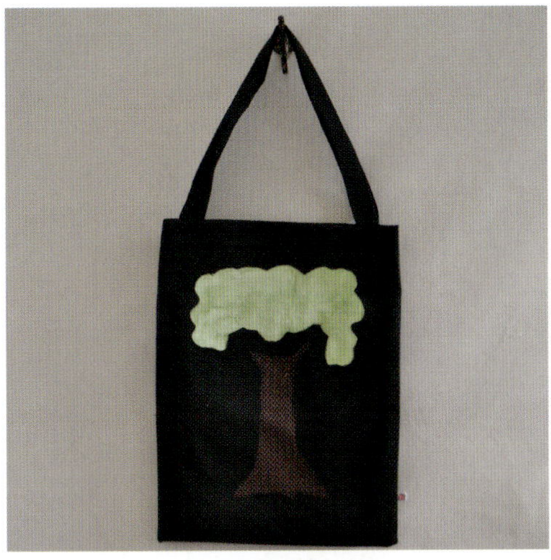 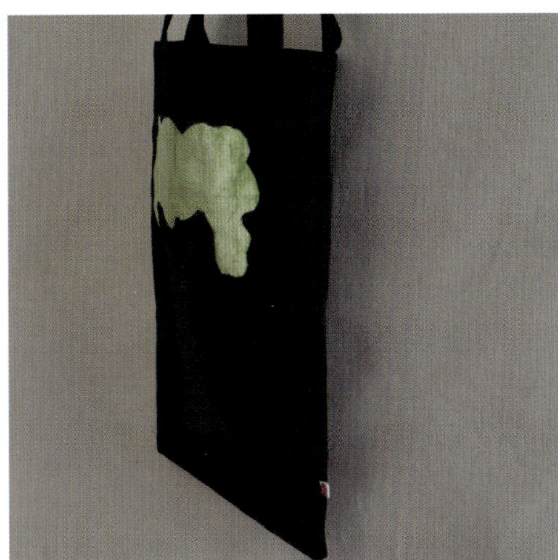 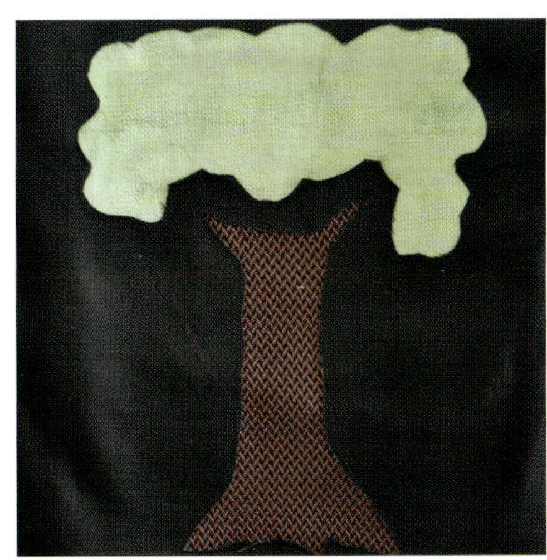

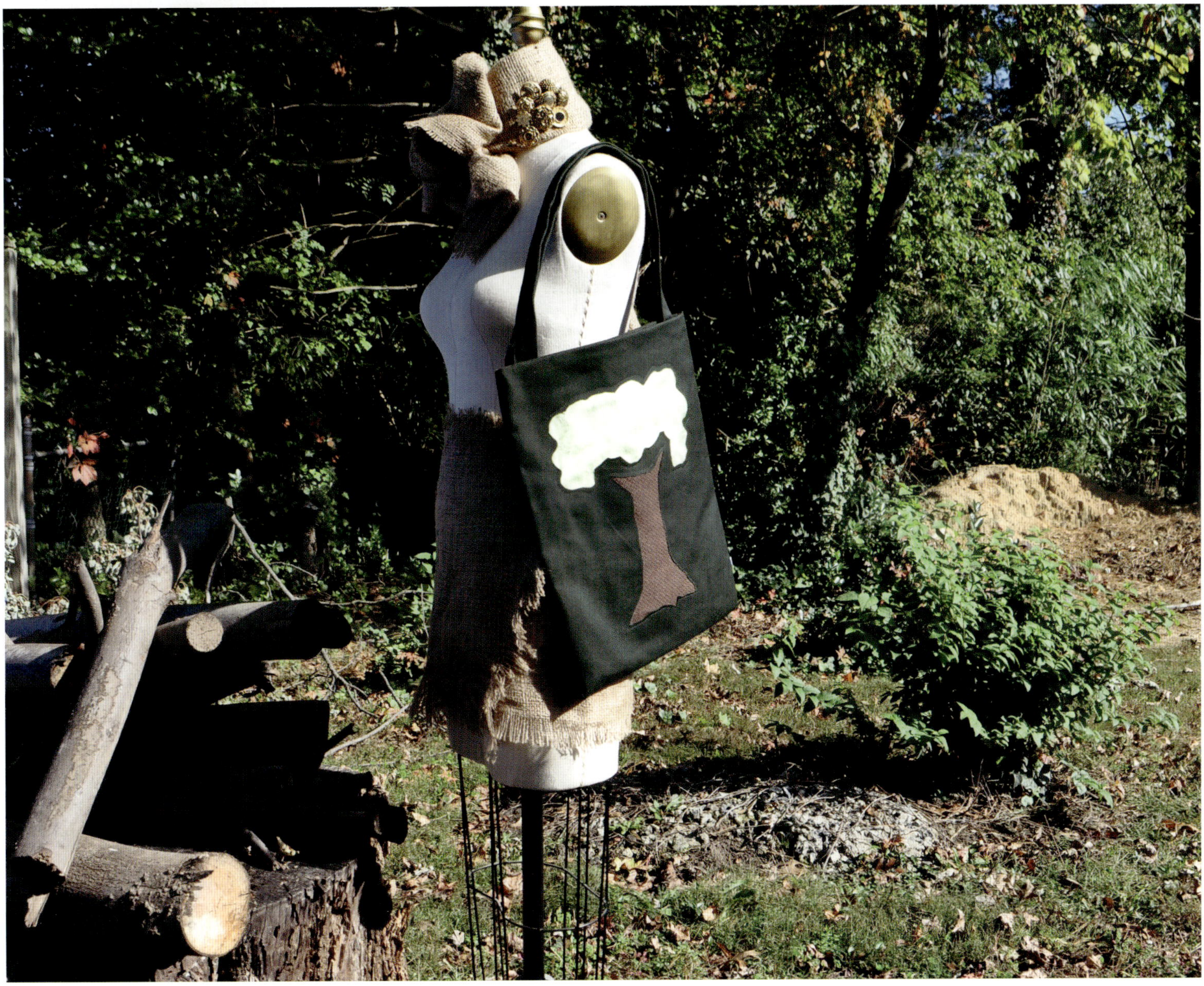

TURQUOISE FIELD BUCKET BAG
DE: Korie Mae Moore

The "Turquoise Field Bucket" bag is handcrafted from vintage brocade fabric, accented with a leather patch pocket, bound by a contrasting blanket stitch and secured with an old-fashioned button.

HUNTER GREEN TREE TOTE
DE: Korie Mae Moore

This tree pattern was constructed with textured brown and black herringbone suiting and textured, velvet-like, vibrant green fabric.

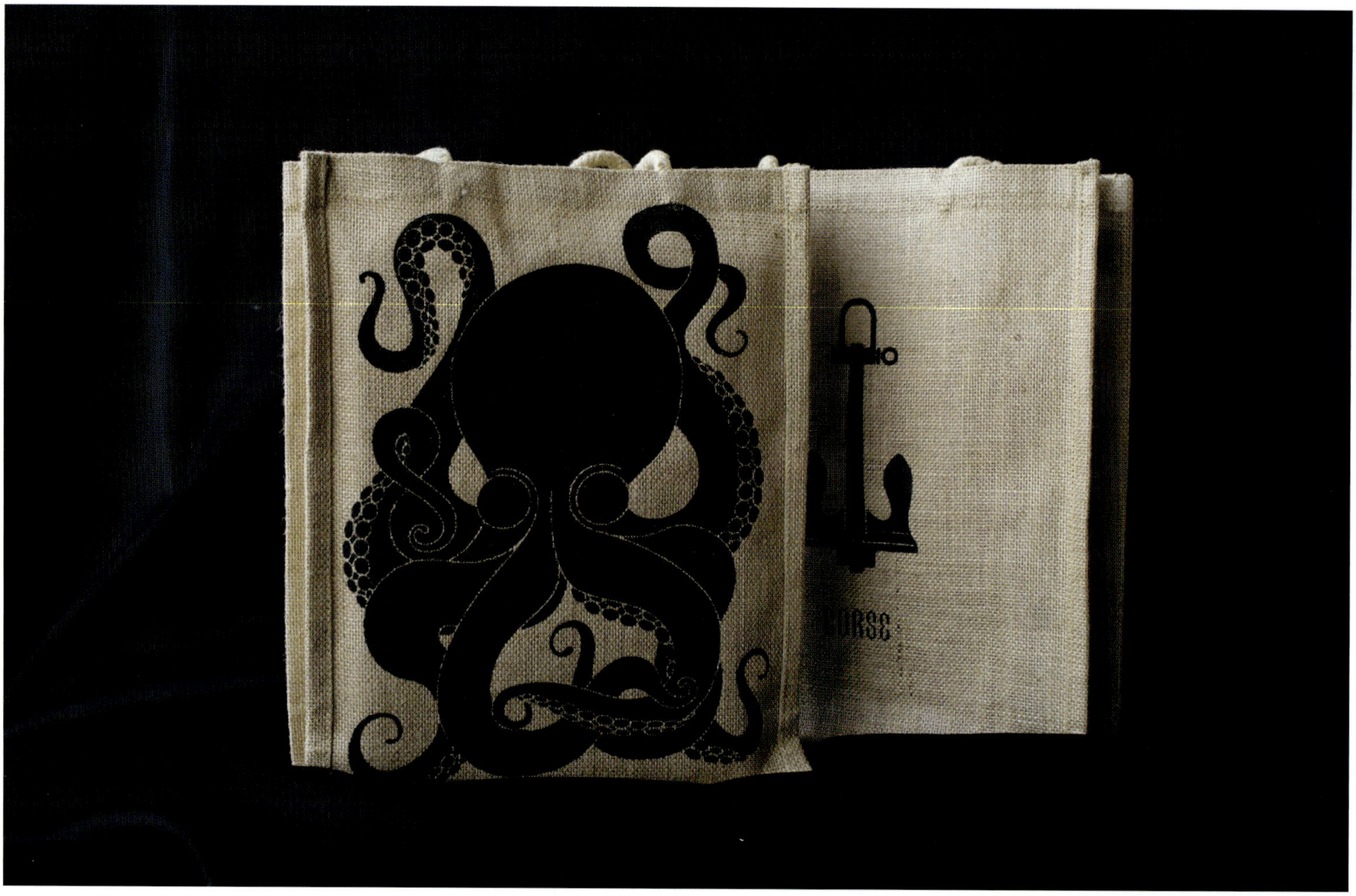

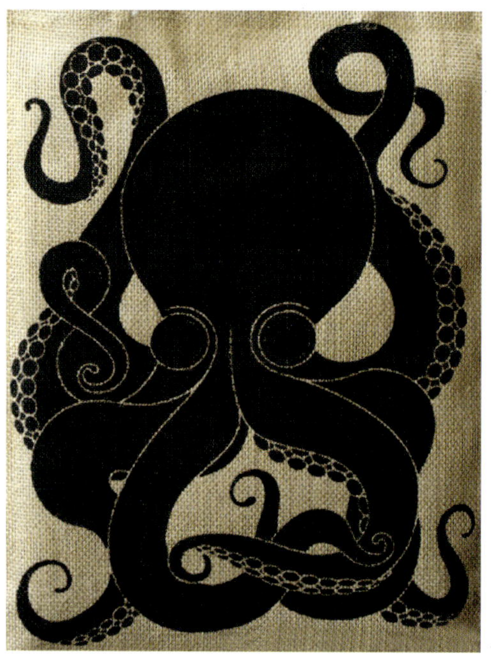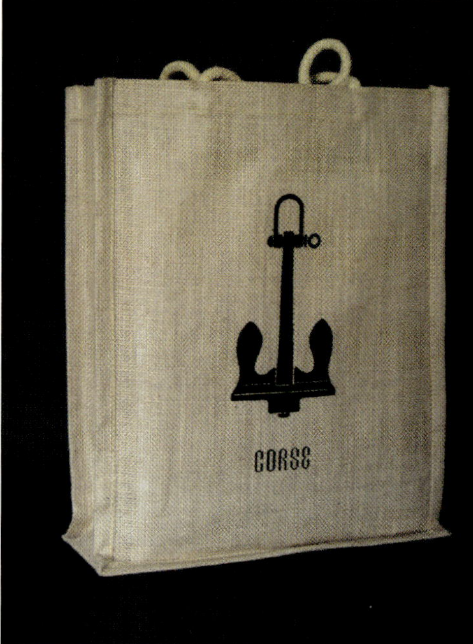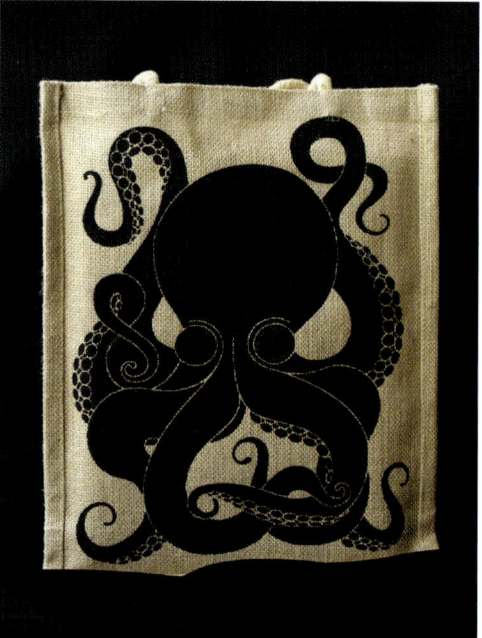

CORSE KRAKEN BAG
DA: Corse Design Factory

Inspired by jute, which is the material for rope that ties boats in the
harbors, this bag was made of 100% natural jute printed with an octopus to
resonate with the marine theme.

RUSTIC BURLAP BAG
DE: Violeta Petrova

Made of lined burlap, this bag is decorated with cotton and handles are made
of braided twine. The complementary chalkboard tag is for personalization.

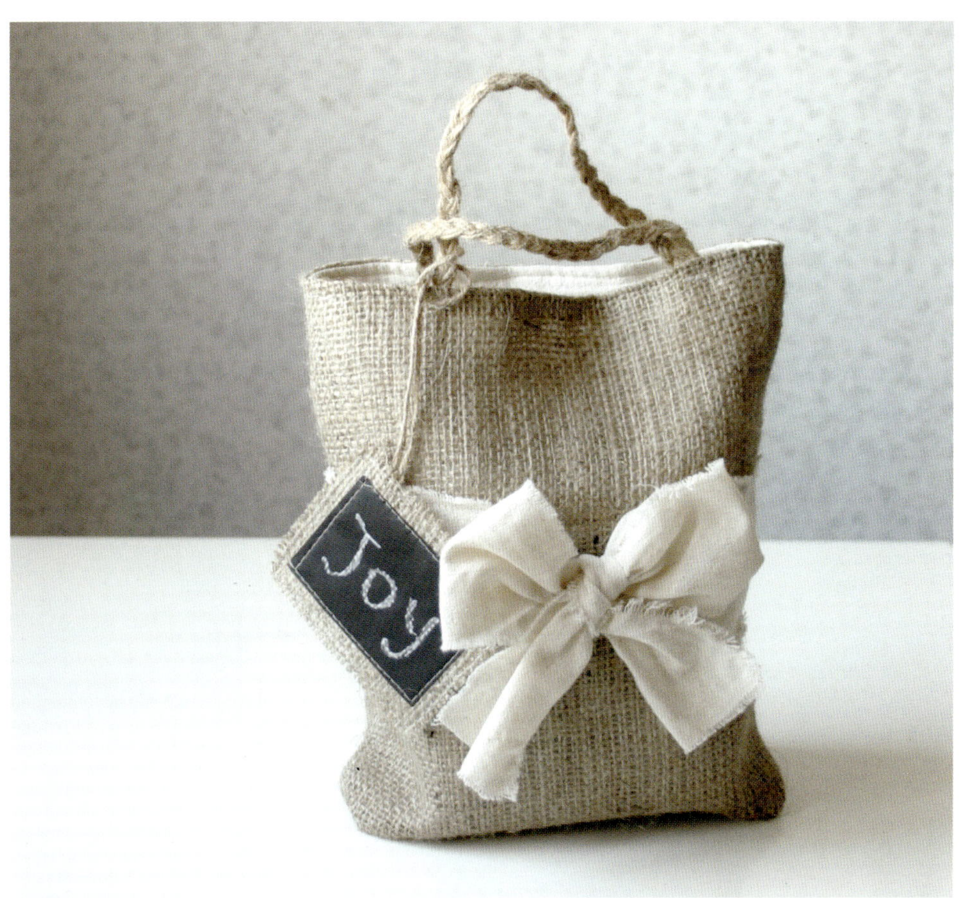

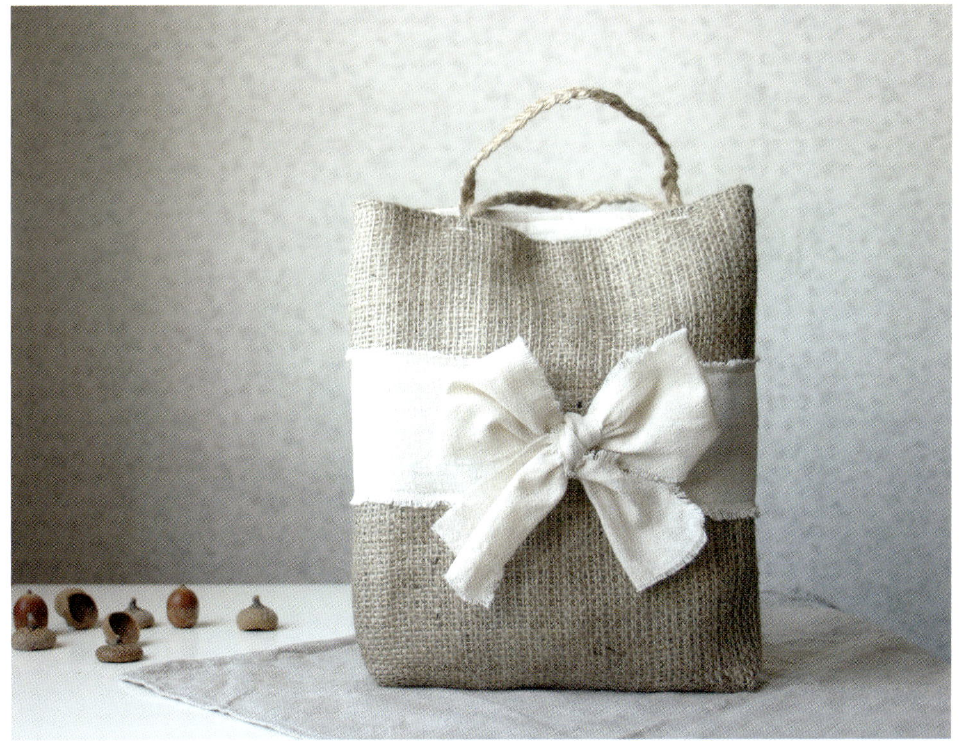

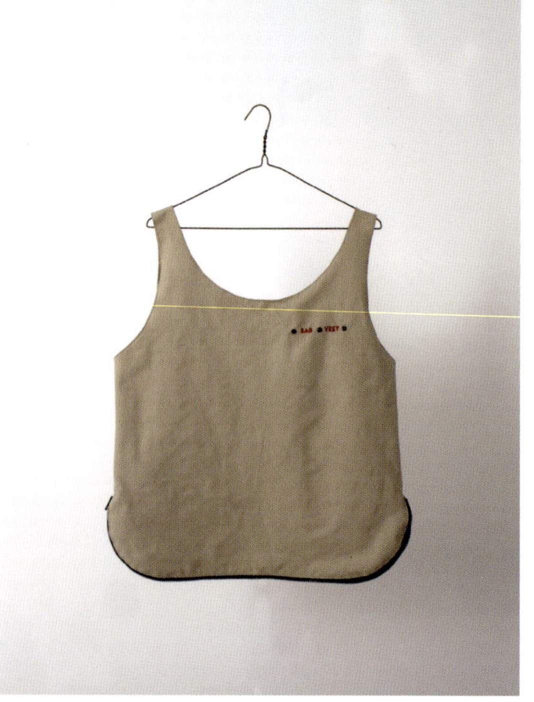

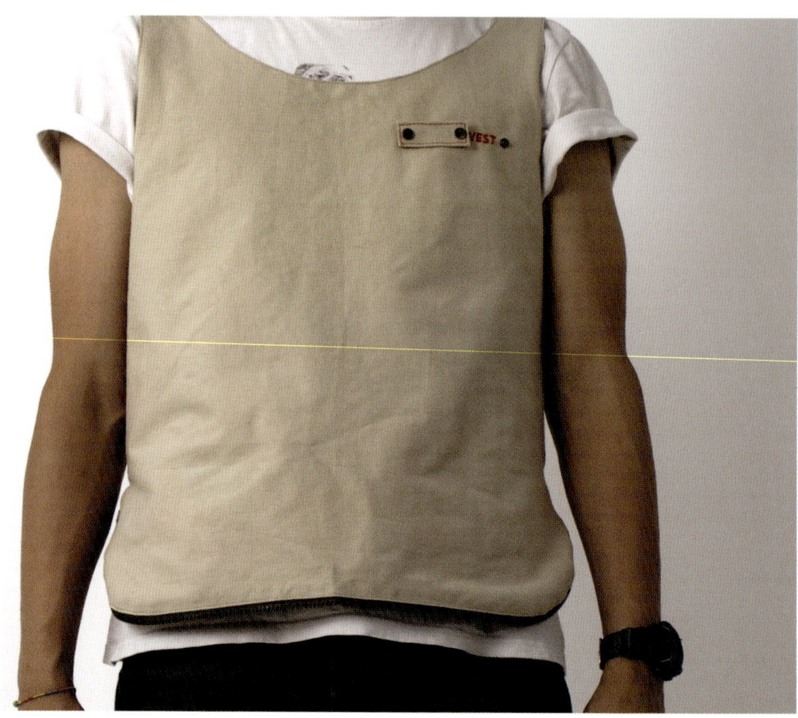

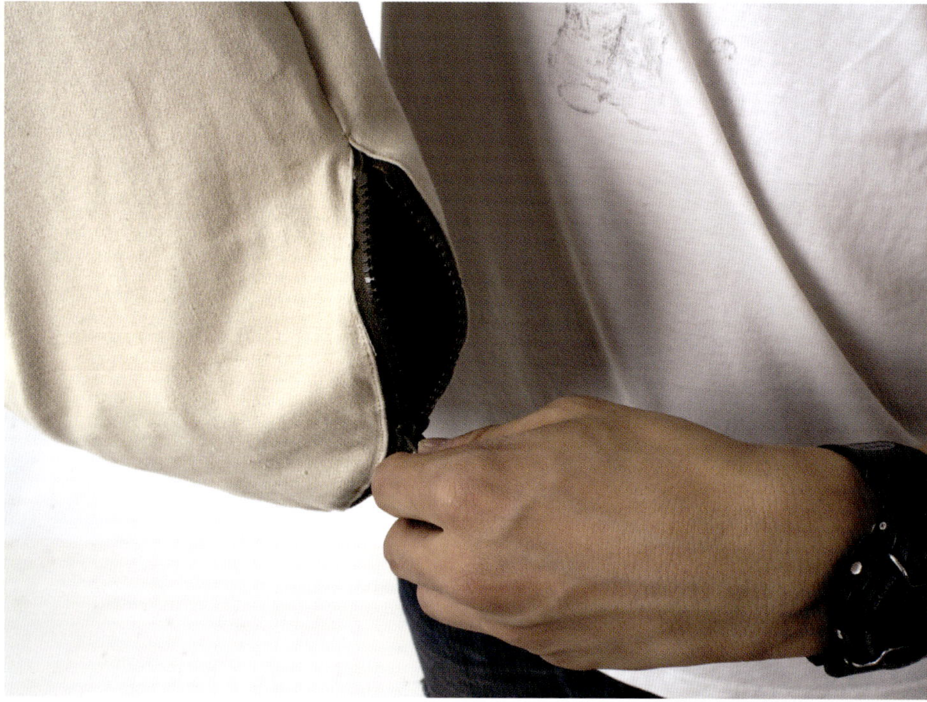

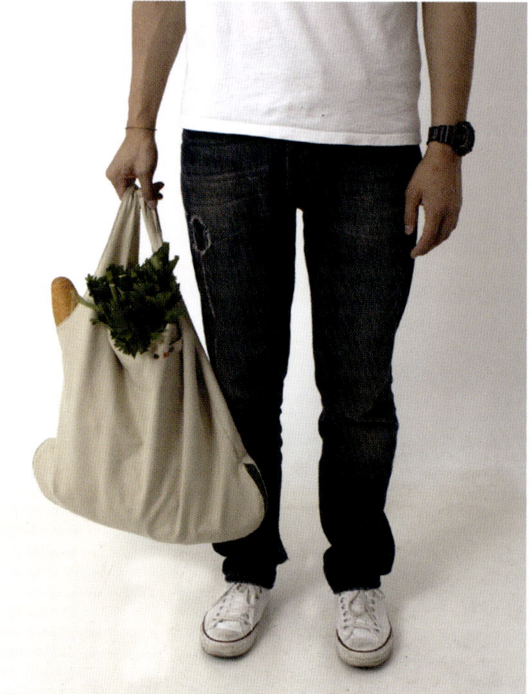

WEARABLE BAG

DE: Kwang-Su Kim

This bag can be converted into a vest using a zipper on bottom.

TANK TOP BAG

DE: Jimmy Lee

Made of thick canvas in shocking orange and dark/light blue, this tank top bag interacts with the contents. A pair of sunglasses can be hung instead of being put inside, creating a playful image.

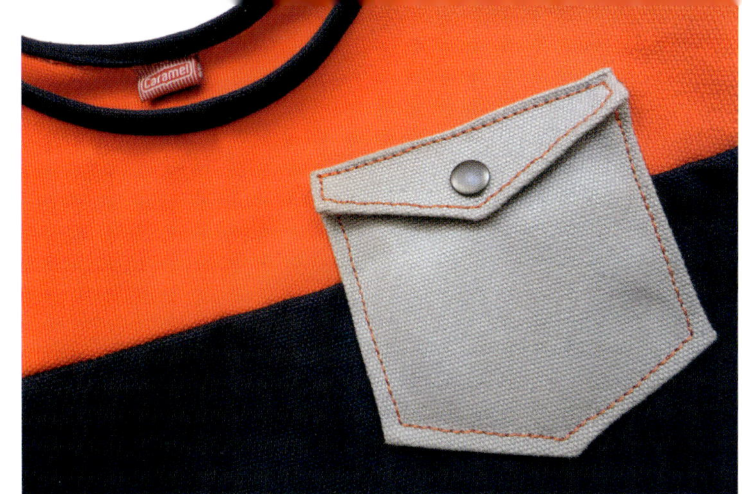
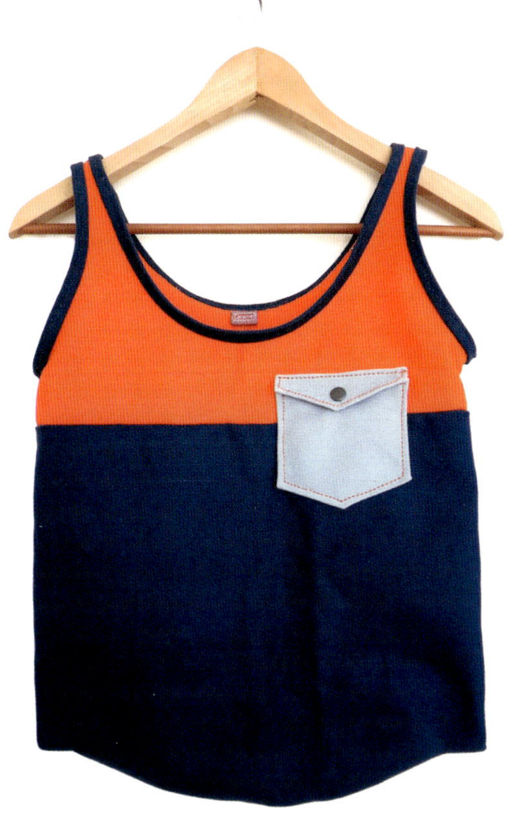
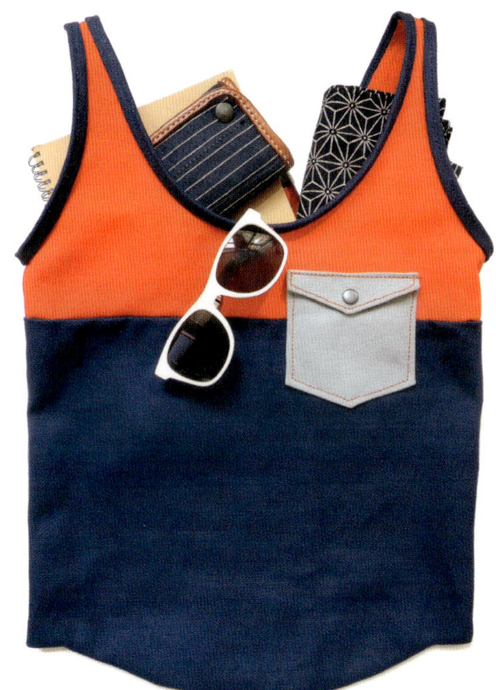
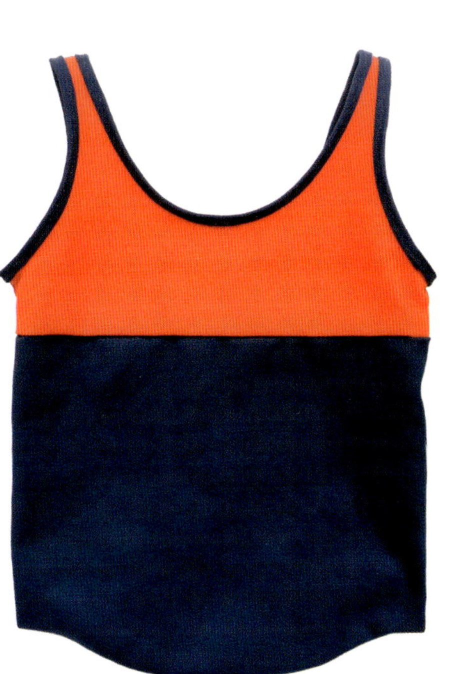

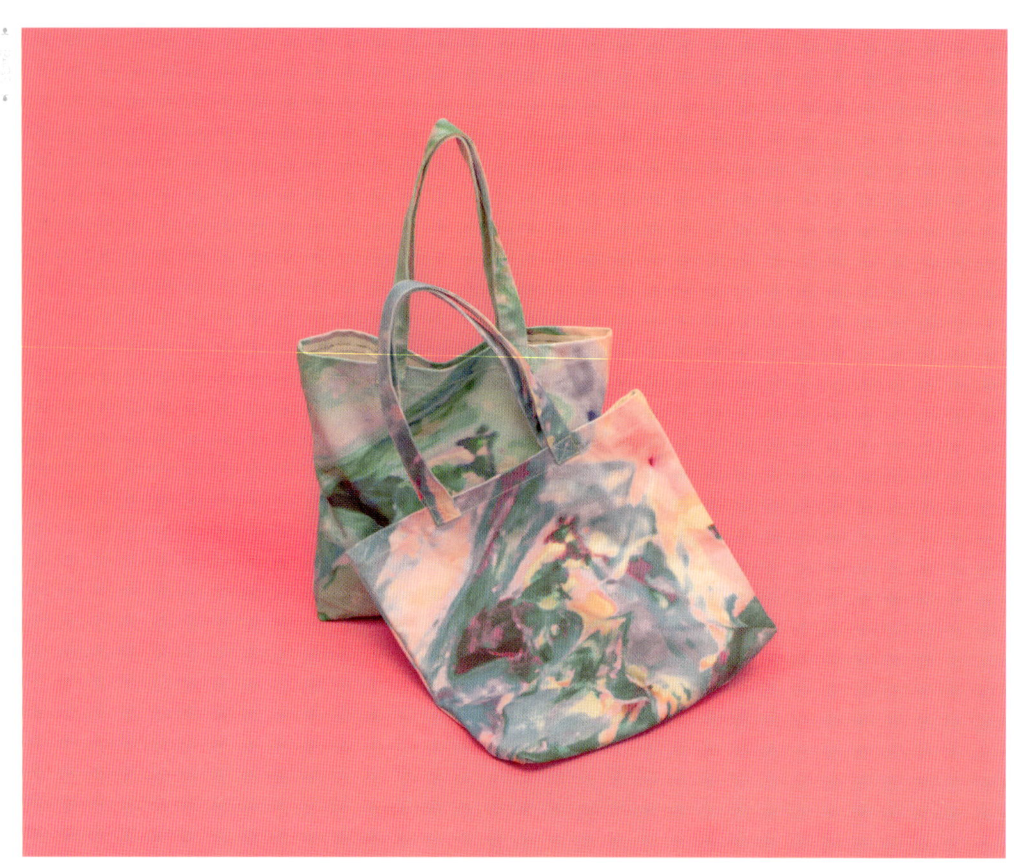

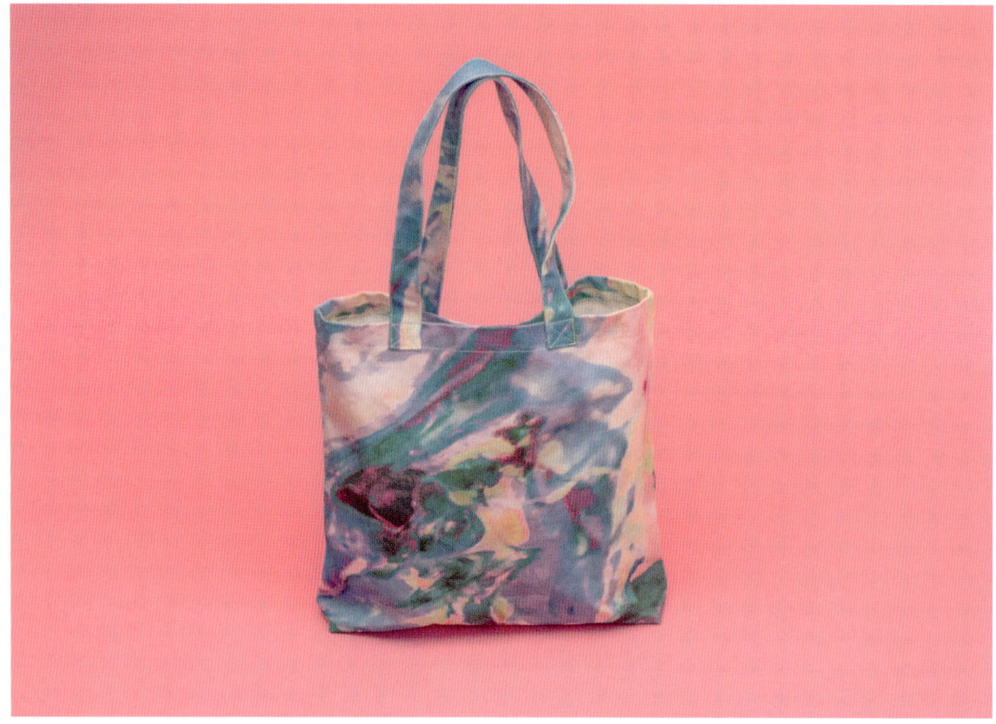

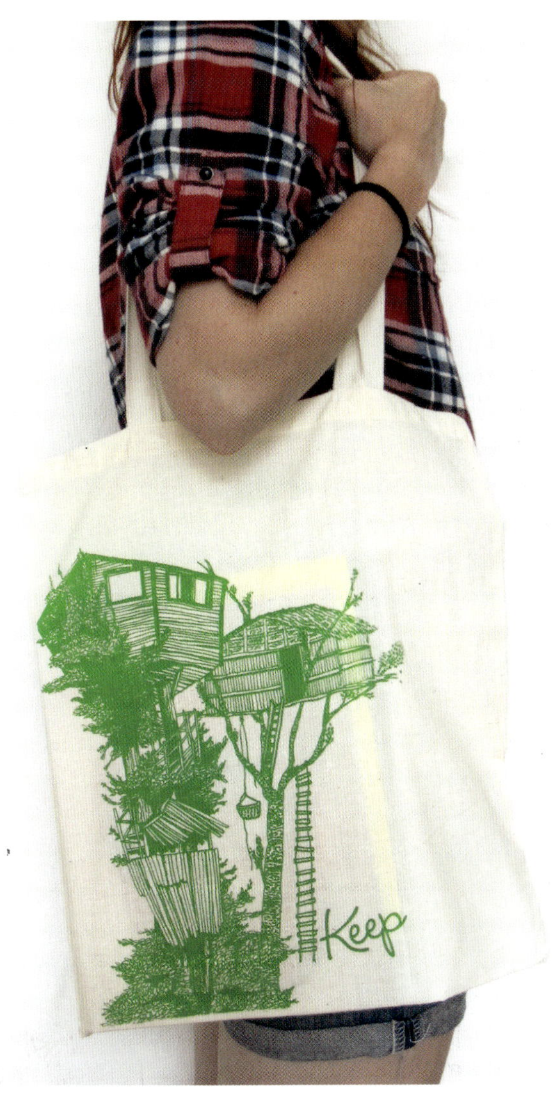

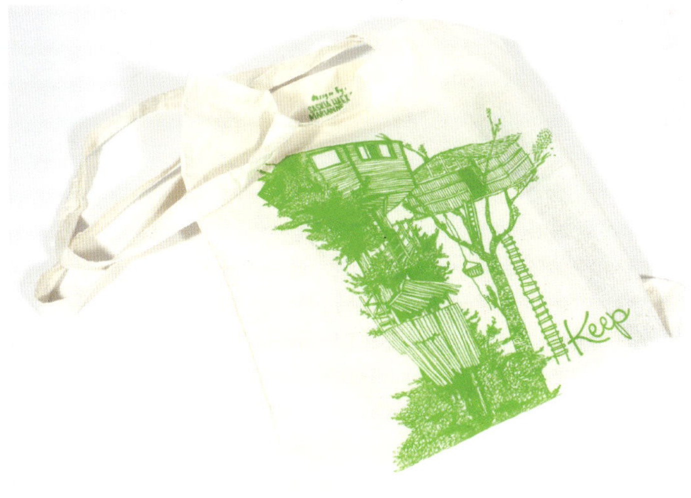

COSMIC TOTES
DA: The Young Never Sleep

Originating from the designer's interest in connectivity and mystery of the cosmos, the bag was printed with an intriguing manipulated photograph of a painted work.

KEEP BAG
DE: Mary and the Locks, Saskia Haex

This bag is a collectable "Keep", with delicate, hand printed patterns in fluorescent green.

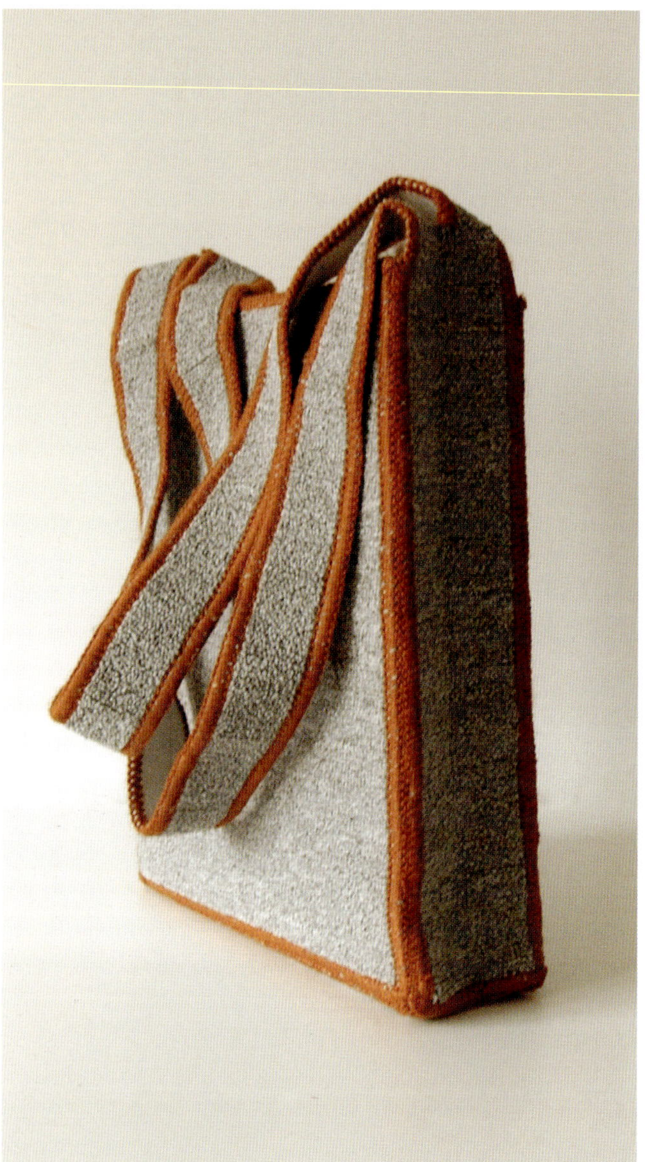

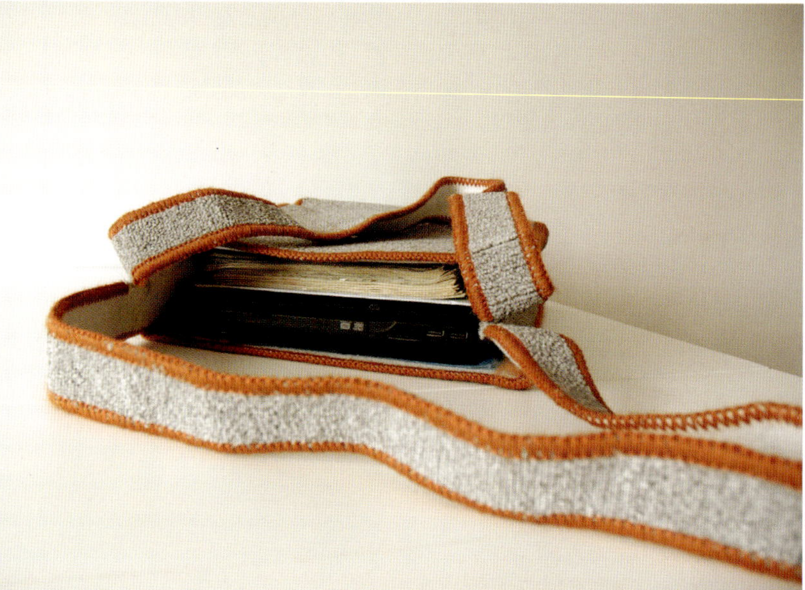

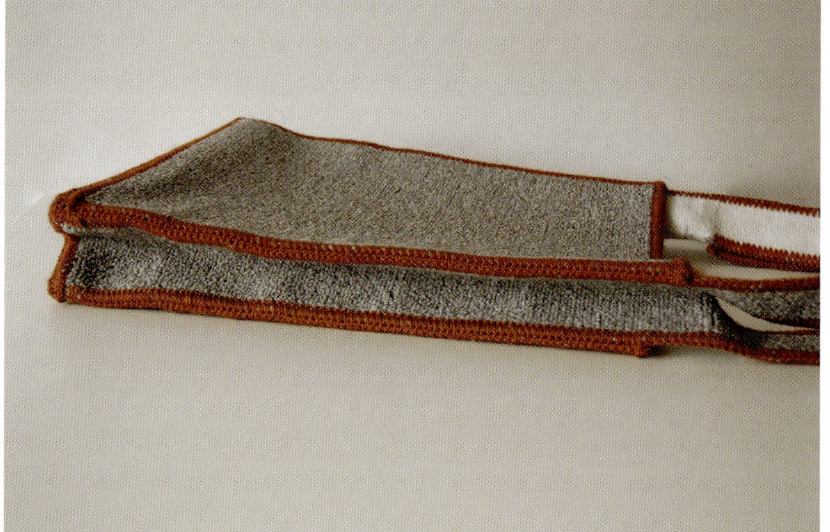

RUG BAG

DE: Ewa Garniec

This bag is made of rug leftovers, creating a raw texture. It can be folded flat once emptied, convenient for transportation and storage.

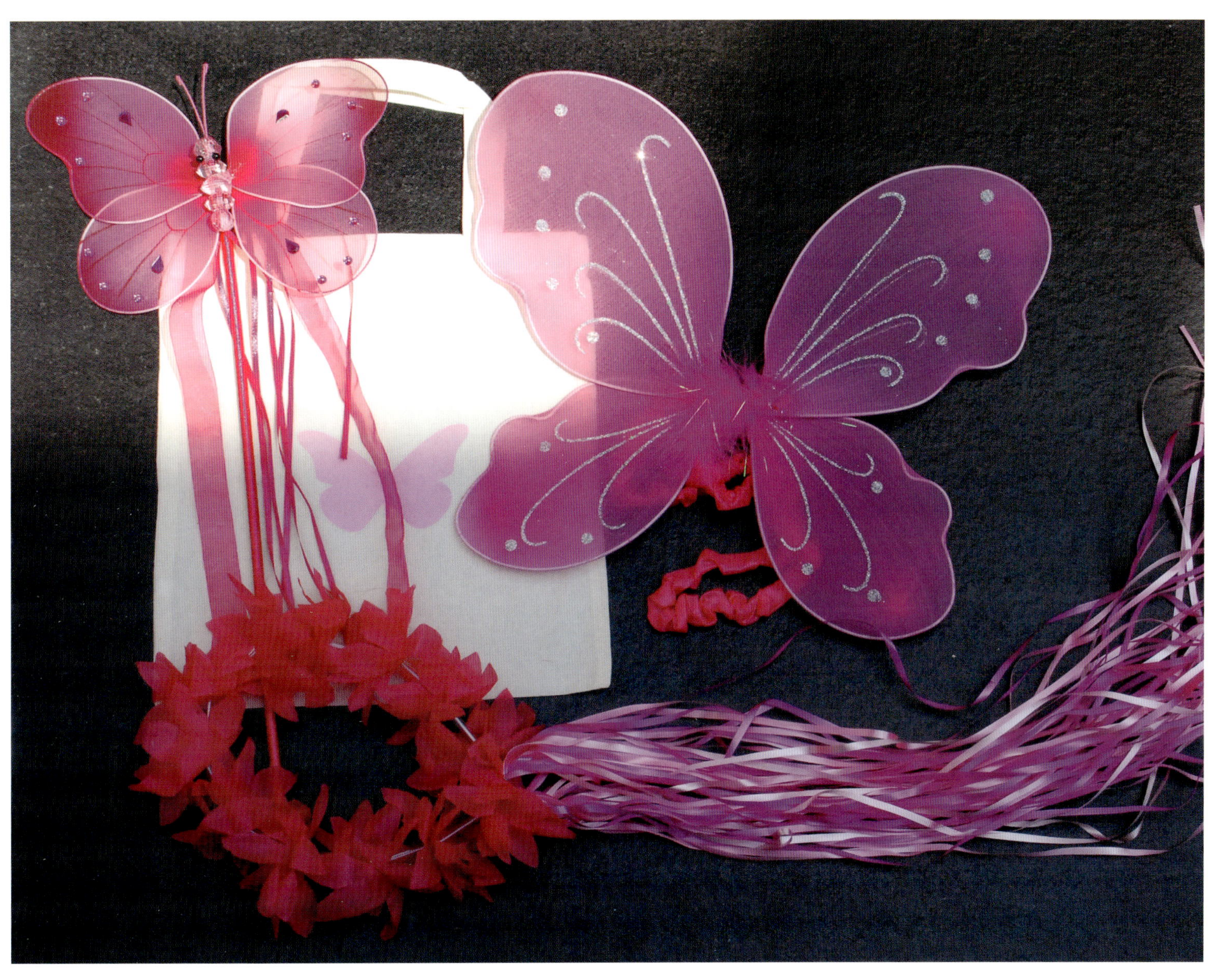

FAIRY GOODIE BAG
DE: Melanie McLaughlin, Ellen Hwang(Celebrating the Big & Small)

Designed as a goodie bag that adds some magical flavor or just as a gift for
children, it is a basic muslin bag silk screened with a pretty butterfly icon.

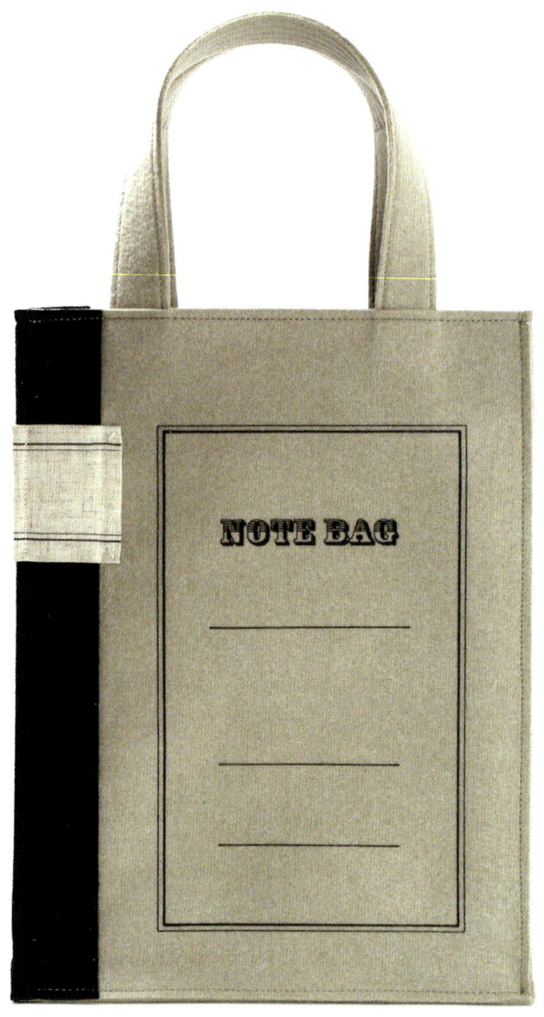

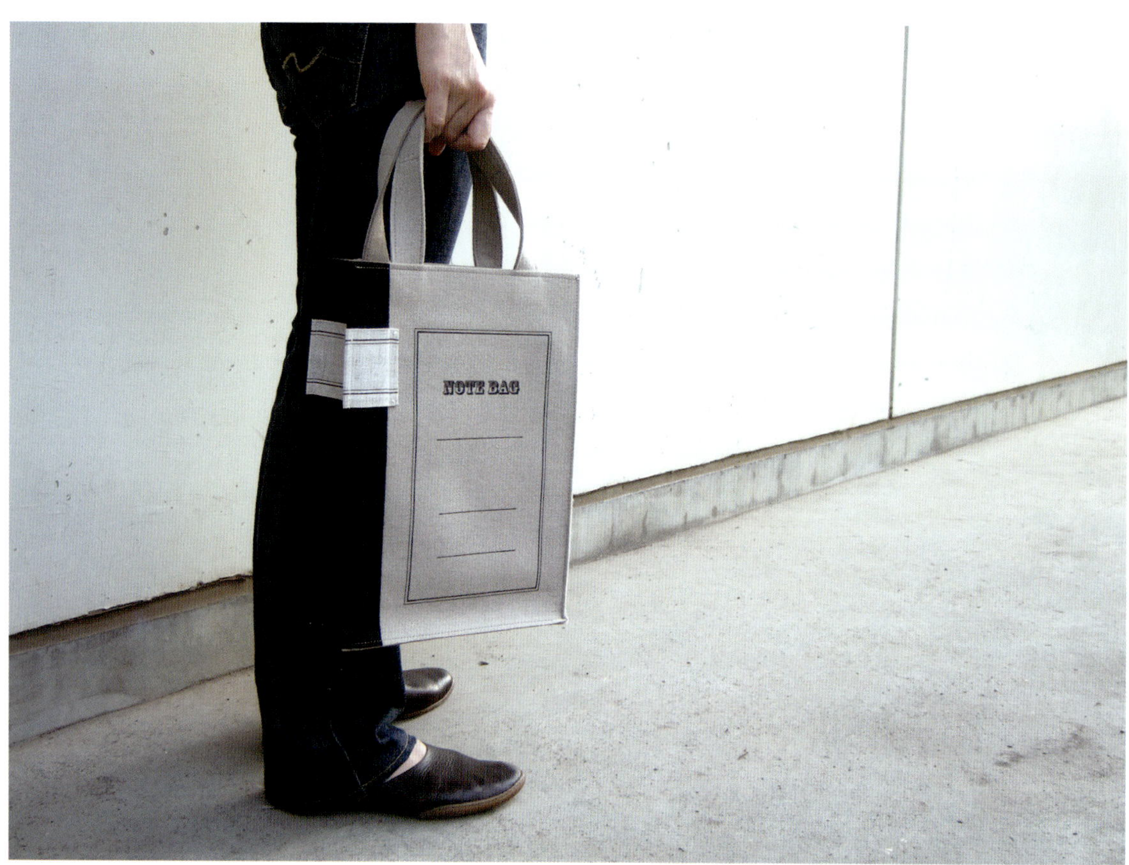

NOTE BAG

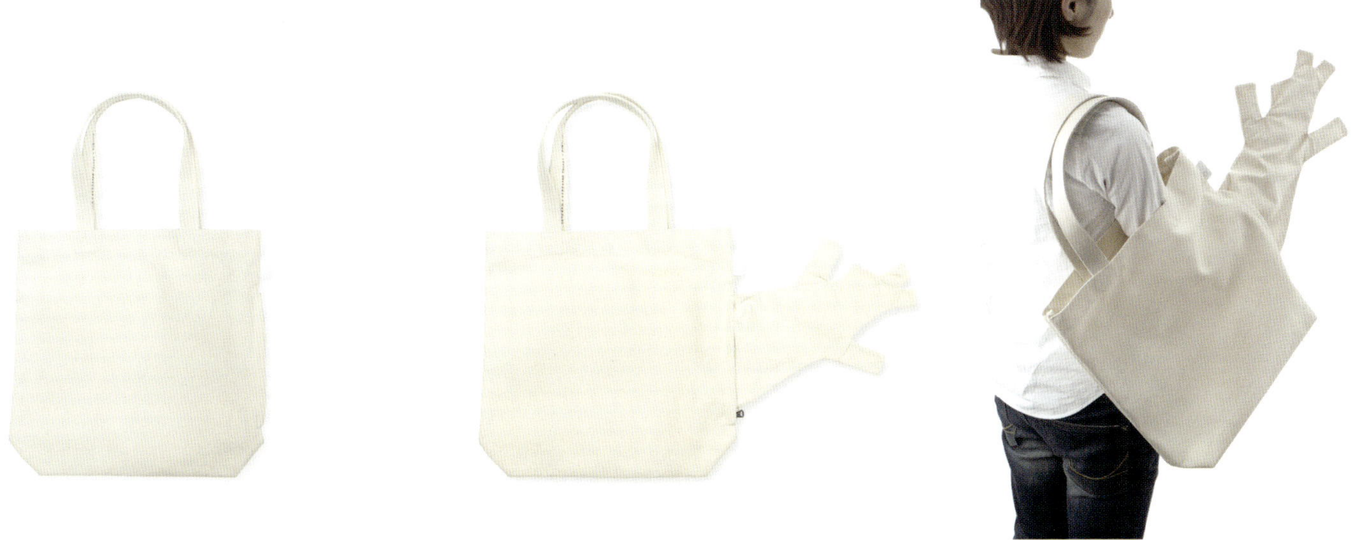

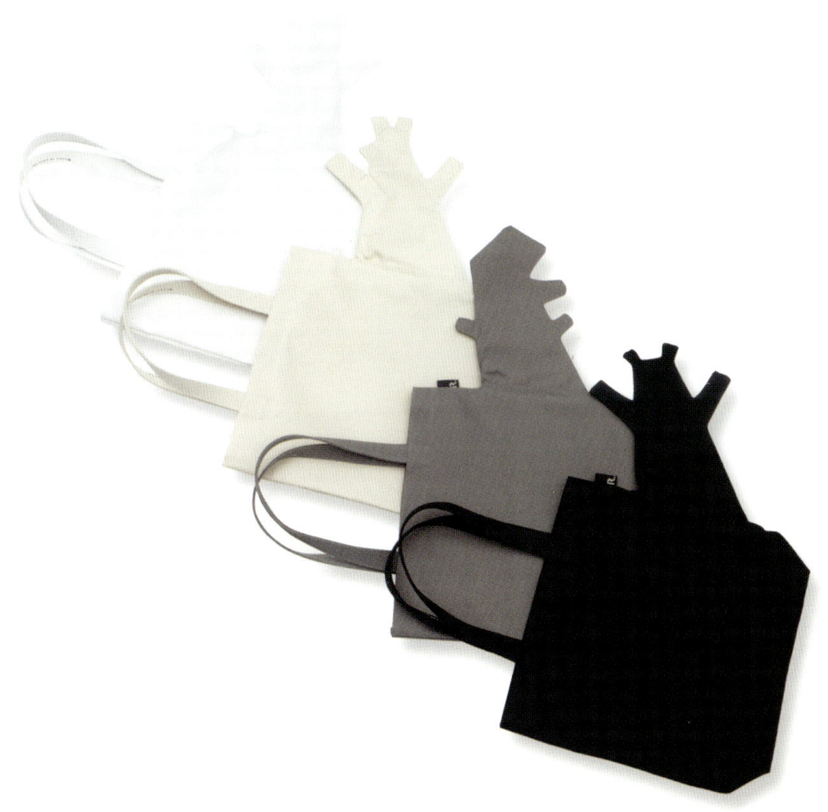

NOTE BAG
DA: Yuruliku Design

The "Note Bag" was inspired by the traditional collage notebook in Japan.

ROOPUPPET
DA: Nendo

Roopuppet is characterized by the protruding pocket, which can be turned
into a puppet. It comes in four versions: a kangaroo, a bear, a human being
and a dinosaur.

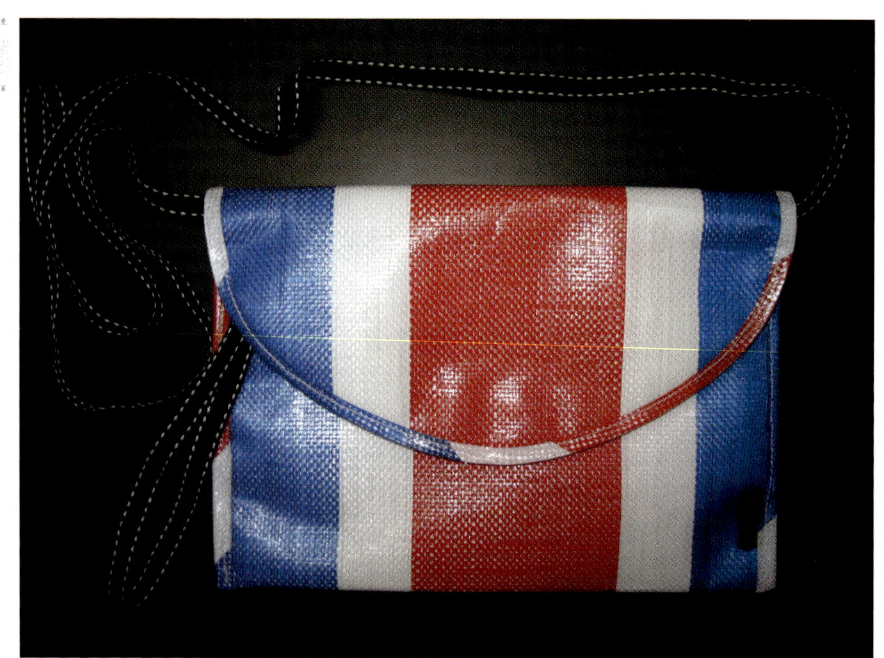

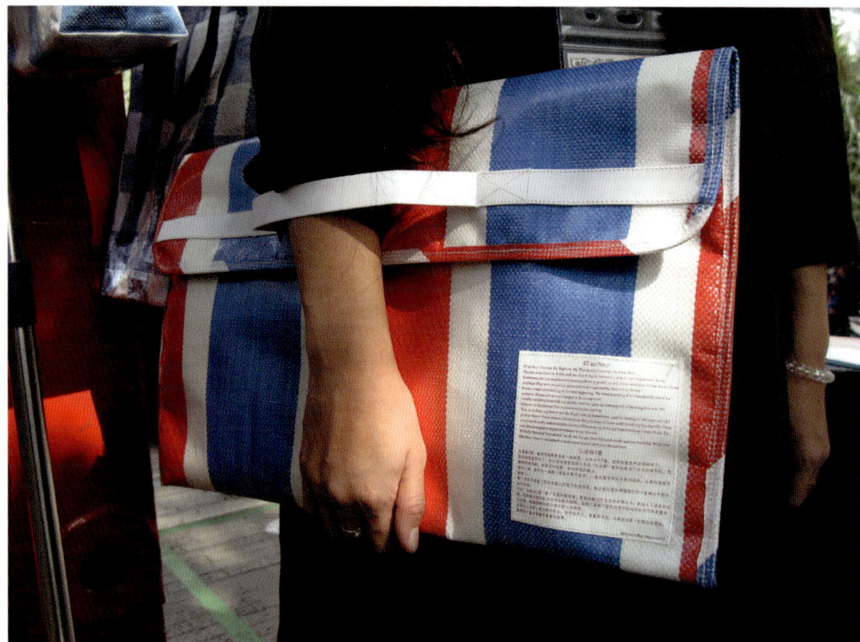

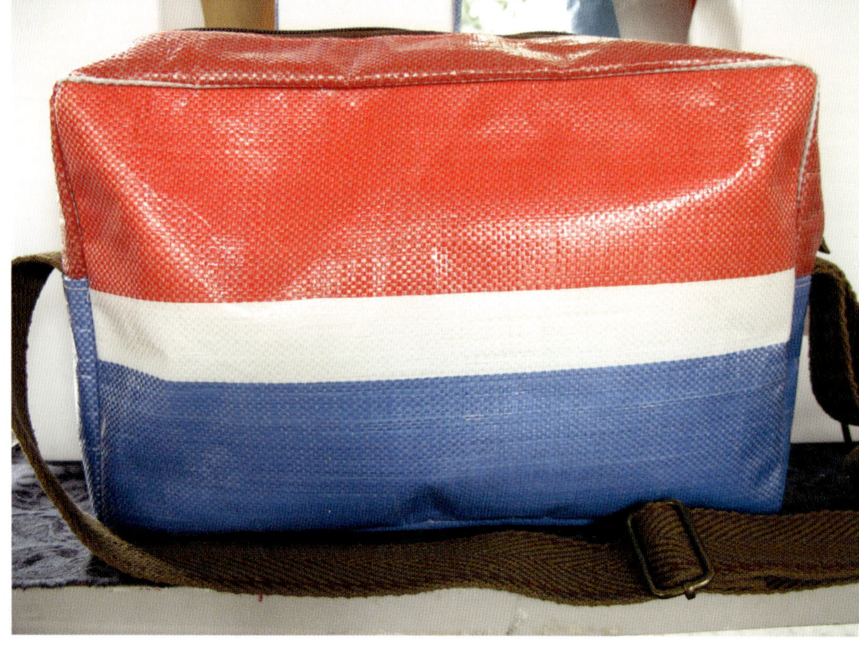

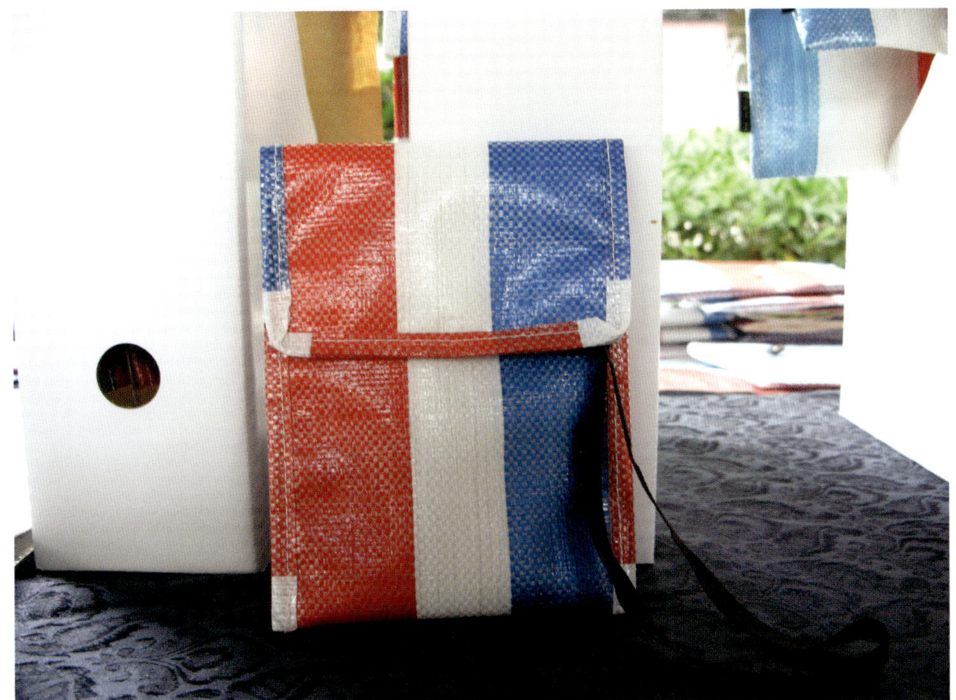
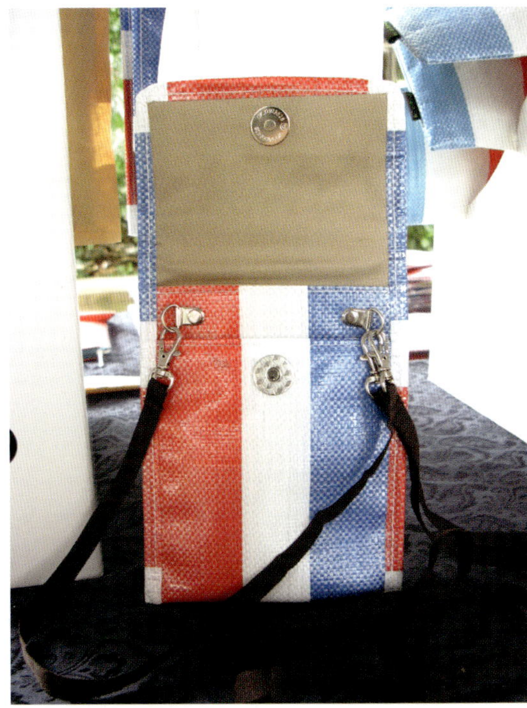
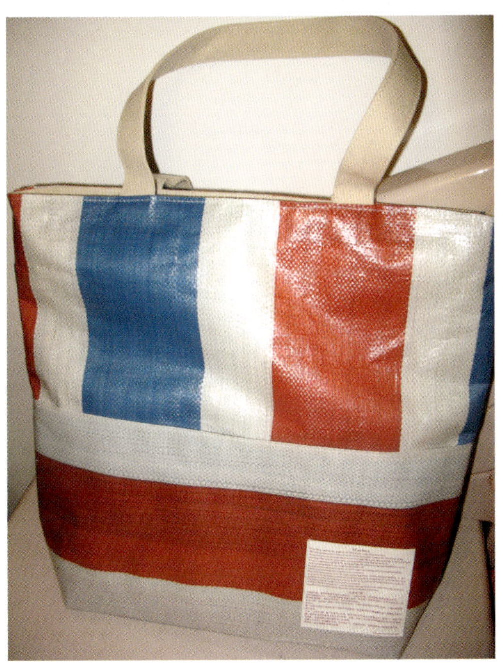
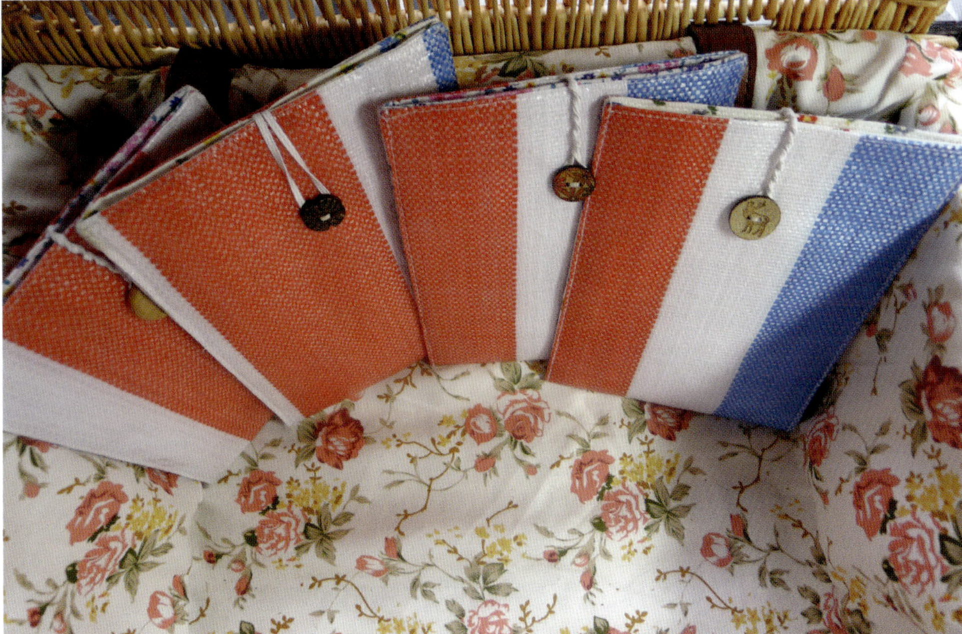

SWATOW STREET 7TH
DE: Hong Han

This series was designed using upcycling from the traditional red-white-blue
bags that can be found everywhere in the designer's hometown Swatow. They
are vintage, ecologically sound, durable, and have a feel of home.

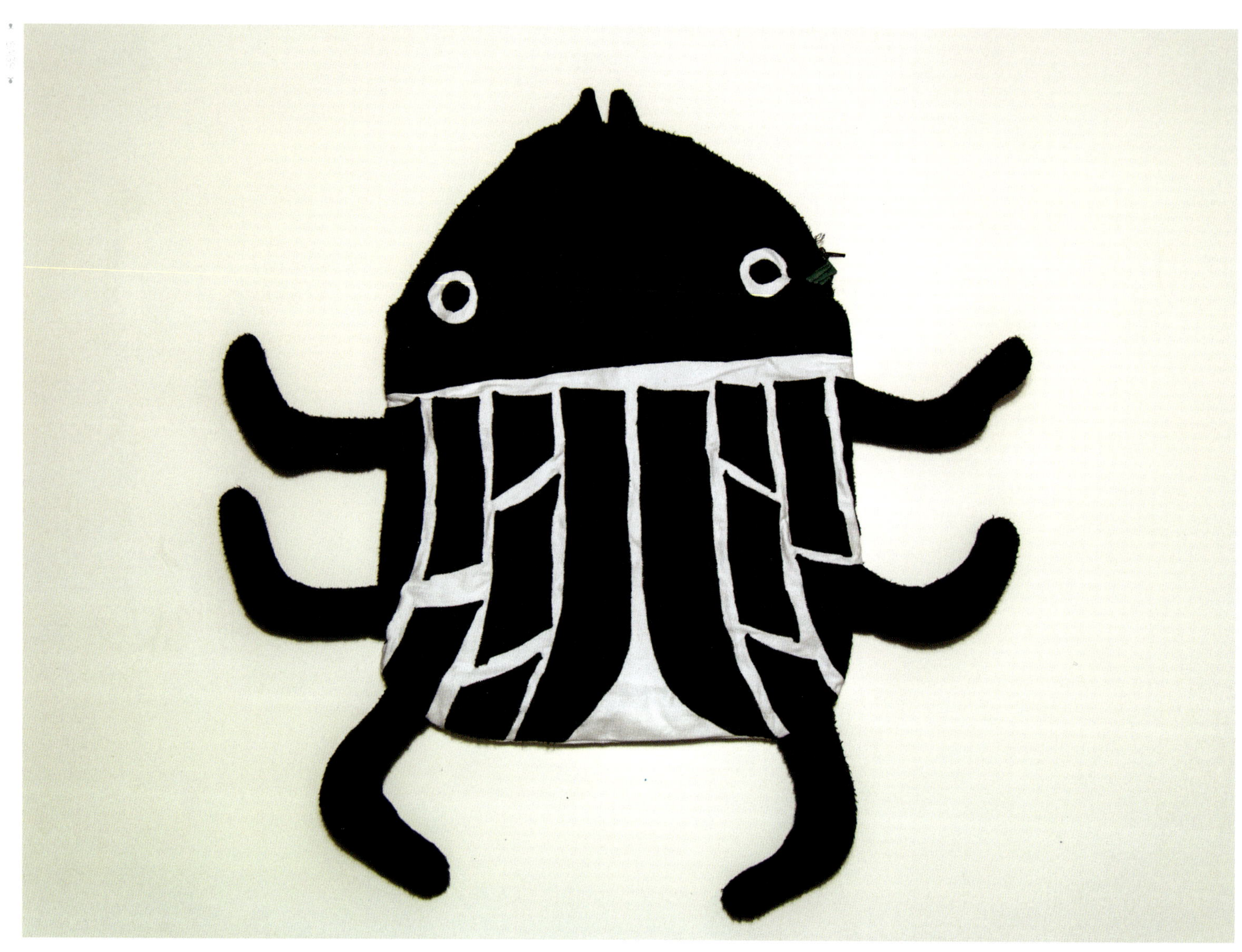

BAG CAT & BAG BUG
DE: Alesia Zawodzinska

In simple black and white, this design is highlighted by the protruding tail
of a cat and the legs of the bugs. The texture of cotton also enhances the
sense of intimacy.

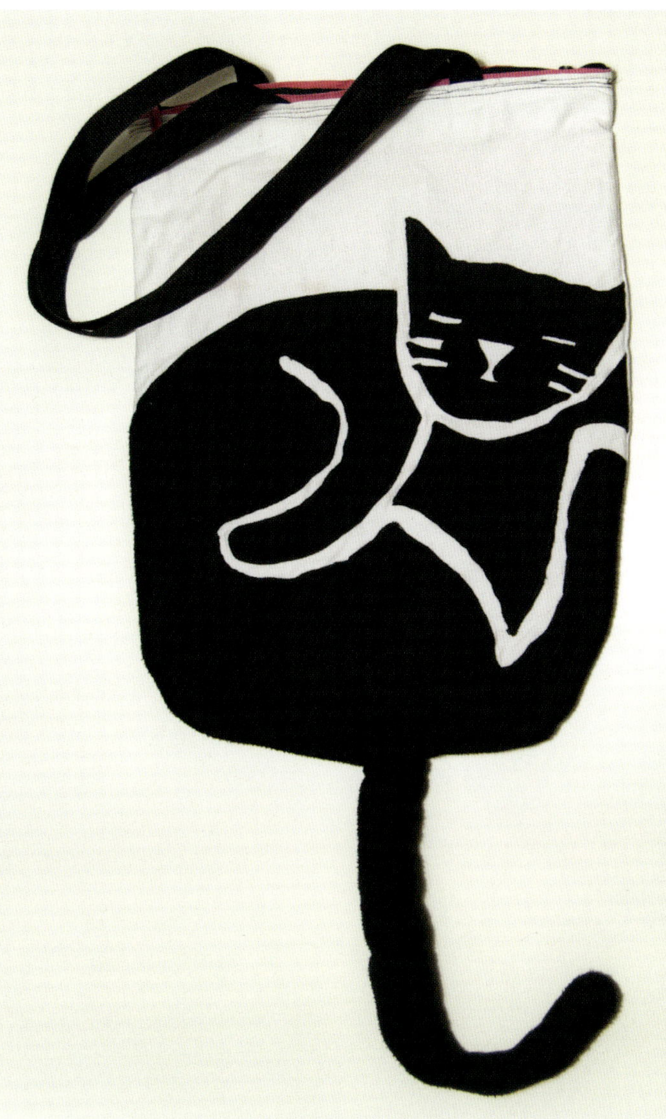

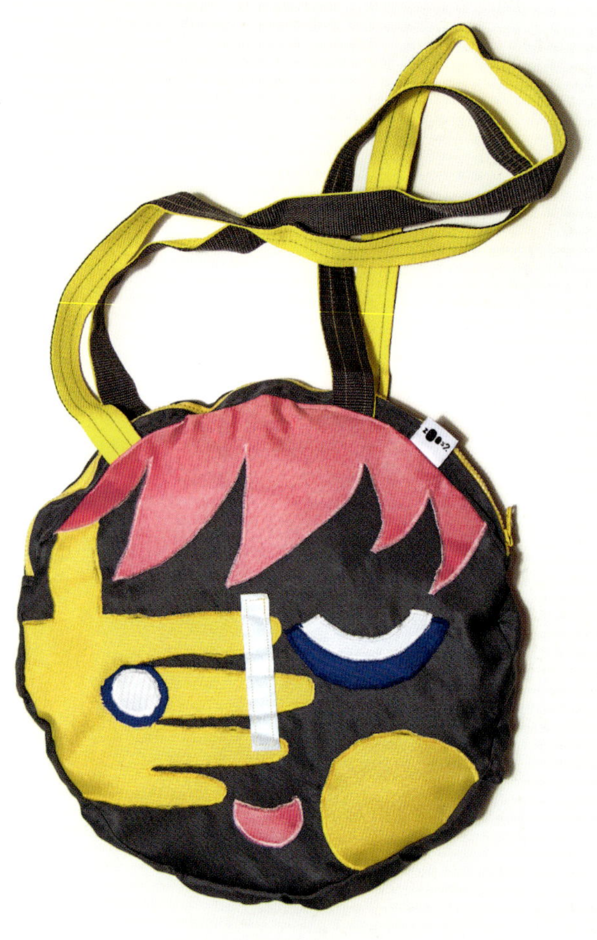

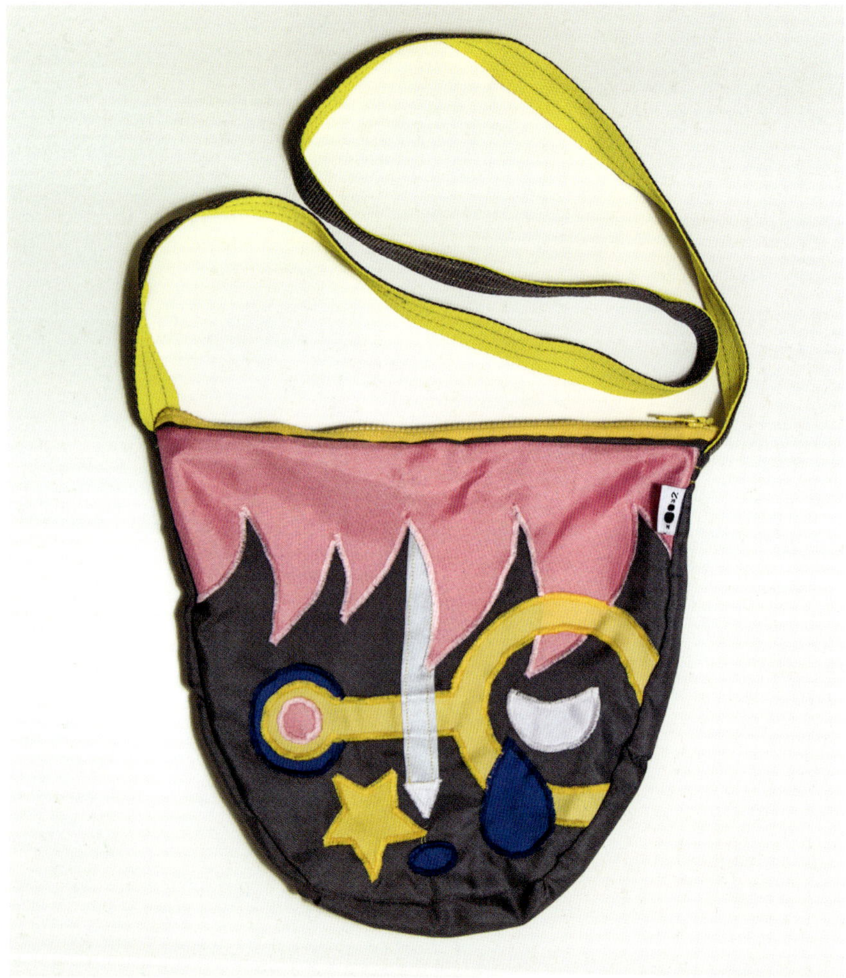

BAG HAND & BAG STAR
DA: Zoo52

Bag Hand and Bag Star are made from Kodura and display faces
with contrasting color combinations and sets of featured
elements. The inside is printed with animal patterns, sewn
with pockets and zips for better functionality.

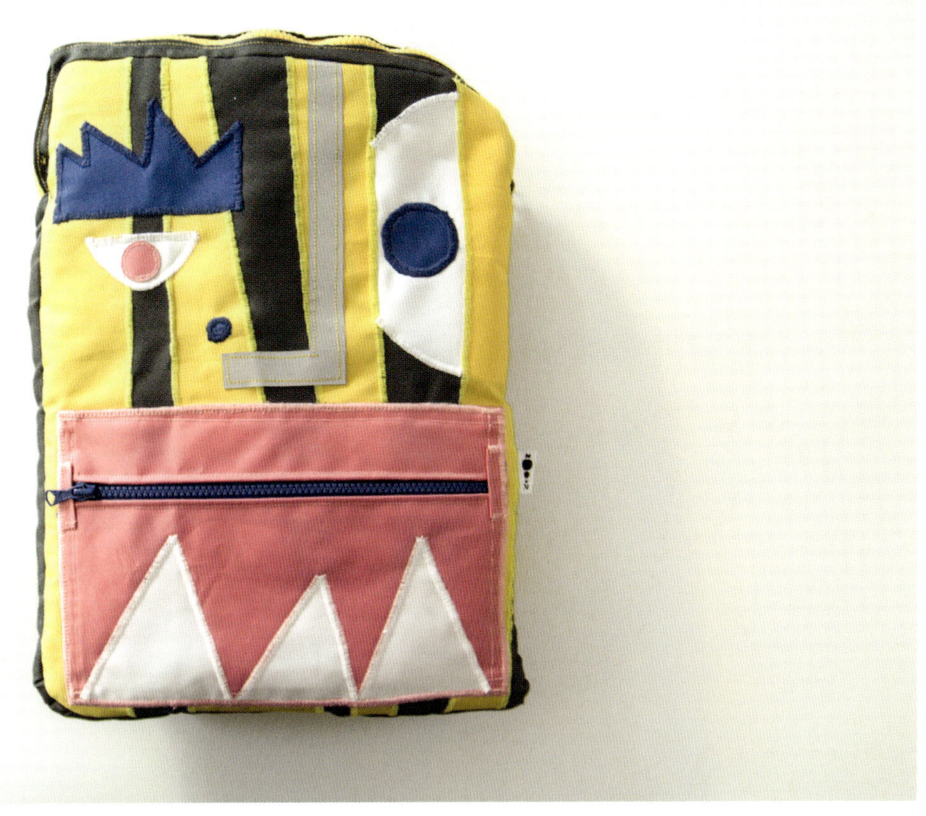

BACKPACK DOMINIK
DA: Zoo52

The "Dominik" backpack has a fun, colorful and unusual
presentation. Made from waterproof fabric, it is stuffed with a
special type of sponge to protect the contents.

KASPER
DA: Zoo52

The Kasper bag features facial expression composed of
geometrical shapes in contrasting palettes, creating a
whimsical feel, yet still highly functional. It is stuffed with
sponge to protect the contents.

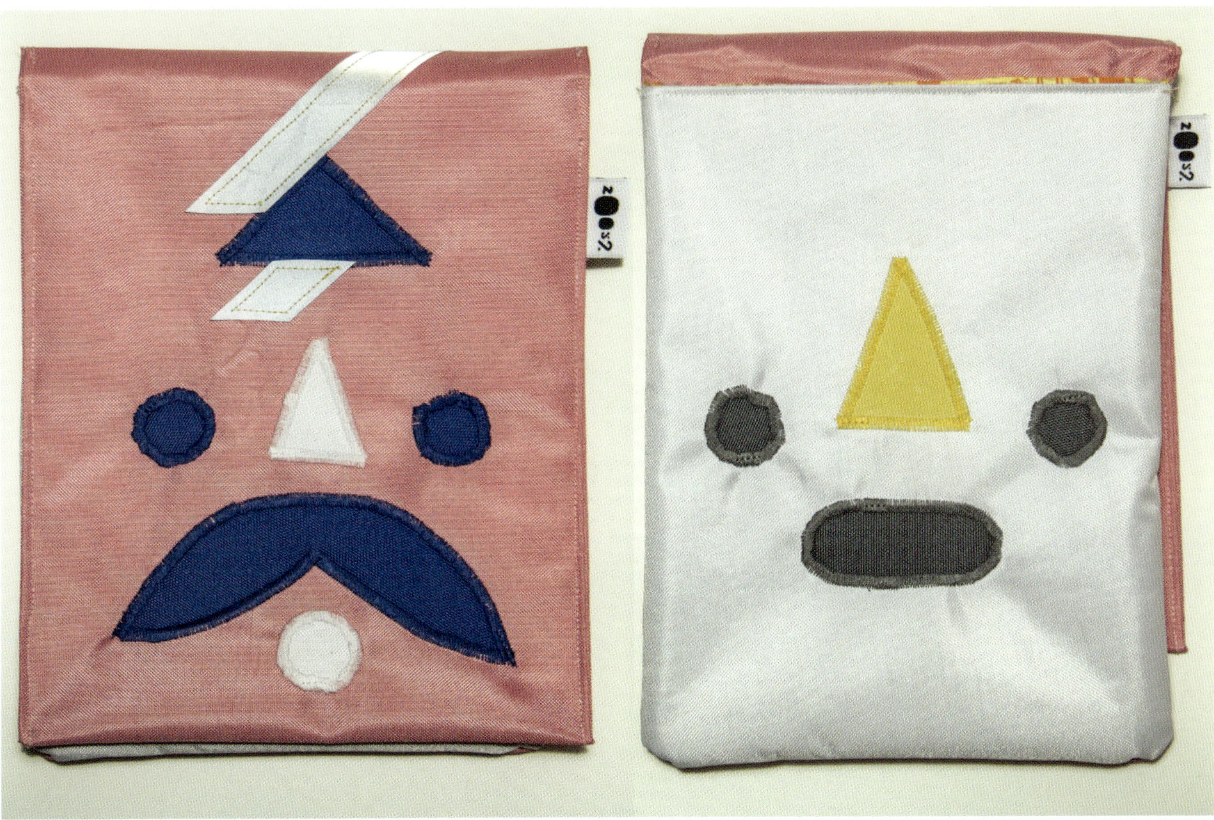

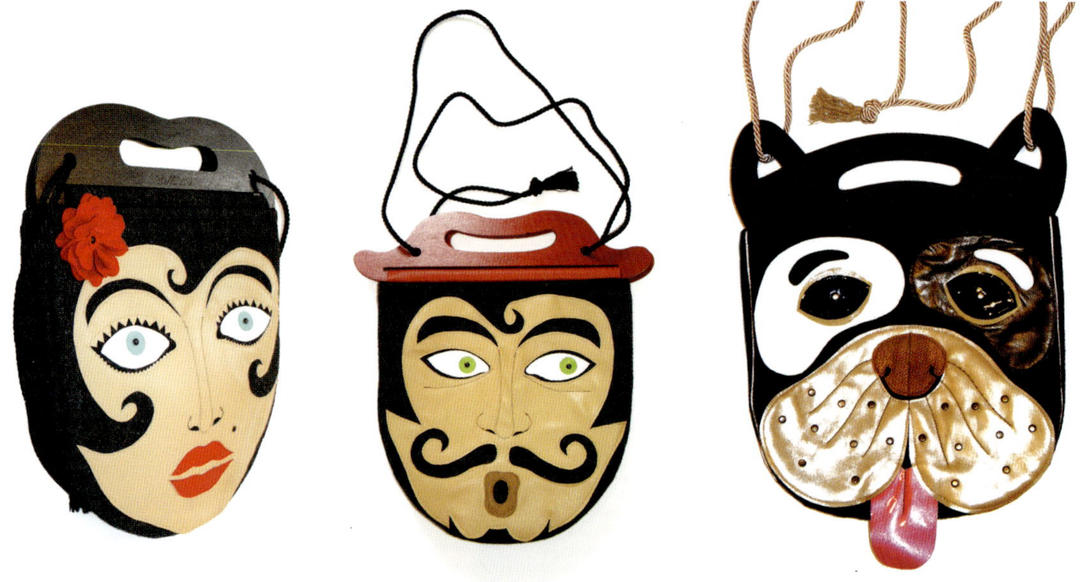

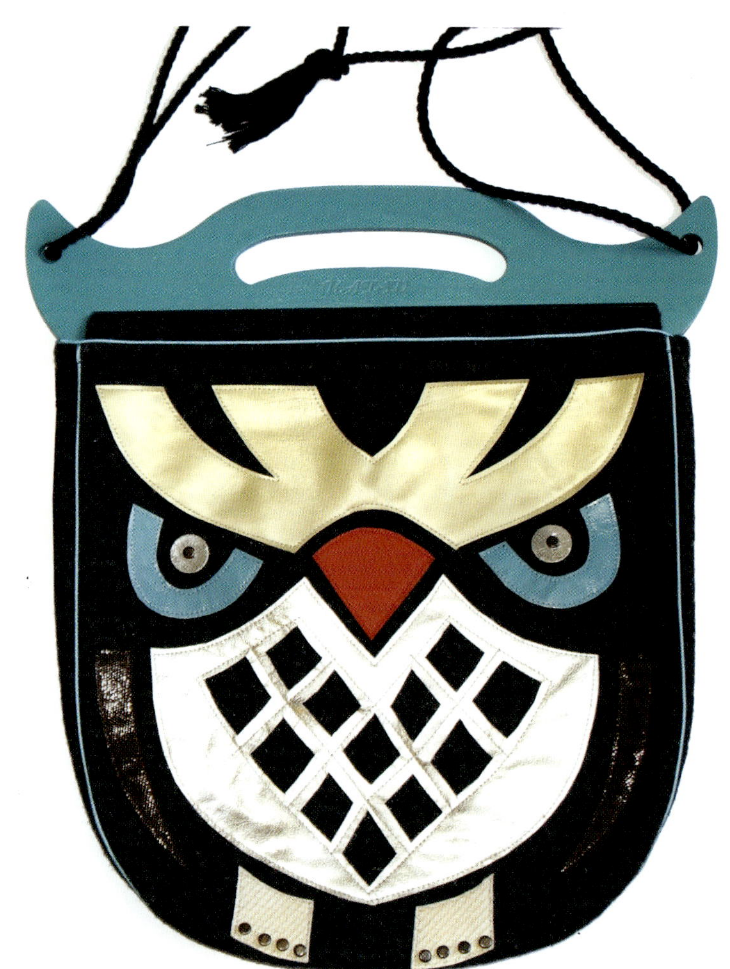

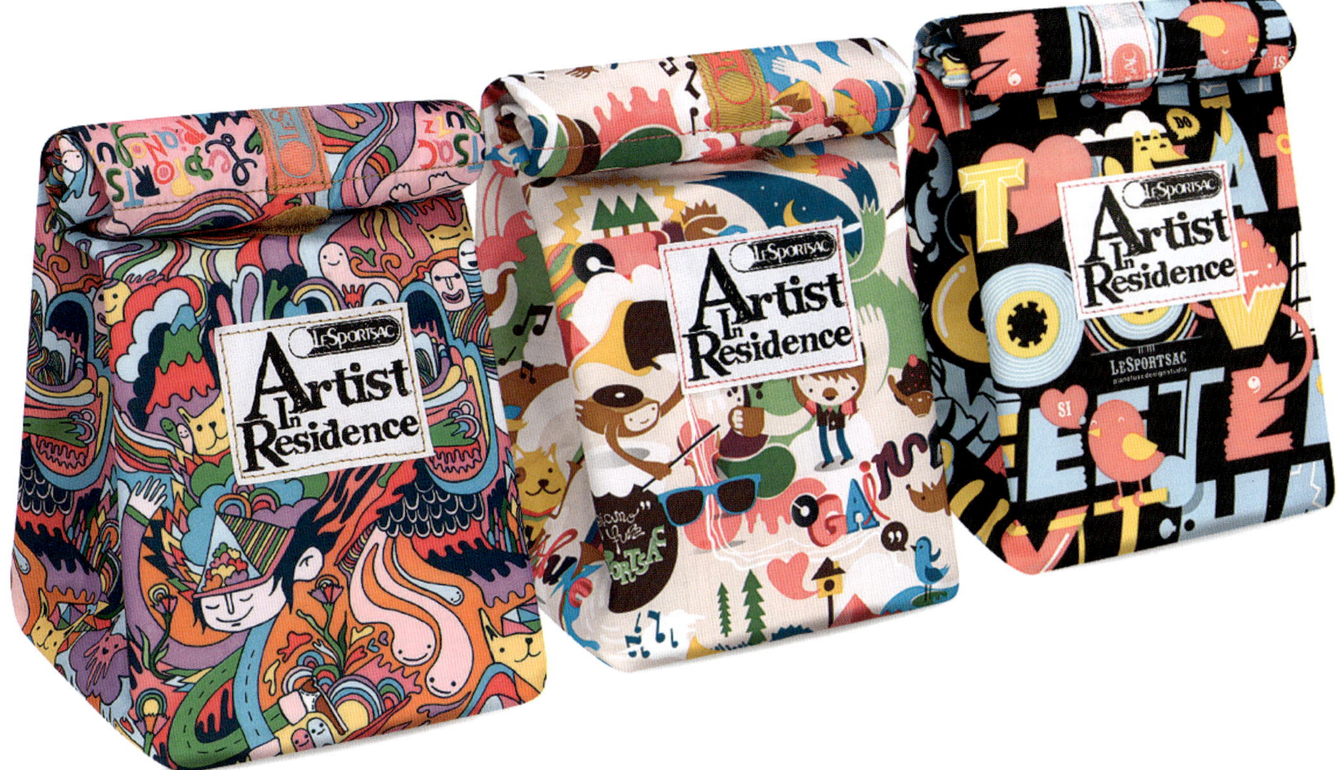

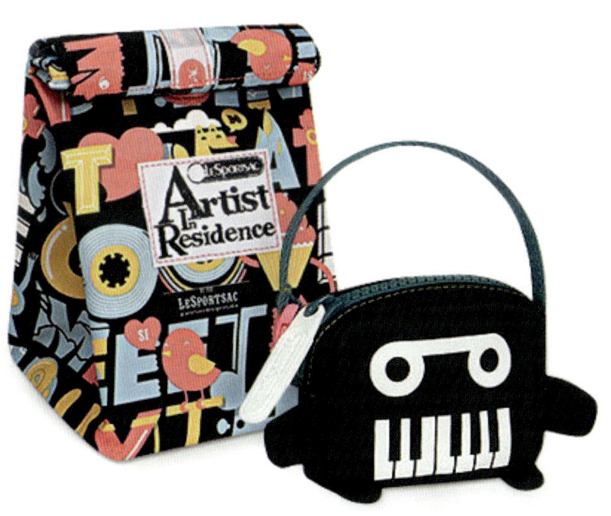

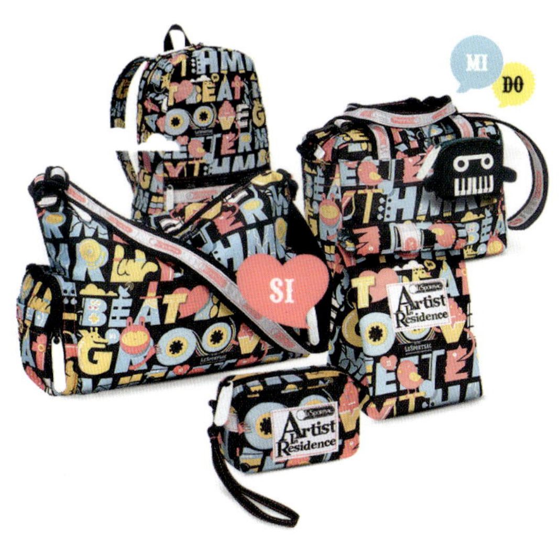

KATSU BAGS
DE: Kasia Sulkowska

This series creates vivid and colorful images of people and animals with
leather geometric shapes, black piping and canvas lining. Each handle was
cut out of 1/8" plywood, painted and sealed to last.

BEAT BEAT
DA: Pianofuzz

The "Beat Beat" bag is printed with illustrations and aims to capture the
moment music is conceived, while still at its most primitive stage before
being recorded.

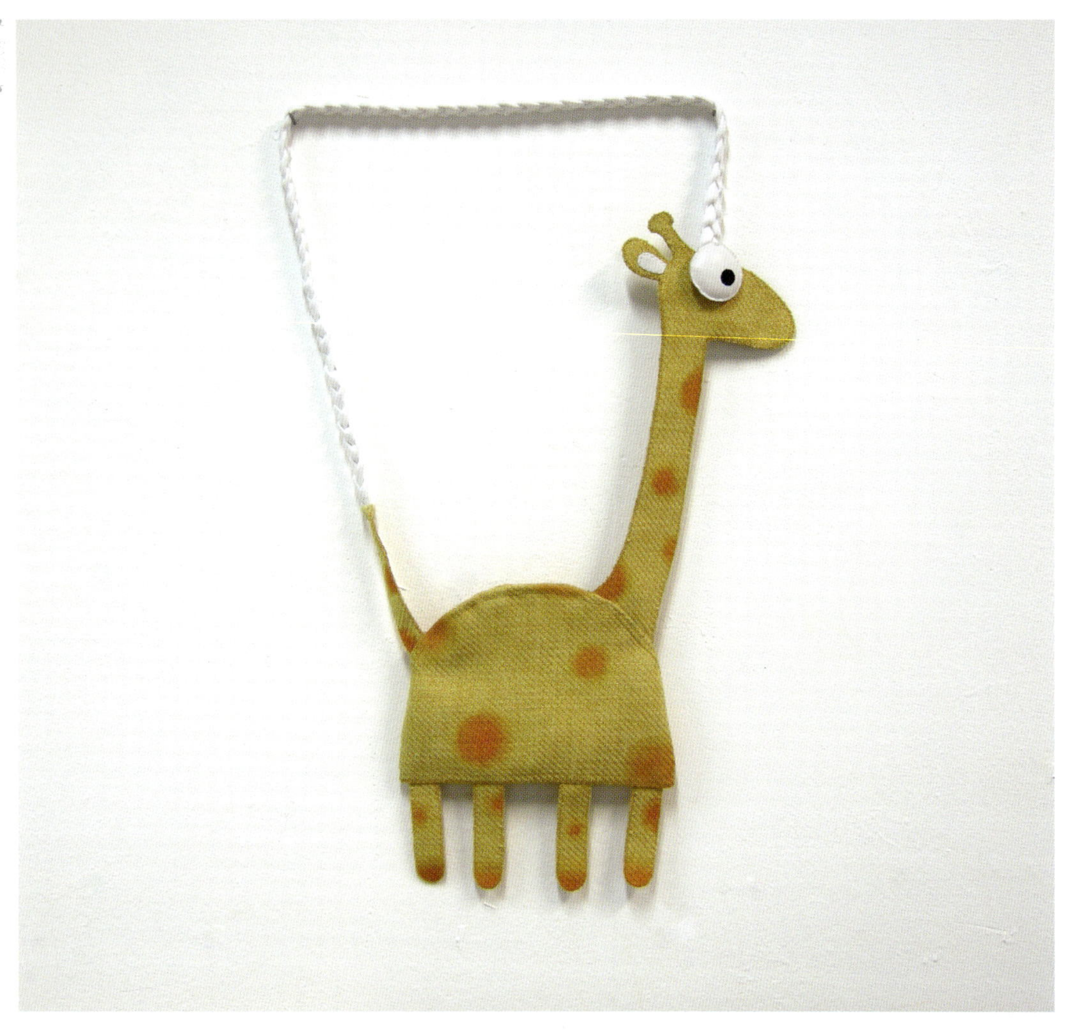

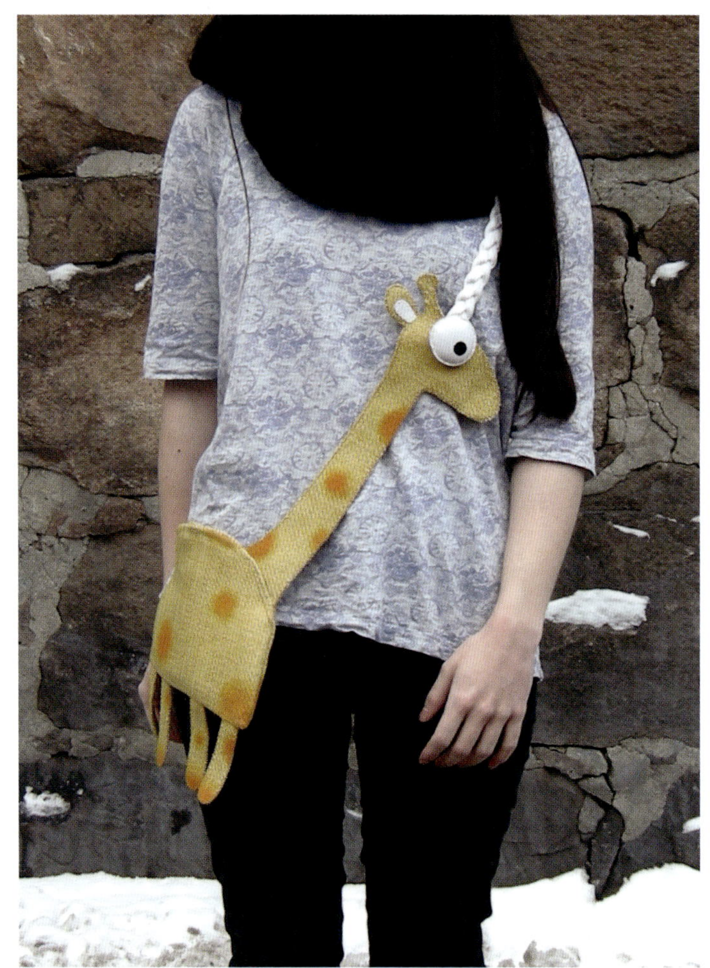

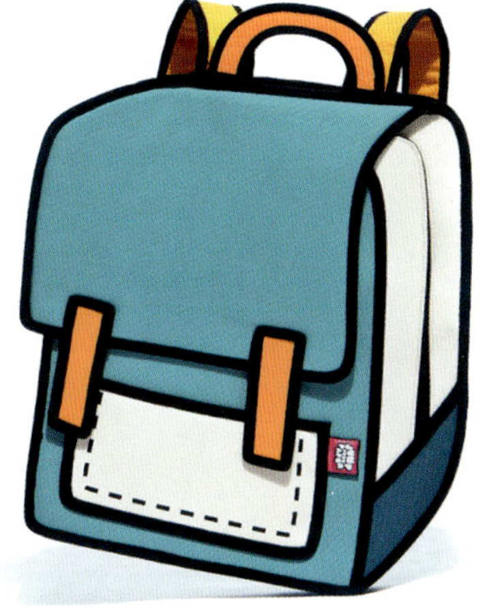

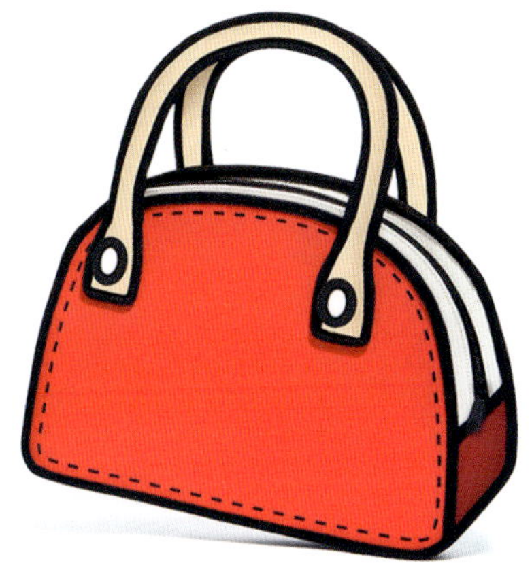

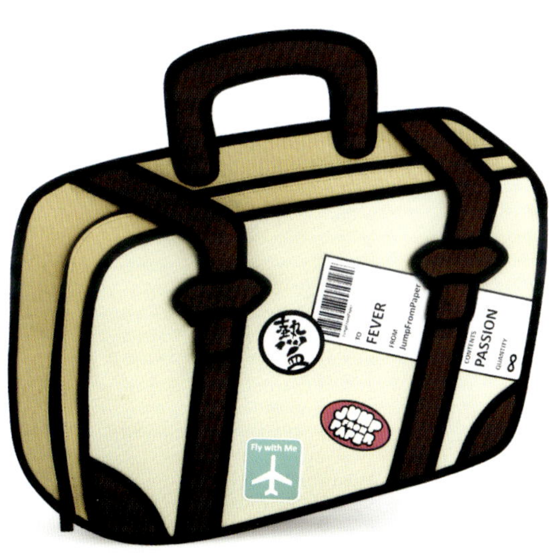

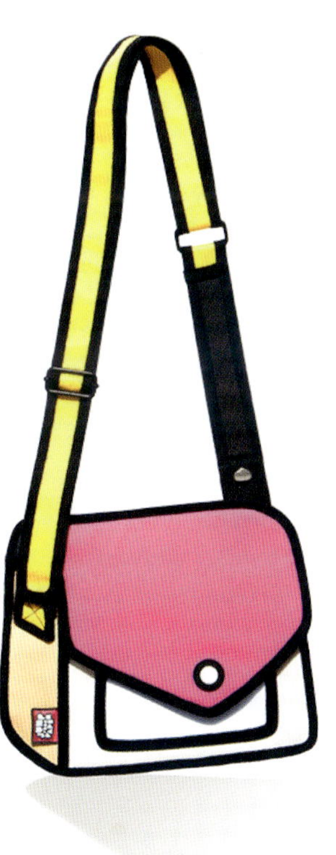

FUN GIRAFFE BAG
DA: Vannes Designs

Handmade and hand painted, the giraffe bag uses the long neck and tail as parts of the shoulder strap.

JUMP FROM PAPER
DA: Jump From Paper

Making a 3D bag look like a childish drawing, "Jump From Paper" stands for the passion to make people laugh, and encourages people to let their imagination go wild.

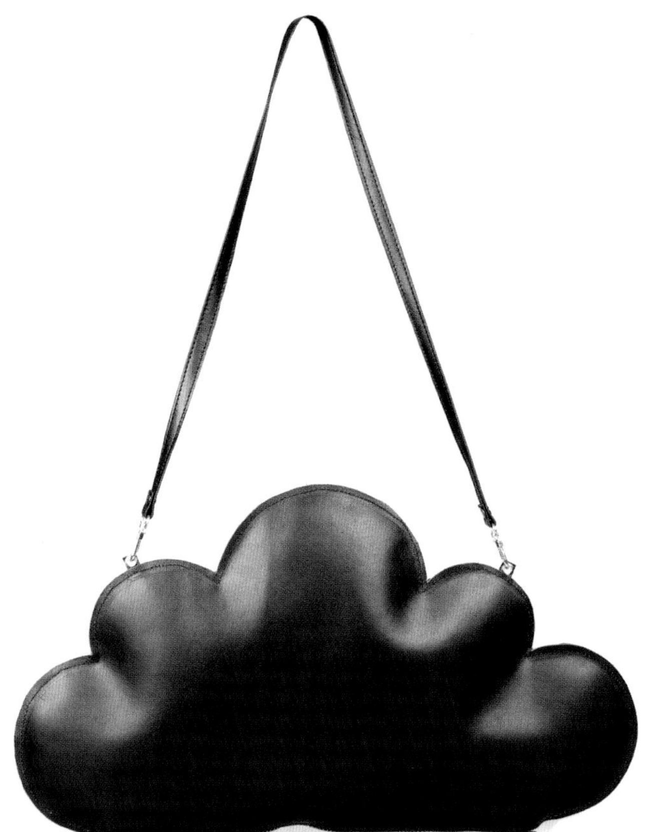 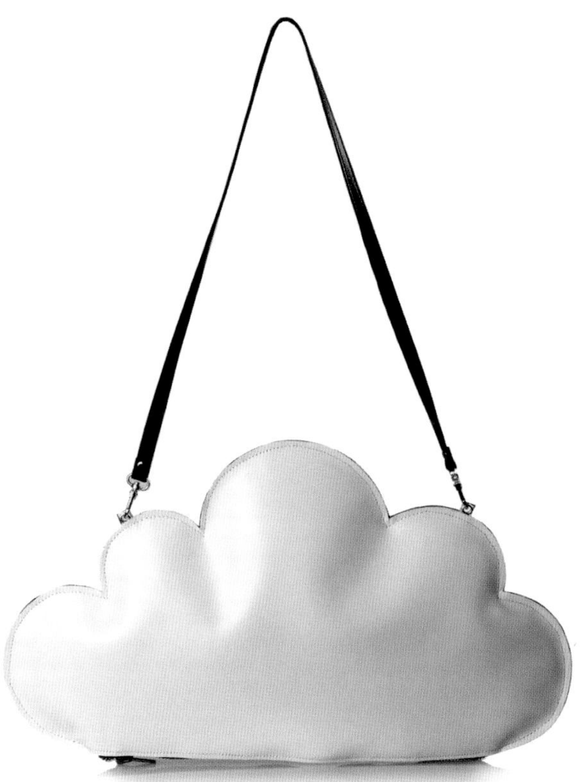

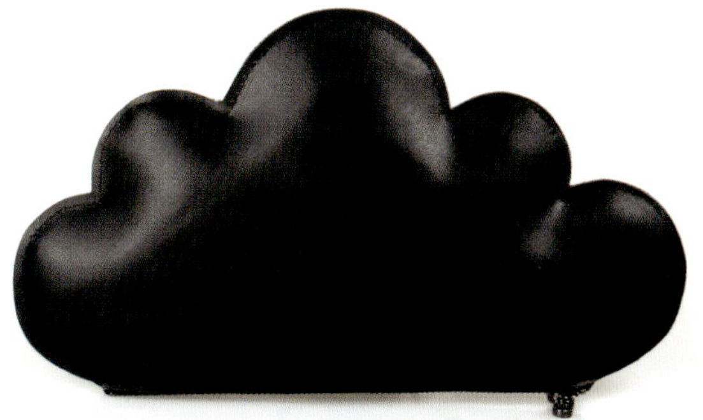

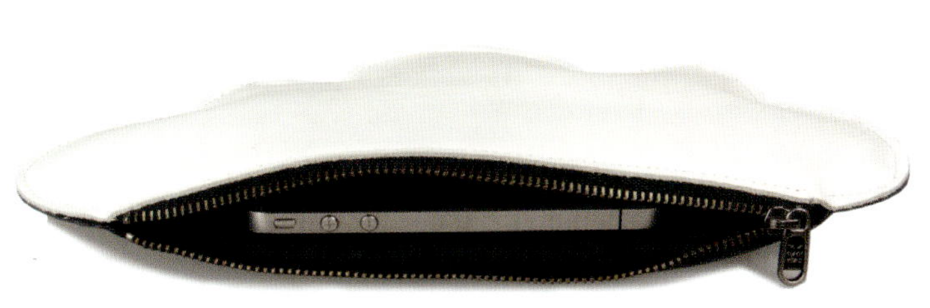

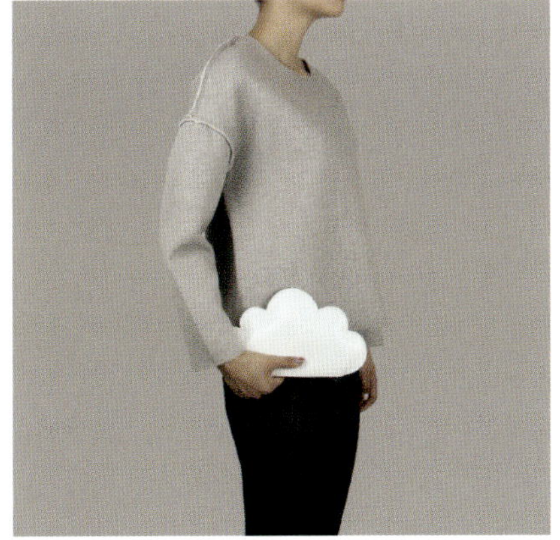

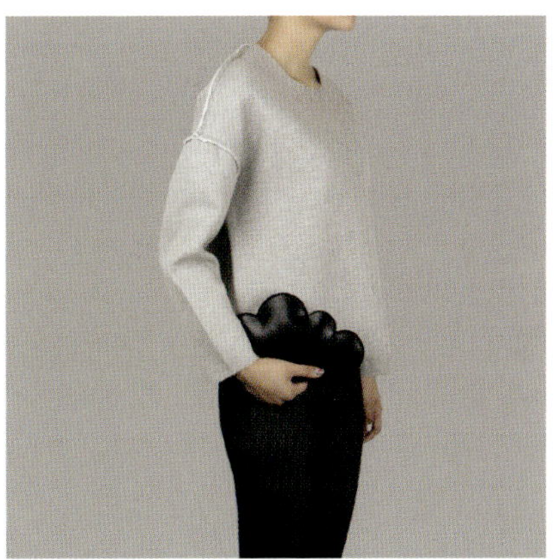

THE CLOUD
DA: Black Head

Created in the shape of cloud, the design enables owner to carry what could have been so
high above the ground - anywhere they want. They come in two colors - one for a clear, blue
sky and the other for a rainy occasion.

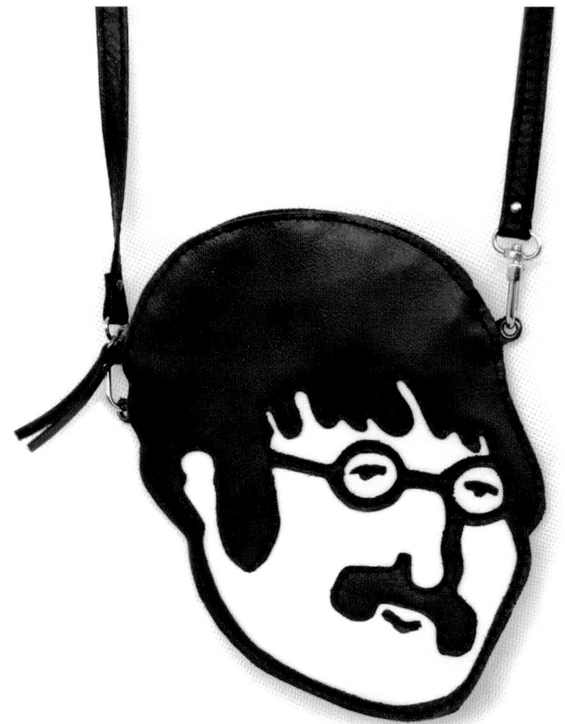

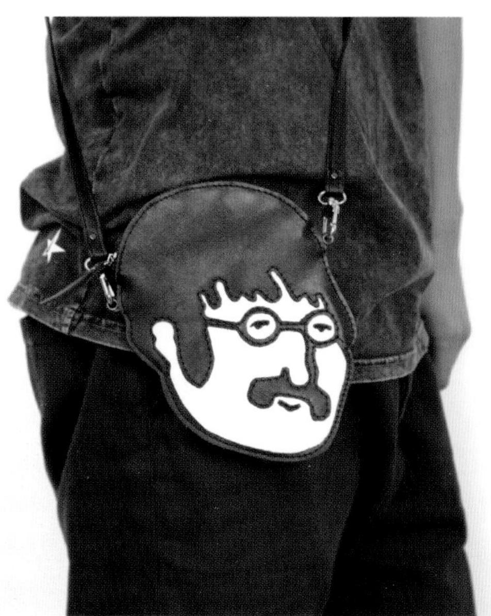

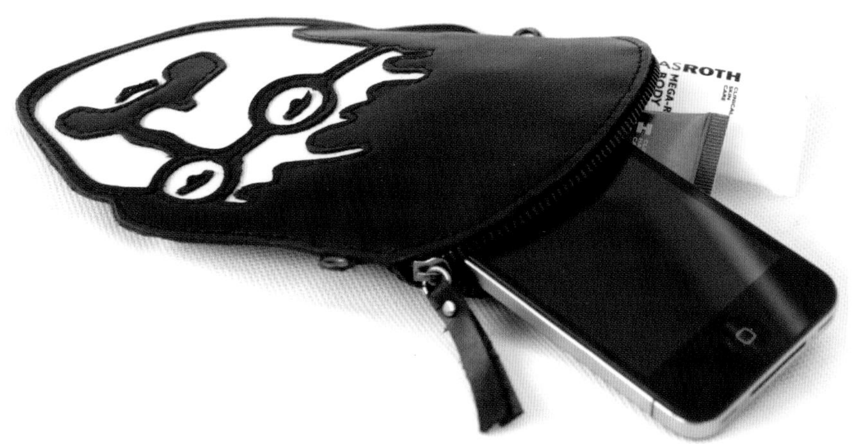

THE BEATLES
DA: Black Head

Wearing a John Lennon cartoon bag is just a cool way to show you love the Beatles or pop music.

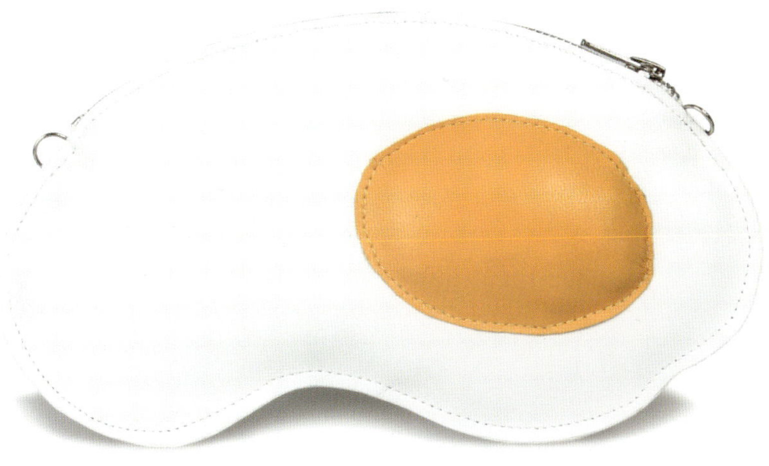

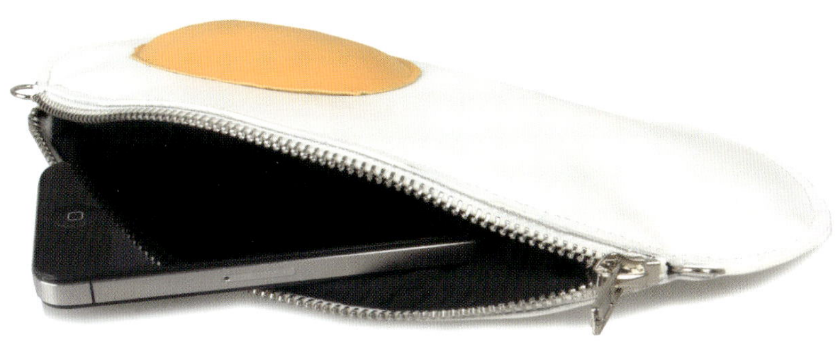

THE FRIED EGG
DA: Black Head

Made of leather, the Fried Egg bag is just a fun accessory to show the owner's playfulness.

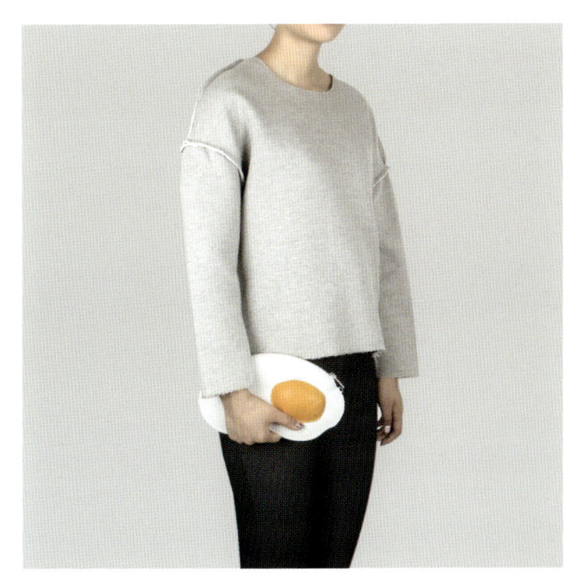

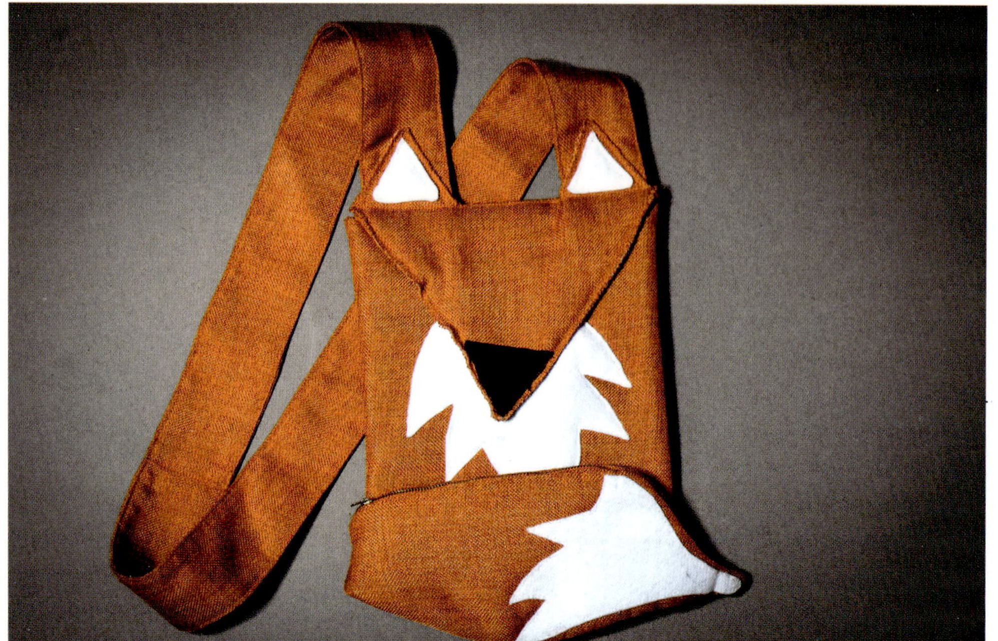

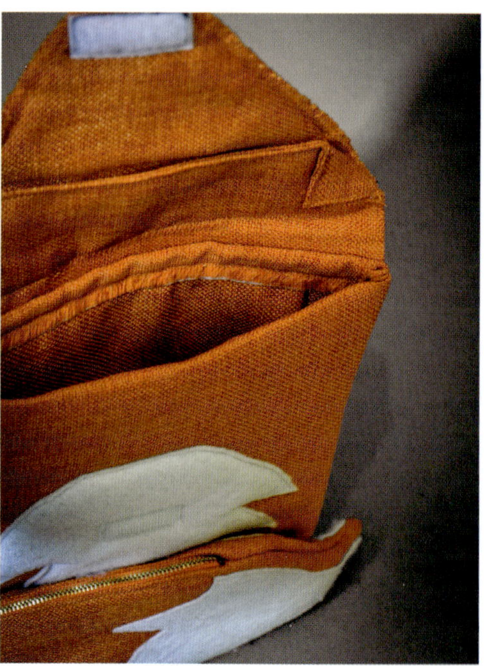

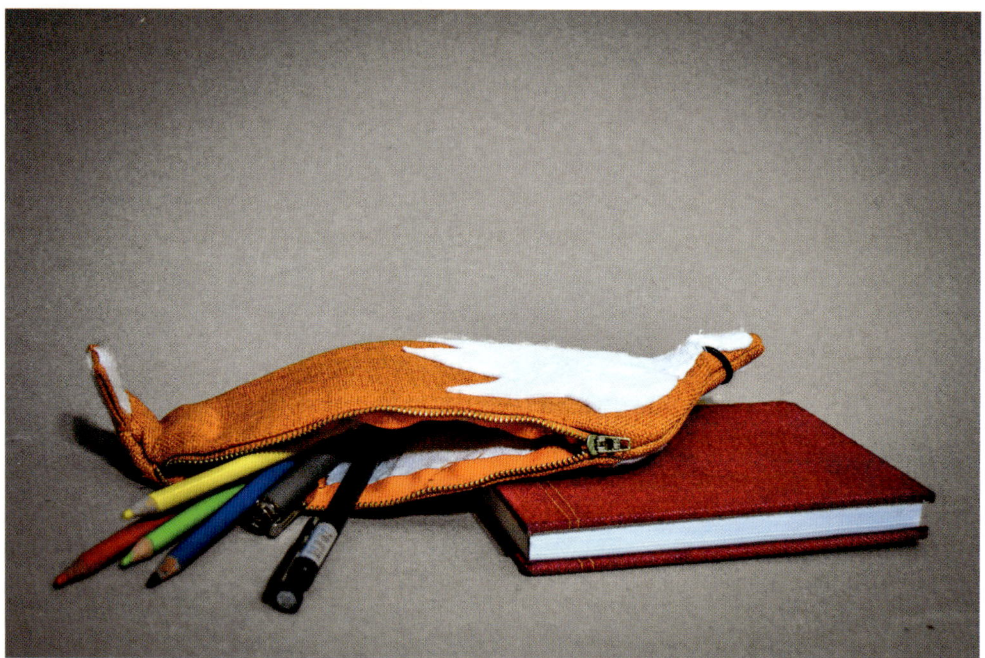

THE FOX BAG
DE: Manuel Ojeda

Based on "the Fox" from The Little Prince, this bag has an interesting
look which is also practical – the nose can be flipped to open the bag
and the tail part is a smaller zipped bag for easy access.

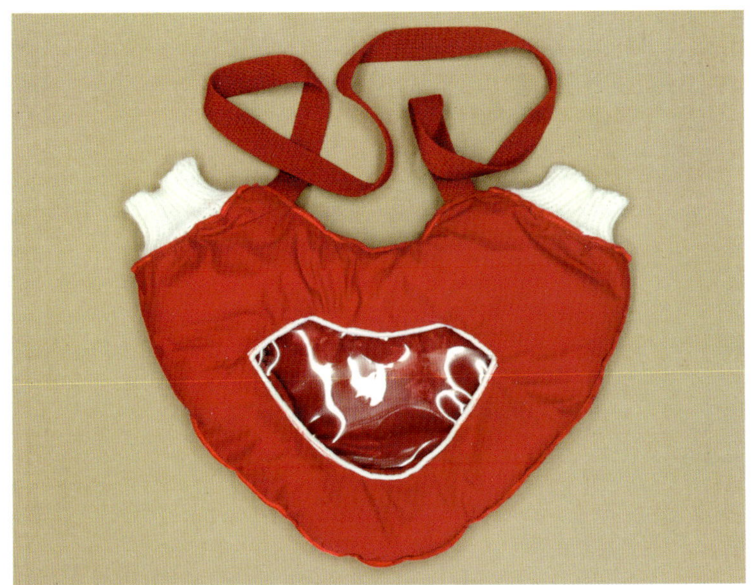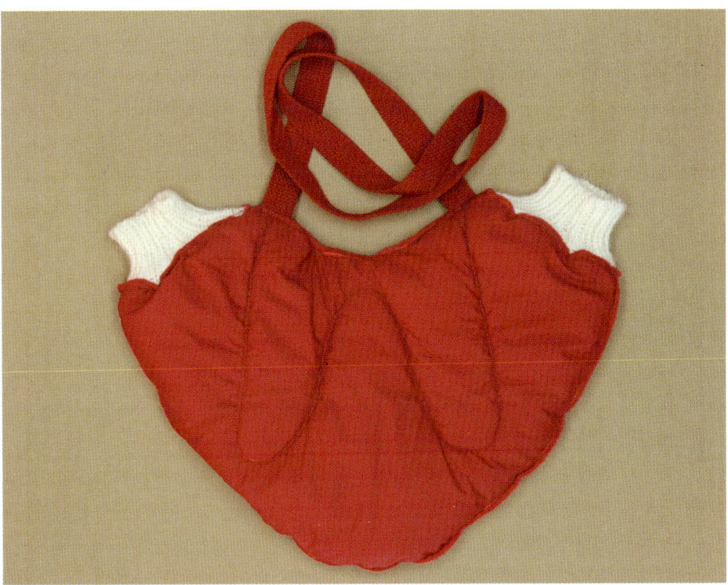

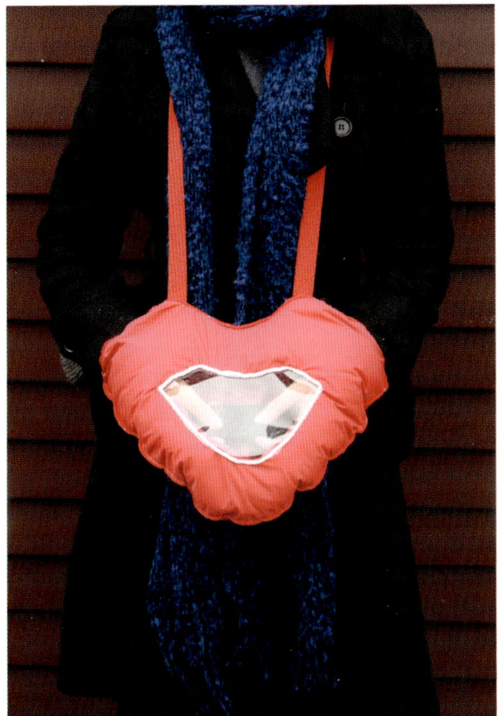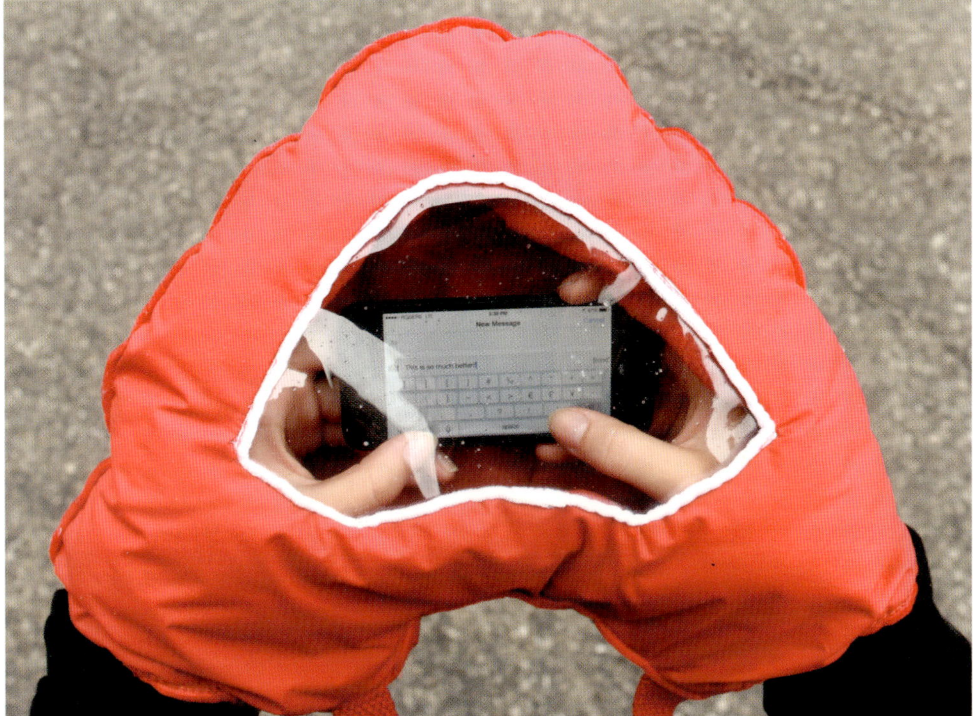

TAHKA THE HAND-WARMER
DA: Clever Maple Inc.

The design enables users to keep on using their cellphone even in cold/
rainy days, protecting the phone well and the uses' hands warm.

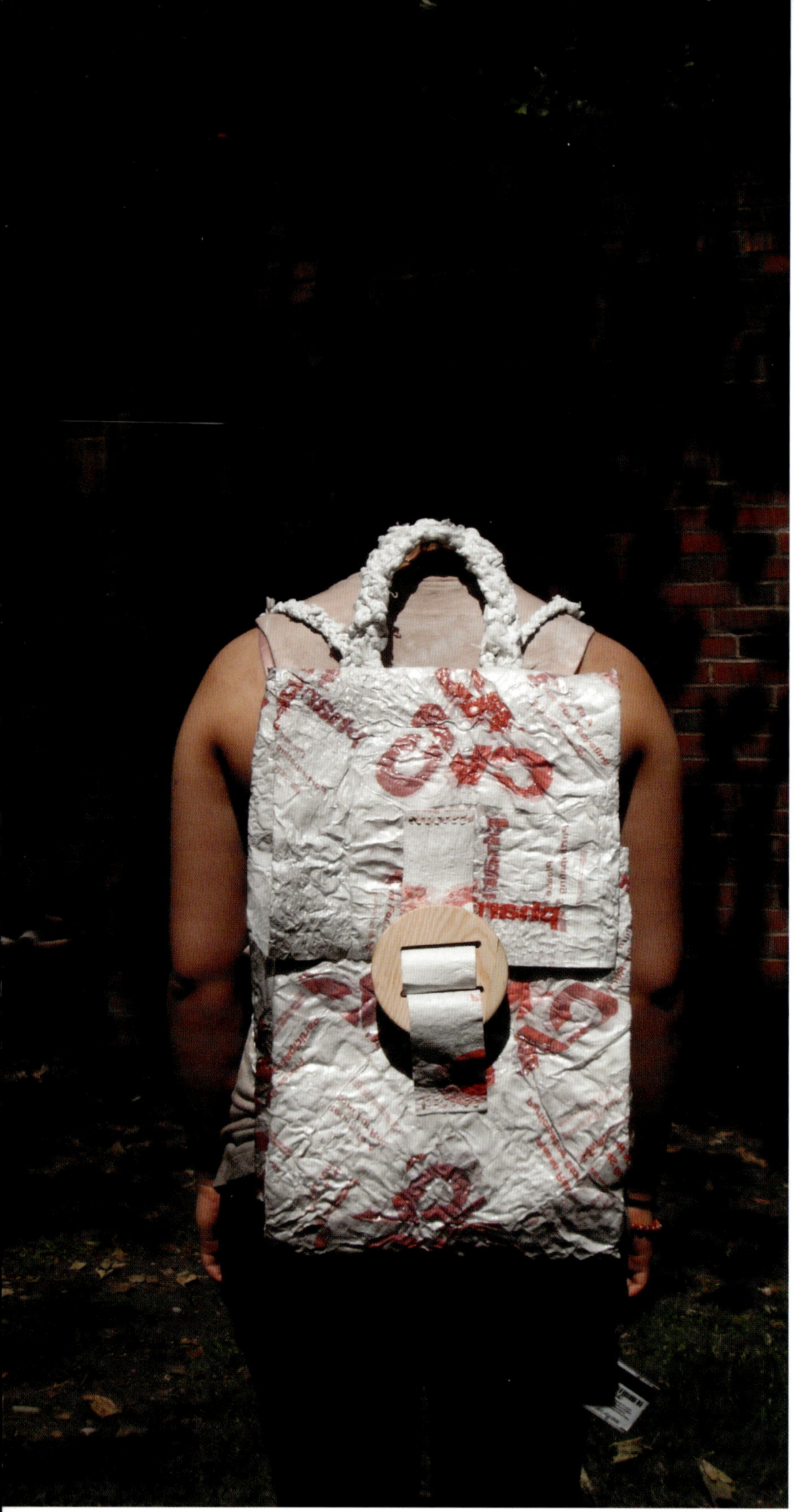

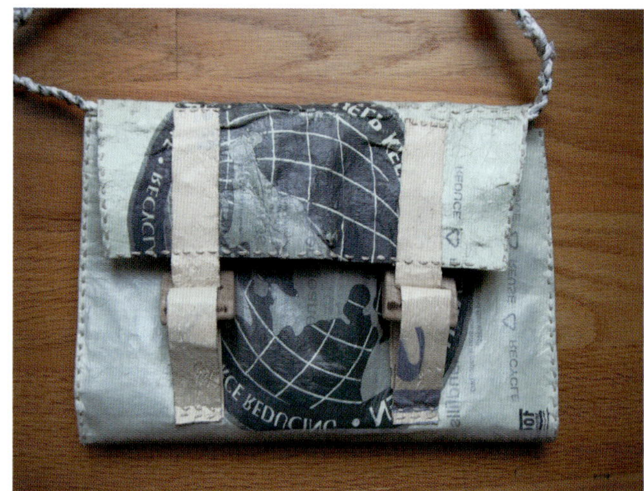

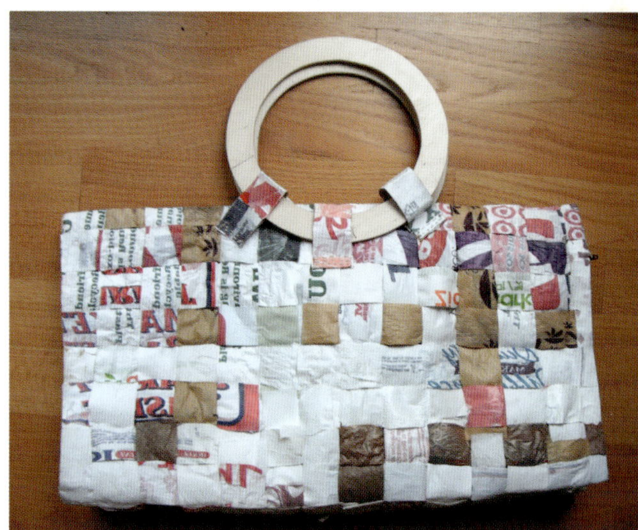

FUSED BAGS
DE: Allison Chen

To create something permanent out of seemingly temporary materials, designer upcyclyed plastic bags by applying heat and pressure to fuse them together layer by layer to get a sturdy material. Designed with this special material the bag has interesting collage patterns.

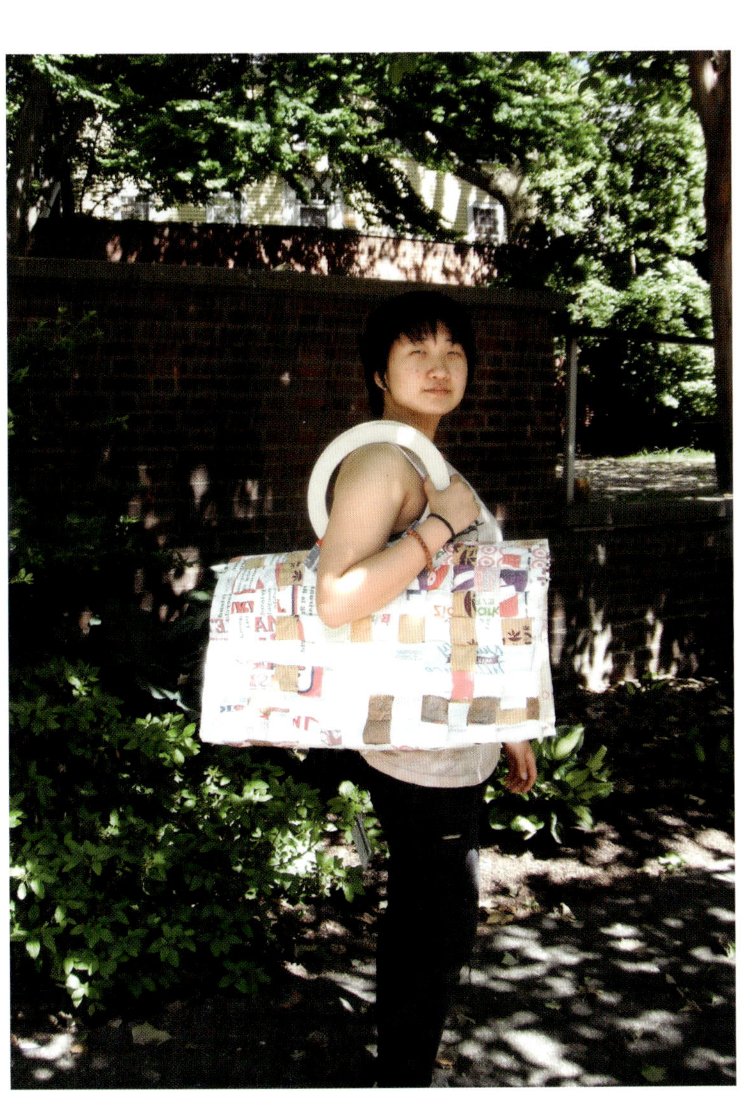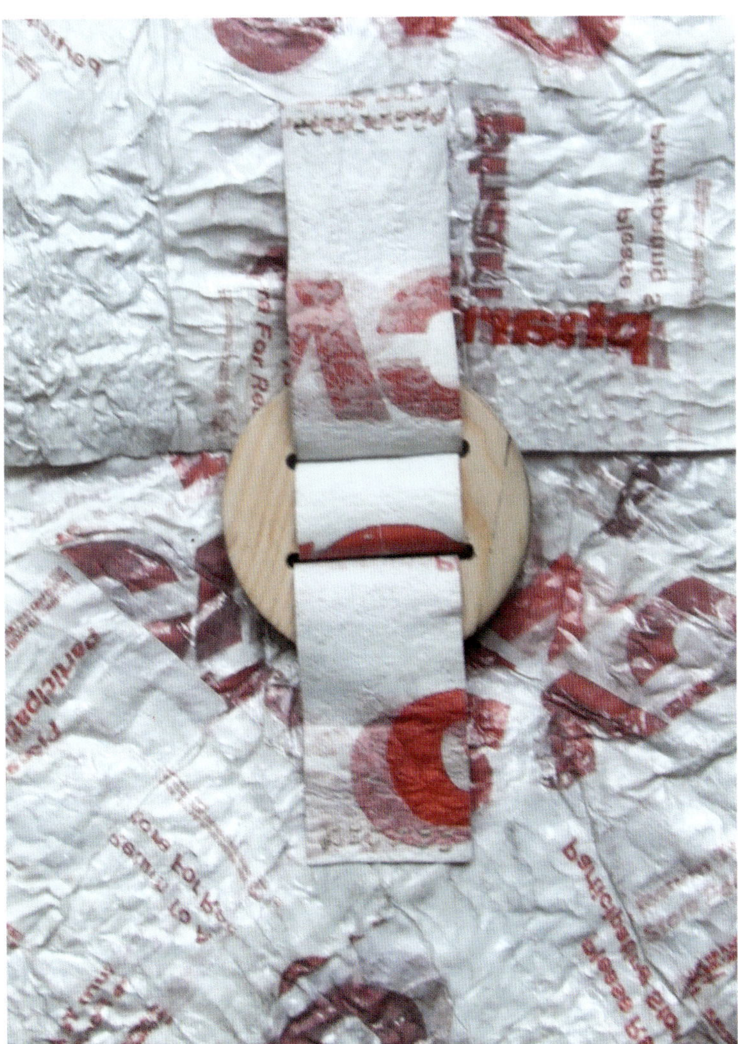

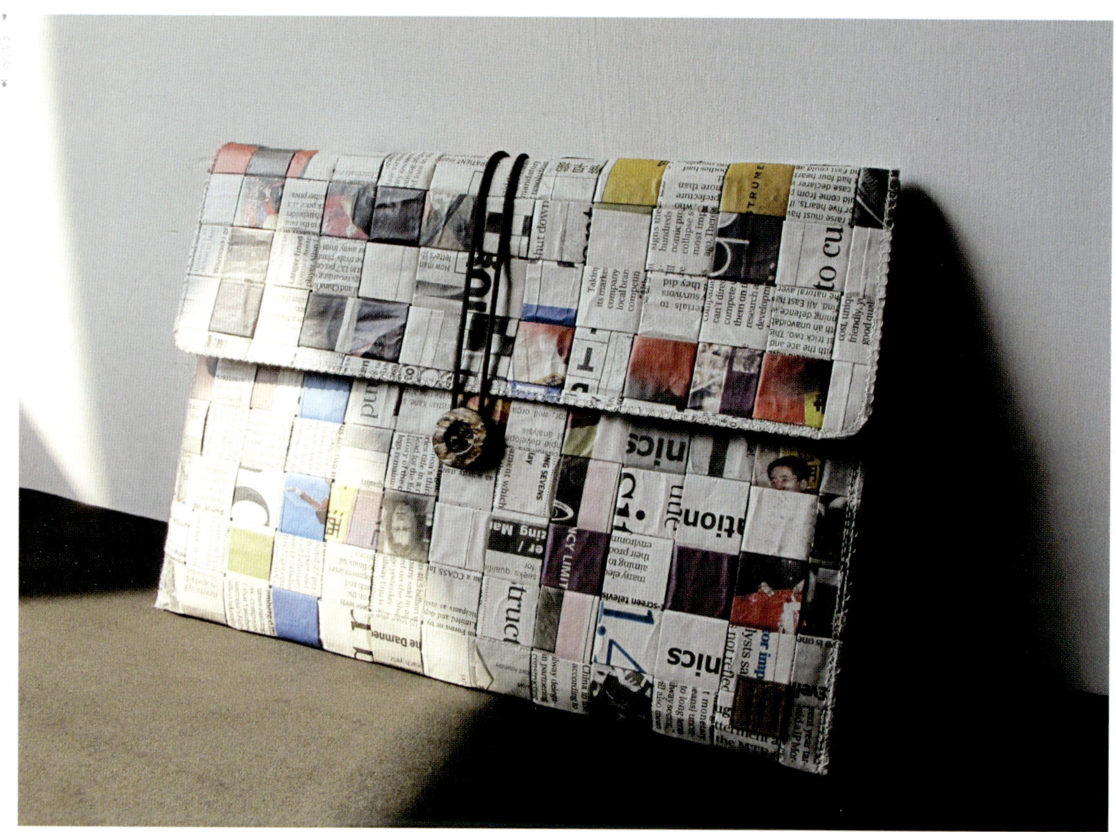

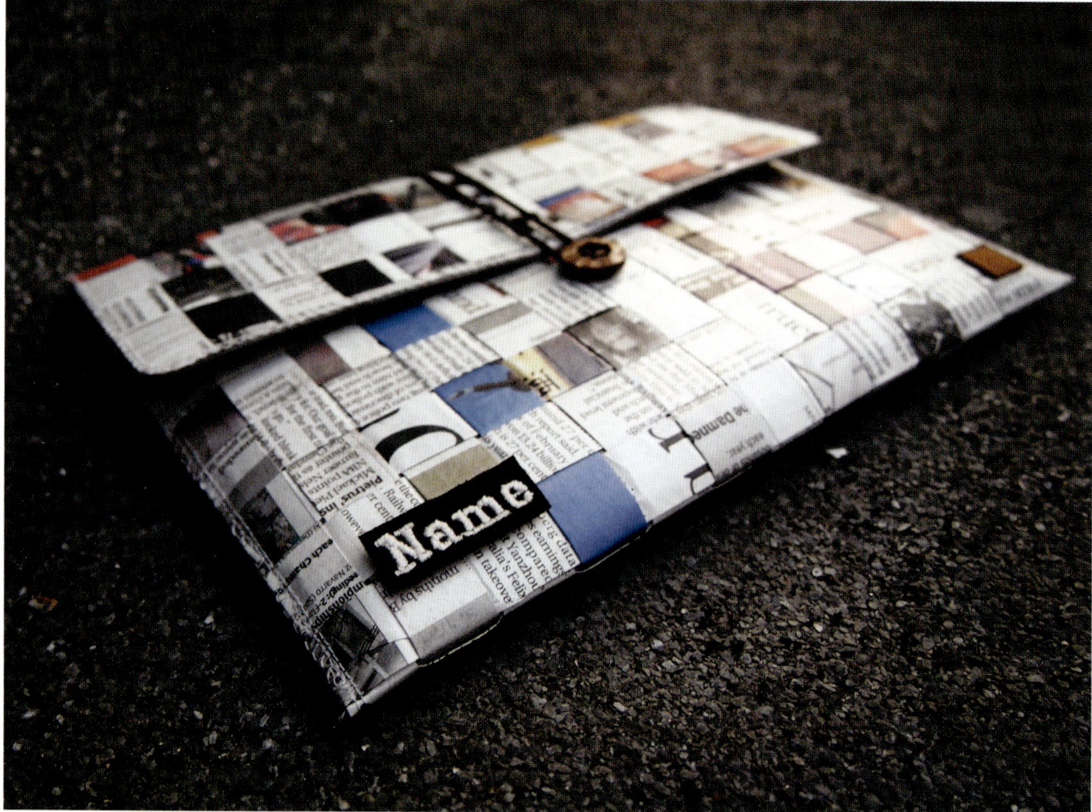

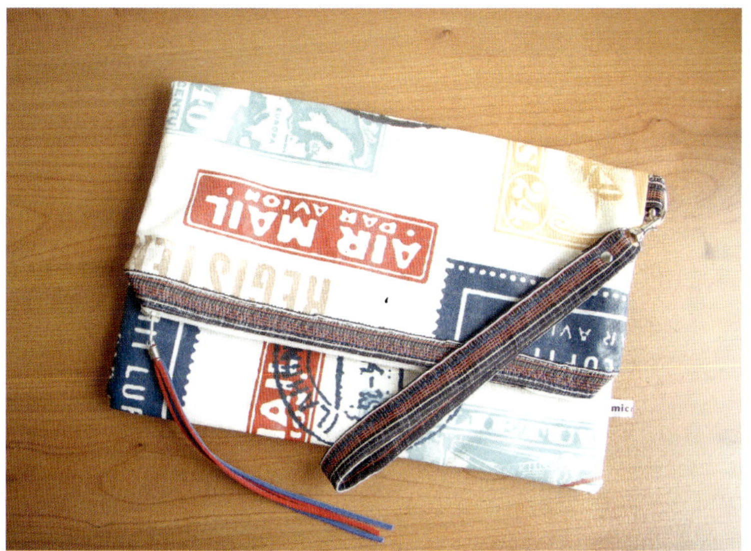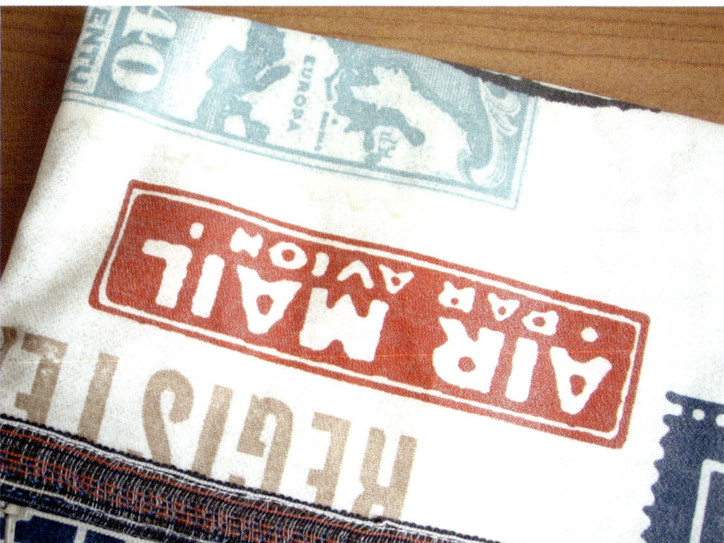

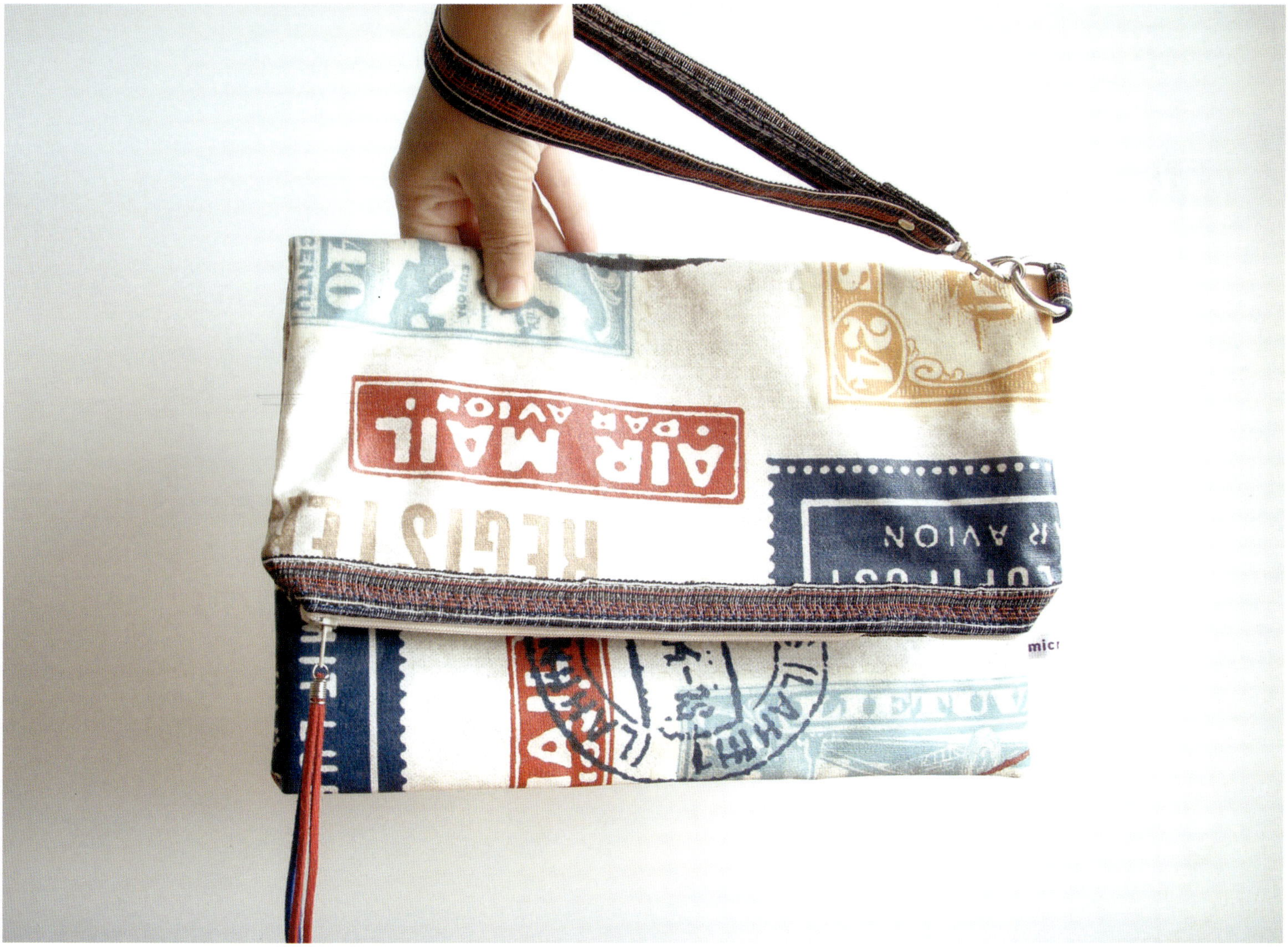

NEWSPAPER PAD

DA: Paralife

Strips of newspaper were woven to be pressed with a PE layer on top to add a waterproof element. The inner cotton lining better protects the contents and provides a softness that improves the tactile experience.

AIRMAIL POUCH

DE: Helena Silva

This design not only folds naturally like a postal bag but also has parts made out of one. The wrist strap and zipper ribbon were upcycled from a real postal bag.

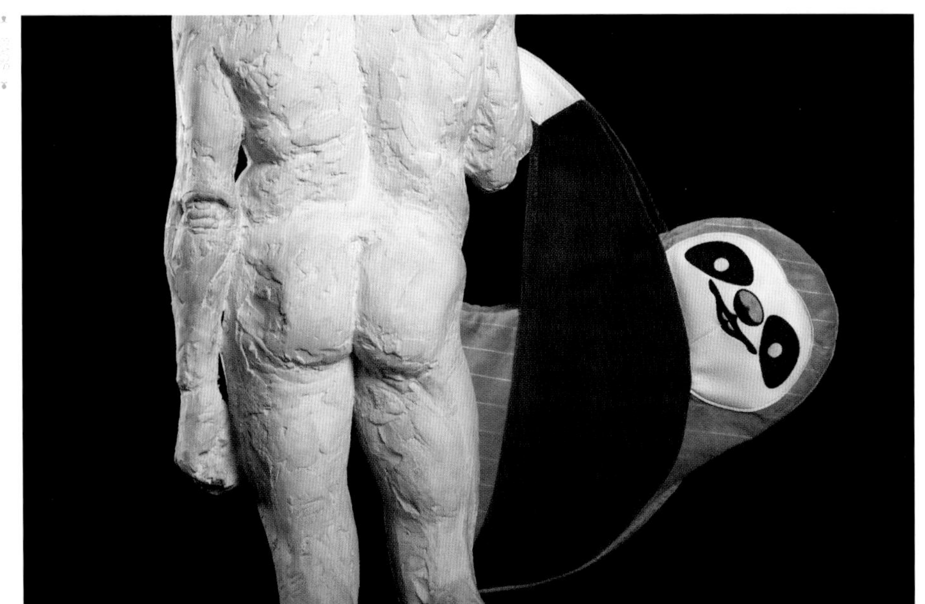

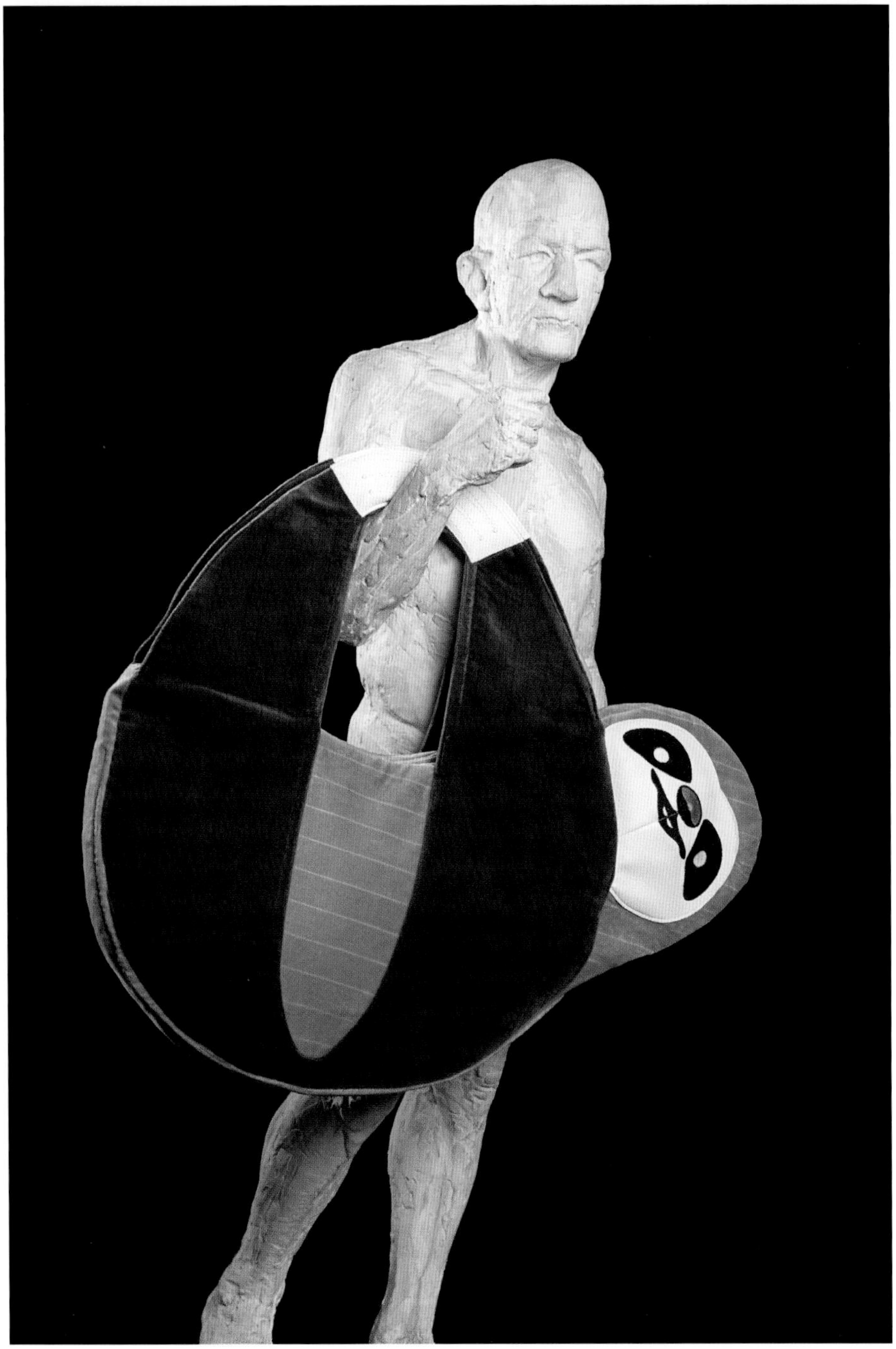

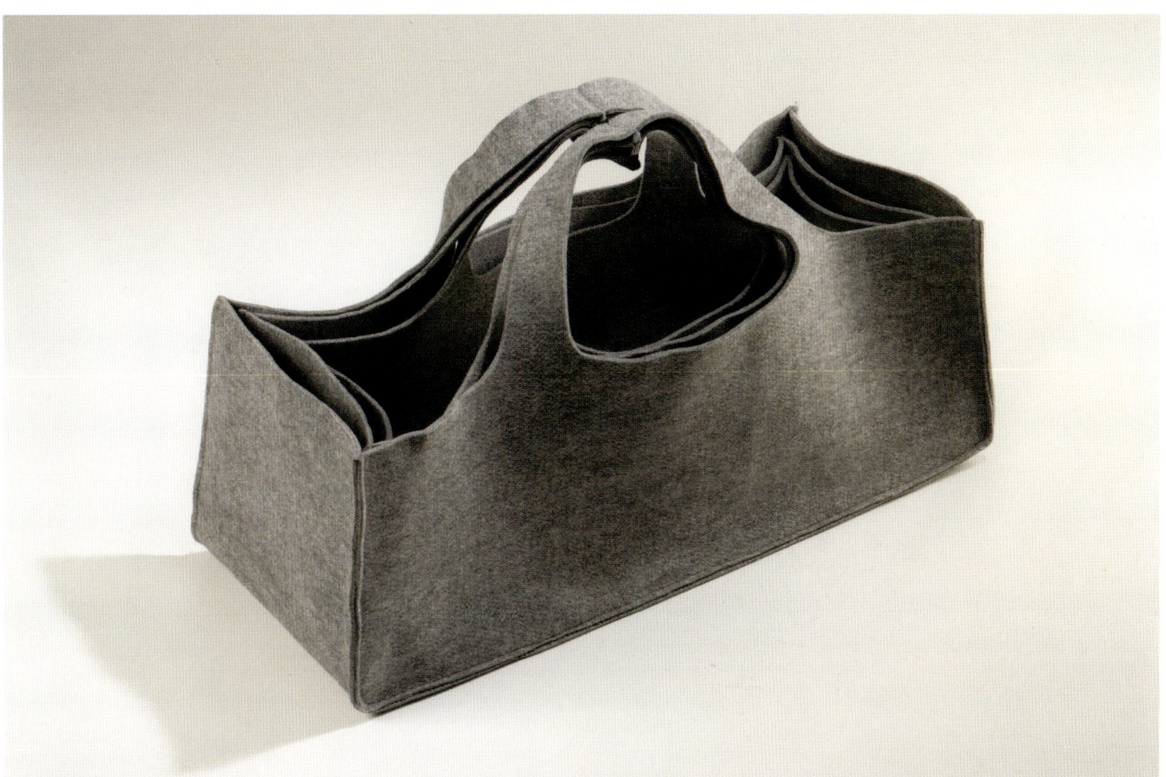

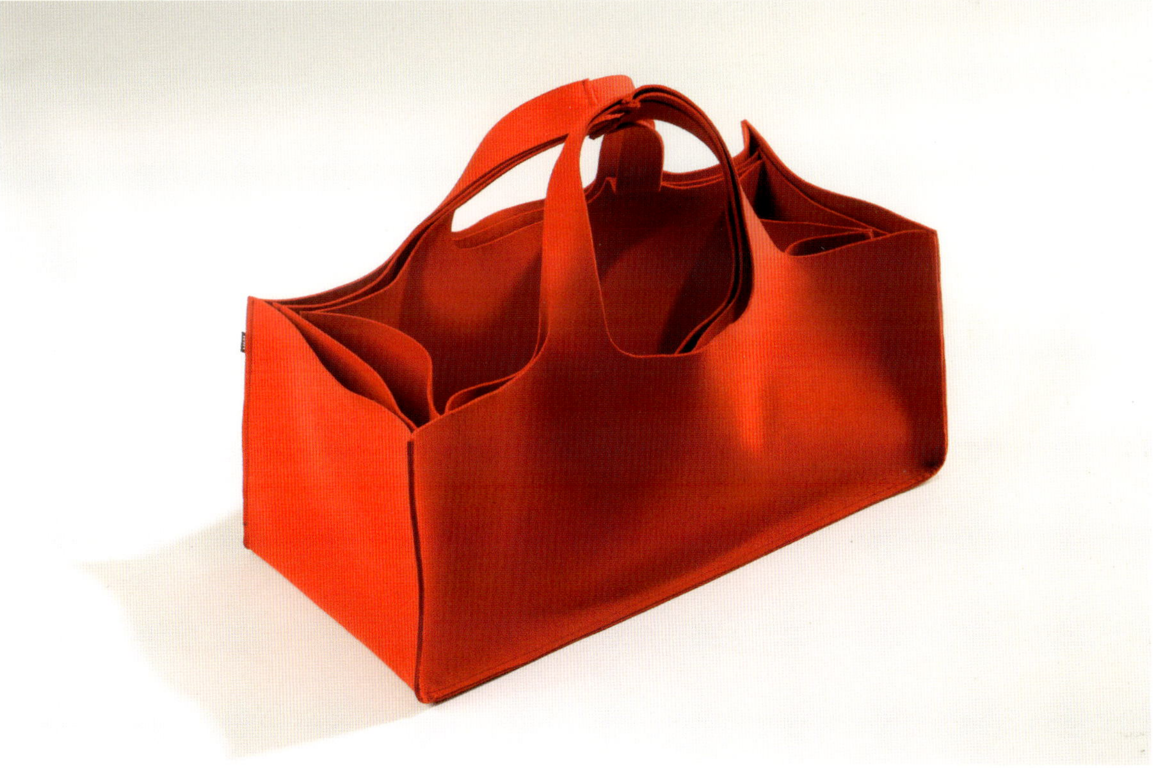

MISTER SLOFF HANDBAGS
DE: Marianna Orsho

Sloth likes to travel but is slow. Marianna was amused by the resemblance between handbags and sloths and the way they both hang upside down, so she designed the character Mister Sloff as a handbag to help him see the world.

TORBUSCHKA
DA: Kaaita

The "Torbuschka" is a clever bag with two smaller bags in its belly like Russian dolls, made of felt upcycled from discarded plastic bottles.

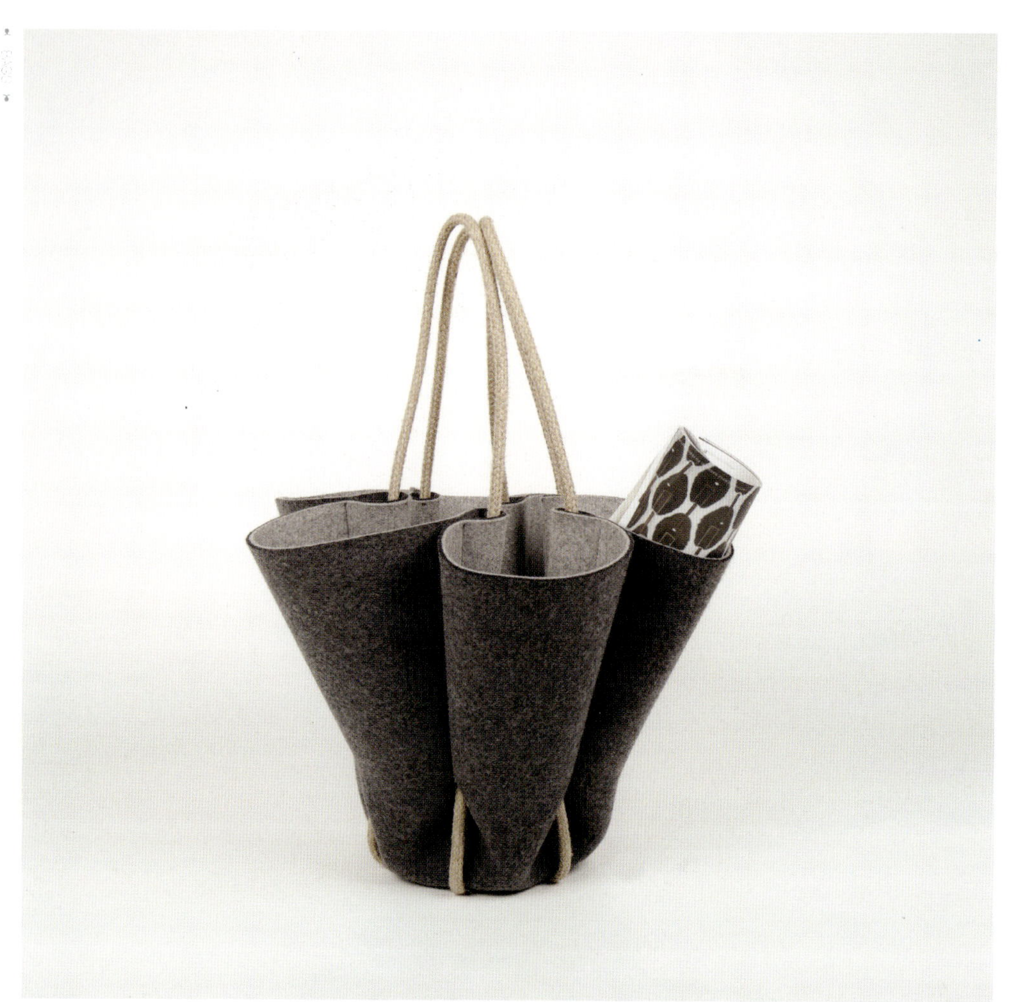

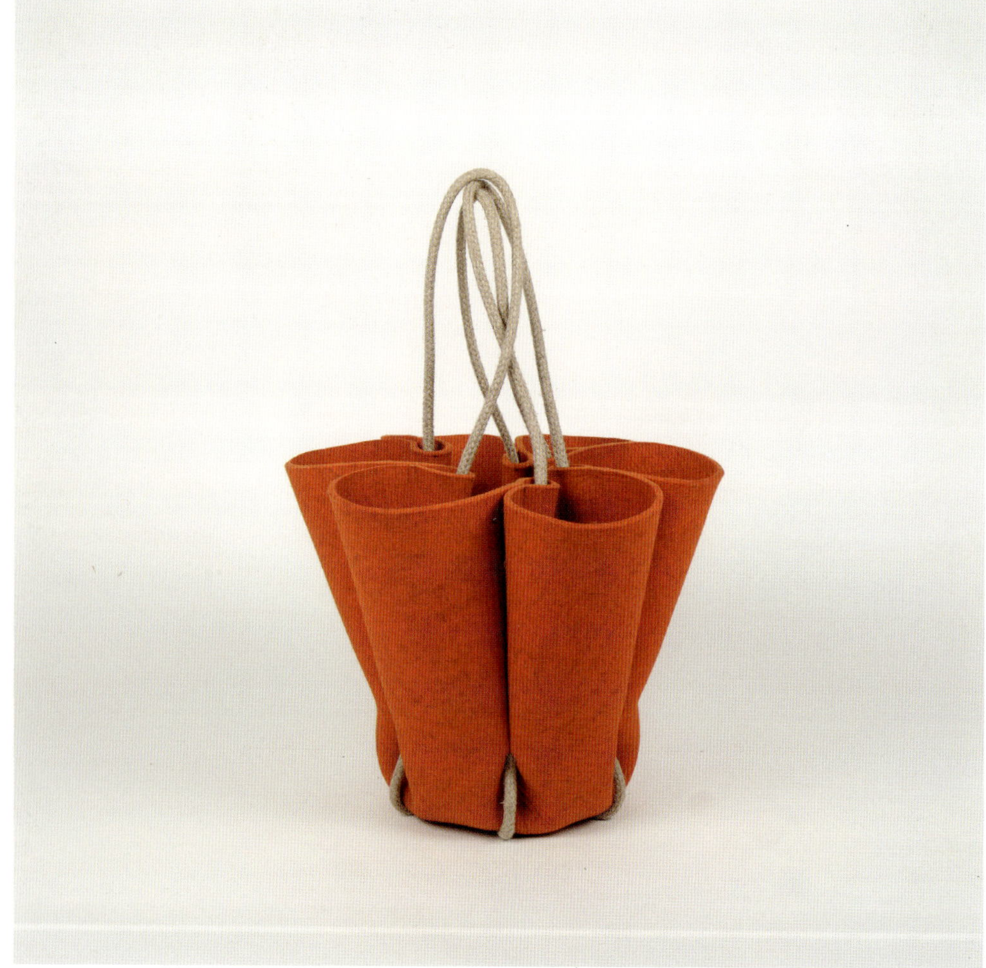

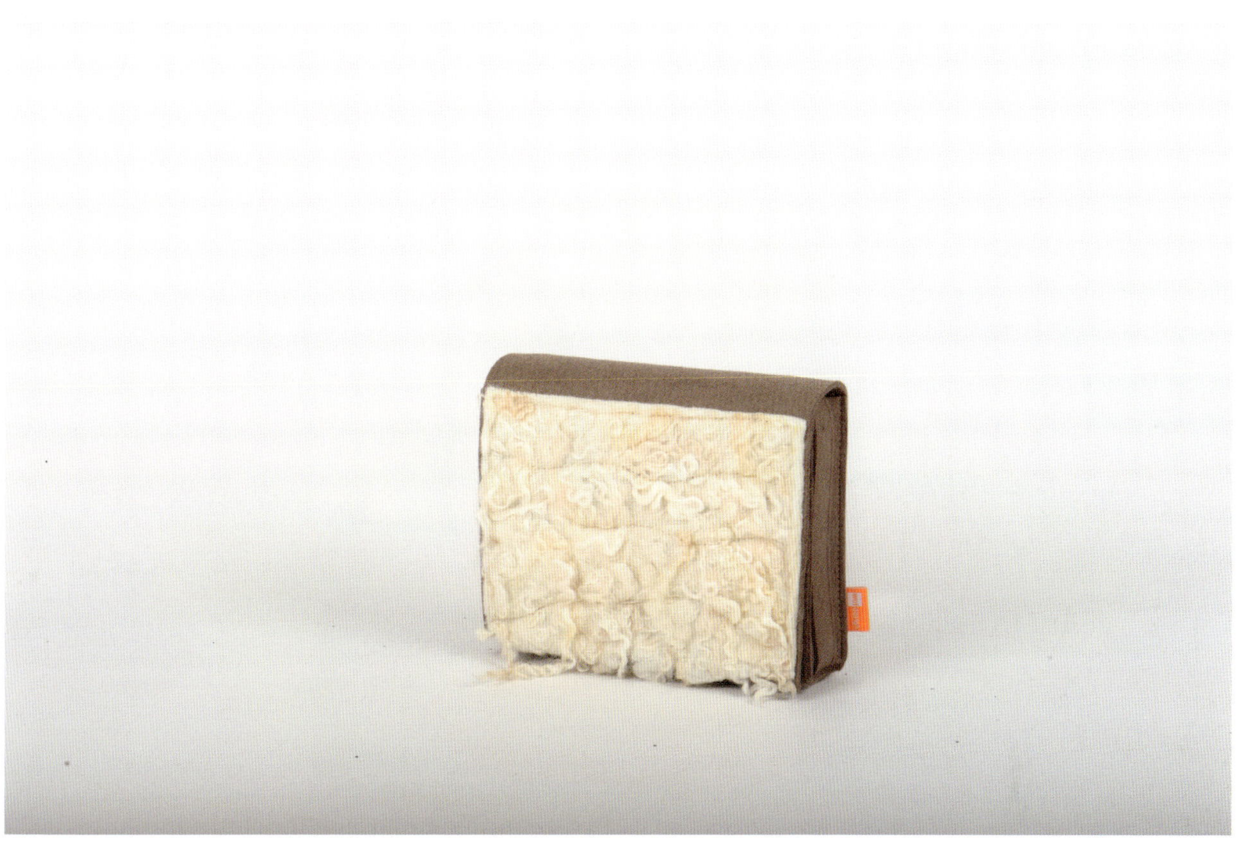

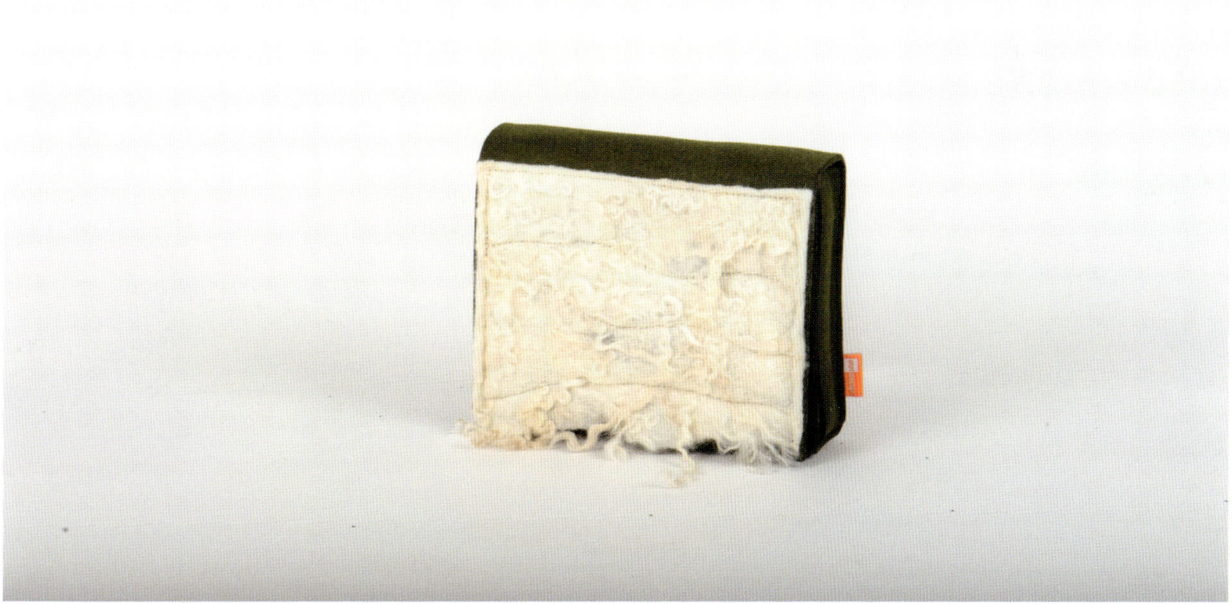

NOMAD
DA: Weidesign

The model on the left features six cylinders folded using only one piece of wool felt, practical for separate storage. The right one is characterized by the fluff in front, while the main body was made of wool felt, which is shock absorbing, water-repellent and flame retardant.

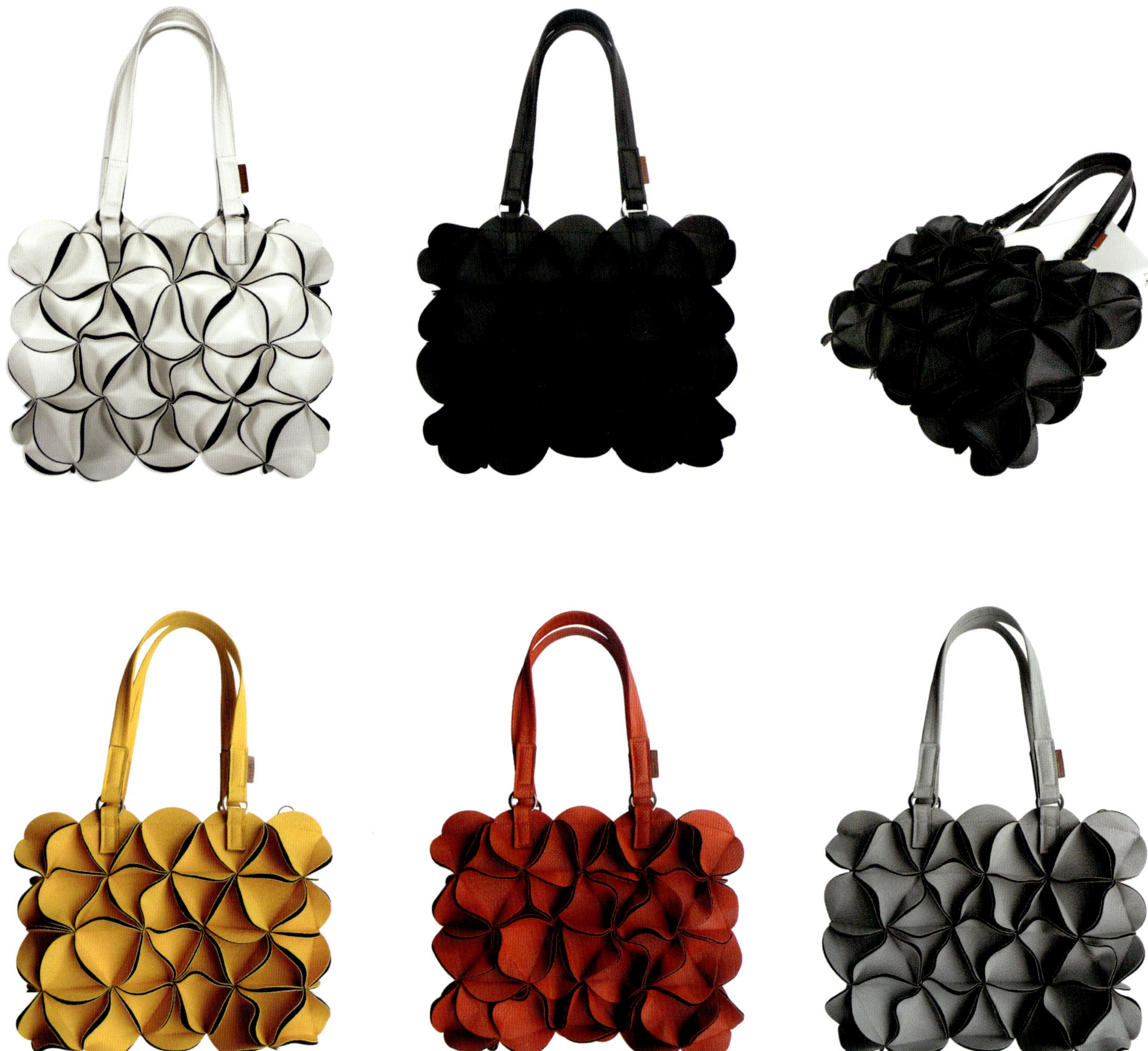

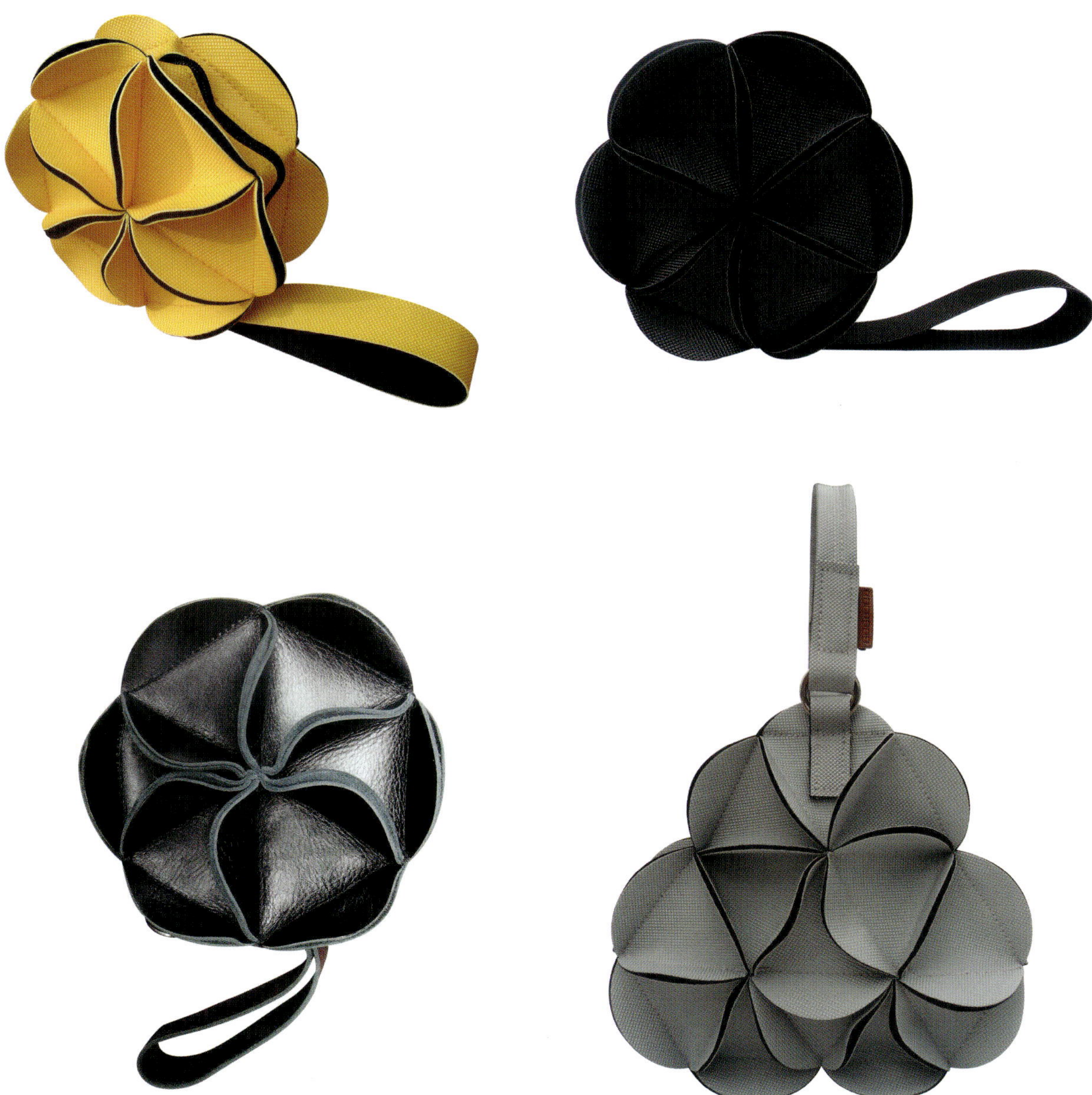

BLOSSOM
DA: Good Job

The "Blossom" series is characterized by small circular modules hand sewn in
a triangle-fold technique that creates a unique floral pattern.

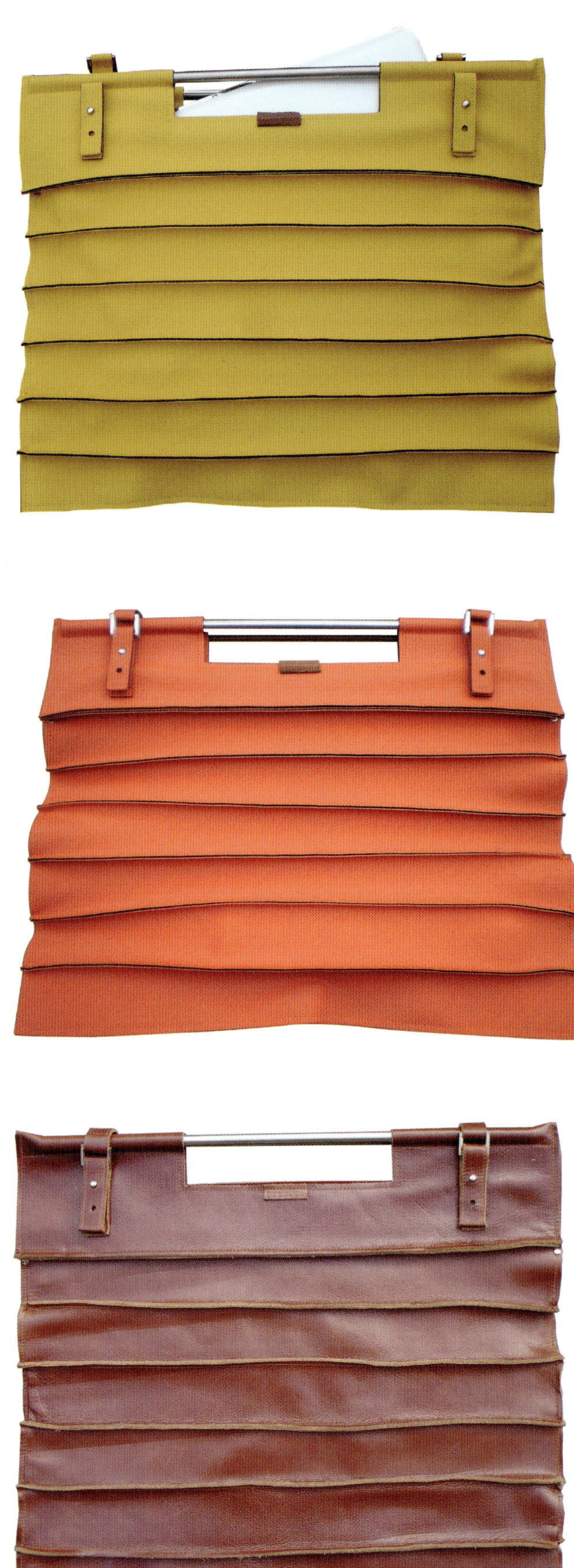
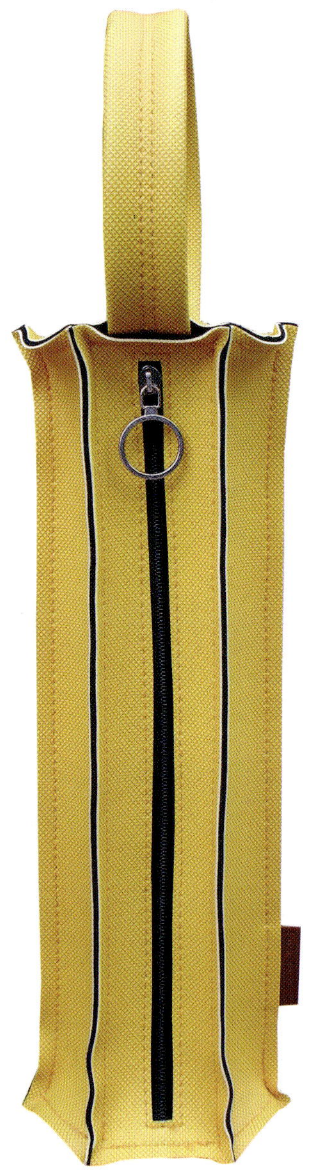

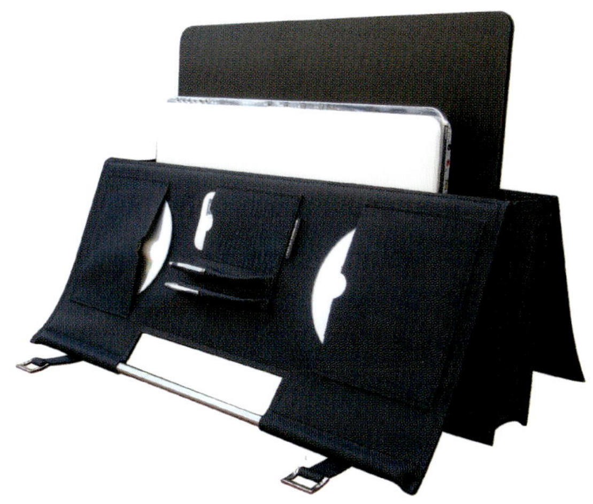

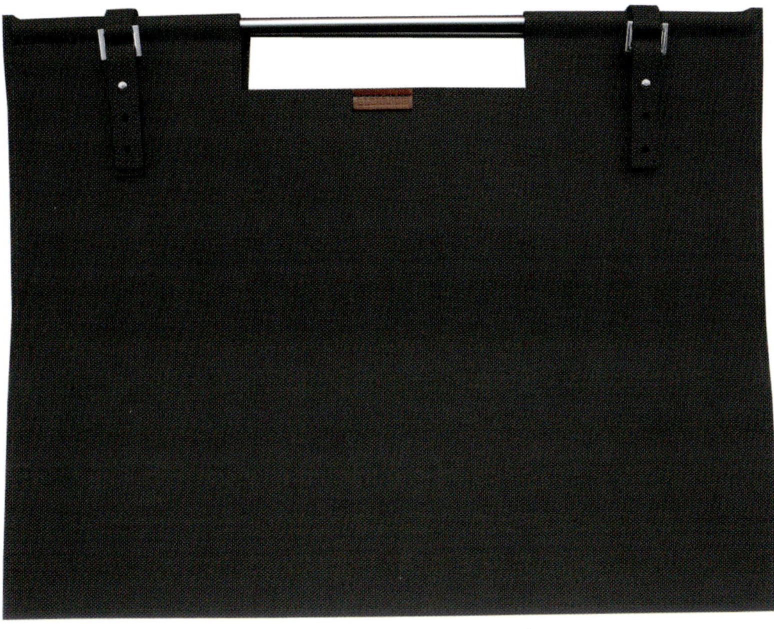

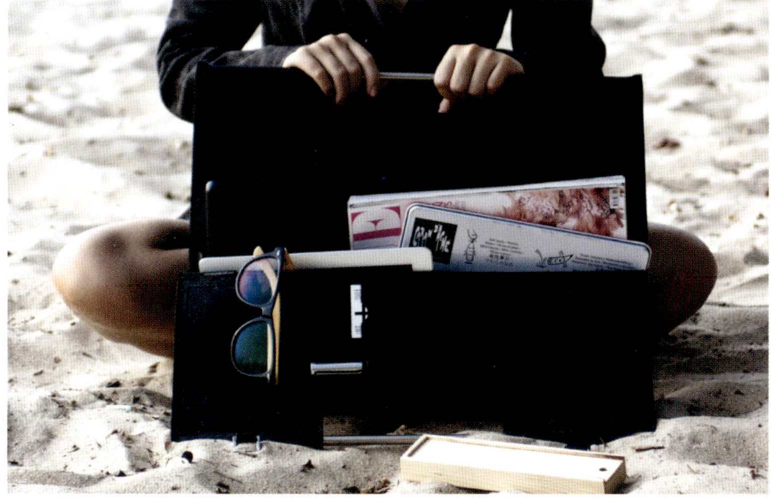

FLUTED
DA: Good Job

Inspired by classical columns, the "Fluted" bag features a distinctively
pleated outside with black lines contrasting with the bright colors.

PROFESSIONAL
DA: Good Job

This design is a "two-in-one" bag that functions as a document bag and a
desktop accessory. In its folding position, the lightweight stainless steel
handle becomes a stable base for the bag.

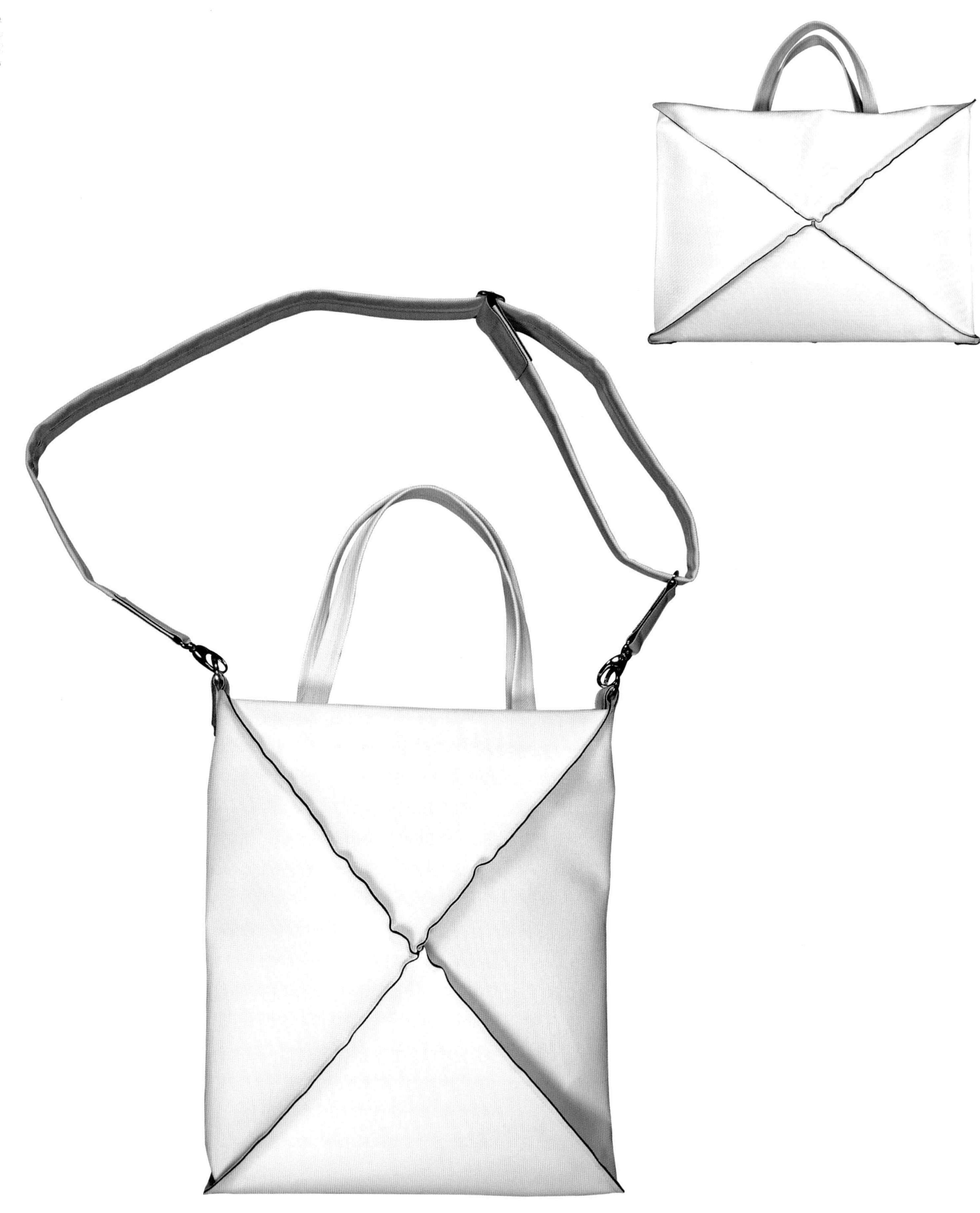

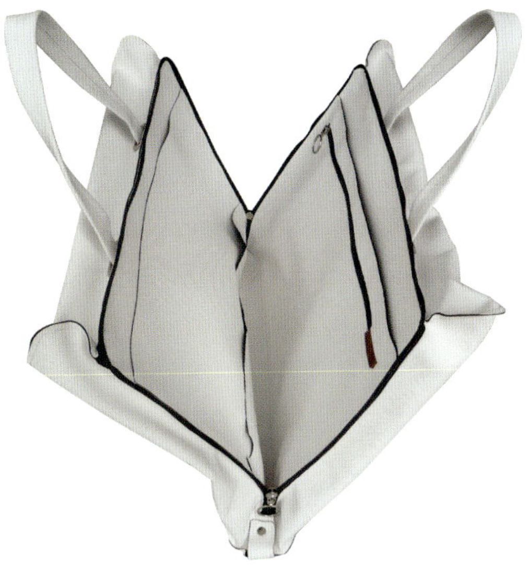

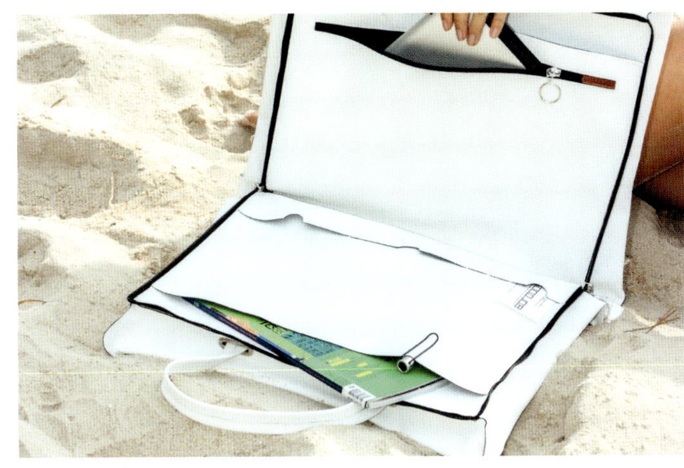

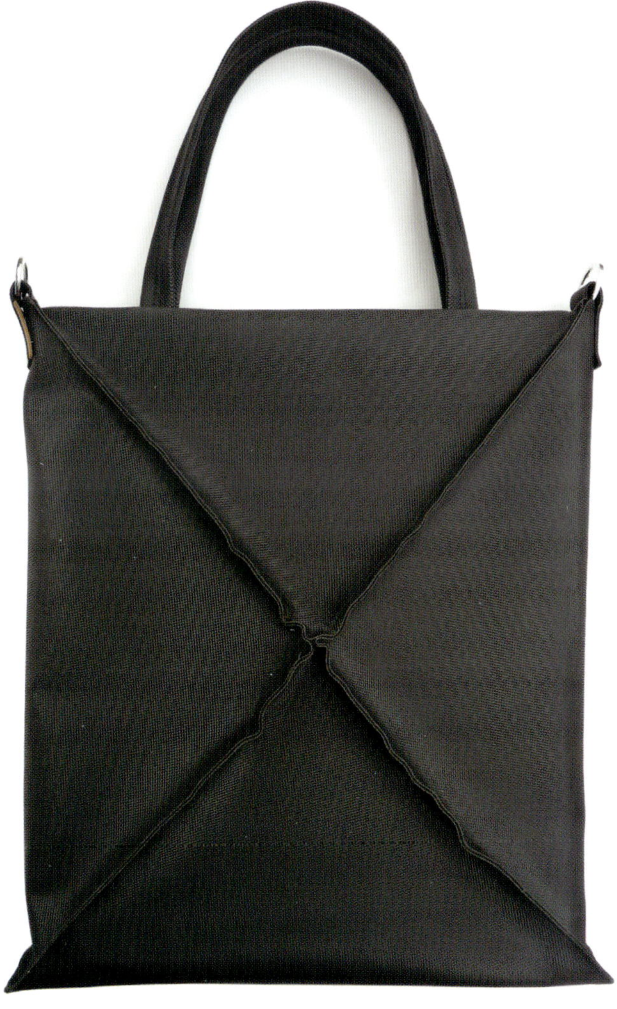

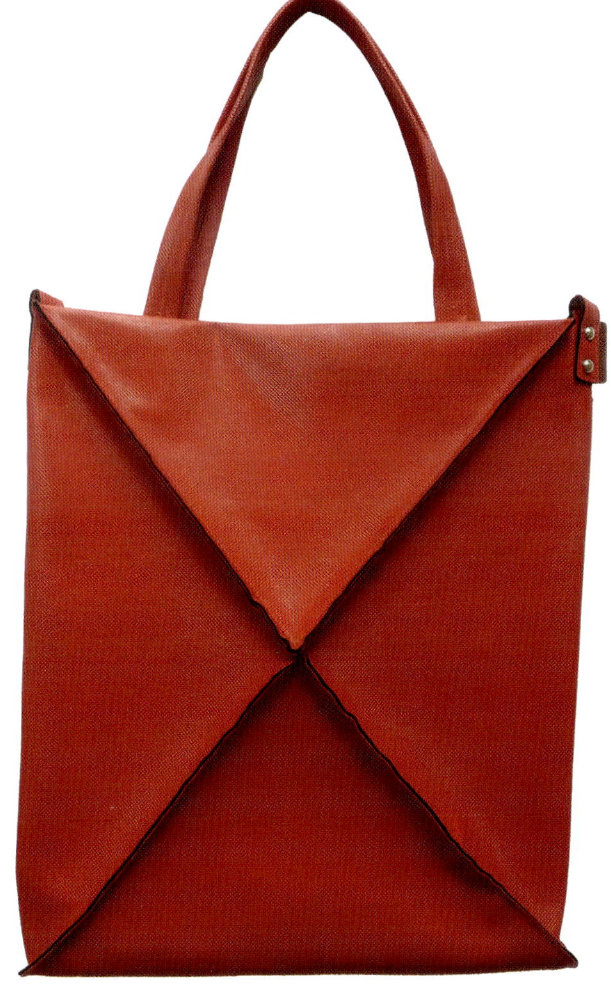

X-PERT
DA: Good Job

The "X" on the front, created with special folding, stands for "X-pert".
With great functionality, the bag opens to reveal layers of compartments,
some of which have zippers to enhance security.

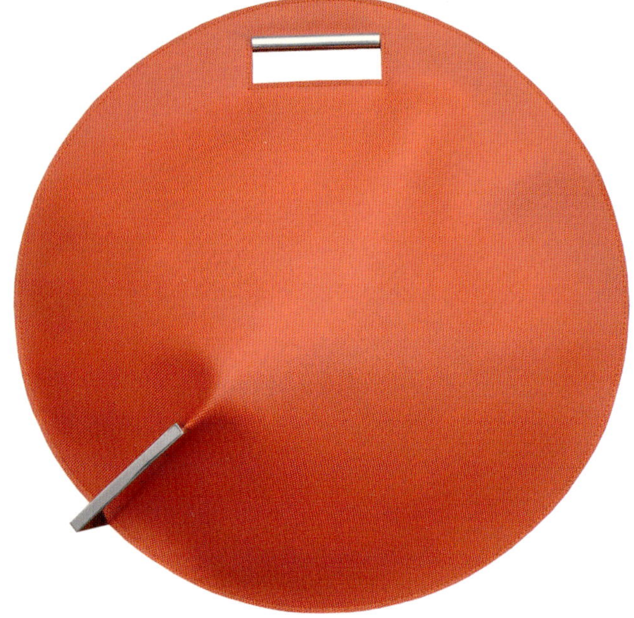
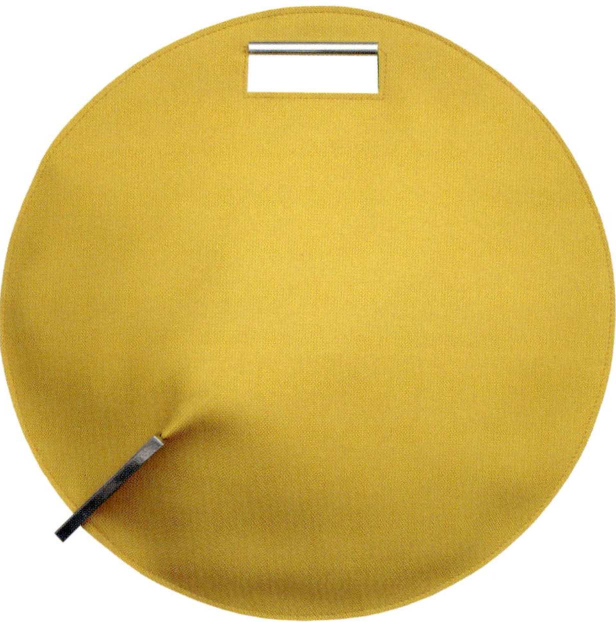
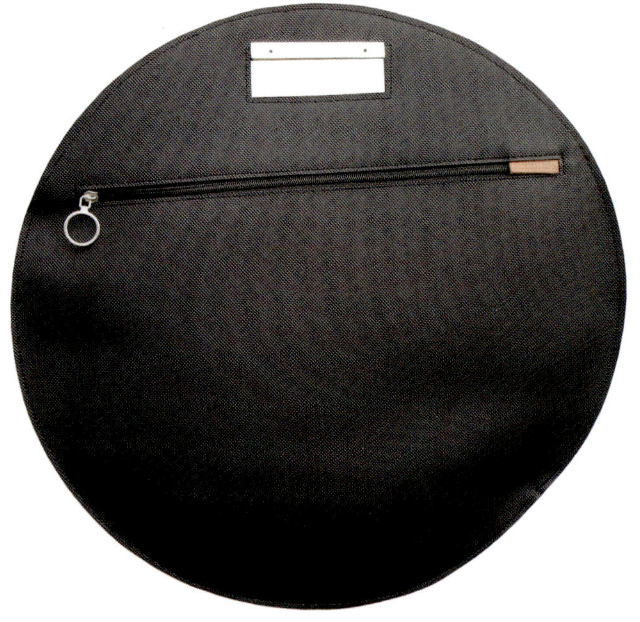
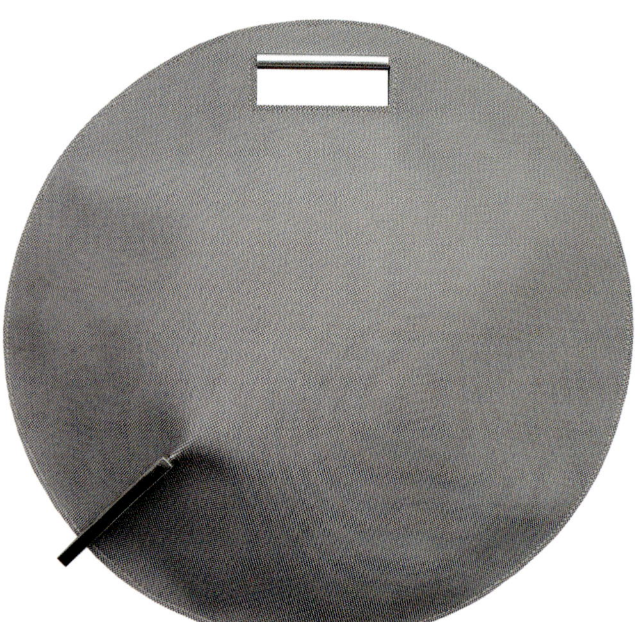

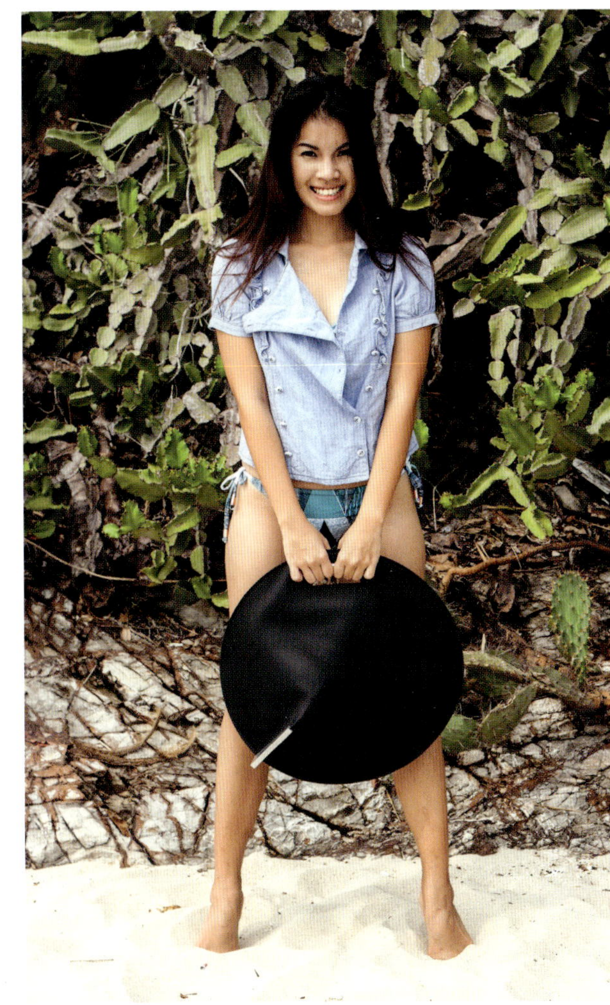

STINRAY

DA: Good Job

The "Stingray" is comprised of two circular flat sheets and the back sheet
lays flat to leave more room between the bag and the carrier's body.
Mimicking the shape of a stingray, the design is a combination of organic
form and modern design.

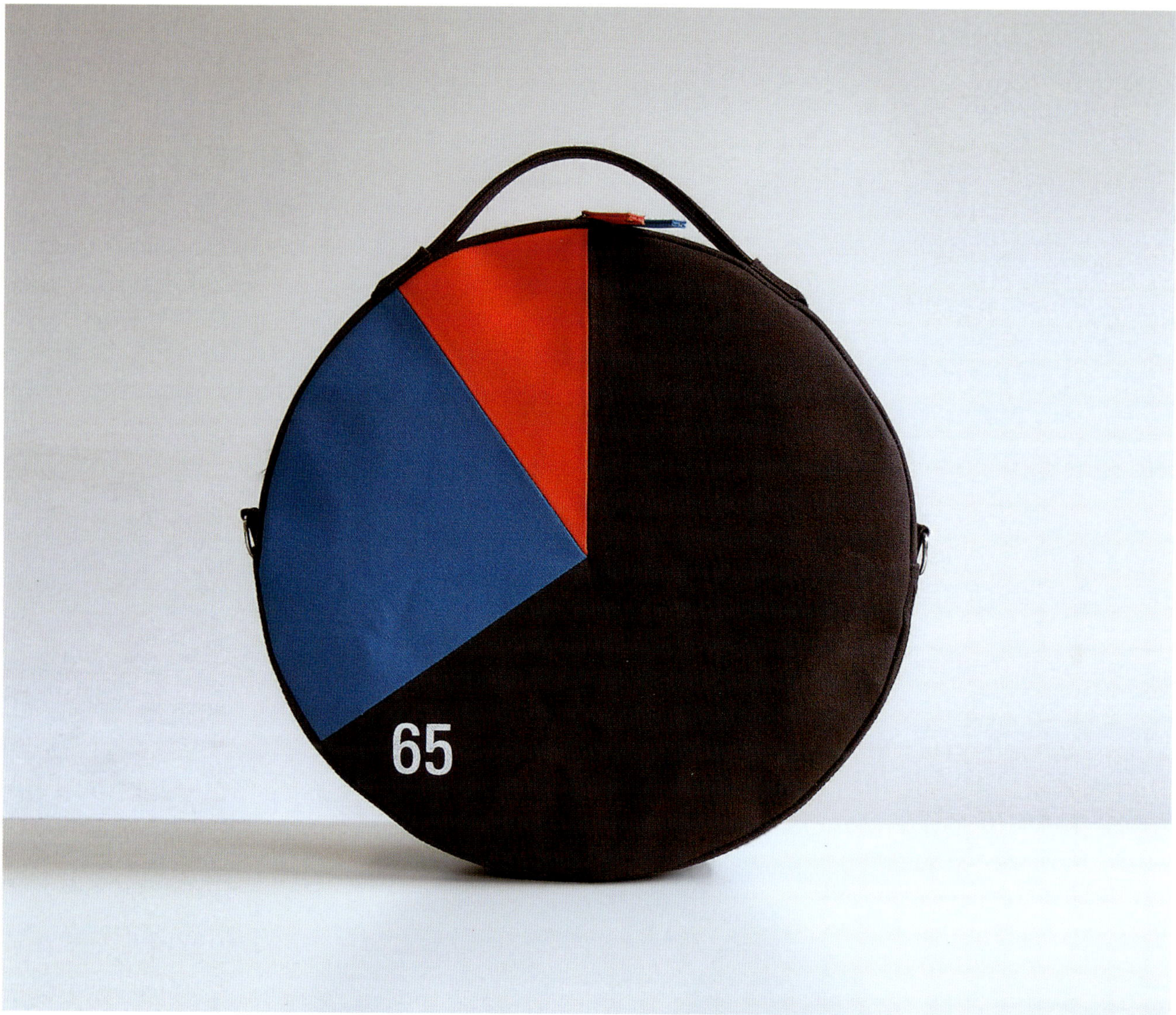

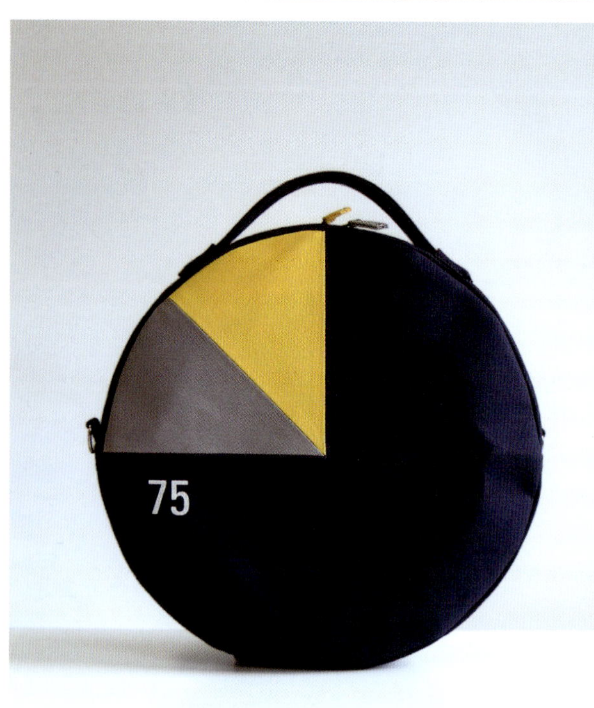
75

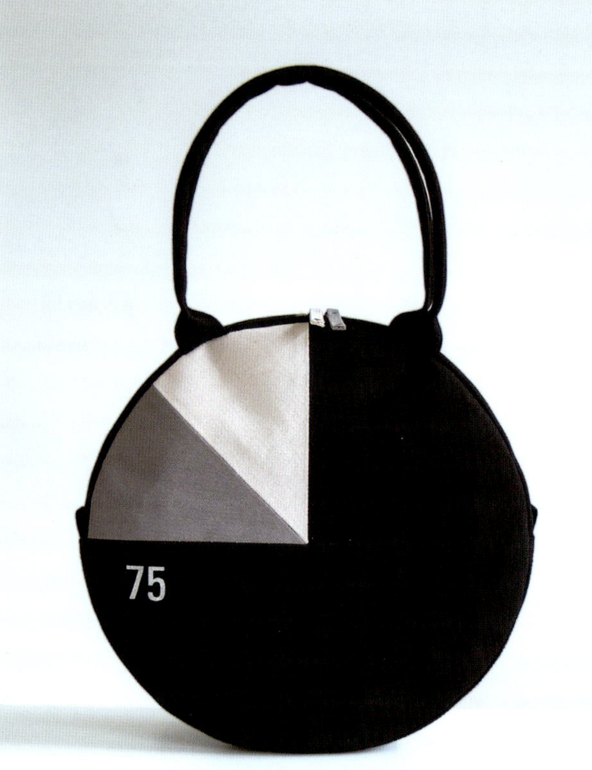
75

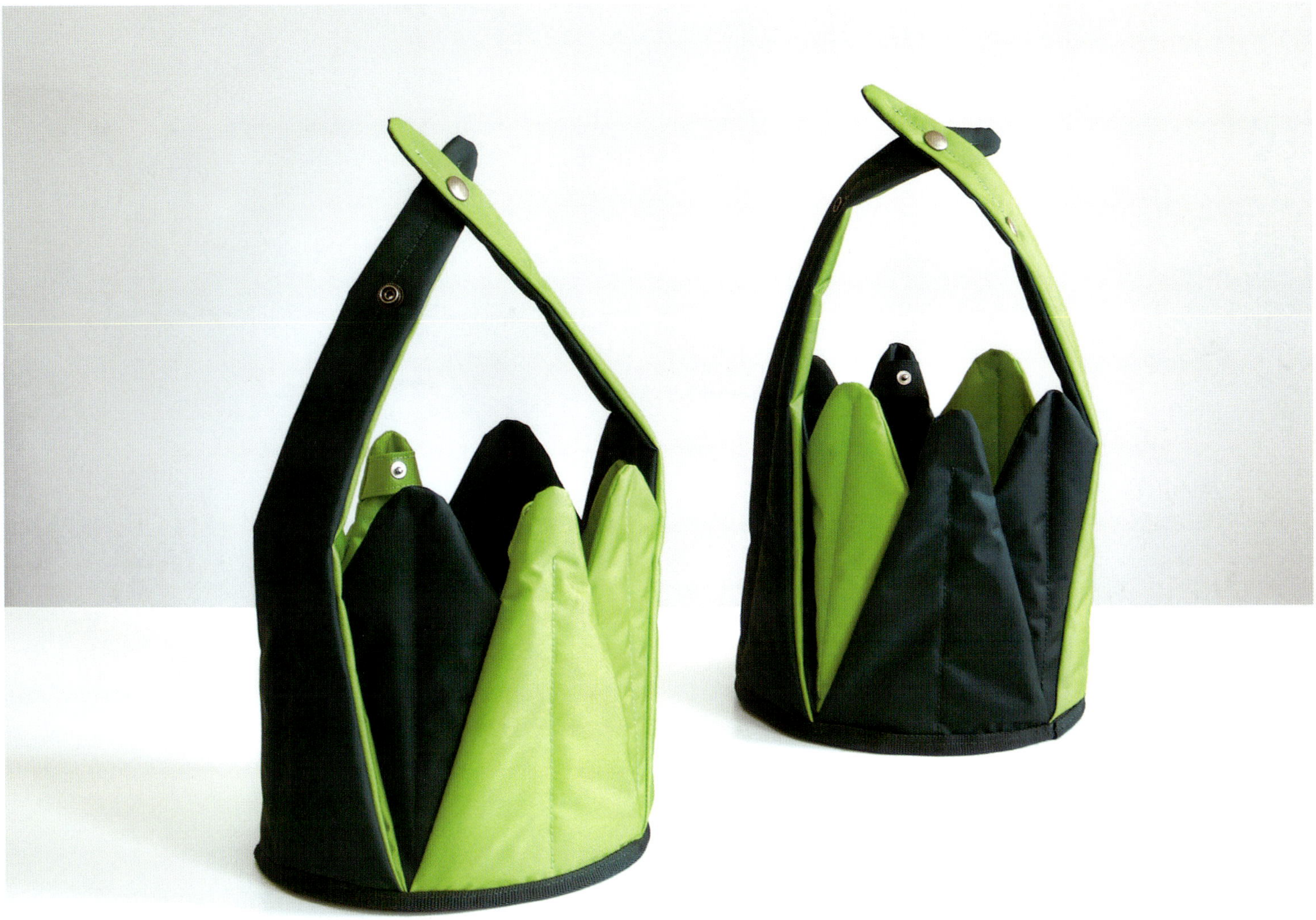

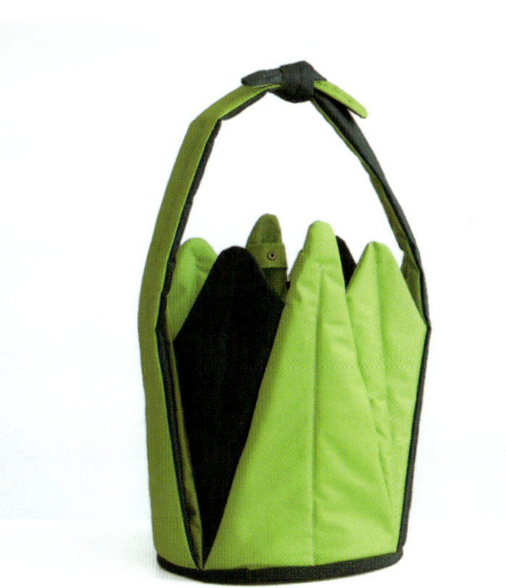

GRAPH BAG
DA: Yuruliku

This pie graph bag was designed with the idea that whatever happens in life can be measured and included in the "pie chart of life."

GRASS BAG
DA: Yuruliku

Designed for the: "Design Everyday Life for Children" exhibition, the Grass Bag has a hidden pocket inside to interpret the concept "Carry your secrets!"

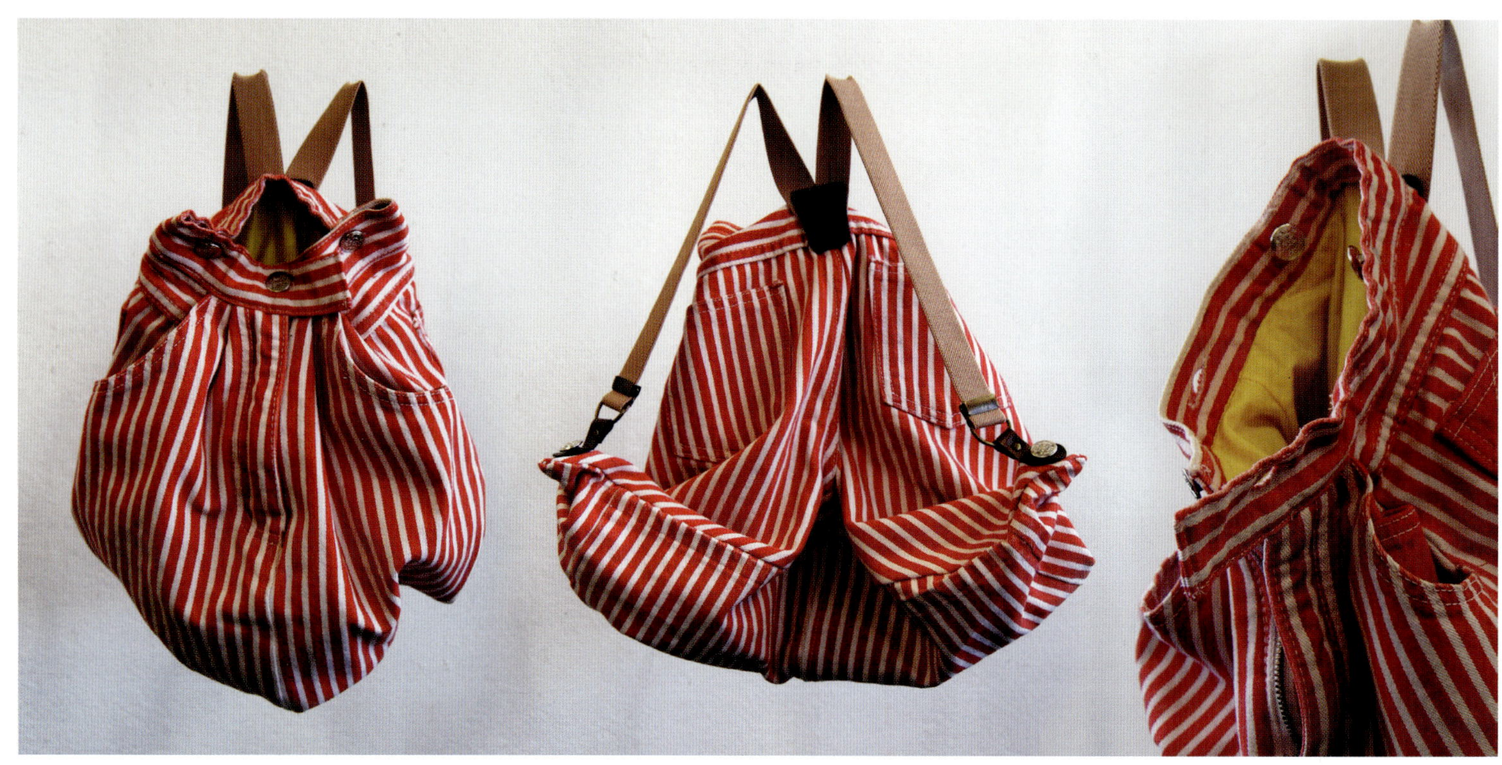

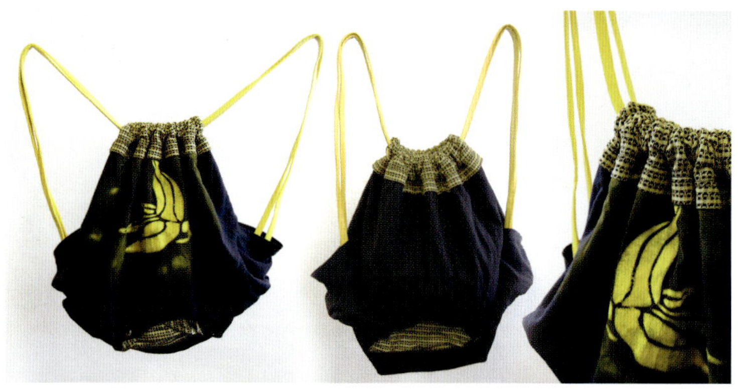

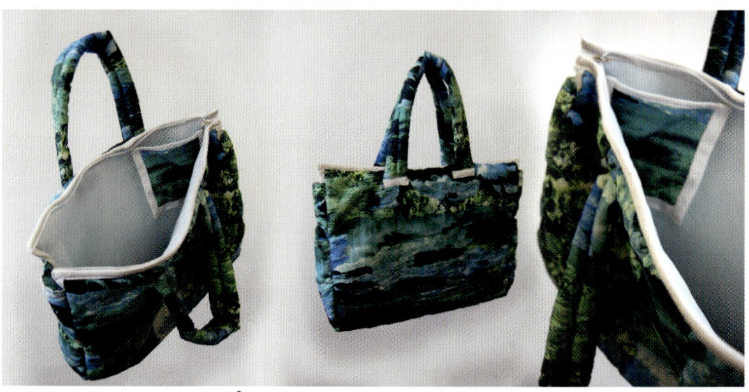

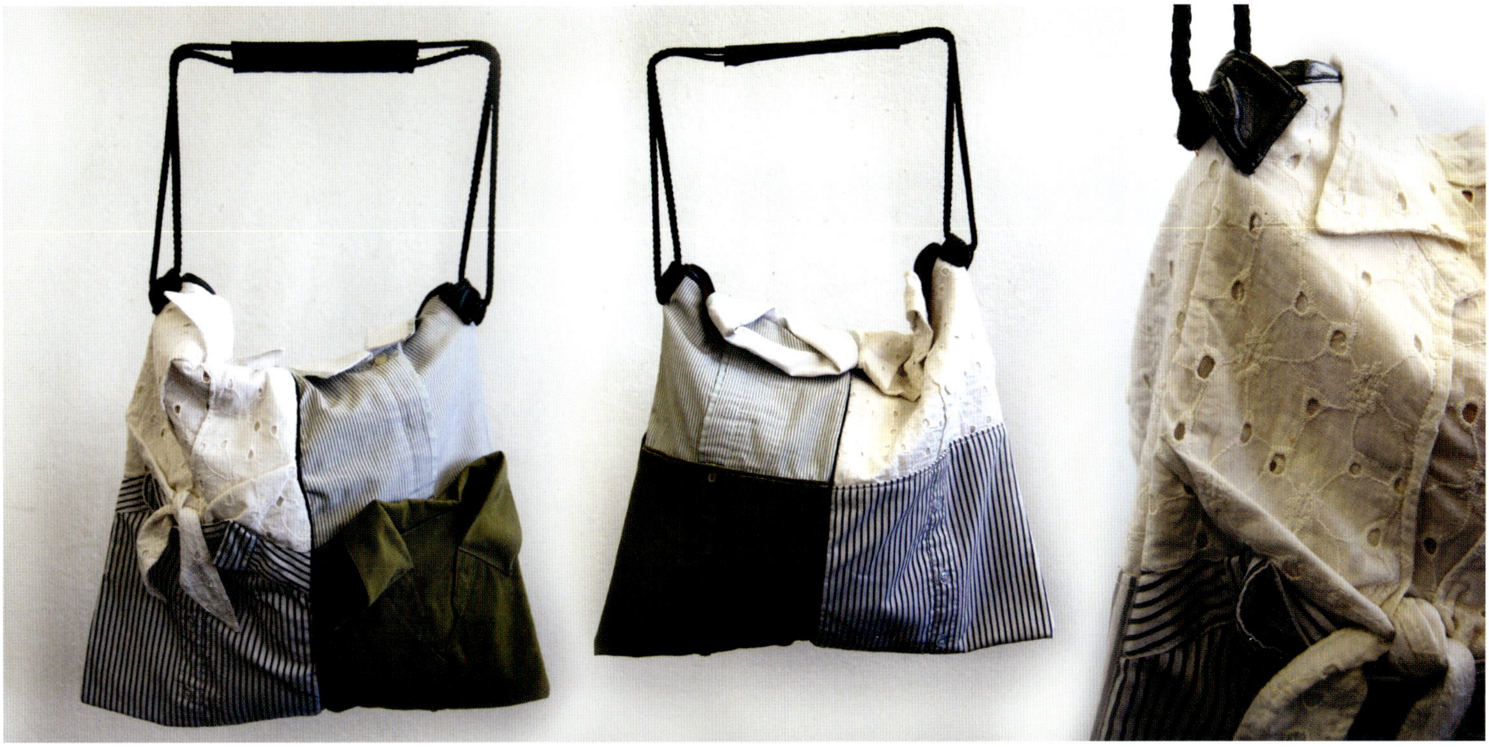

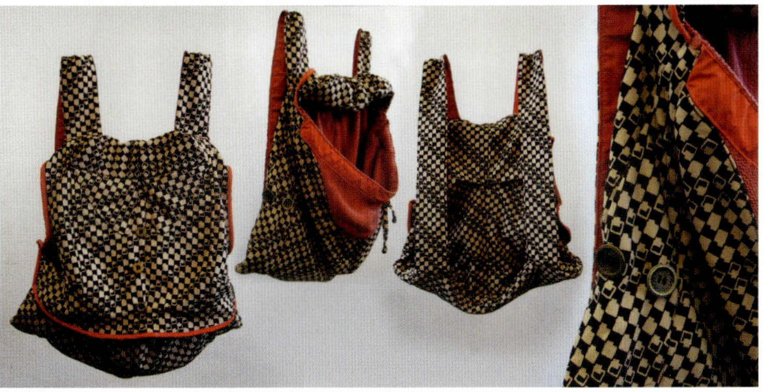

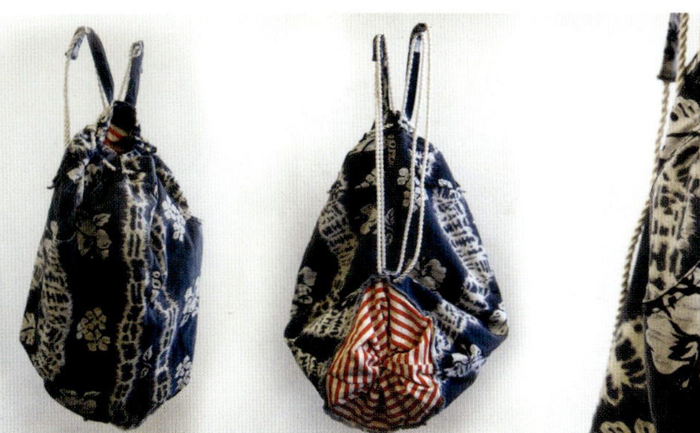

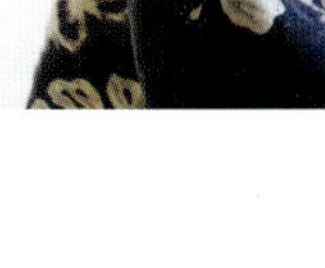

UNTITLED BAG
DE: Agnes Varnai

The "Untitled" bag is a series in which each piece is unique in the material
they are created from, ranging from designer's childhood clothes to items
found on the street. The bags are not subject to any trend, but bestowed
with their own character as well as great functionality and comfort.

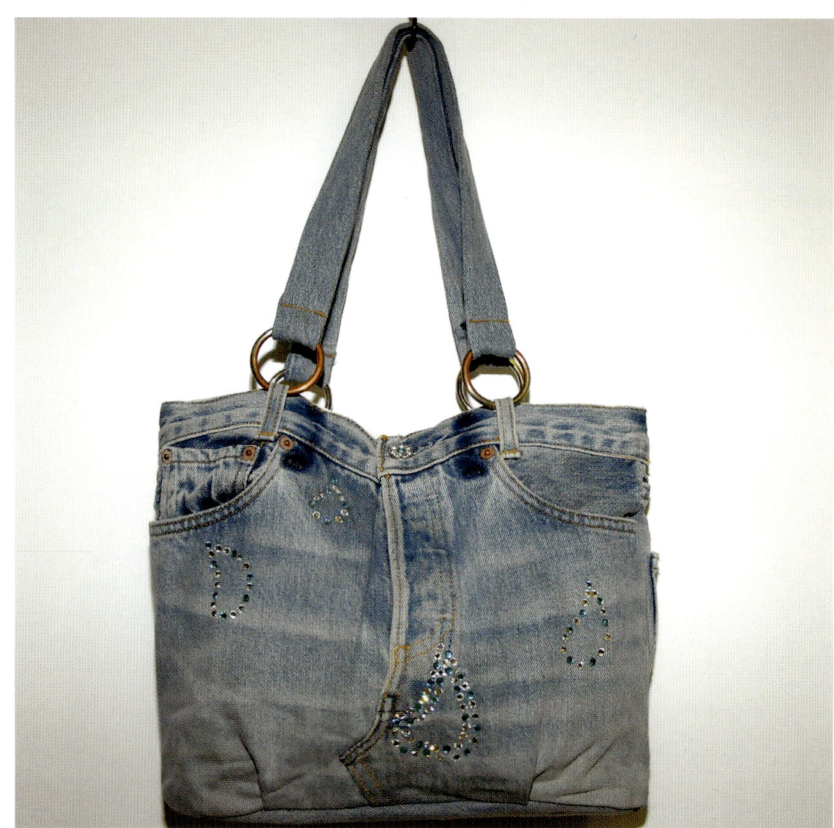

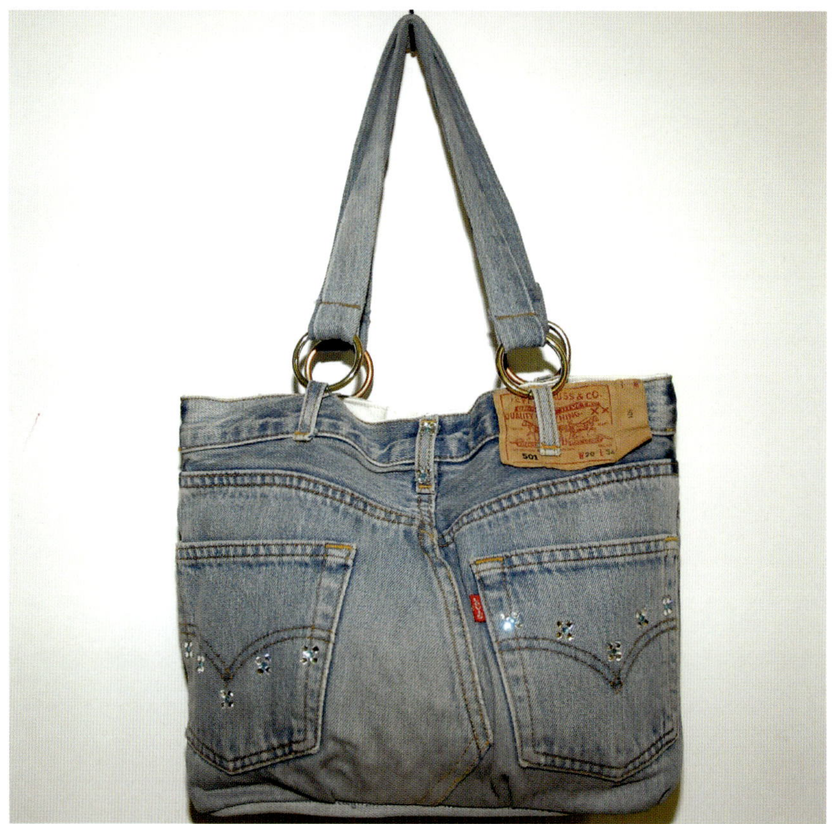

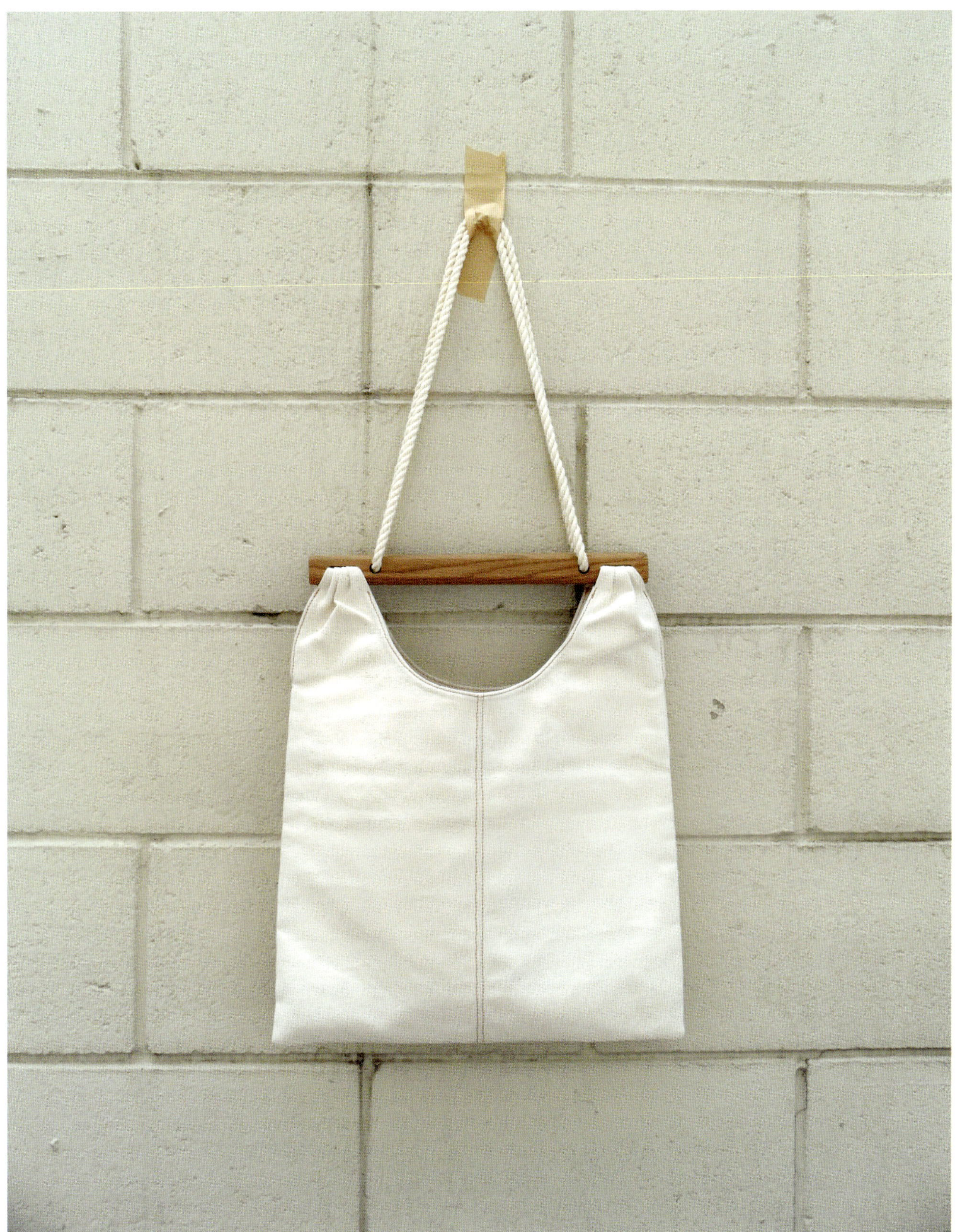

JEAN BAG

DE: Liat Avshalomi

This bag was transformed from a pair of jeans, with the original back pockets retaining their functionality, and the lining recreated with different fabric and inside pockets.

TWO WAY BAG

DA: Way Down Deep

The "Two Way Bag" was intended to ignite a spark with two differing materials, so it used canvas with a wooden handle. It can be carried as a shoulder bag or a cross-body bag.

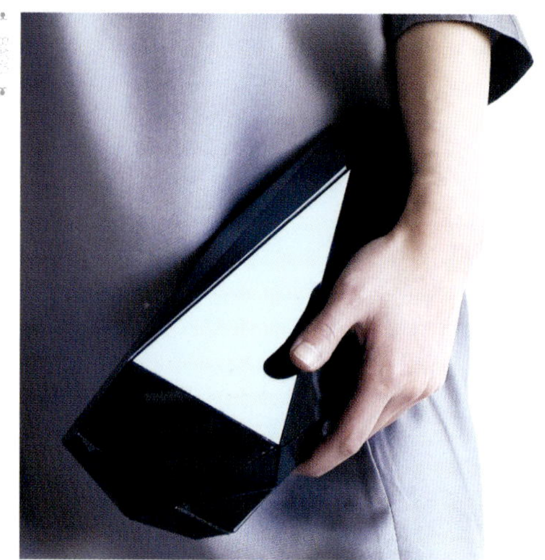
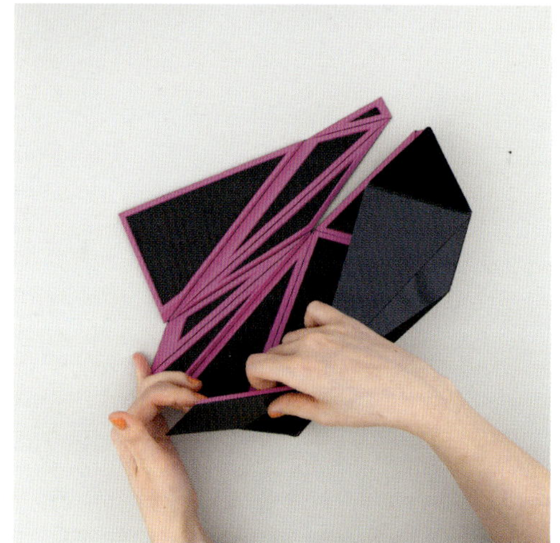
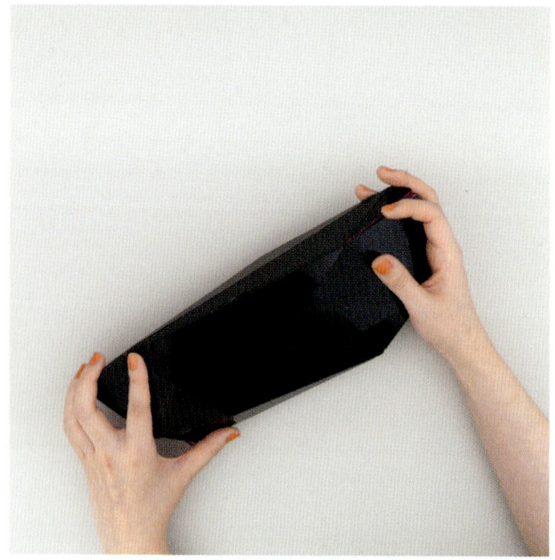
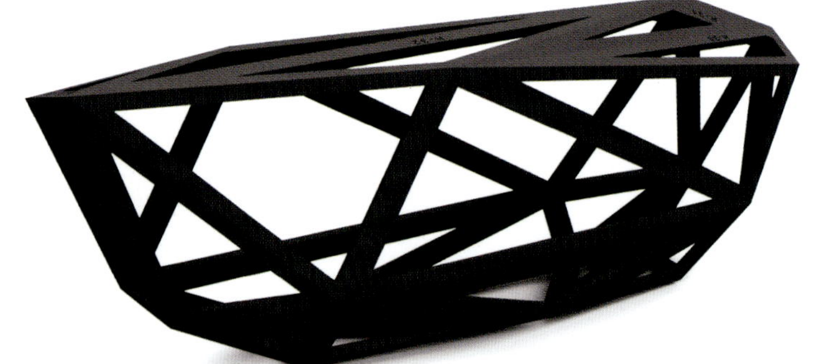
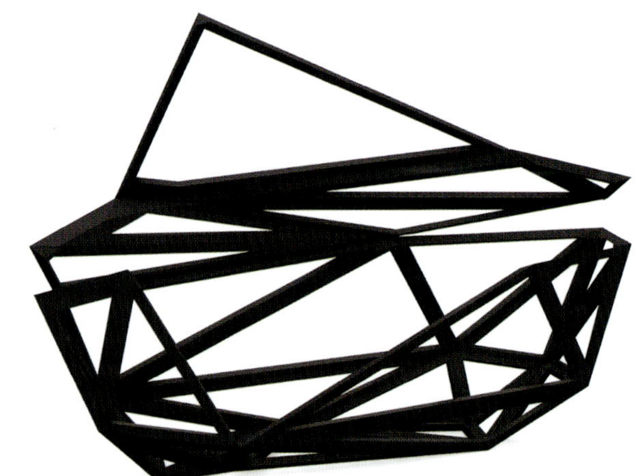
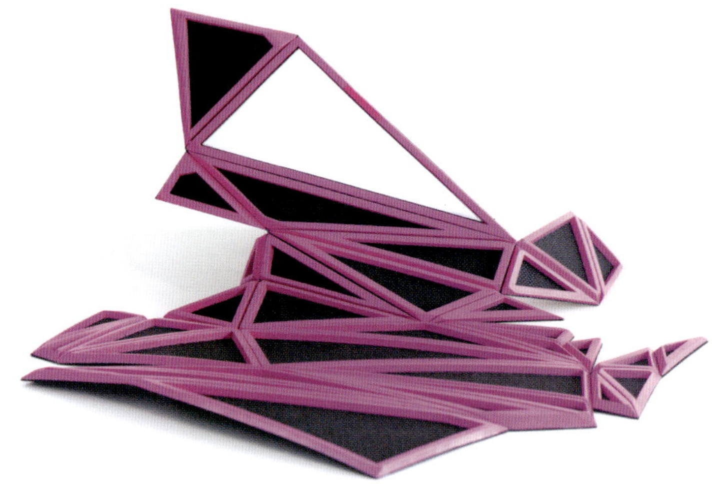

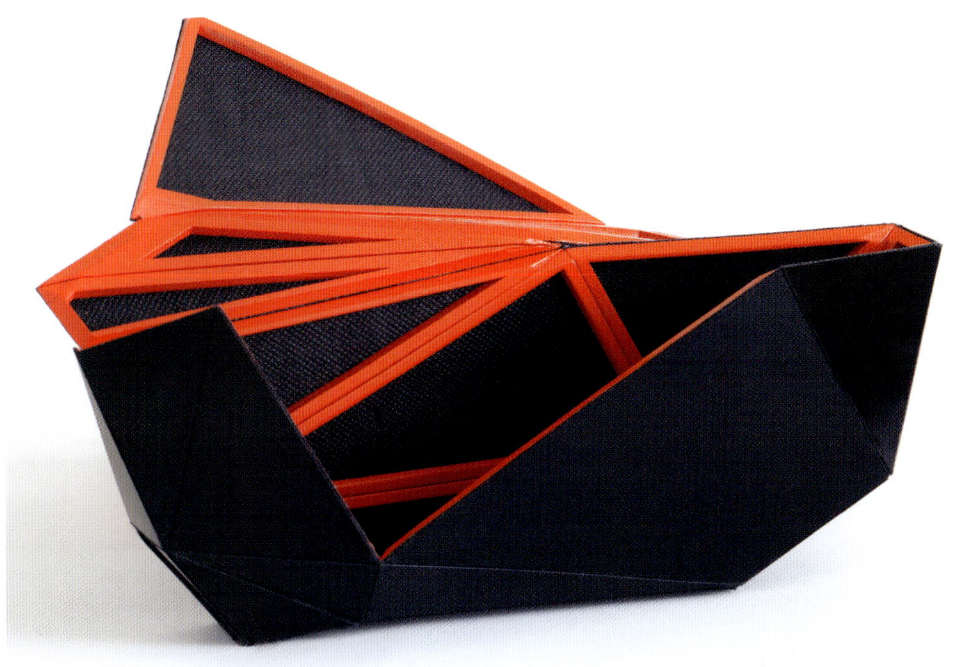

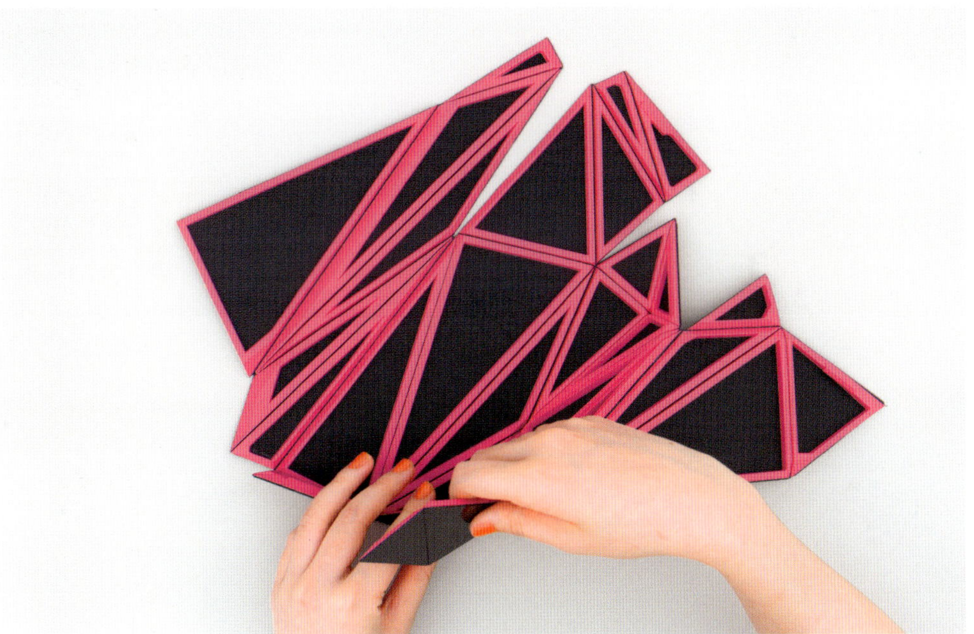

ORISHIKI
DE: Naoki Kawamoto

'Orishiki" is an idiosyncratic carrying device composed of triangular segments in different shapes and sizes. It can be folded like origami and wrap thing like "furoshiki" - a kind of traditional Japanese wrapping cloth.

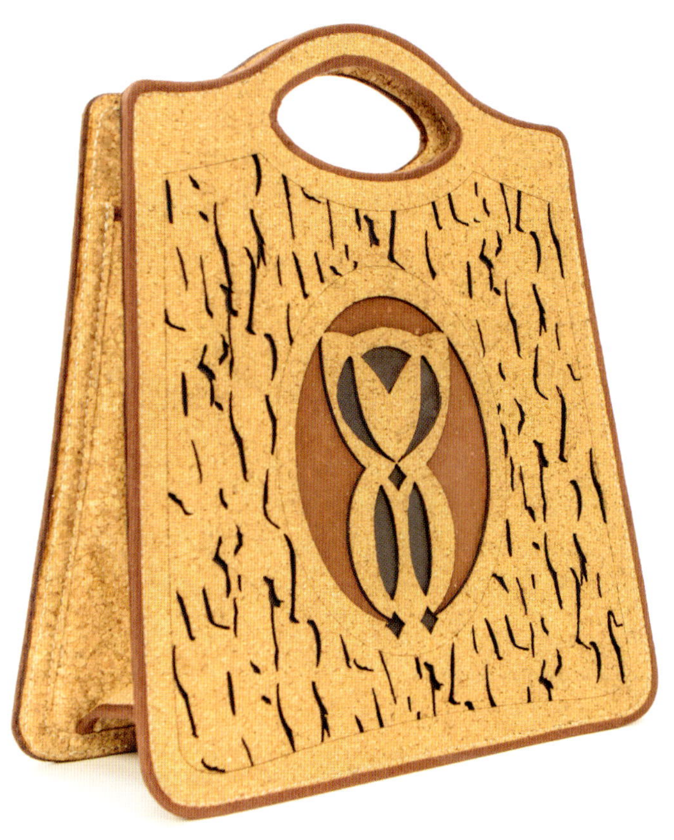

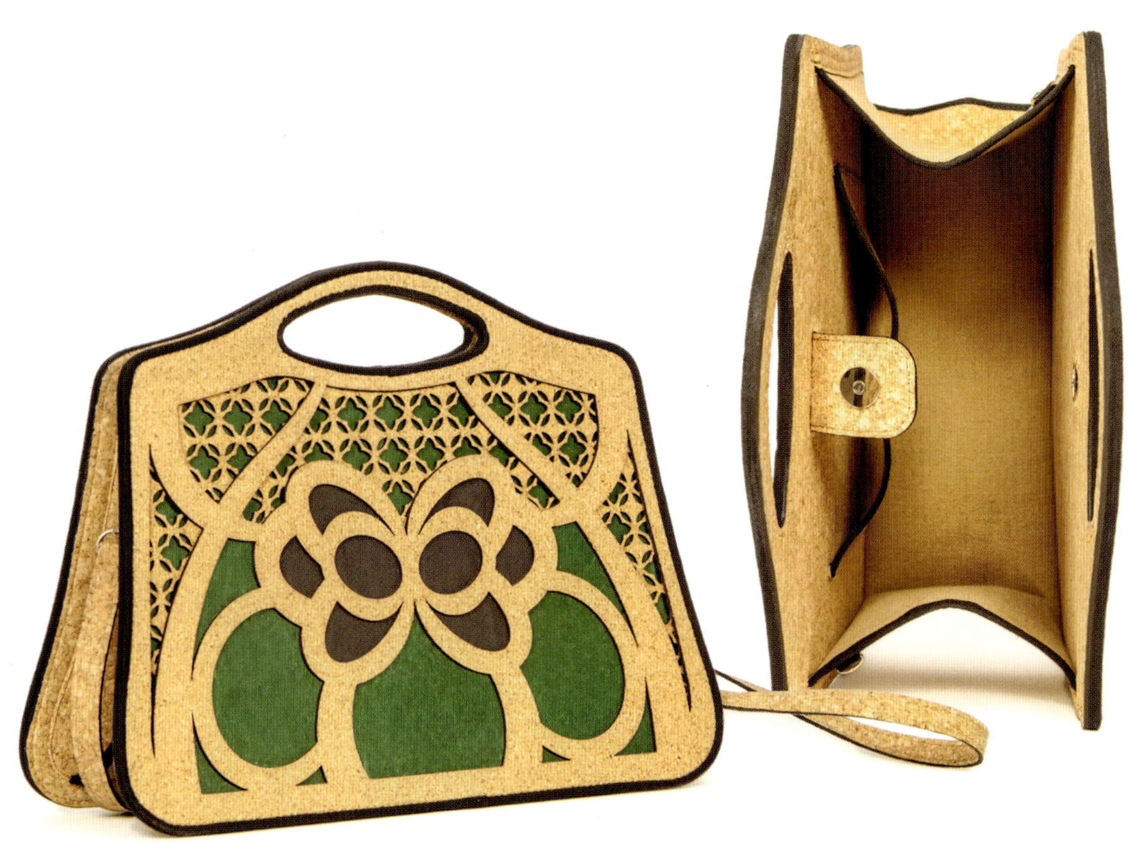

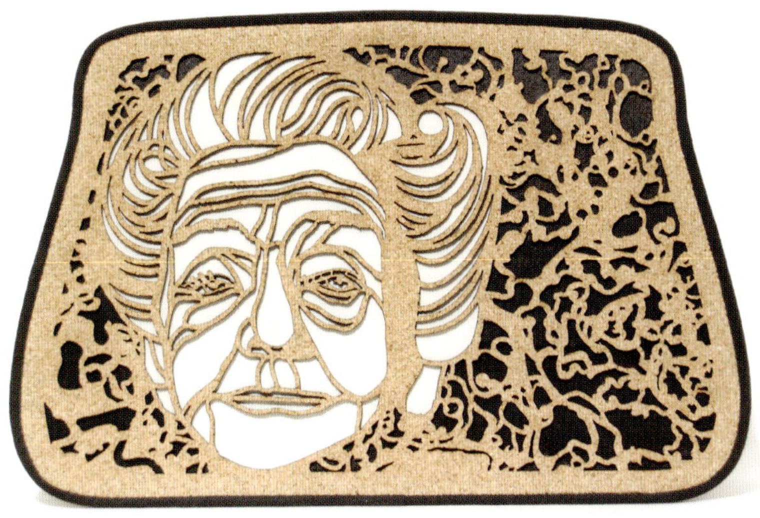

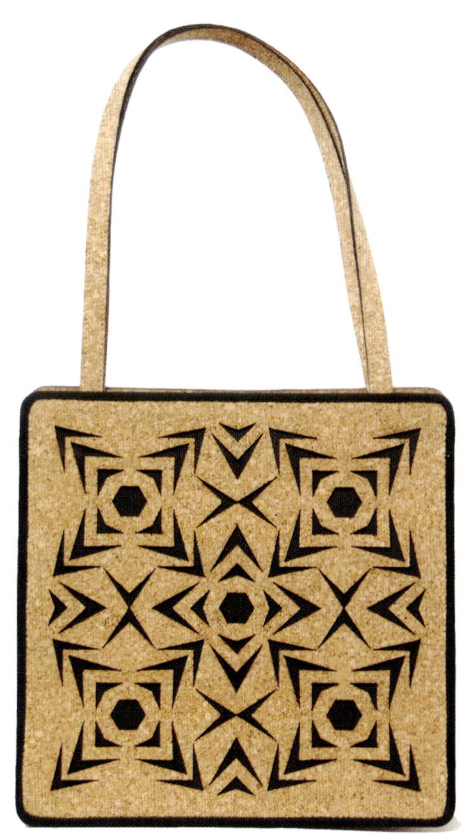

TRASFORMAZIONE EST-ETICA
DE: Silvia Massacesi

Made from natural cork and recycled cellulose fiber, this series features various patterns, whose presentation exploits the visual contrast created by these two materials. Illustrations on the bag was designed by Daniele Geniale.

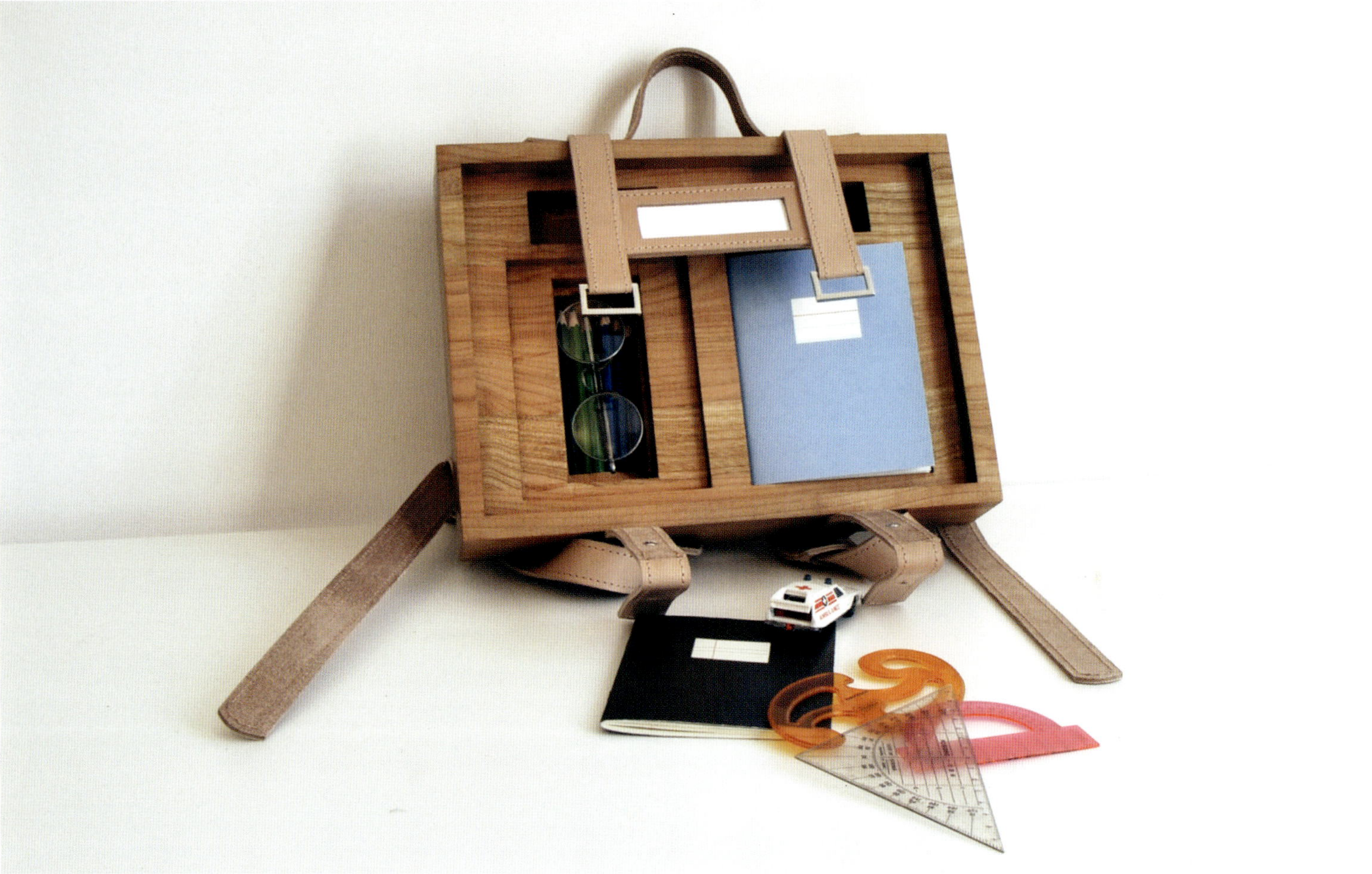

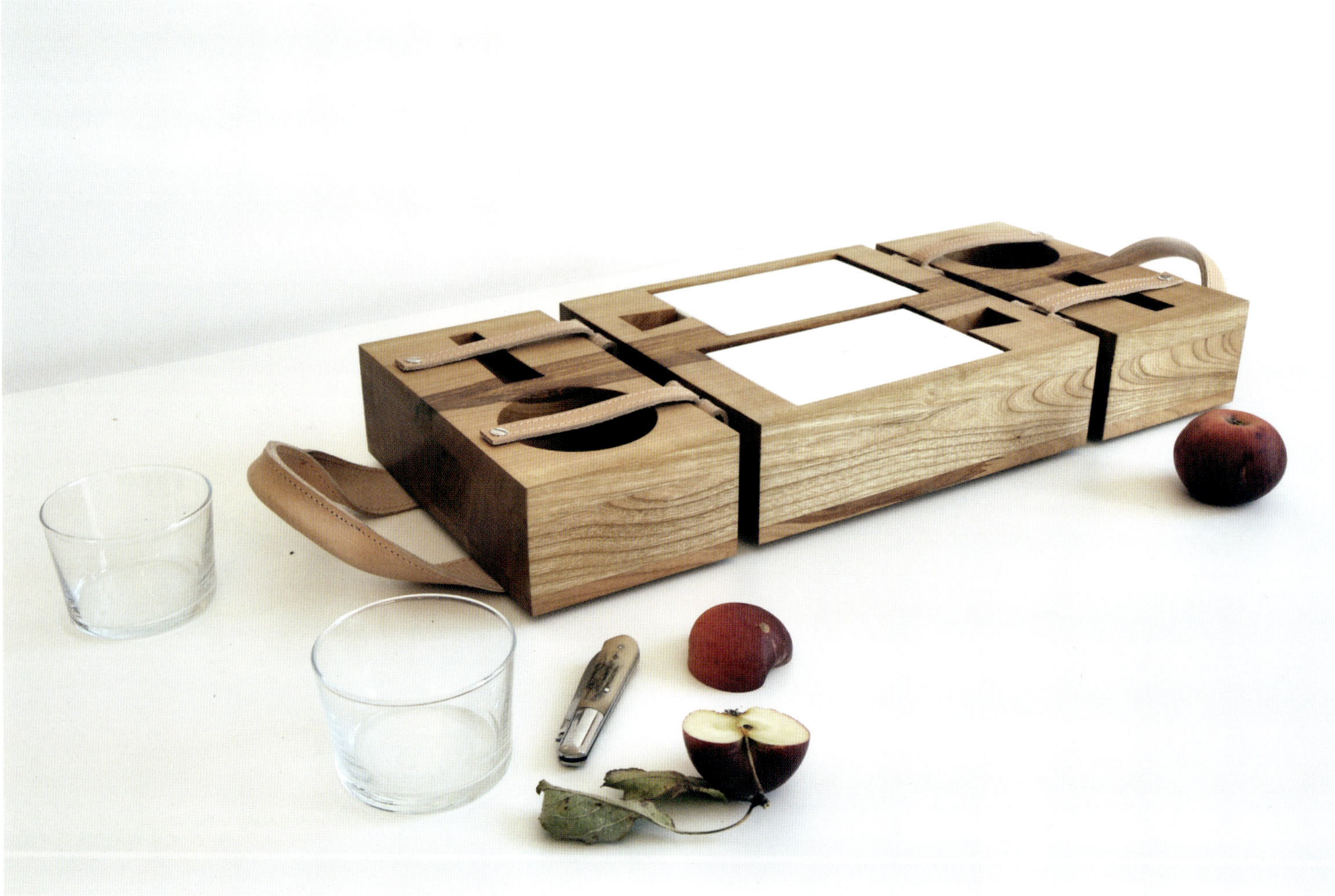

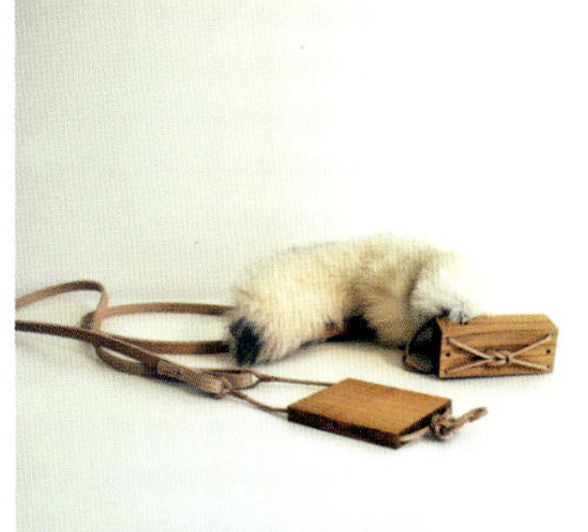

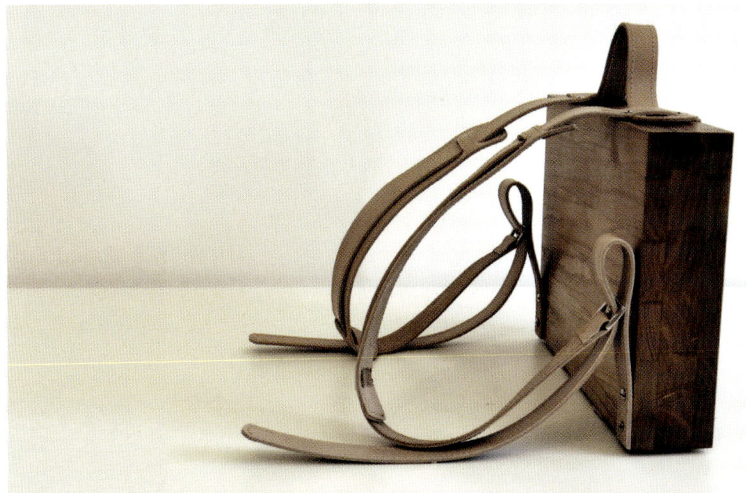

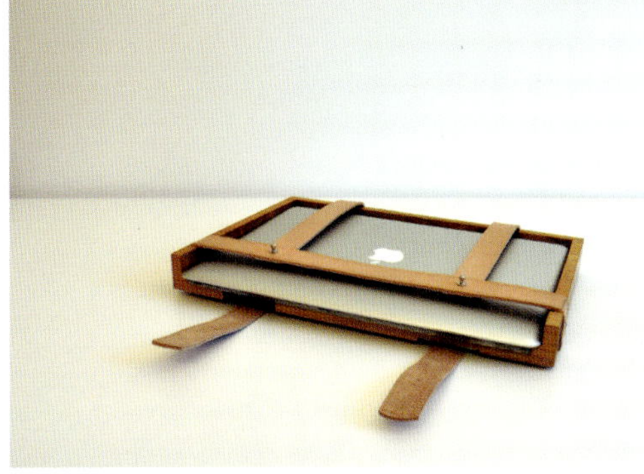

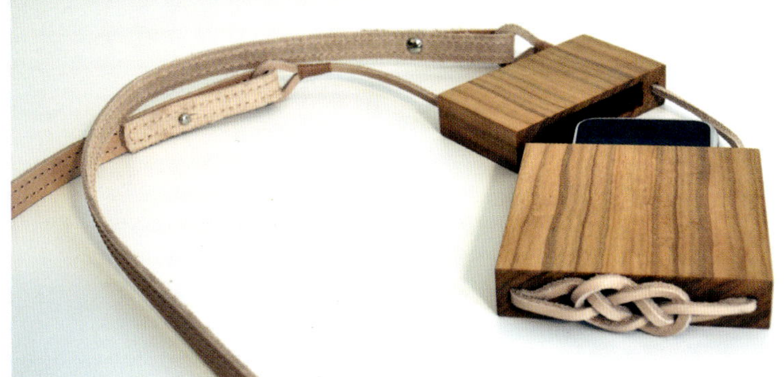

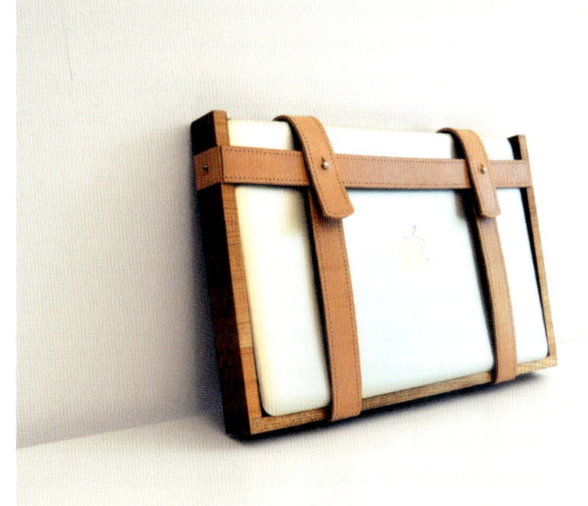

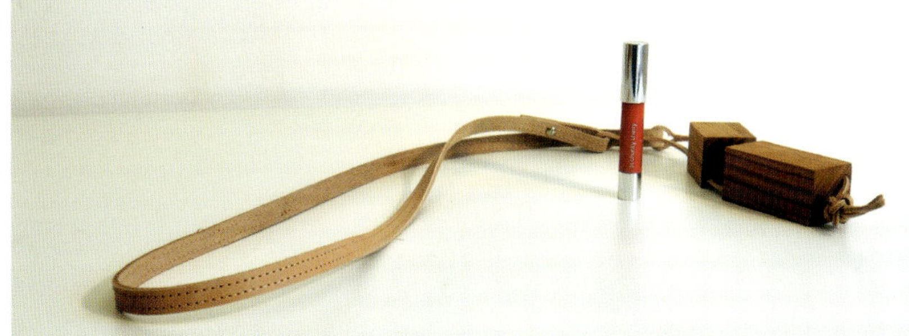

BOX COUTURE
DE: Dombon-a-tanya, theBetaVersion

"Box Couture" is an experimental concept mainly made of wood. It can be
easily assembled as integrated container or dissembled into parts to carry
objects in different sizes and shapes.

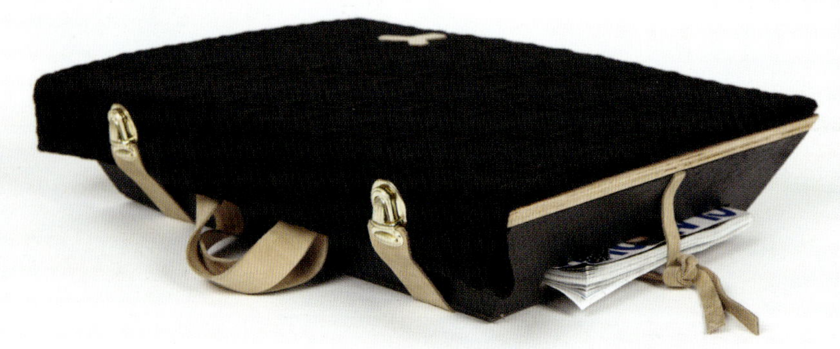

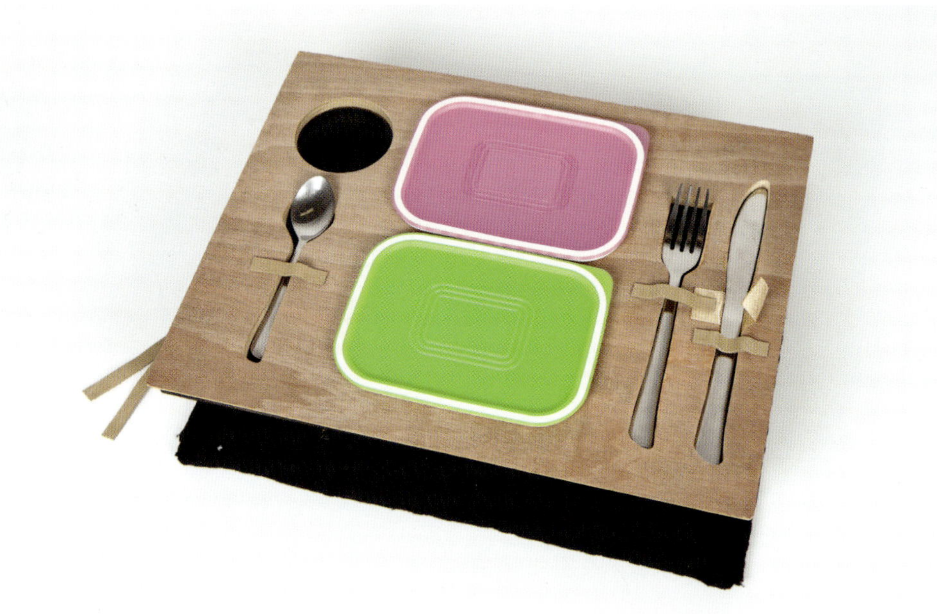

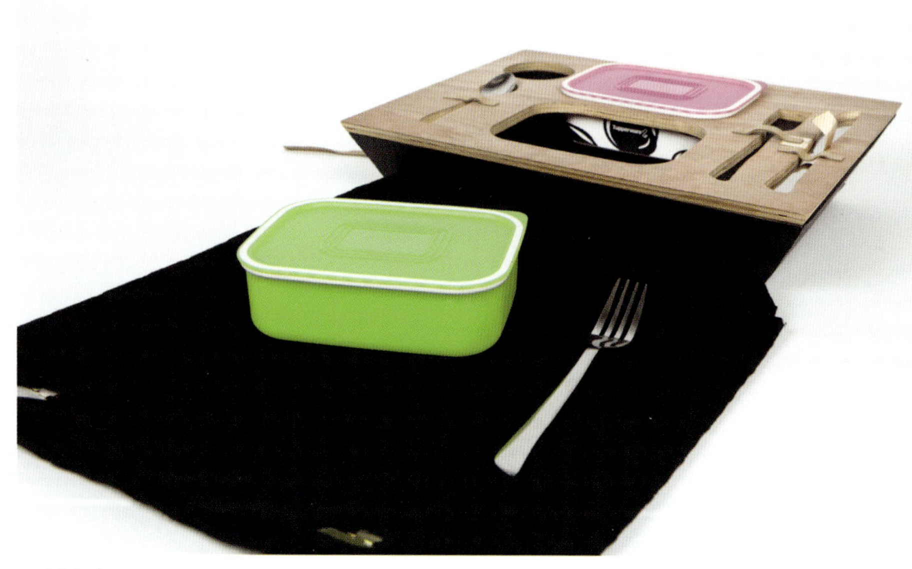

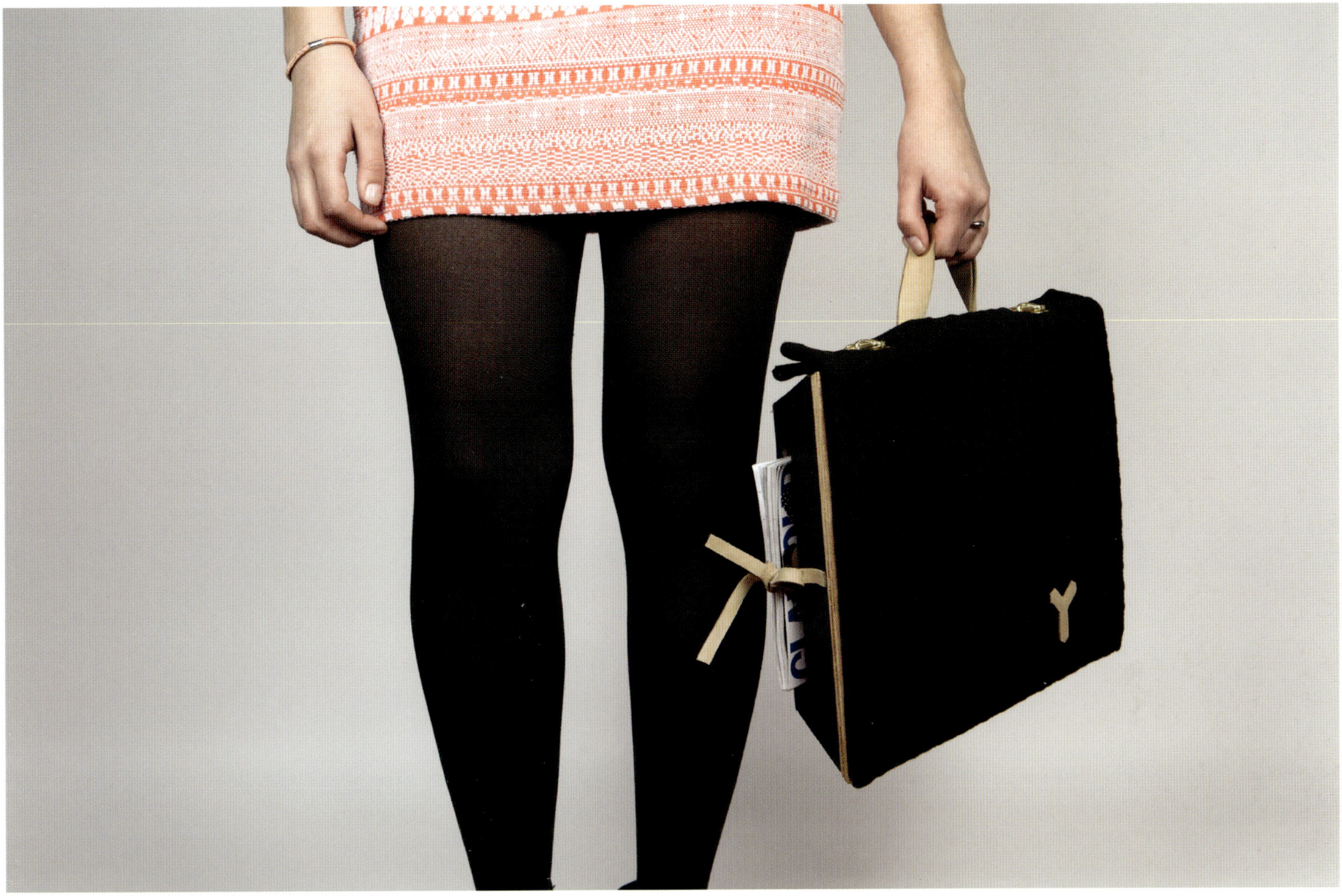

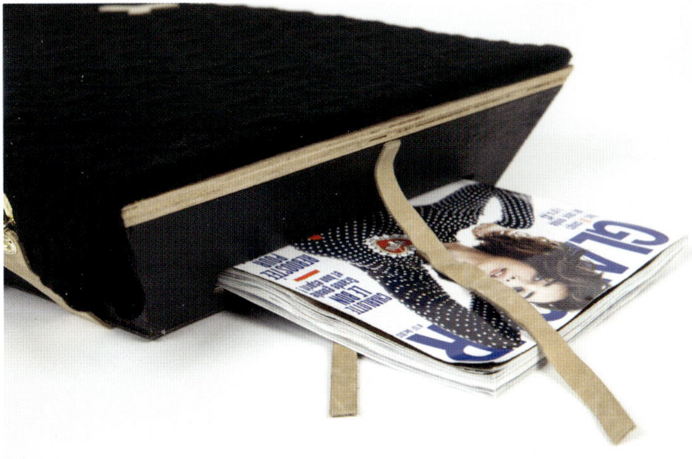

DESAYUNO

DE: Yona Cossard Guennoc

"Desayuno" includes a timber frame for lunch essentials that enables users to carry their lunch. When unfolded, it works as a tray for dining or the cover can be used as a tablecloth. There is even a slot for a magazine.

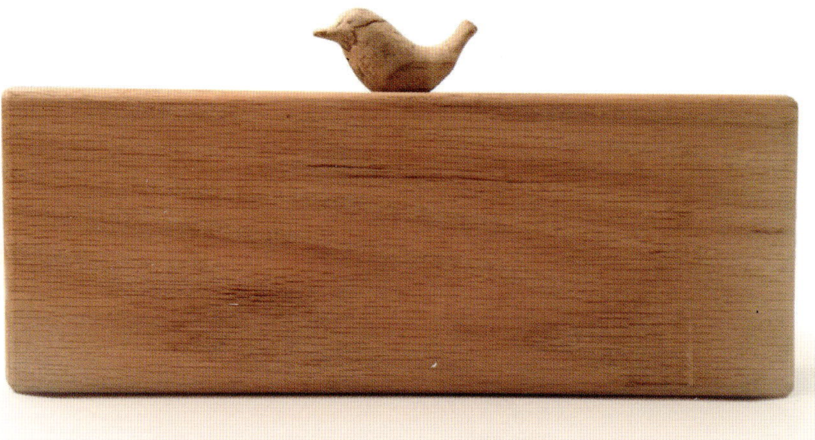
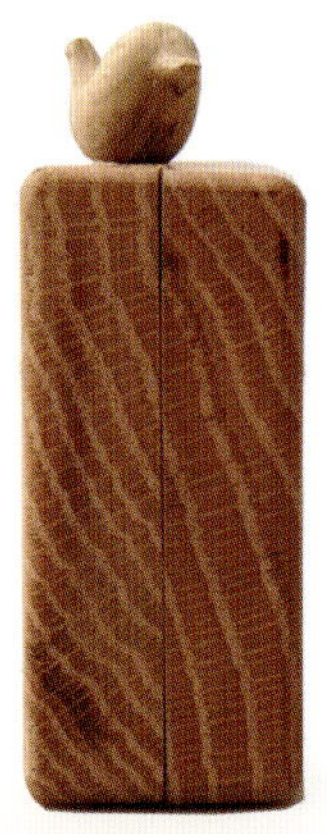

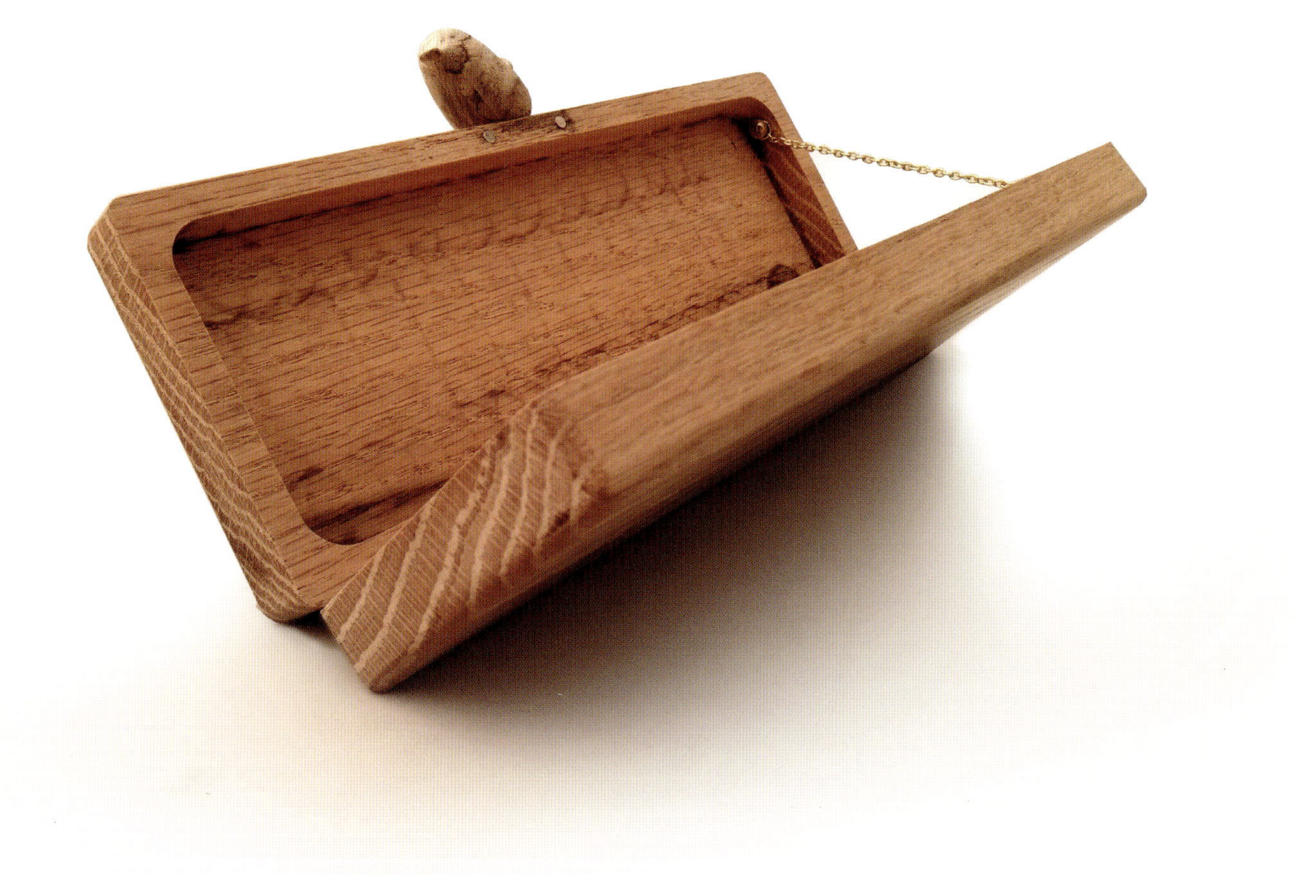

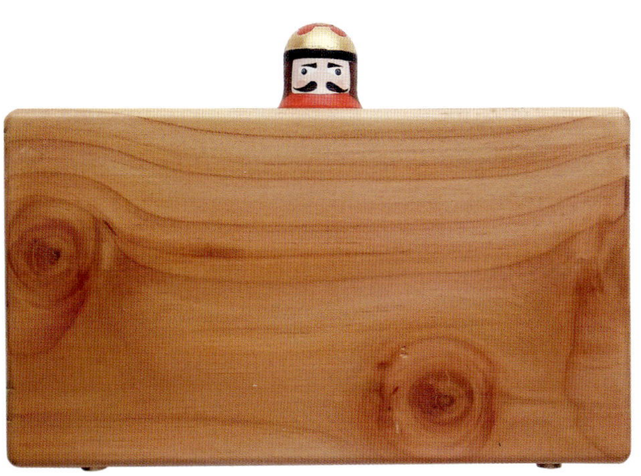

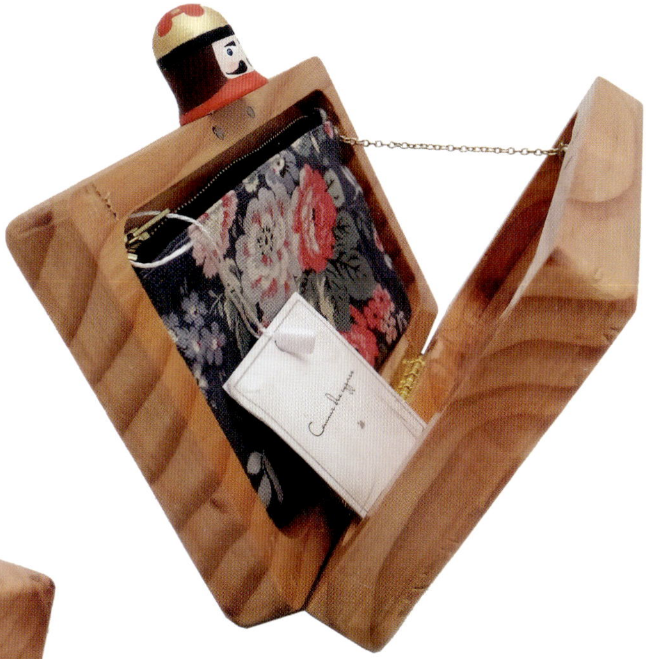

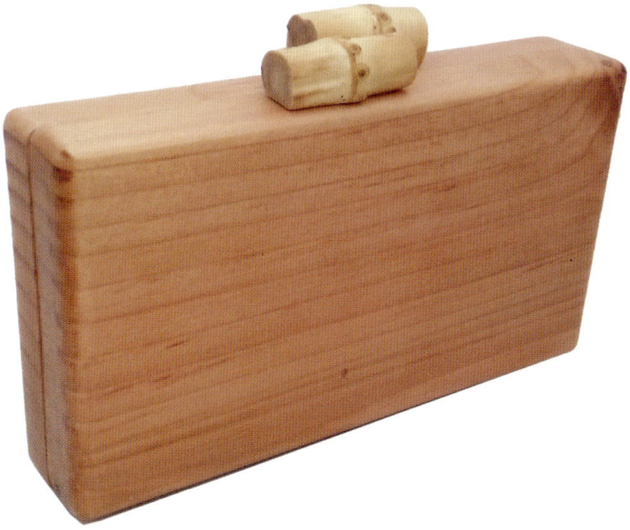

WOODEN BAGS
DA: Comme Des Cygnes

This wooden bag series is adorned with varied wooden dolls that act as the open/close mechanism, with a chain to better control the bag's width when open.

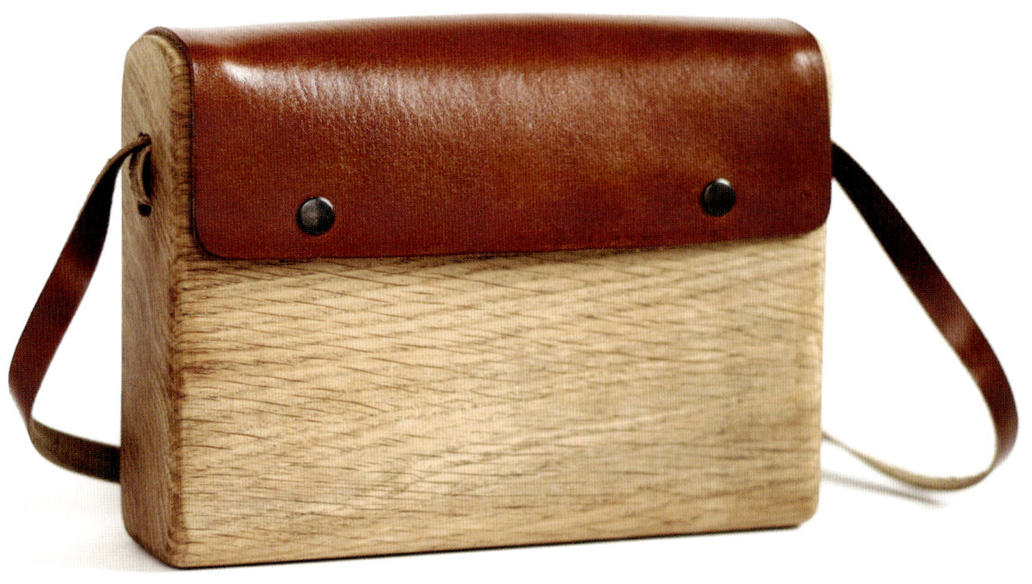
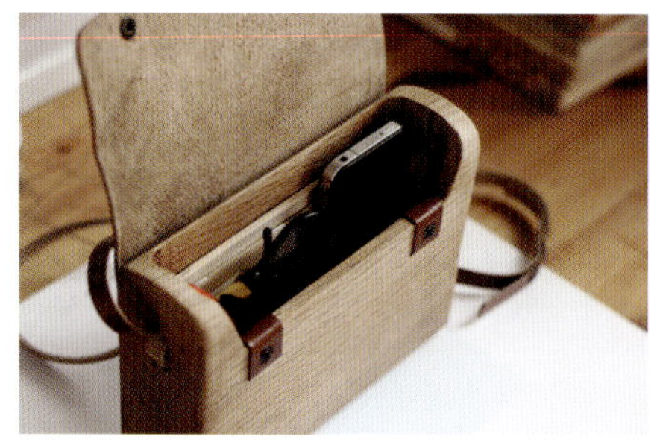
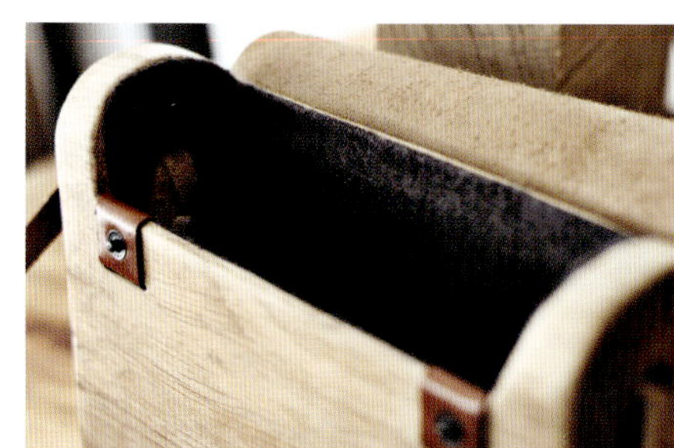

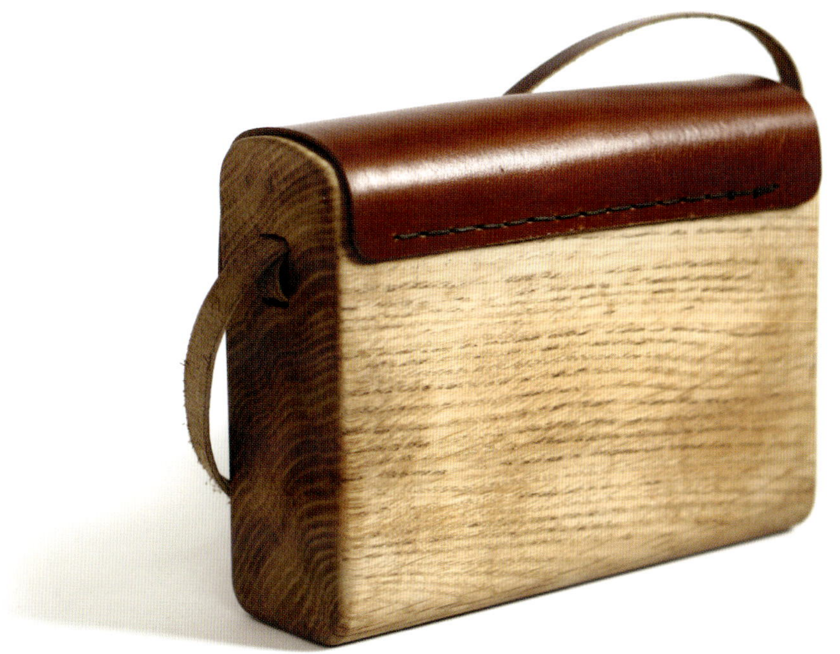

OAK BAG
DA: Haydanhuya

Handmade using one piece of oak wood, the bag has a lid made of vegetable
tanned leather. Each bag is carved with a unique ID on the backside.

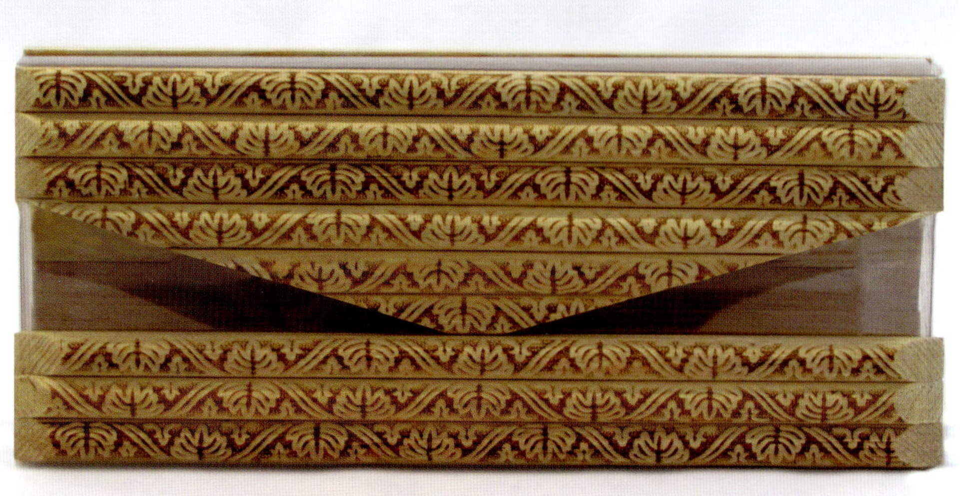

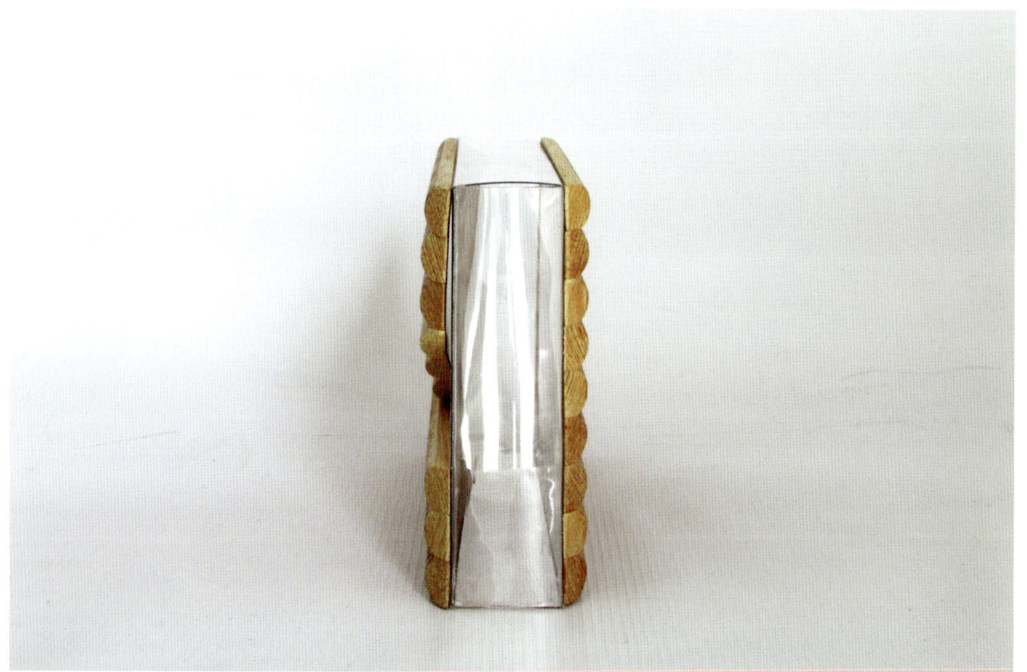

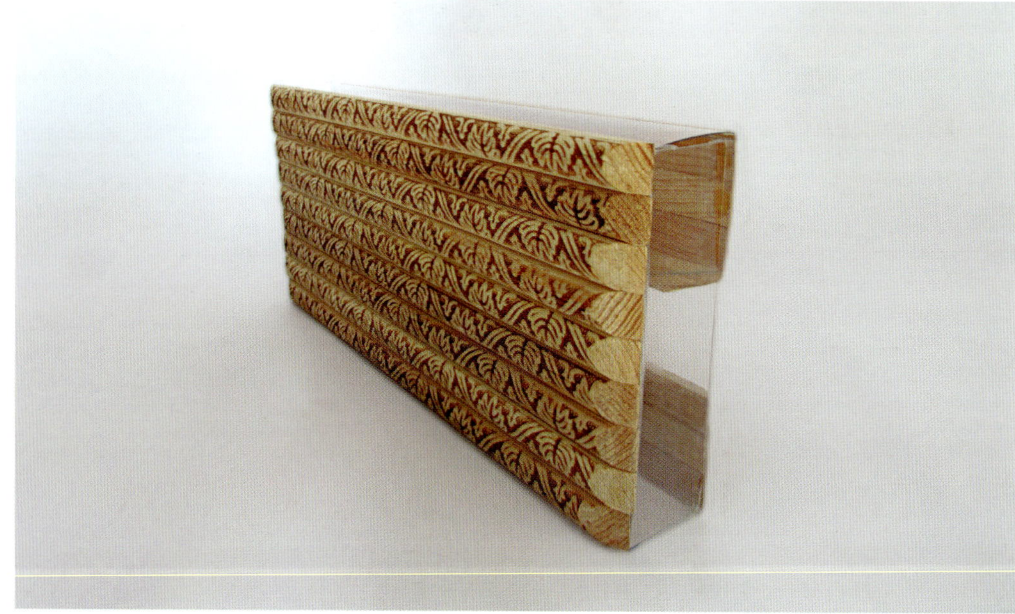

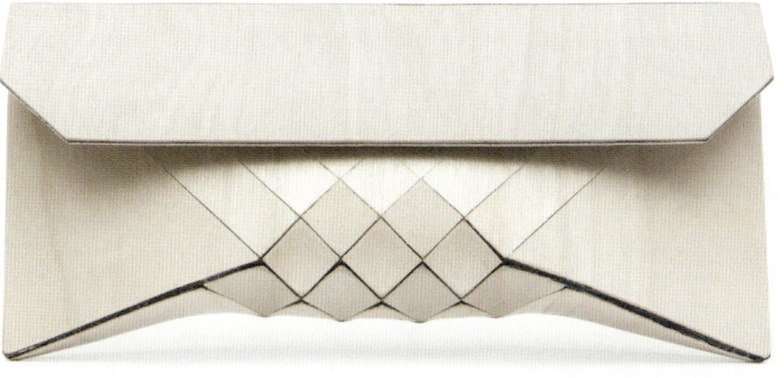

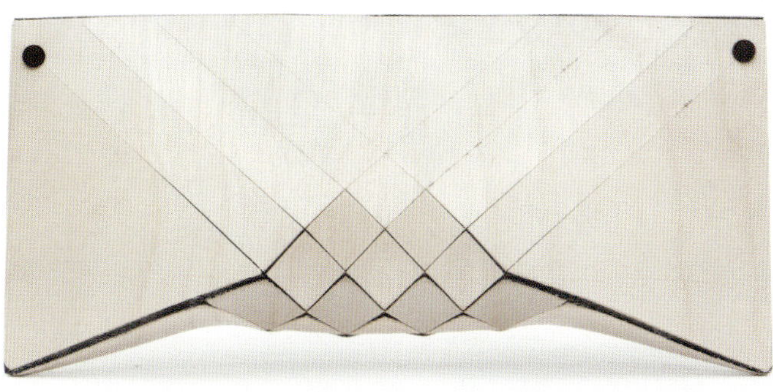

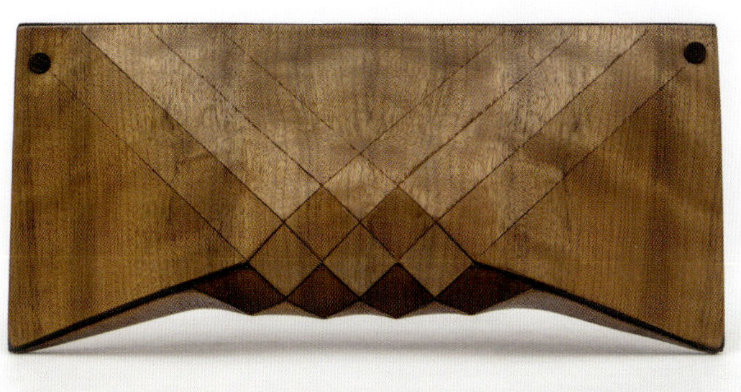

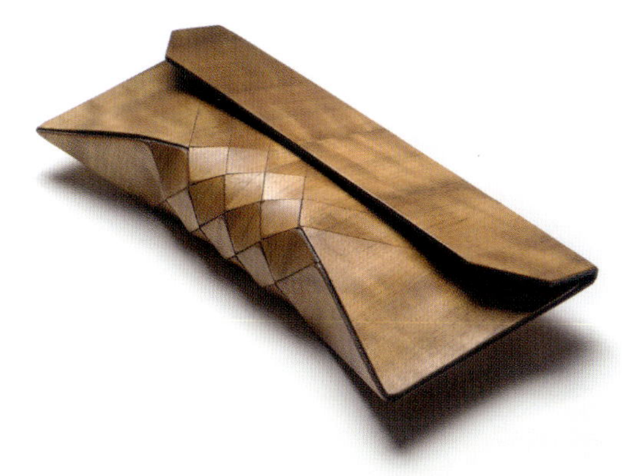

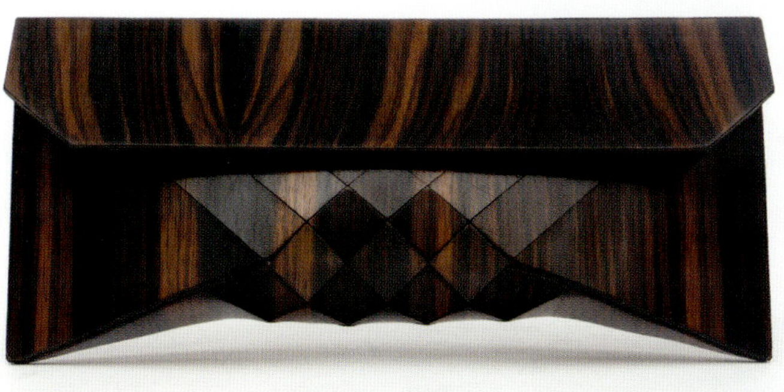

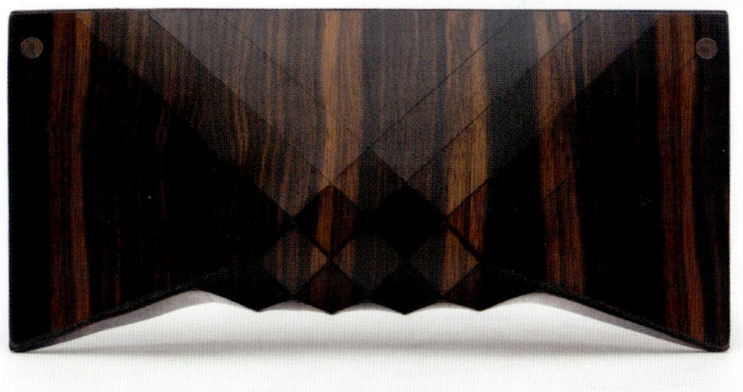

WOODEN TRANSPARENT CLUTCH
DE: Mónica Villarreal

Using plastic and wood, the designer tried to create a comparison between the modern (plastic) and the antique (wood). The opaque surface shows the beautiful cutting and engraving on the wood.

WEARABLE WOOD CLUTCHES
DE: Tesler Mendelovitch

This series originated from experimentation on making hard material soft and vice versa. Turning a wooden surface into a soft textile, the designer created a bag with geometrical underbelly for a comfortable grip. All the wood pieces were chosen to individualize each model.

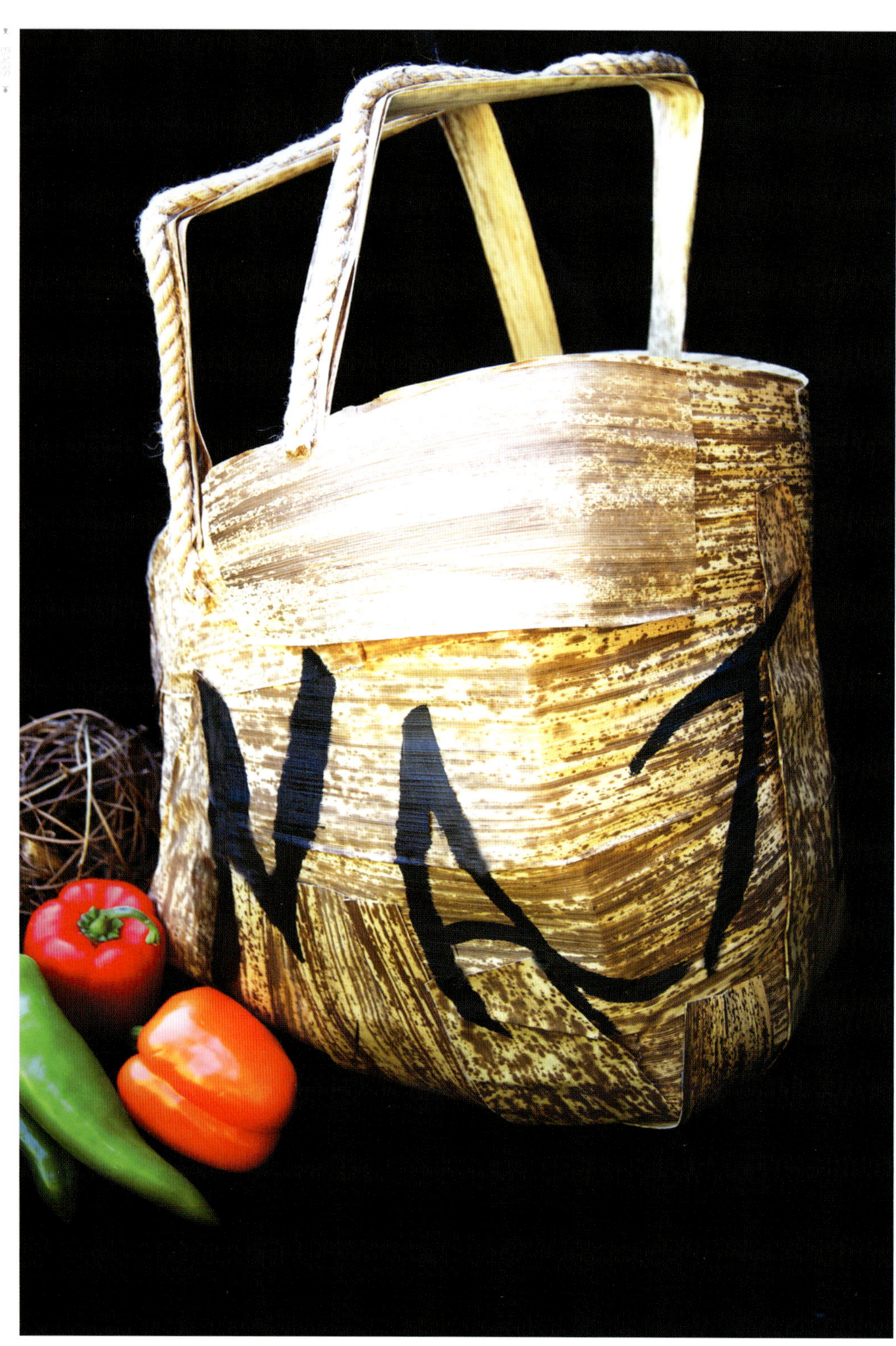

BAGS

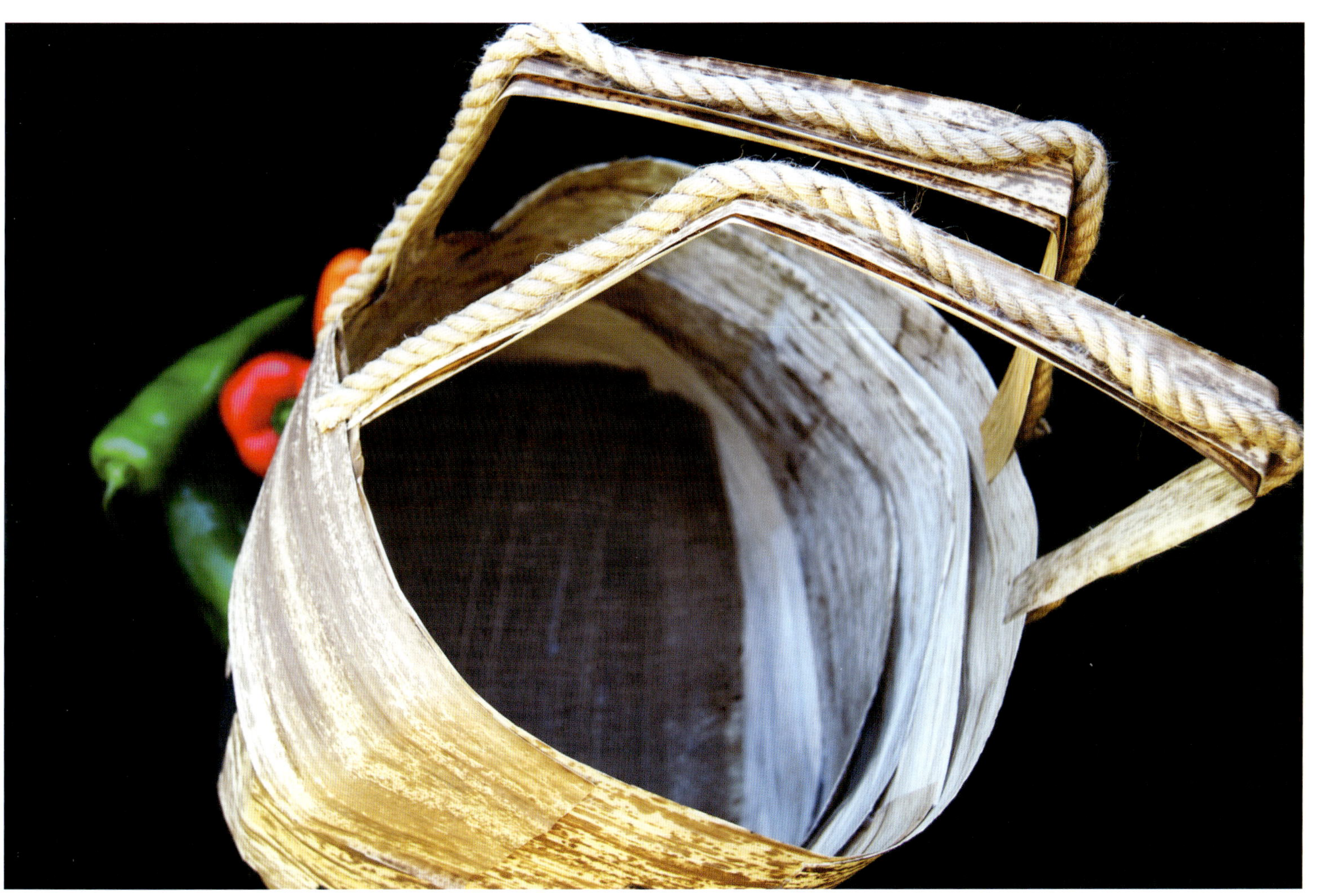

NATURL

DE: Somia Saadat

The "Naturl" shopping bag was made of materials obtained from nature, like
dried bamboo leaves, rope, and burlap.

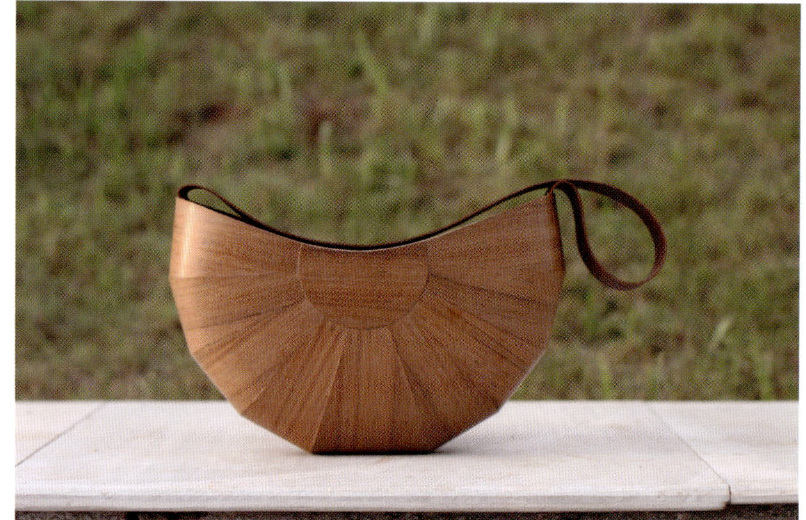

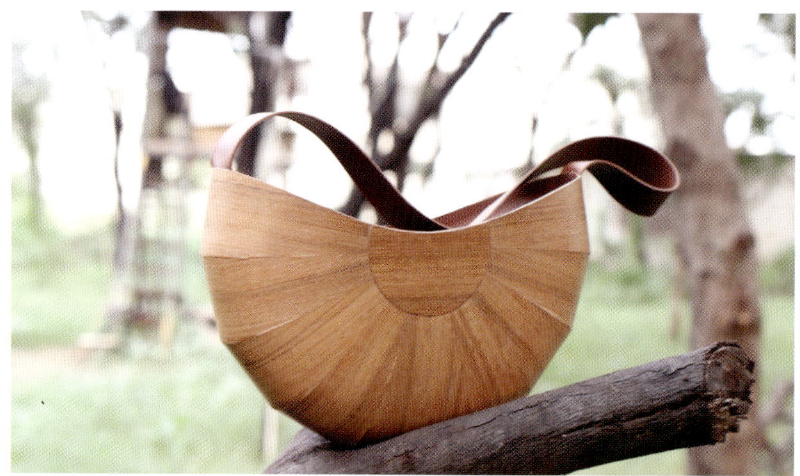

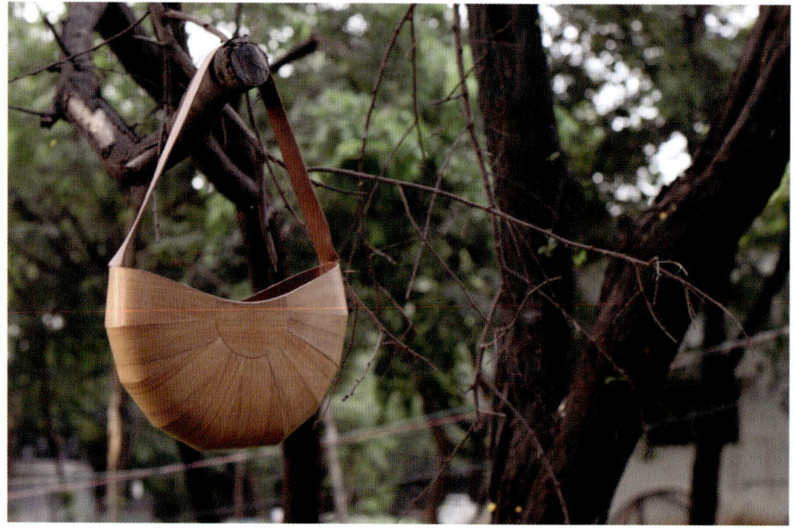

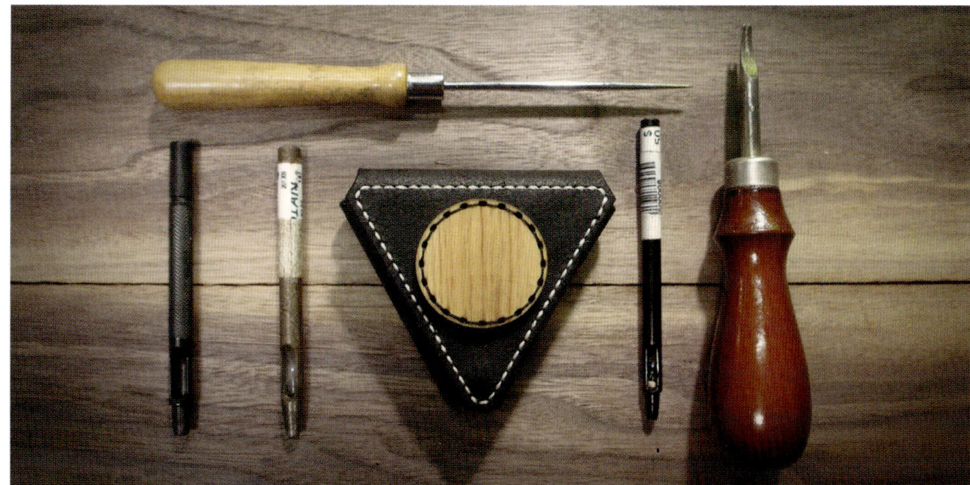

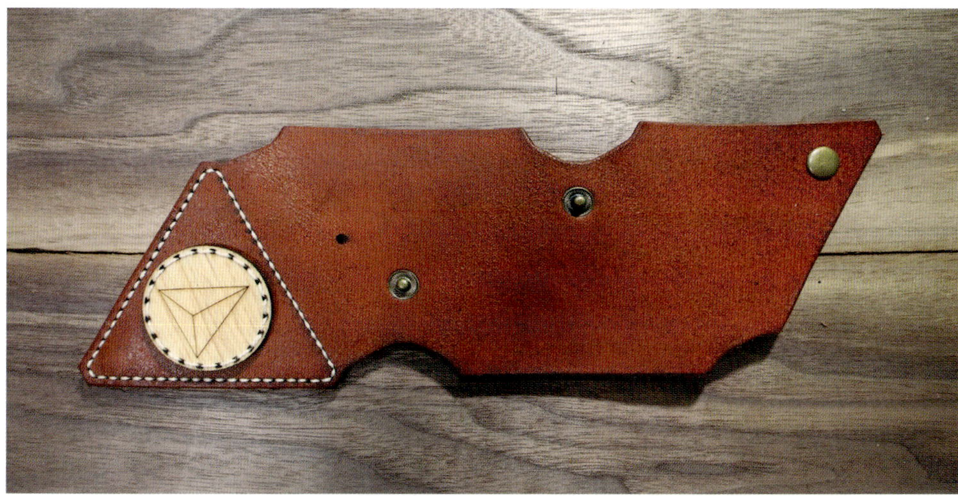

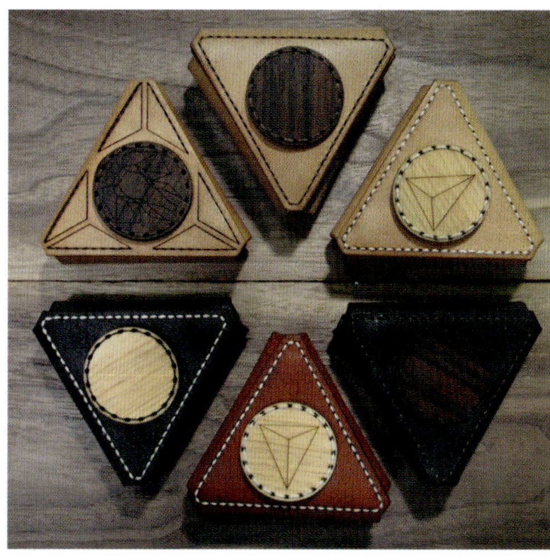

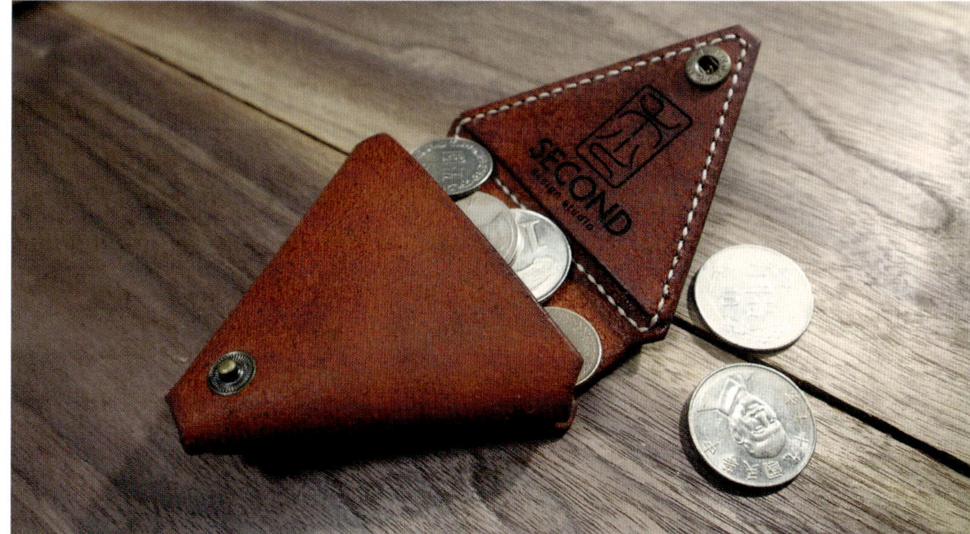

LE VENETTE
DE: Archana Ishwar Patil

Created using strips of teakwood wasted during furniture production, Le
Venette used heat bending to obtain the unique shape, and the patterns were
digitally designed, then dry pasted on the surface.

TRIANGLE
DA: Parsec

The "Triangle" was made of two materials with "warmth" – scented wood and
cowhide. Laser cut with patterns and utilizing heavy stitching in addition
to the traditional button, the design is a sturdy and nostalgic.

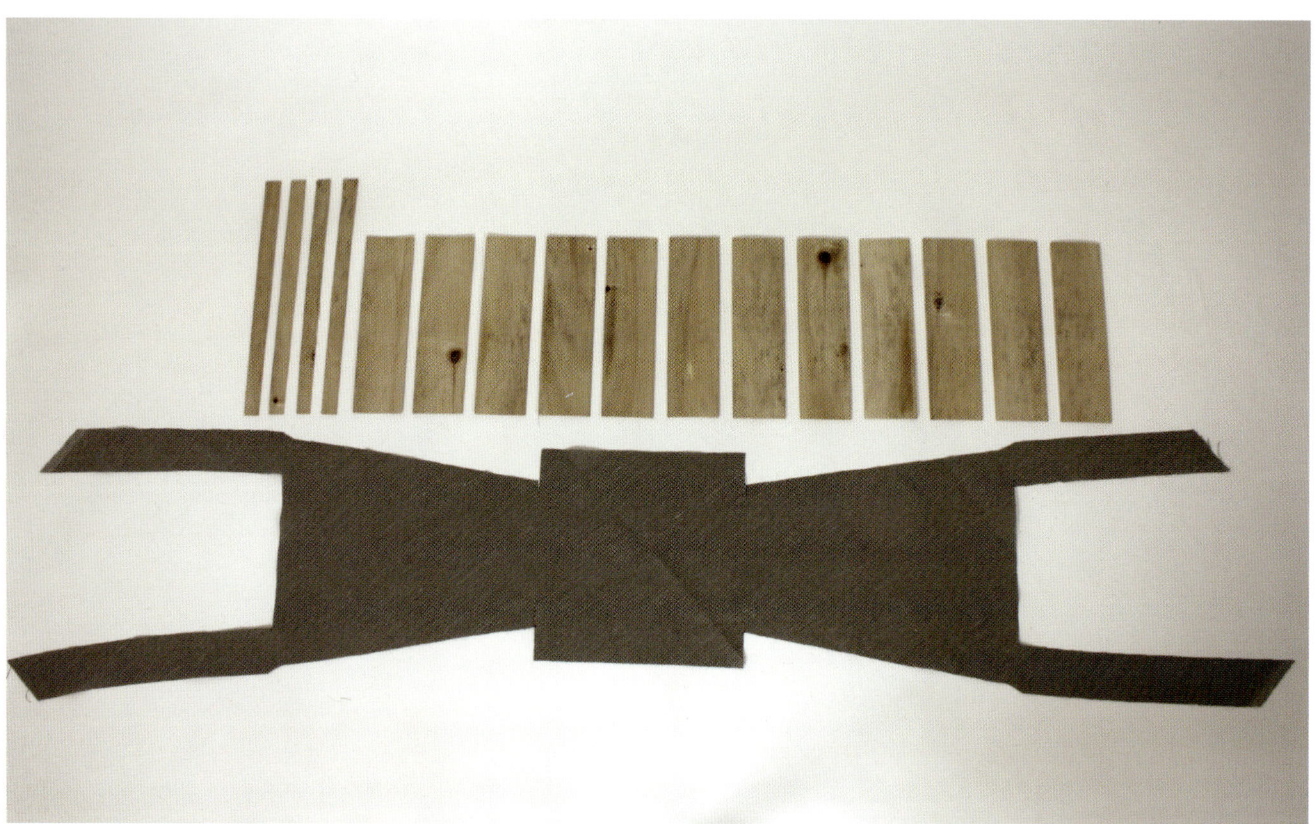

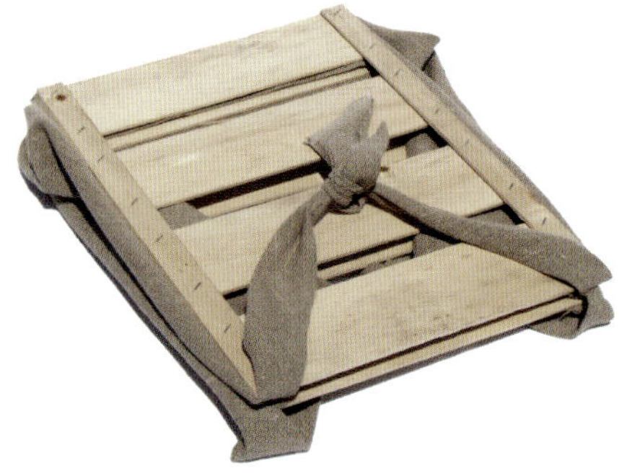

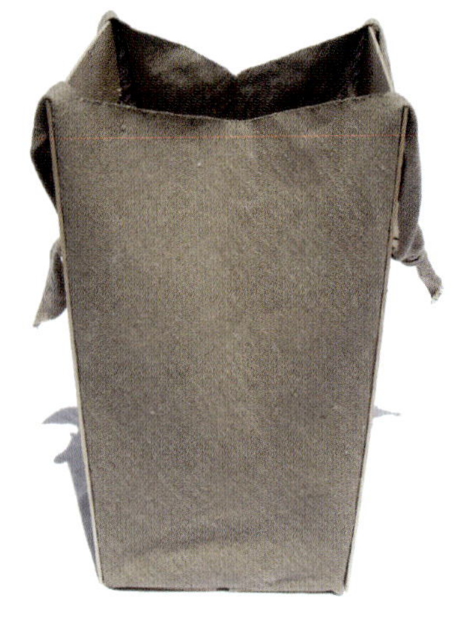

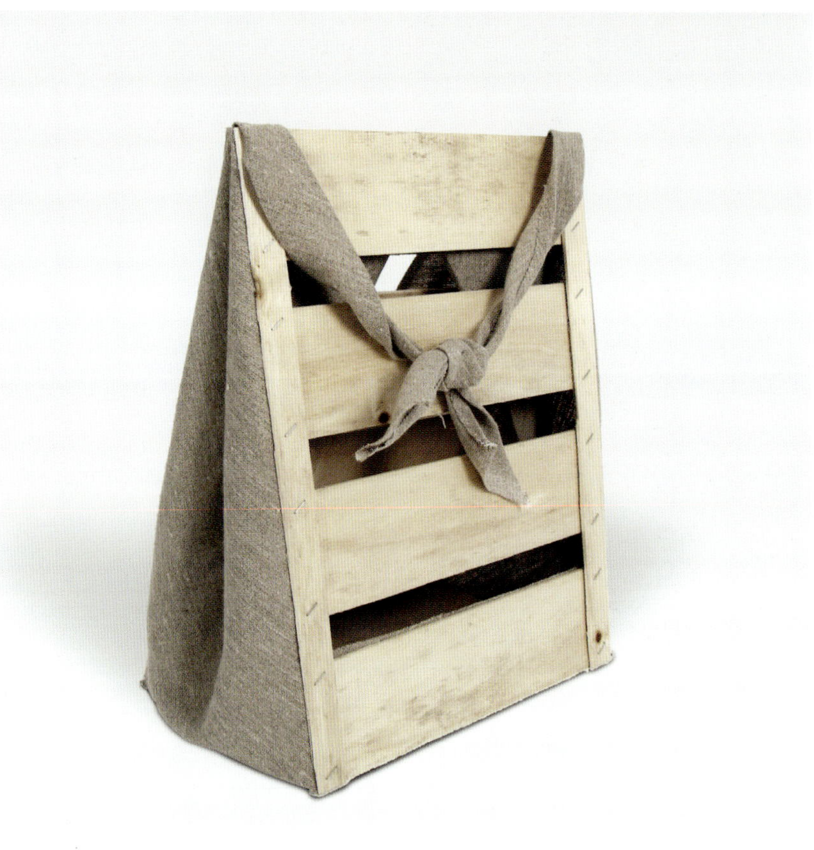

ECOBAG

DE: Arthur Kenzo, Francois DMD

Using a traditional lightwood crate and linen fiber, the design is ecological and easy to produce.

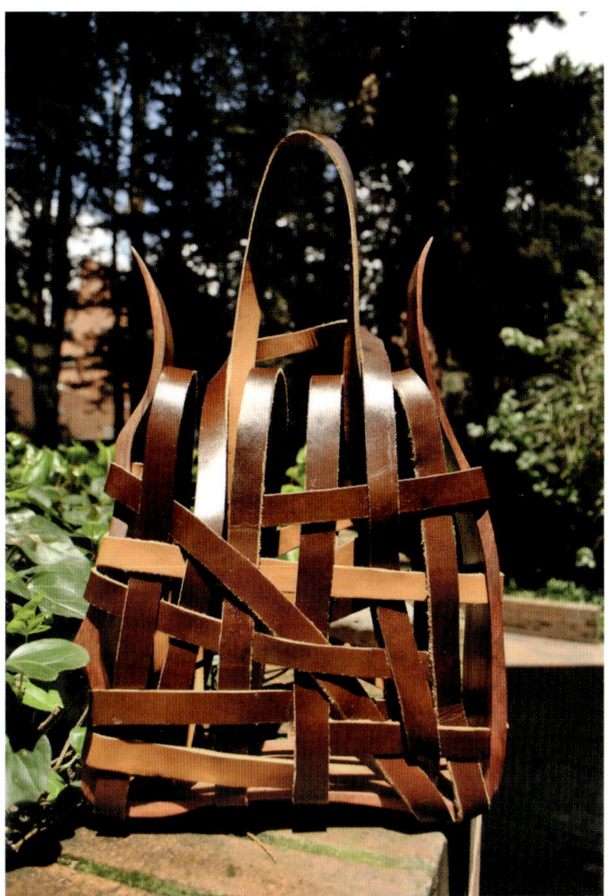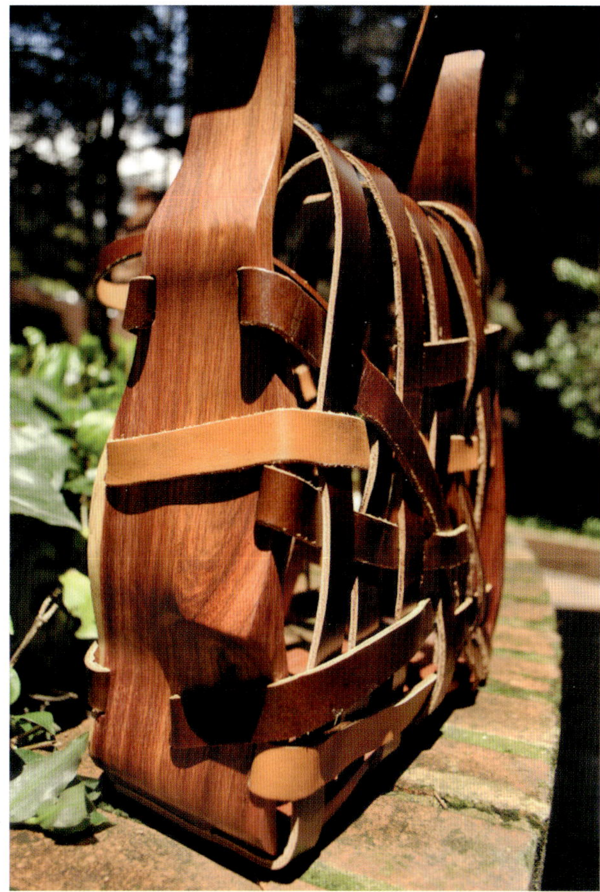

BLIND STRINGS

DE: Vivian Pérez

As an abstract representation of a rational mind that comes from the designer's inner perceptions and thoughts, this design uses wooden and leather strings to symbolize the strength that keeps everything in one's mind in place.

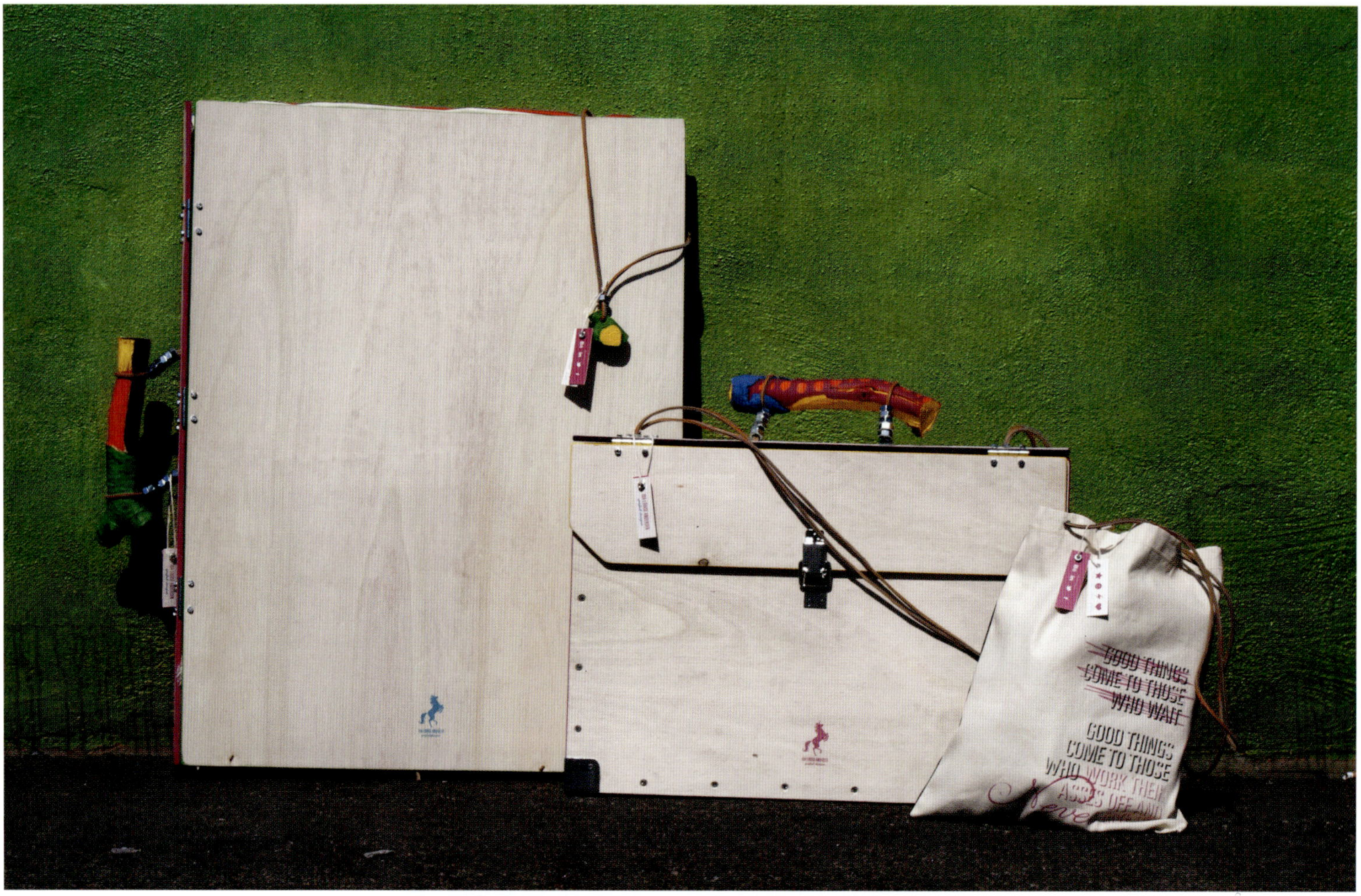

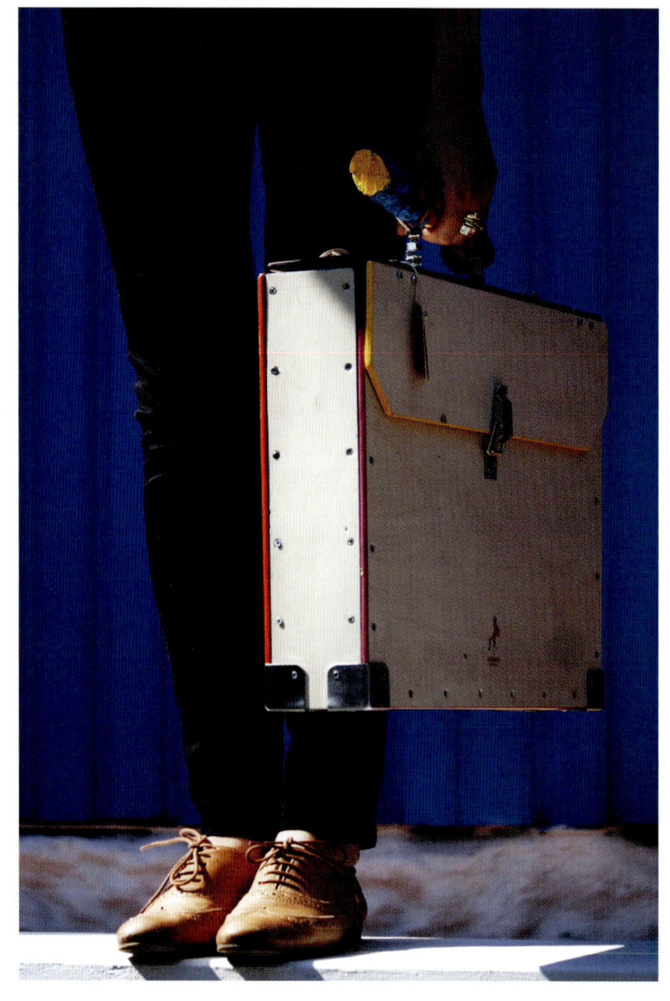

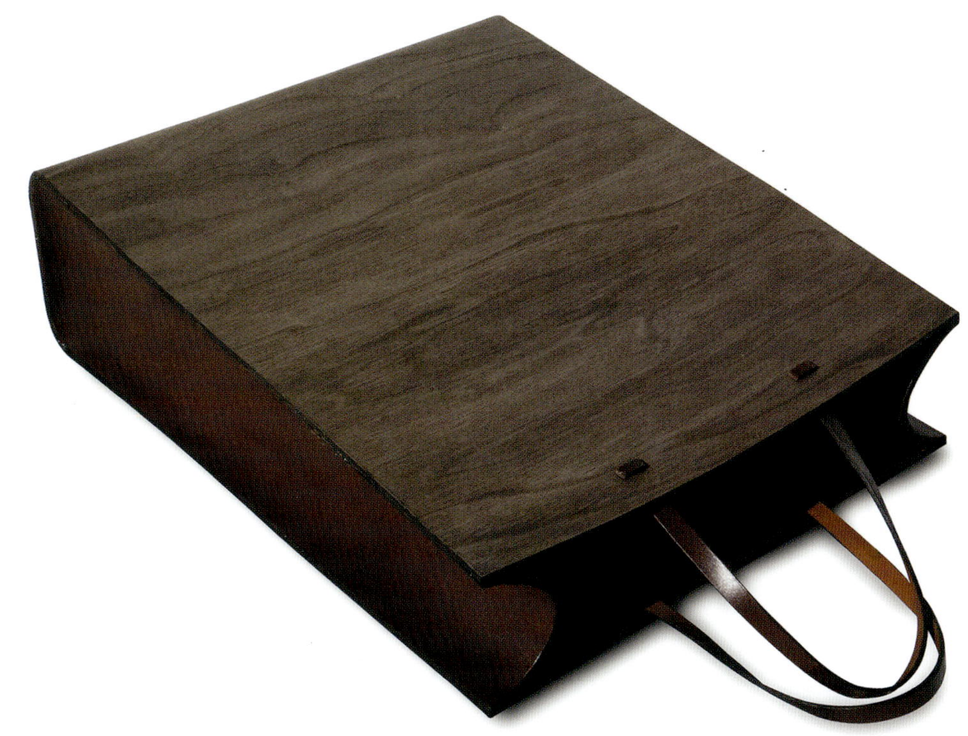

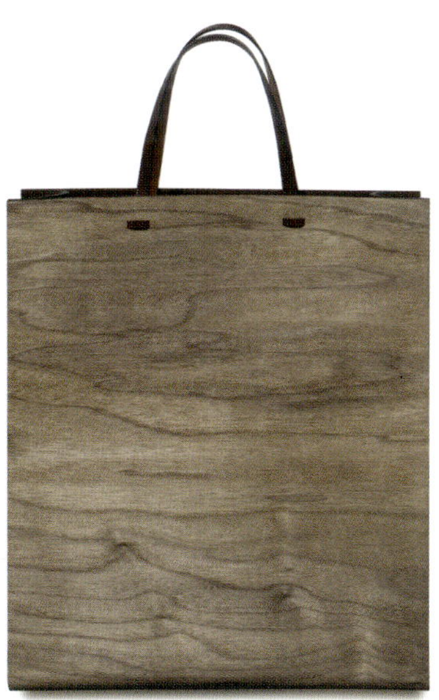

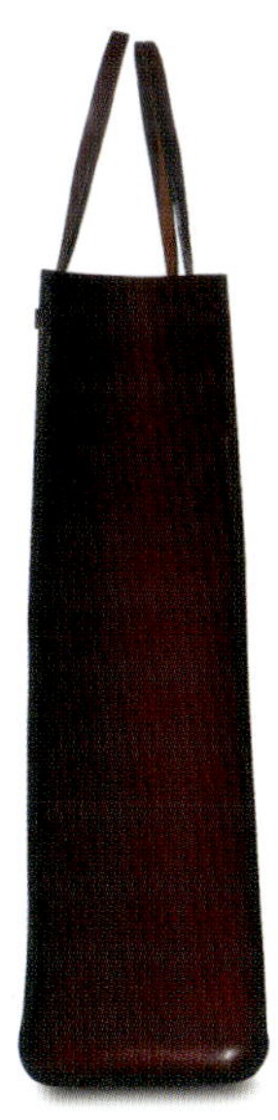

IDA LOUISE ANDERSEN
DE: Ida Louise Andersen

Created using wood, which represents designer's love for handcrafted goods, this bag was painted with bright colors on the borders and has a colorful handle. The unicorn drawn on the front indicates a magical feel.

OWL
DA: Oscar Joya Aguilera

The "Owl" combines walnut wood and cowhide leather, giving it a strong look and durable quality. These material will also change with usage, gradually become a unique piece changed by the owner's own touch.

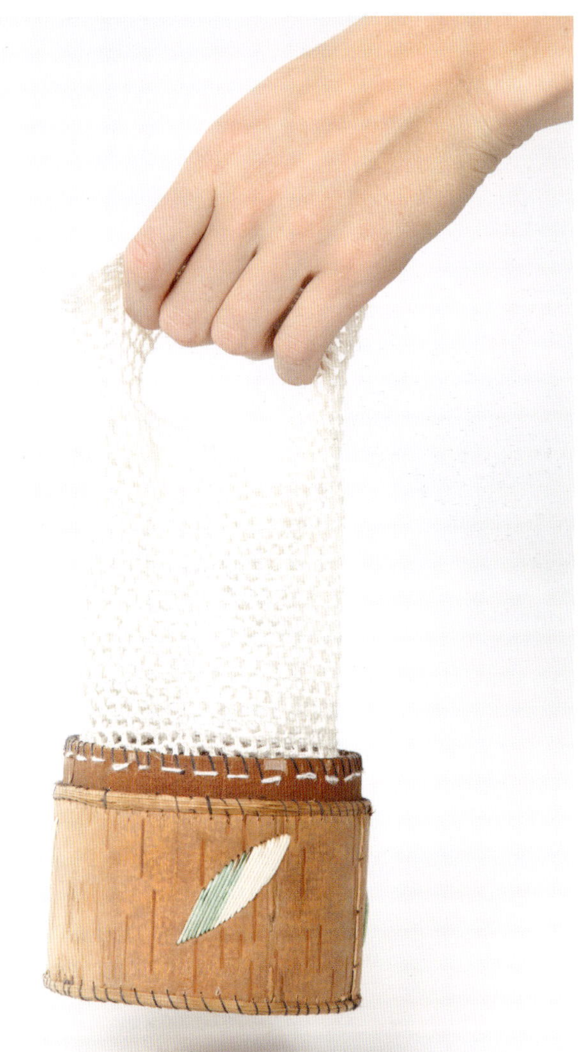
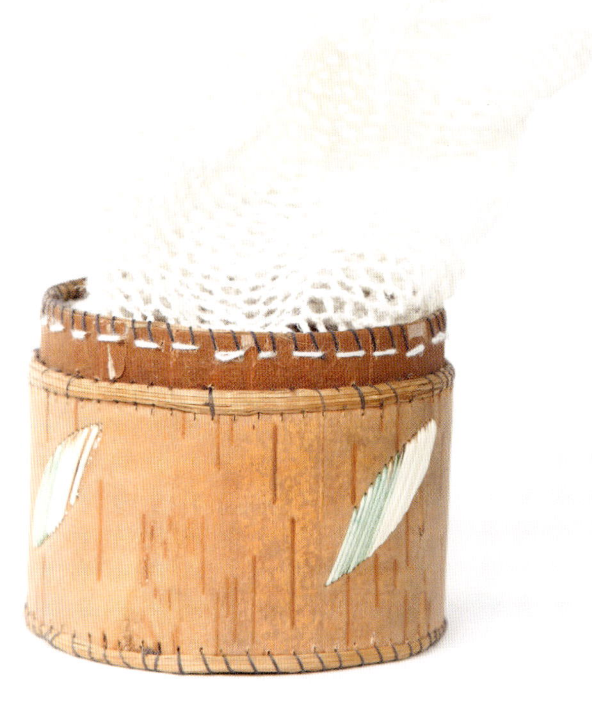
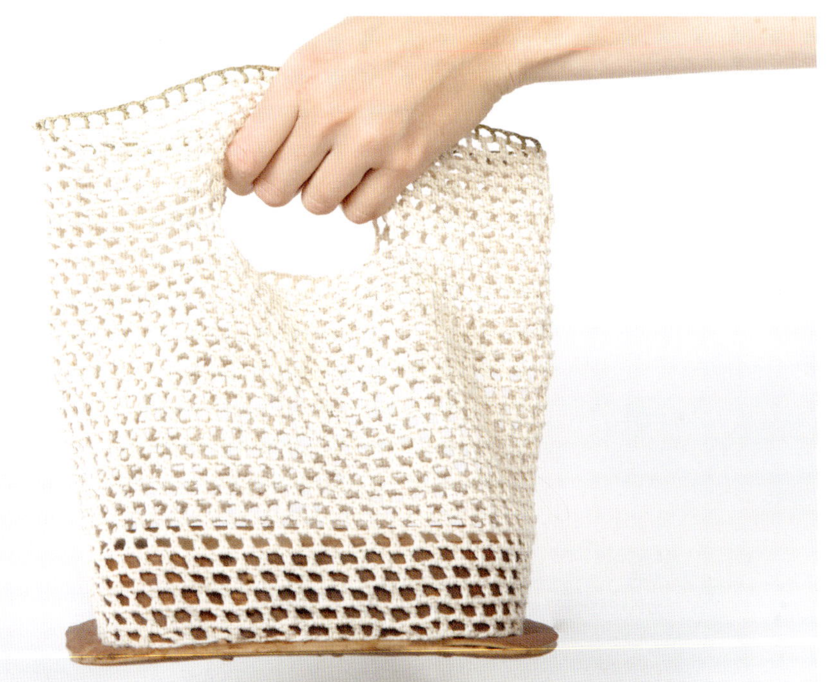
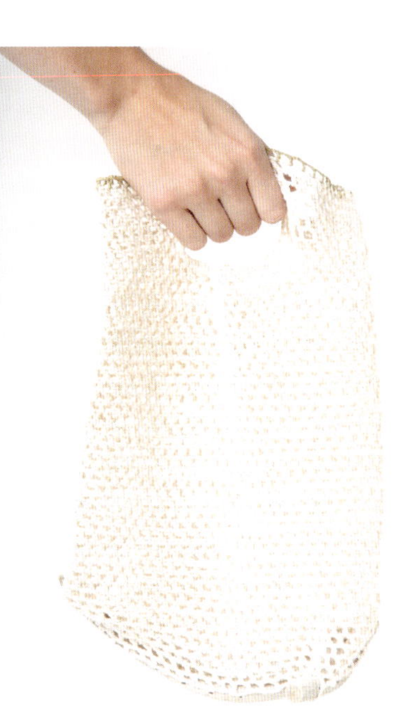

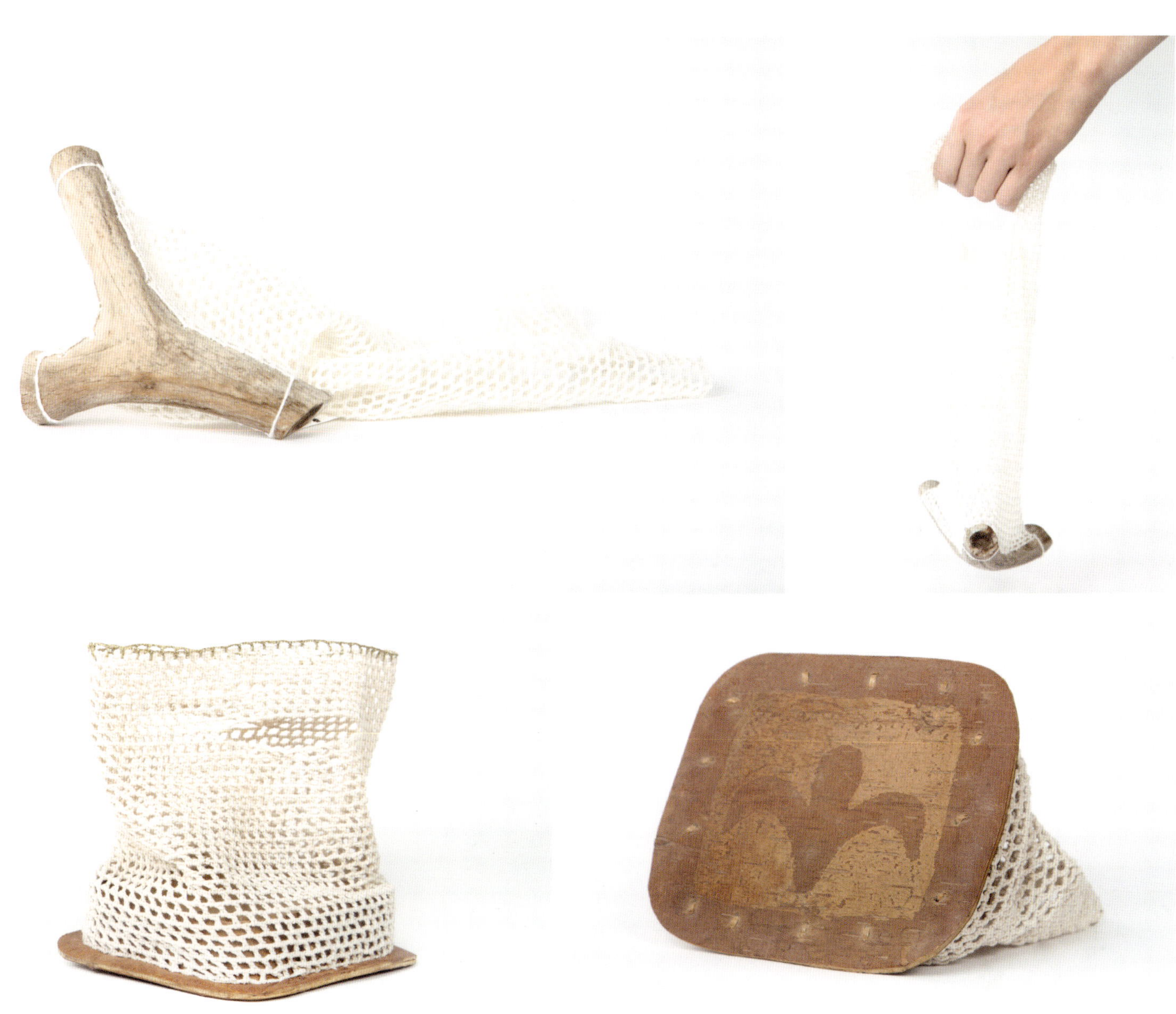

GROCER'S SAC
DE: Tabitha Osler, Sprayfun

Inspired by the traditional grocery and Canadian First Nations artifacts,
the designer assembled hand crocheted sacs with various carrying vessel:
birch bark baskets, antlers and more.

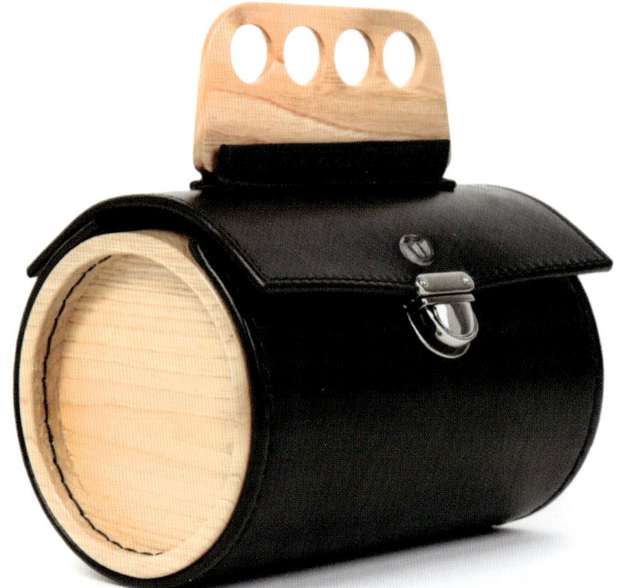

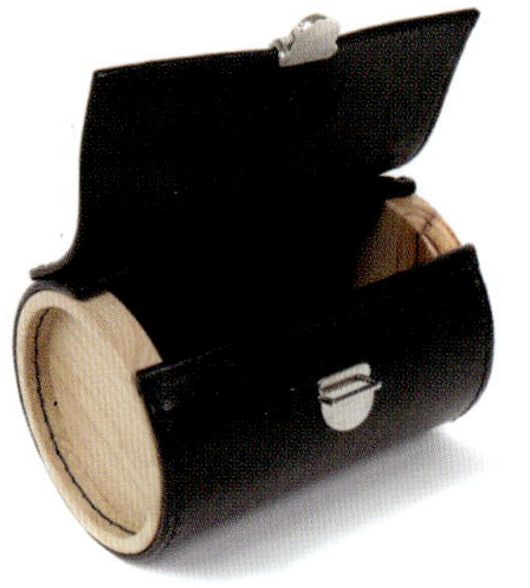

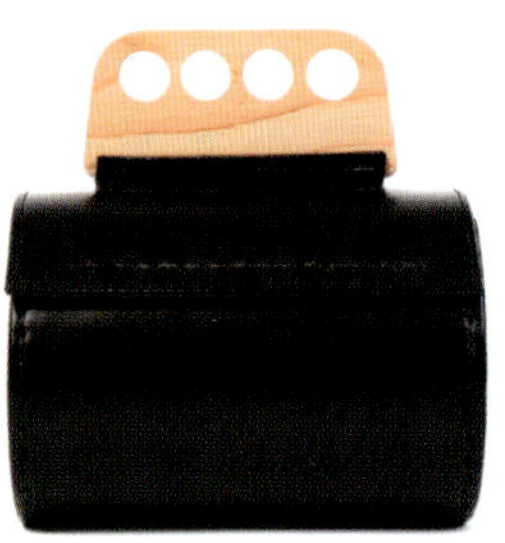

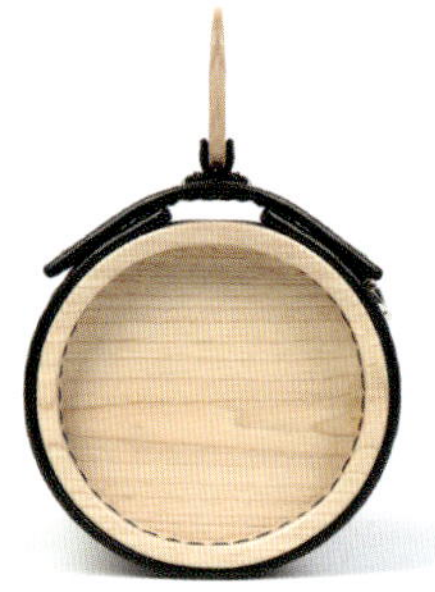

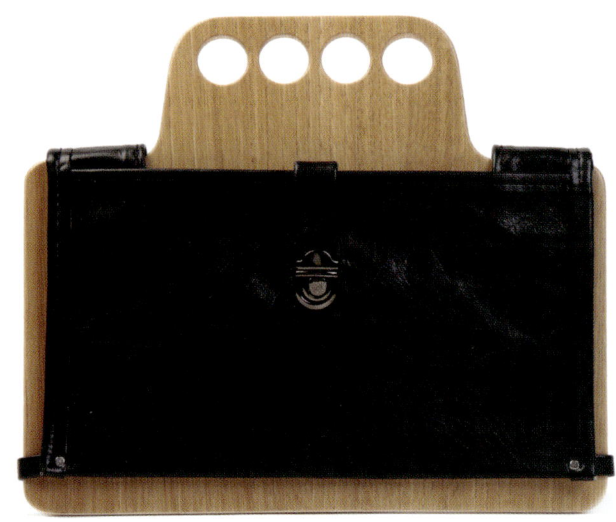

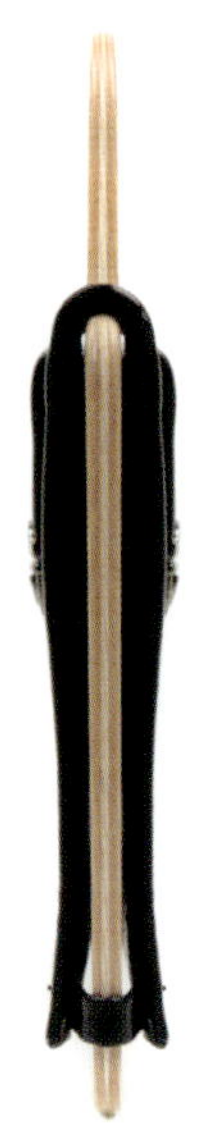

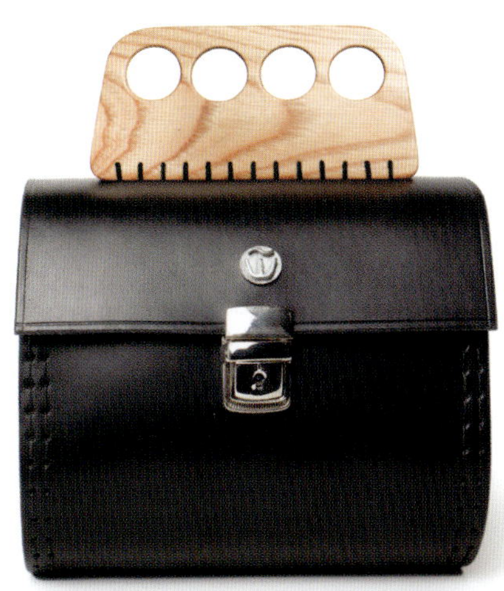

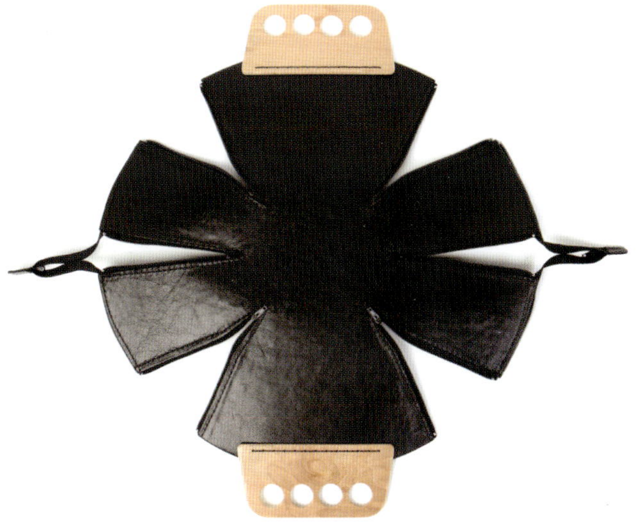

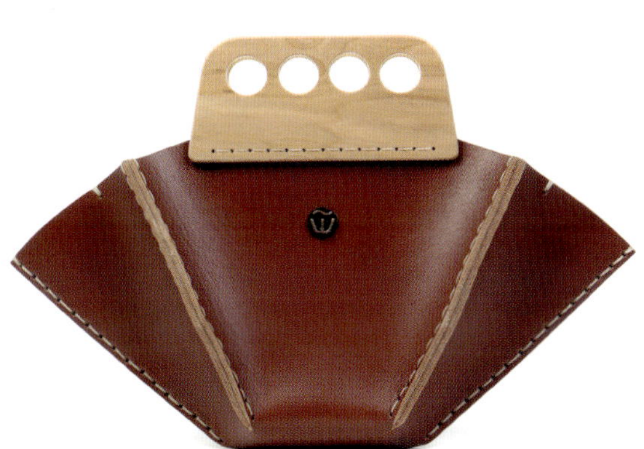

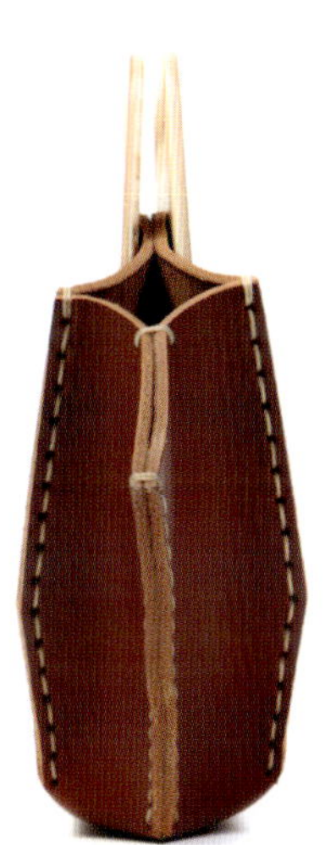

WONDERWOOD COLLECTION
DA: Assaad Awad

The WonderWood series uses pine wood in different ways as a part of bag
structure, with the beautiful contrast of hand stitched wood and leather.

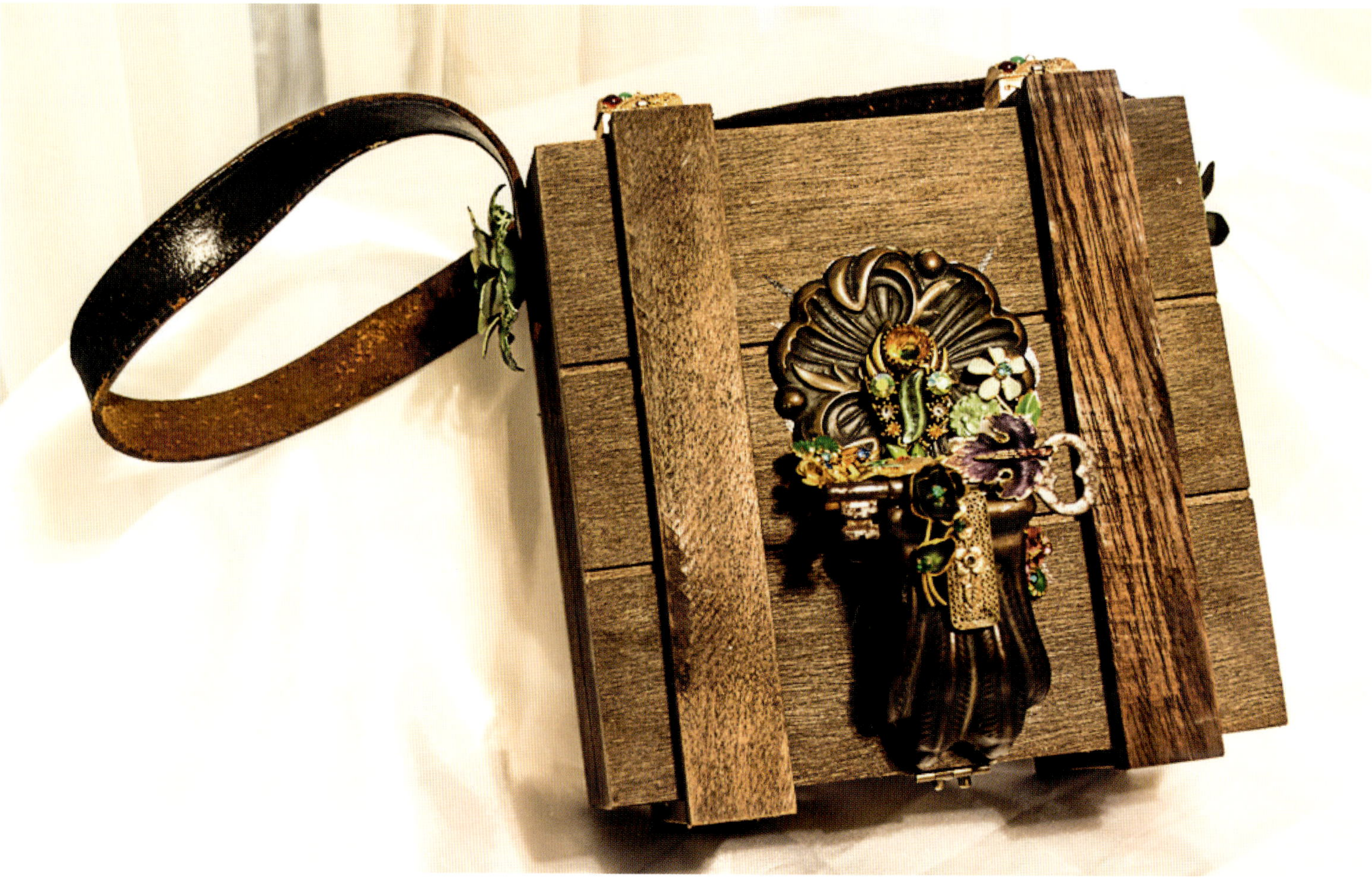

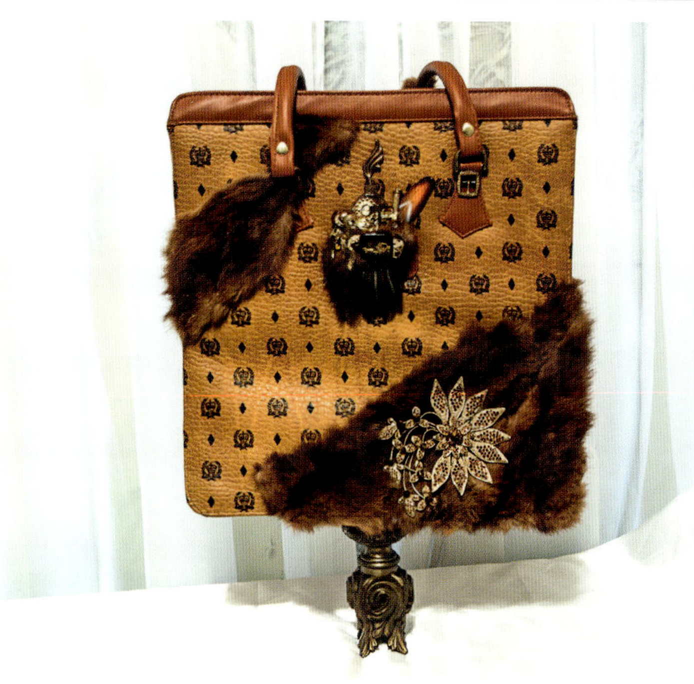

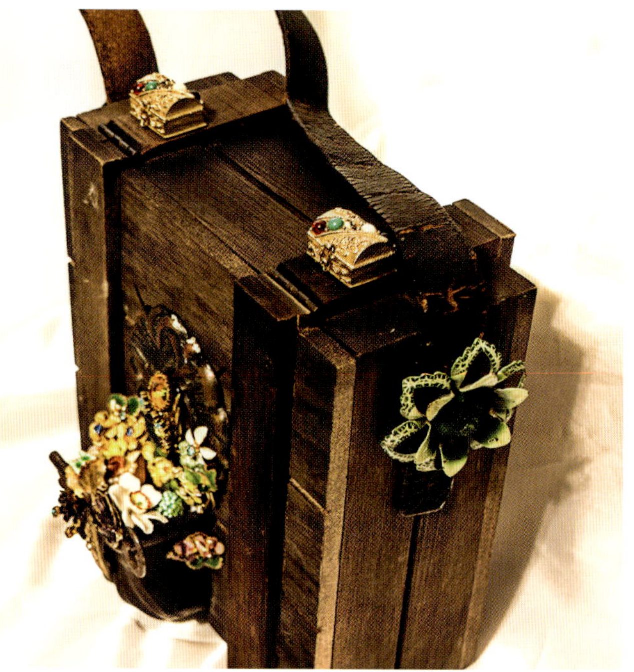

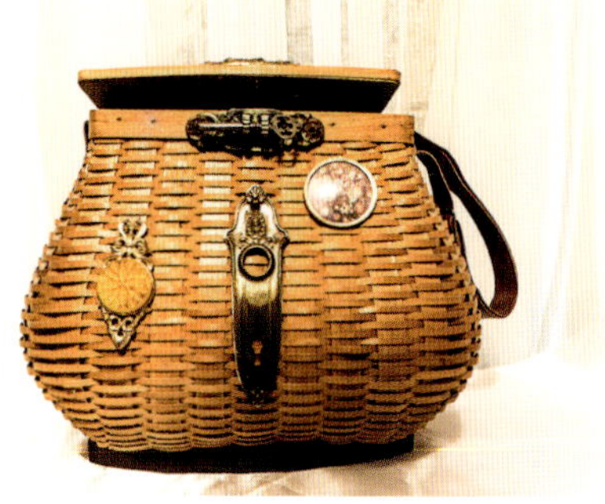

THE TREASURE WOODEN BOX PURSE
DE: Marelle

The works of this collection include ordinary handbags, wooden cases or baskets adorned with vintage jewelry pieces created by Marelle, turning them into artworks with stories.

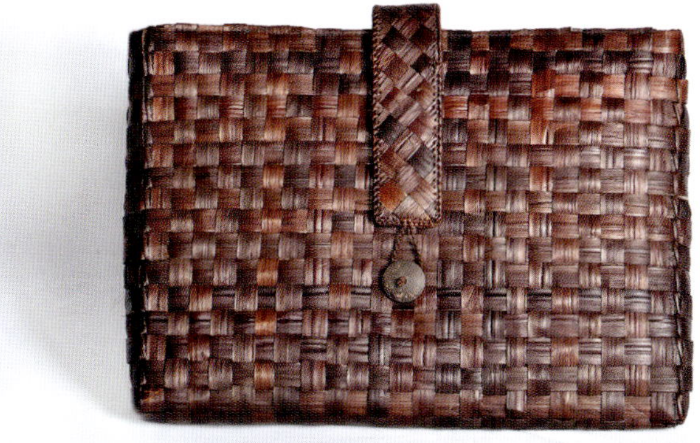

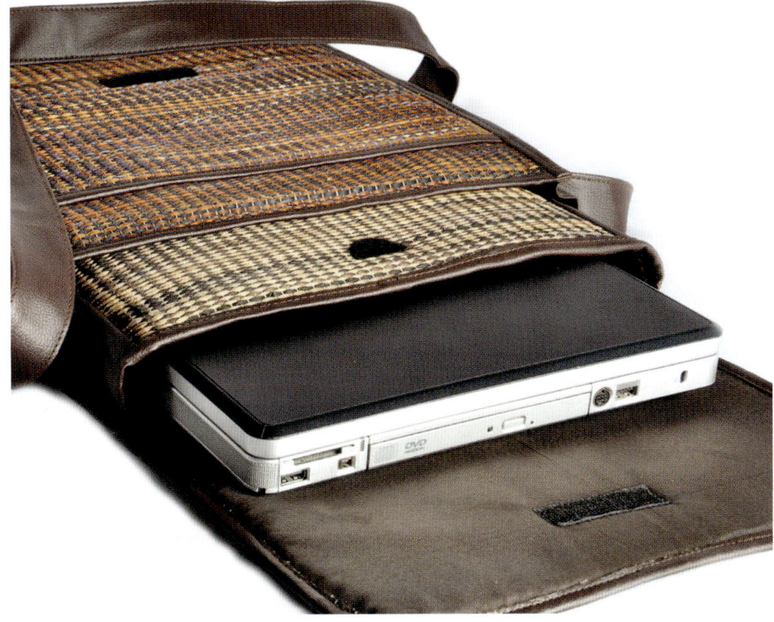

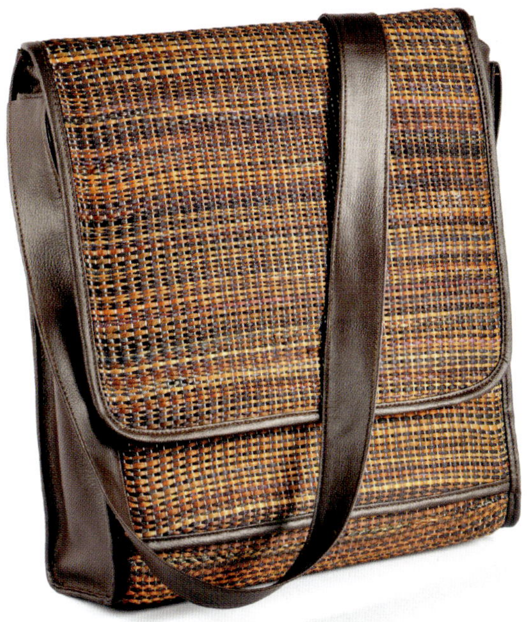

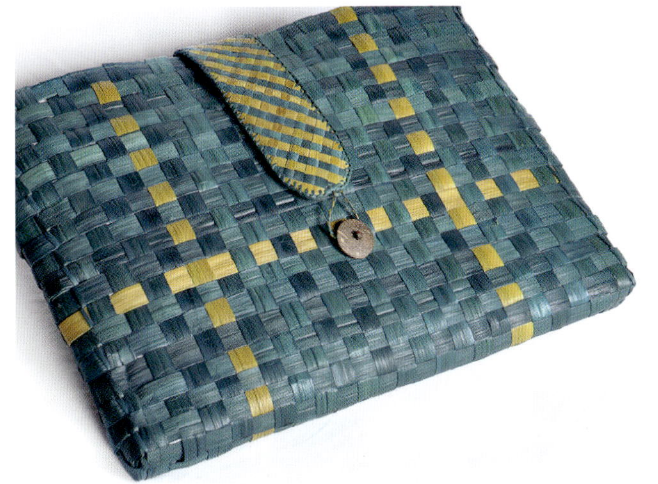

COLORFUL HAND-WOVEN BAG
DE: Durgesh Khatri, Maulshree garg

Hand woven with screw pine leaves that had been dyed in various colors, this
series has a glimmer and texture that reflects an Indian essence.

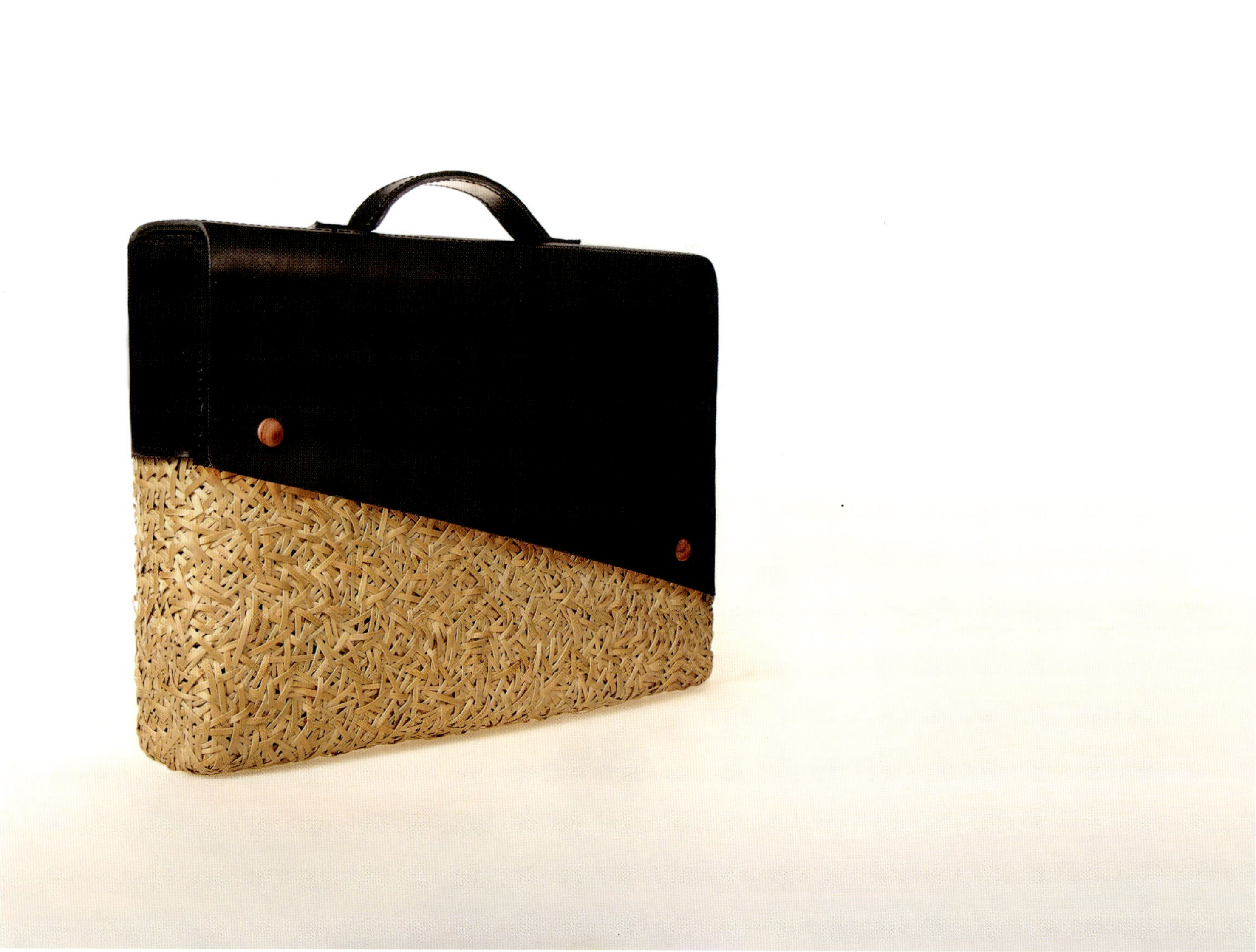

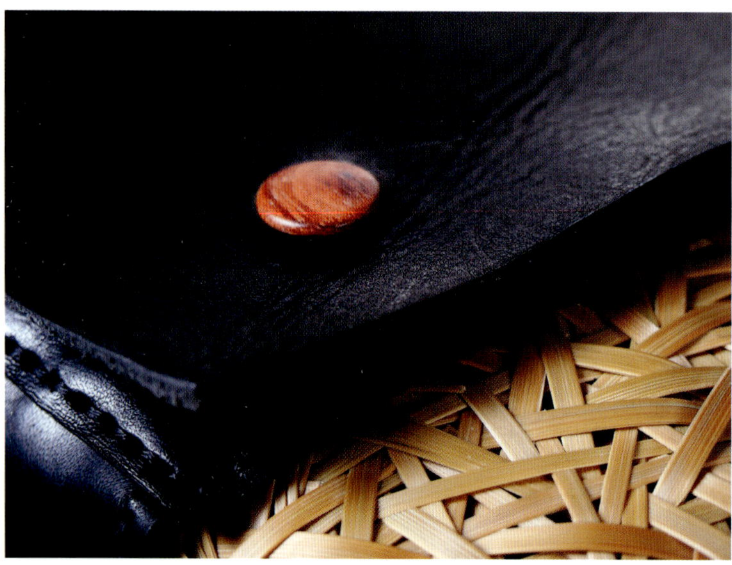
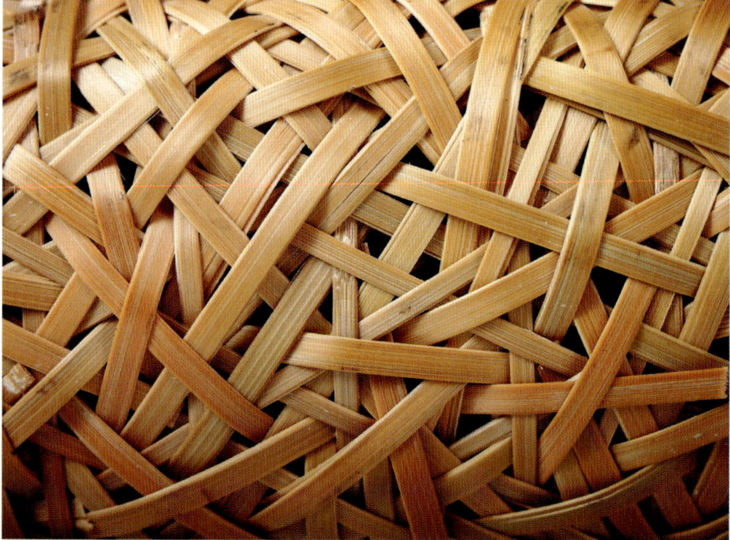

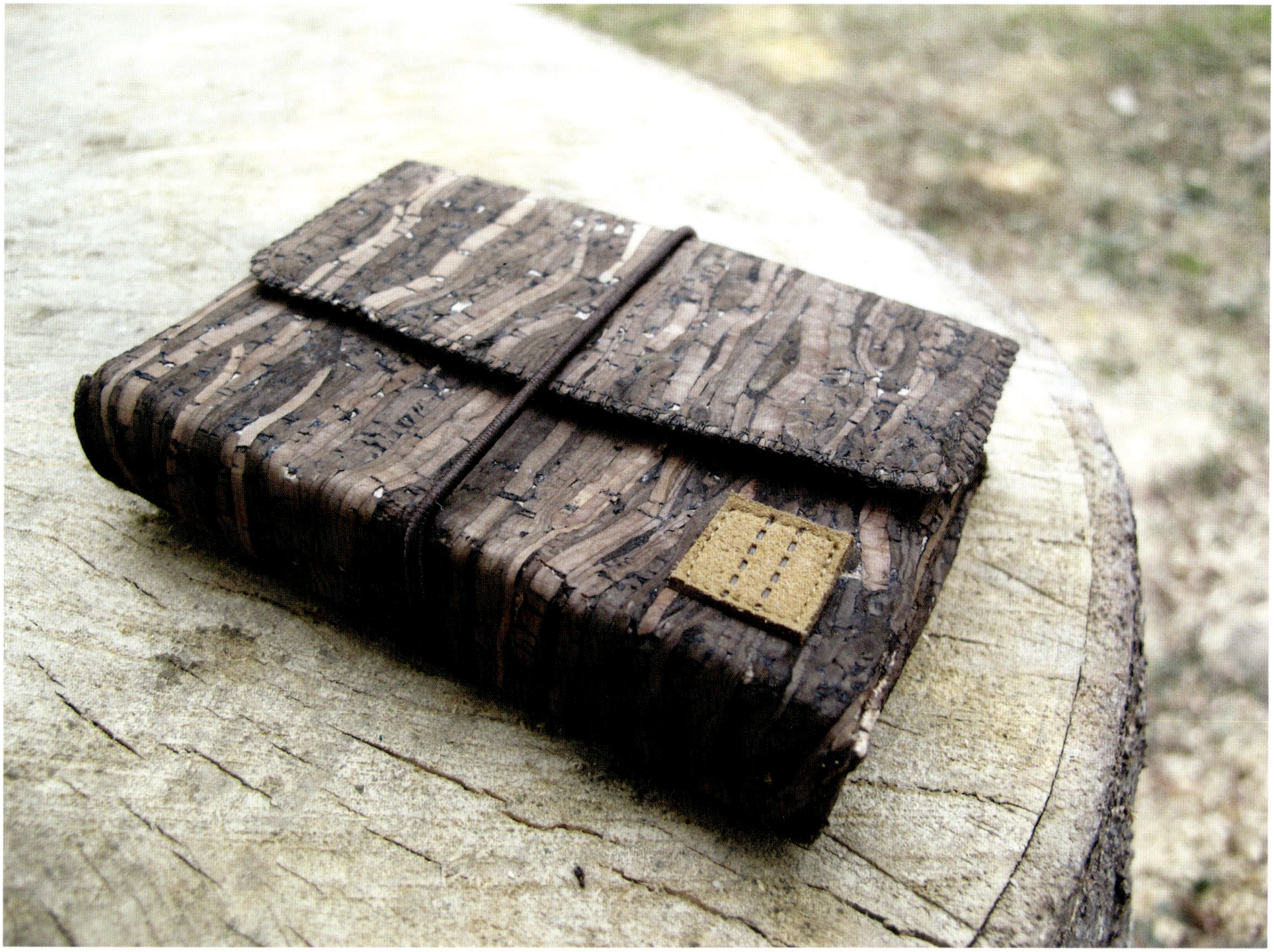

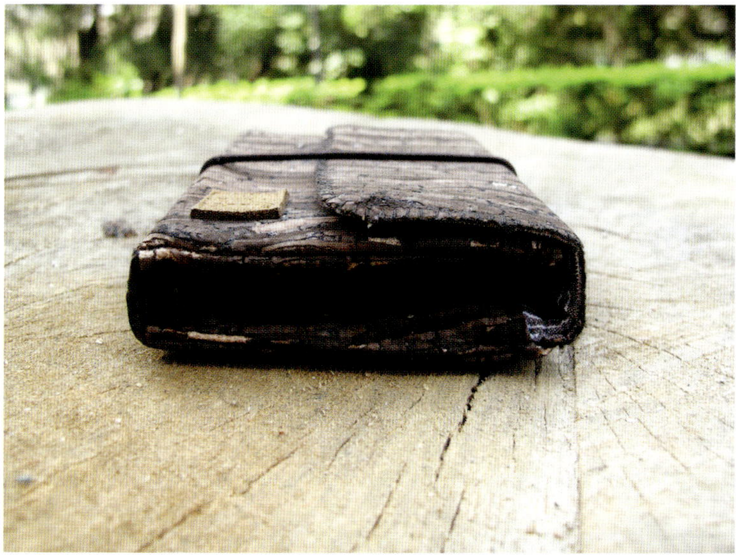

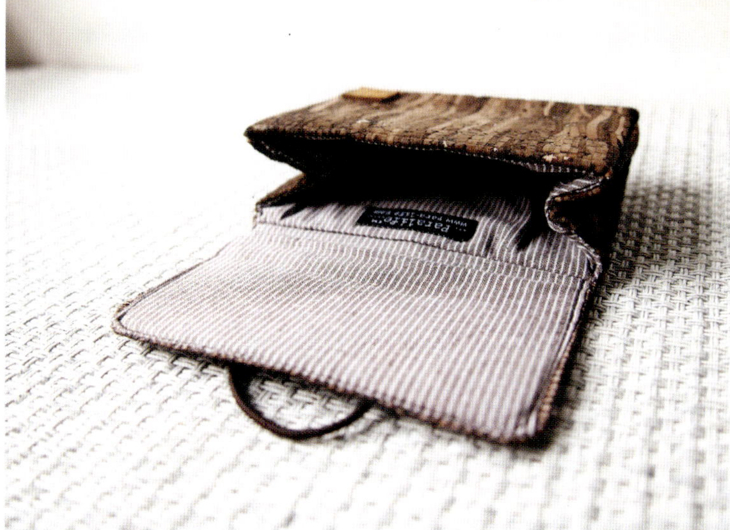

WOODEN GRAIN PURSE
DA: Paralife

This design used corkwood as the exterior surface for its unique and fine grain, which has a soft texture after being pressed on a thin cloth. The lining is cotton for better protection of the contents.

THE BALANCE
DA: Drii Design

Integrating bamboo weaving and leather craft, the design is a beautiful fashion piece to represent the spirit of the craft. Moreover, the flexibility and tension of the bamboo weaving can protect the contents.

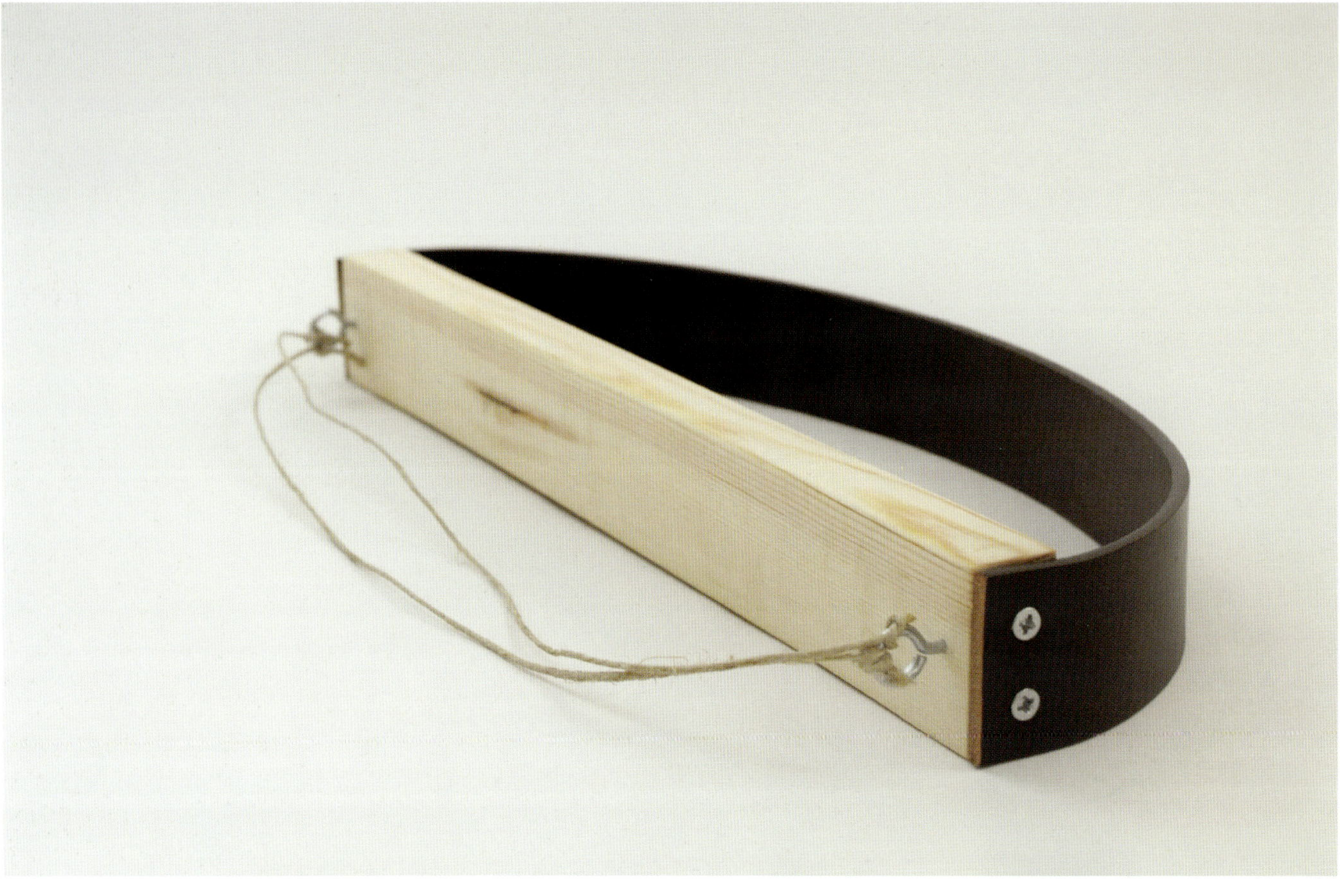

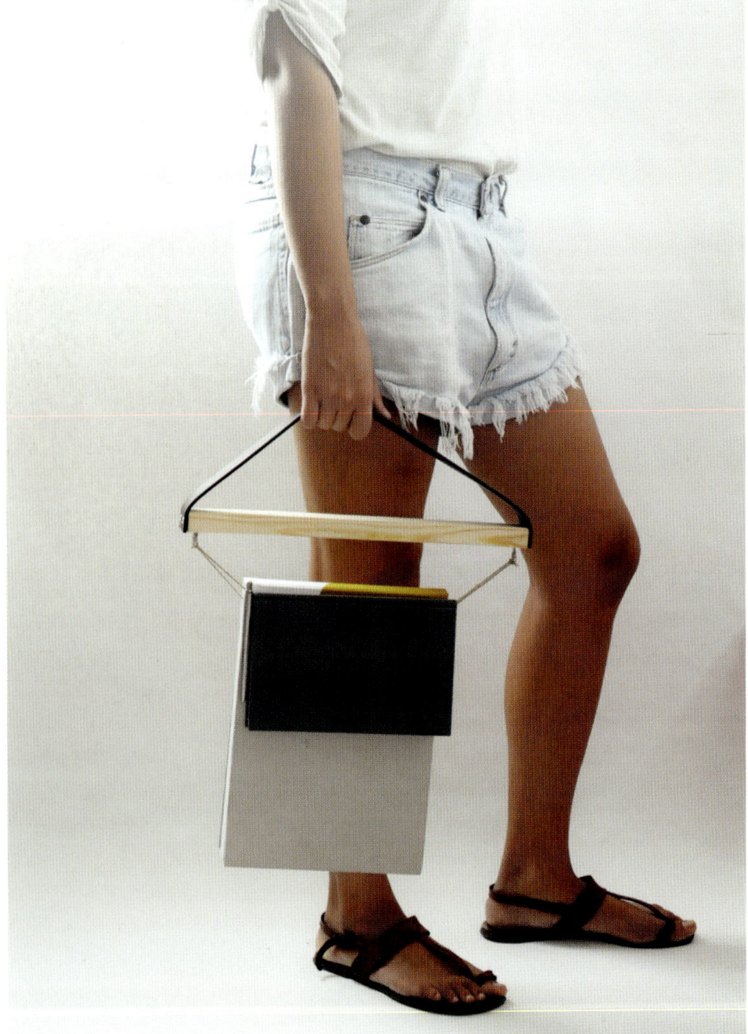
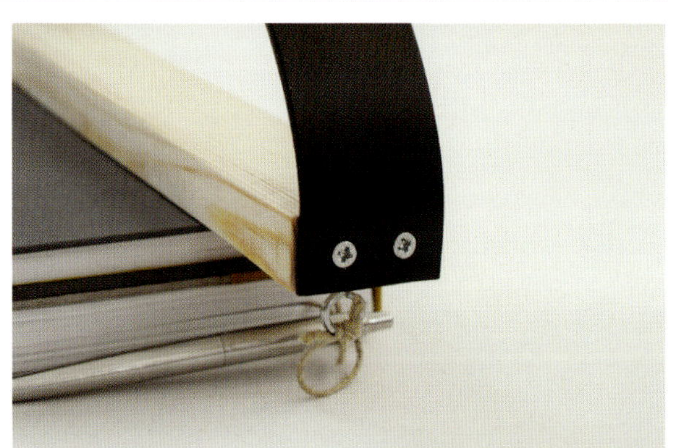
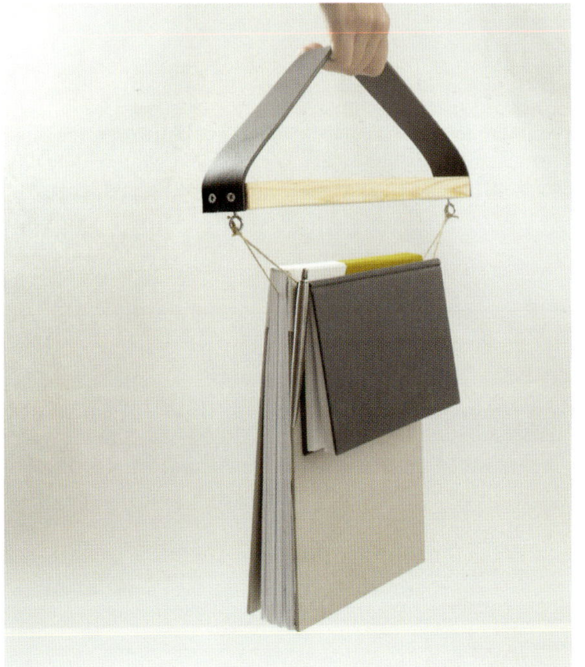

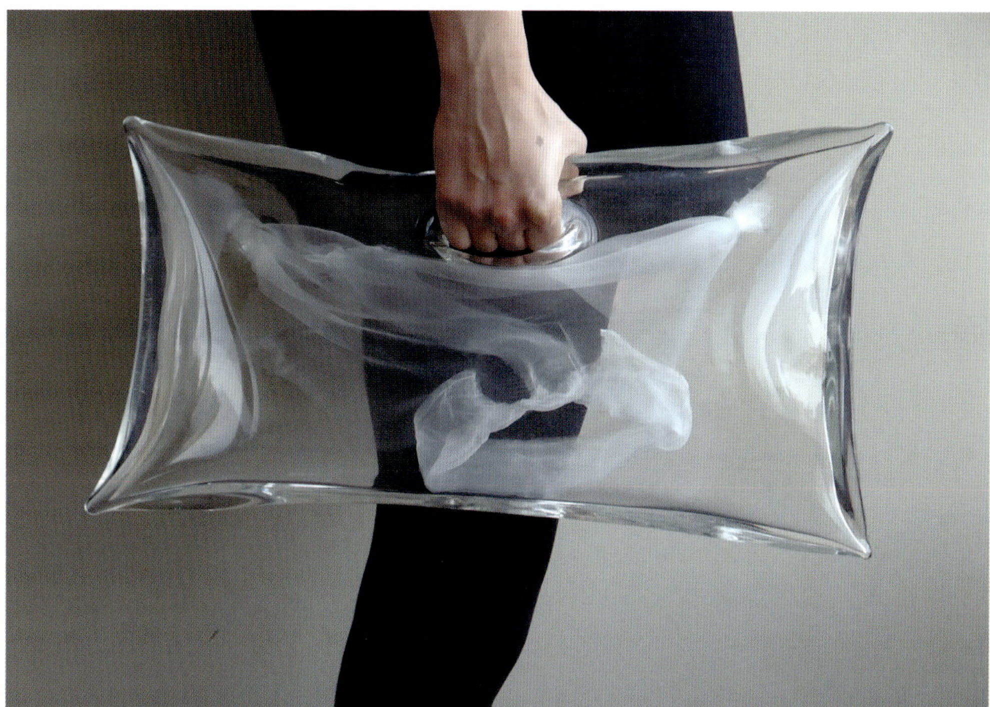

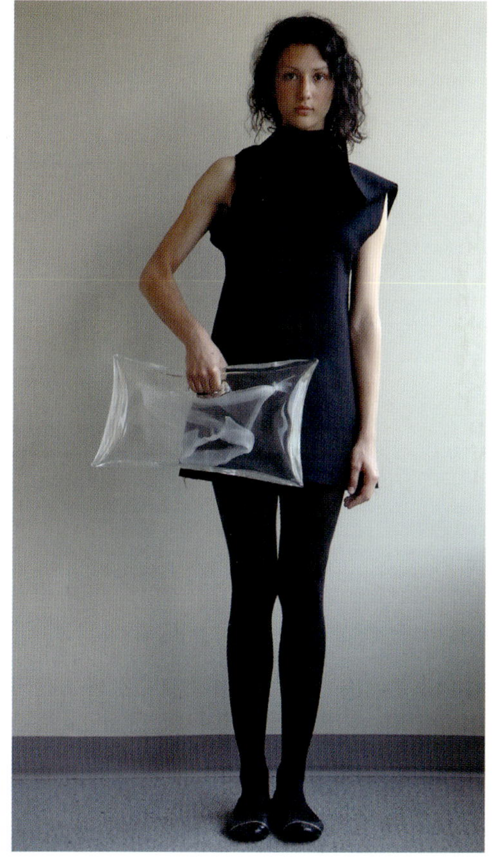

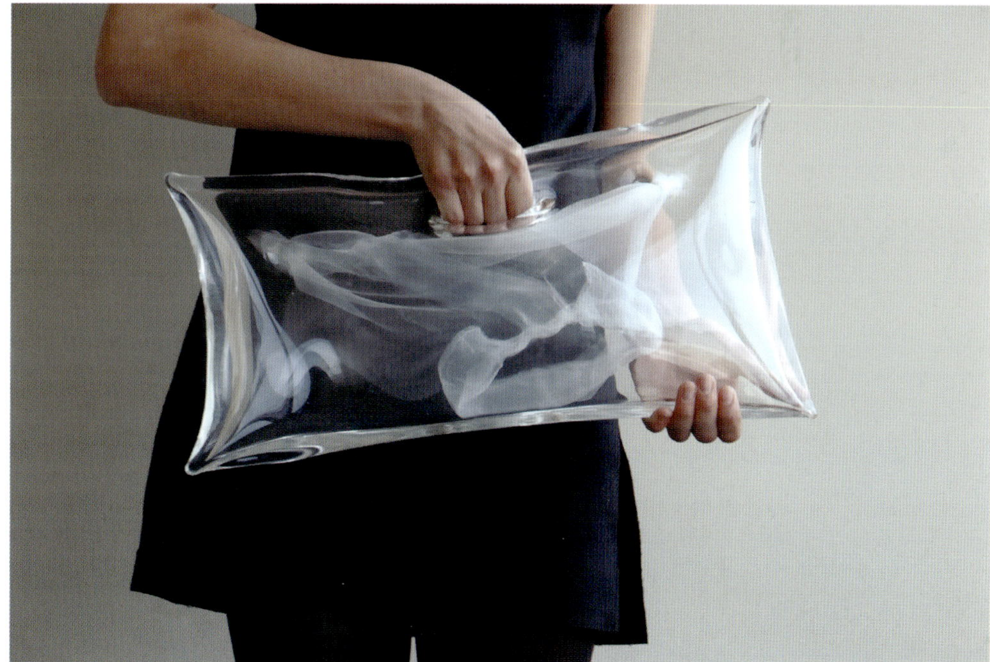

HANG BAG
DE: Michou Vasilis

Offering a different way to carry books, this design enables the user to store and retrieve books easily. Strings can be added as desired.

GLASS HANDBAG
DE: Ying Gao

Paradoxically using a bag significantly heavier than its contents, this project aims to explore the nature of and the relationship between accessories and their content through this aesthetic and transparent piece.

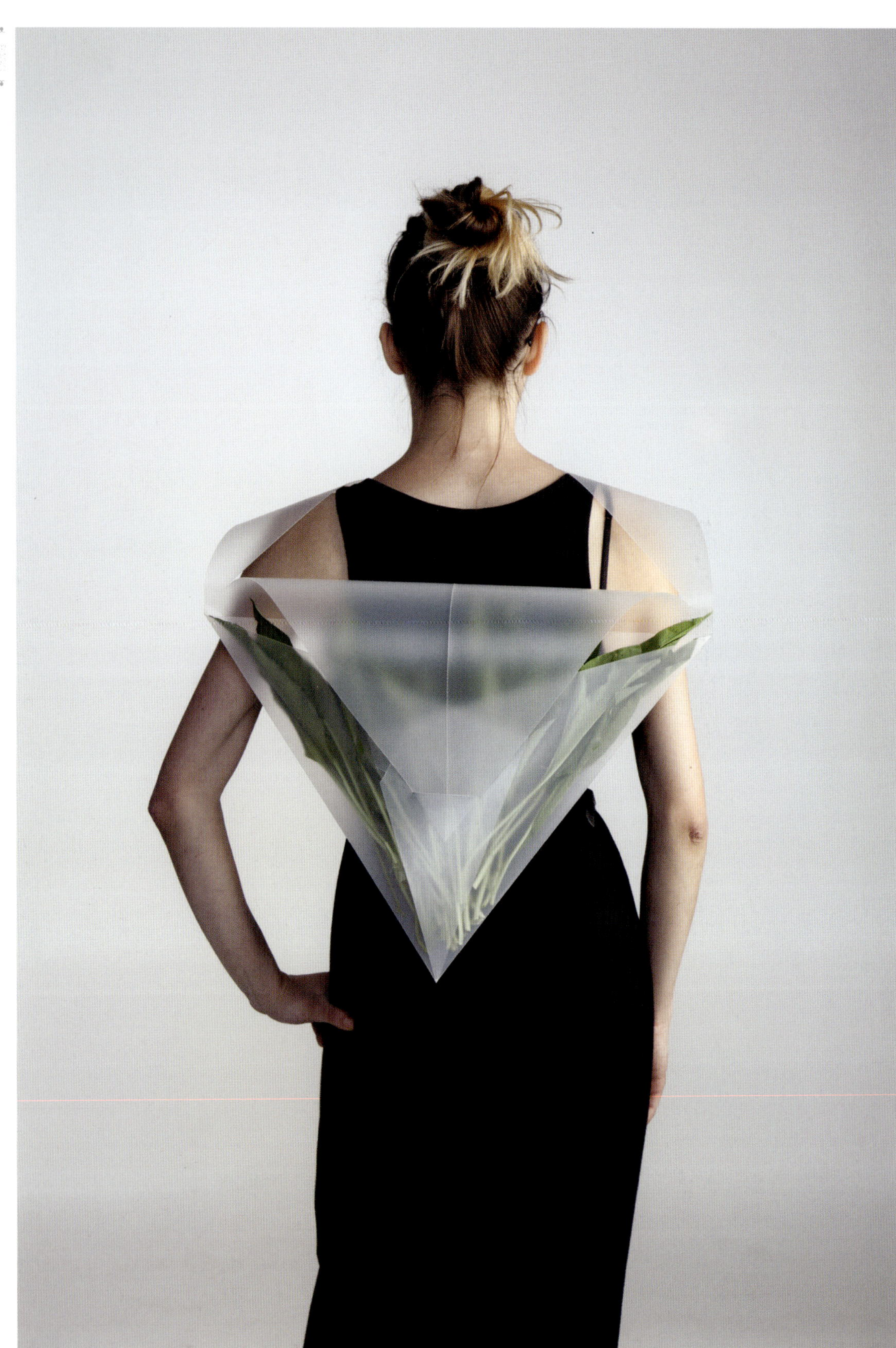

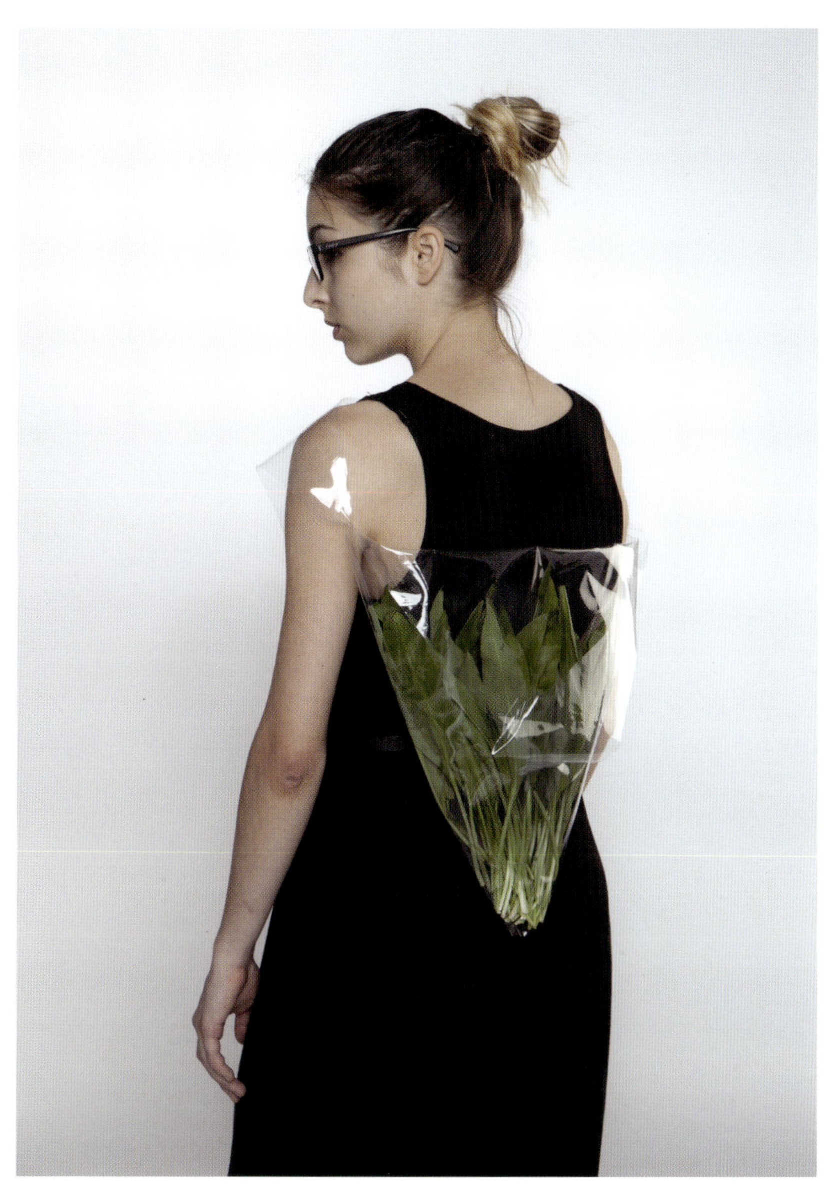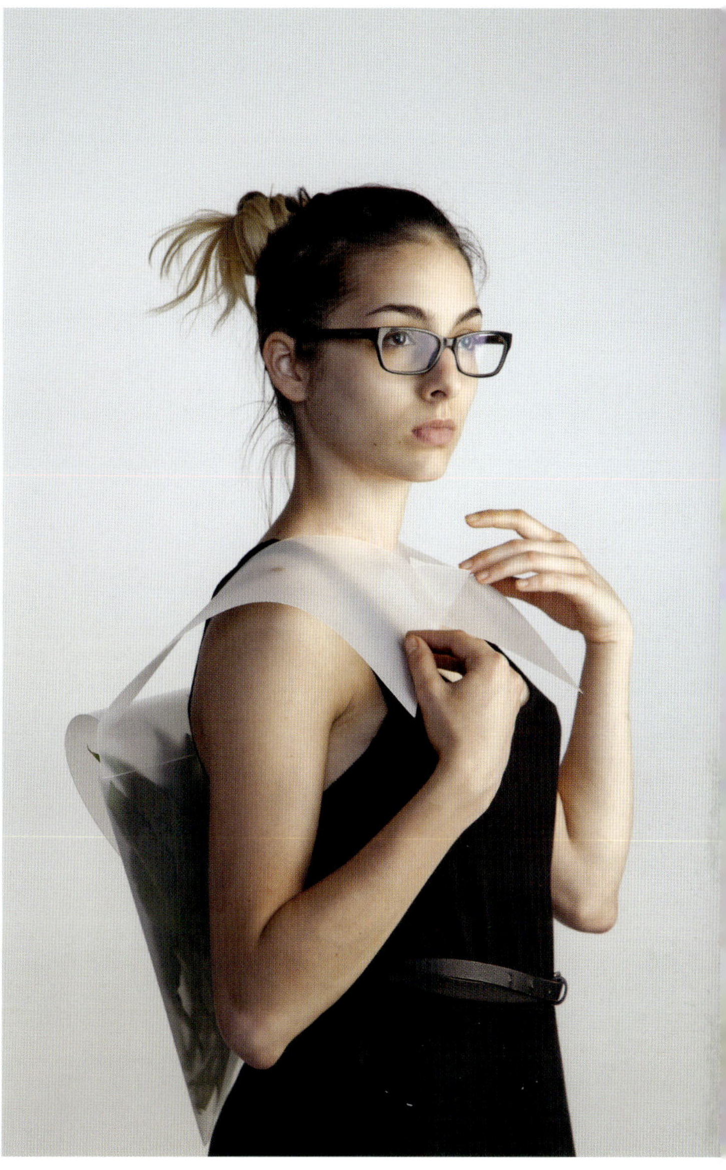

PLASTIC BAG DESIGN
DE: Nora Kovács

This series was made of very light, transparent one-piece material - plastic,
which was folded and stitched to create a special triangle shape.

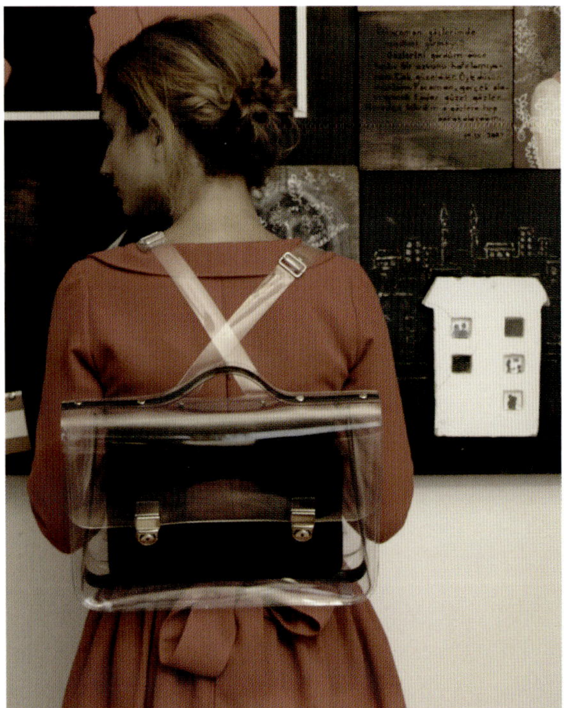

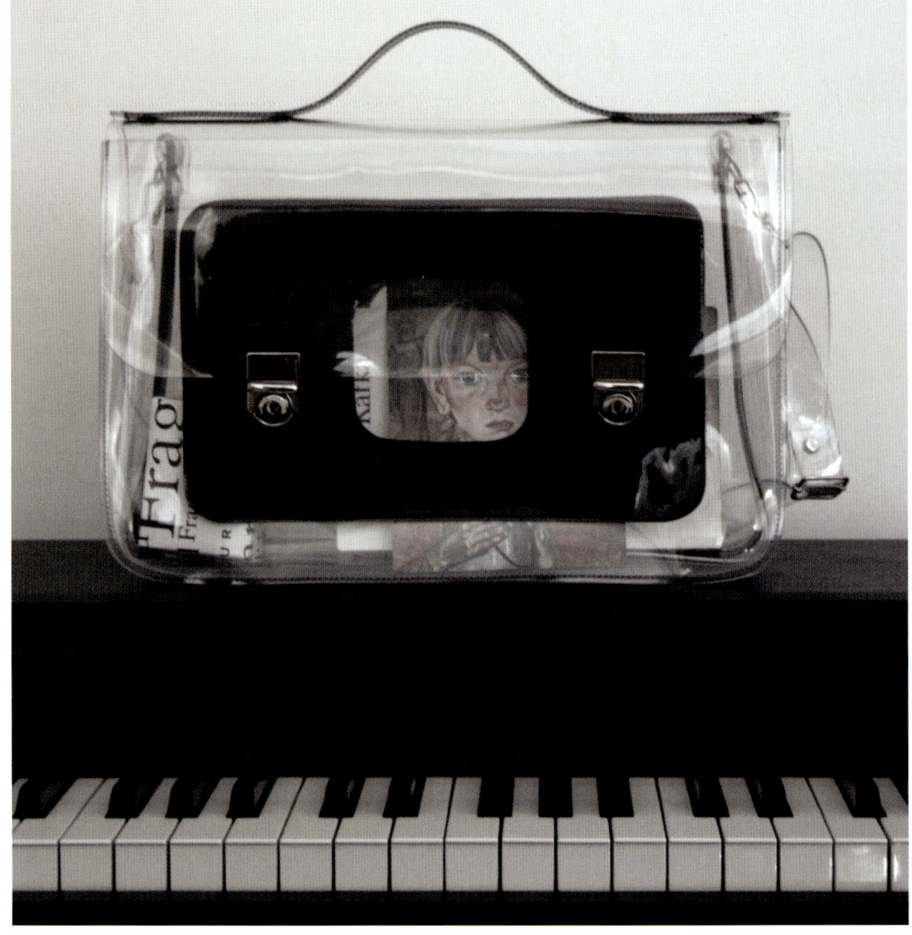

KAFKA

DE: Yegane Dilek

The "Kafka" allows users to decide what to show and what not to show
the public with two color sections. The white part is crystal clear for
visibility while the black part is translucent to only reveal contents
vaguely.

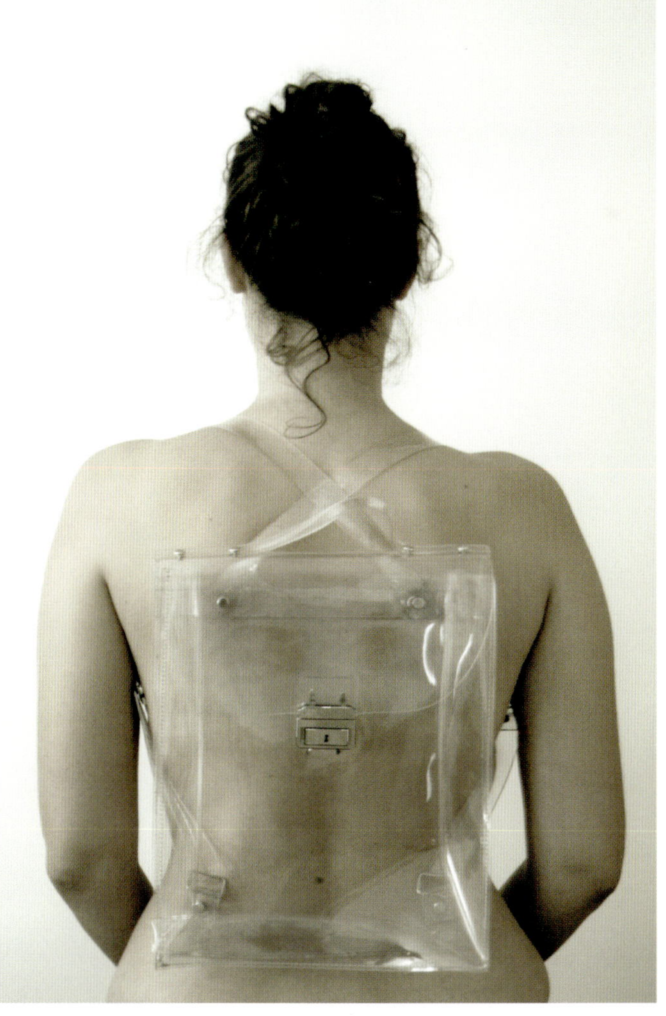

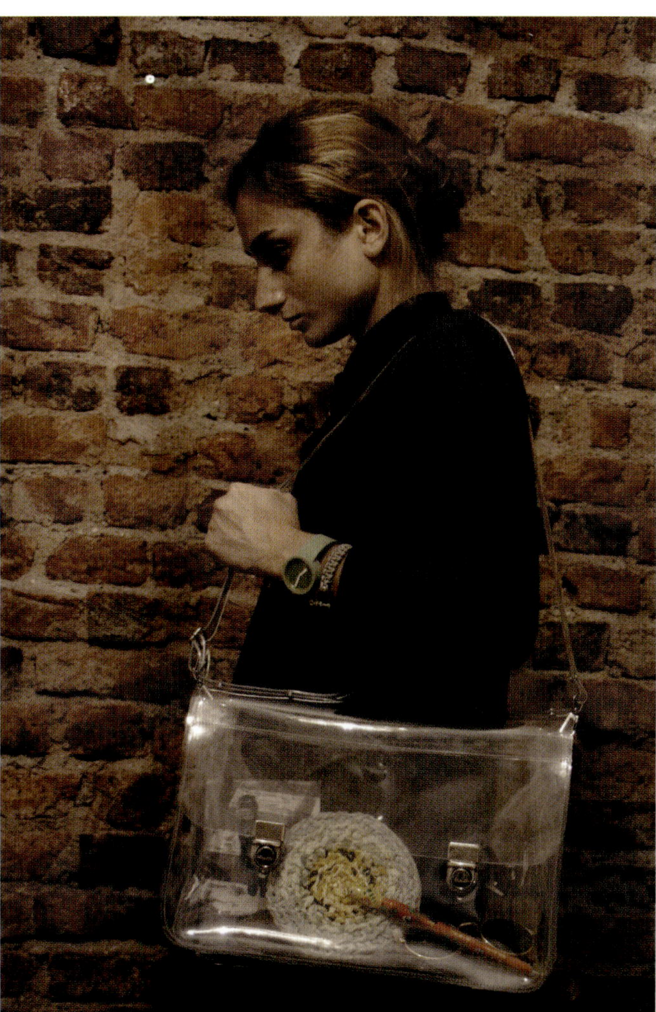

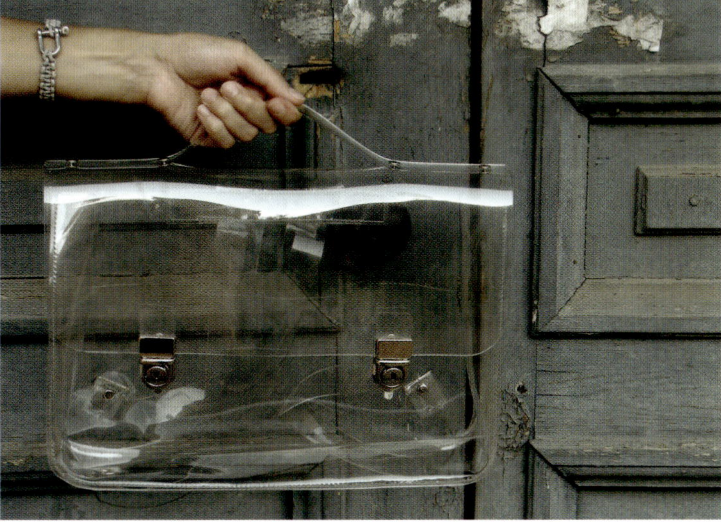

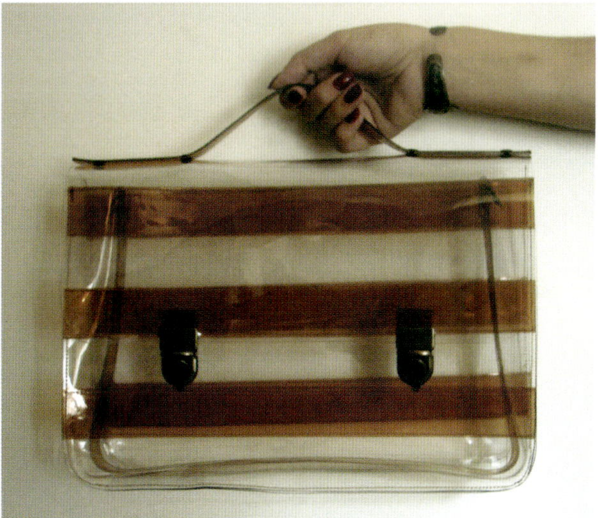

GHOST BAGS
DE: Yegane Dilek

Ghost Bags aim to eliminate color incompatibility of bags and outfits by offering a totally transparent bag made of PVC, whose appearance changes with the contents.

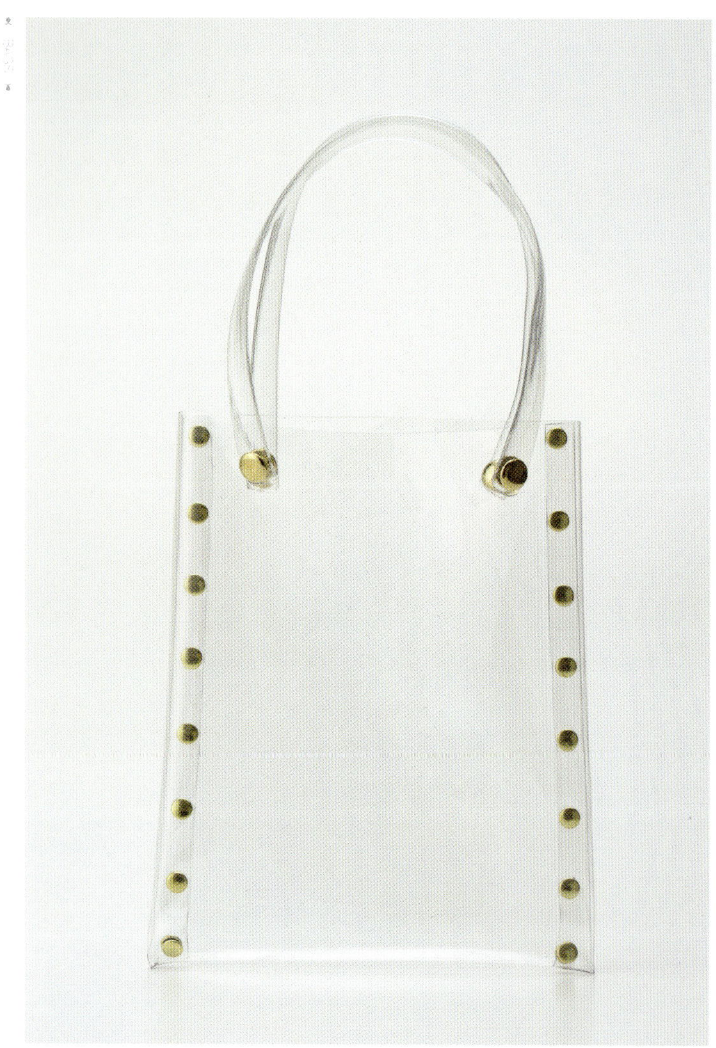
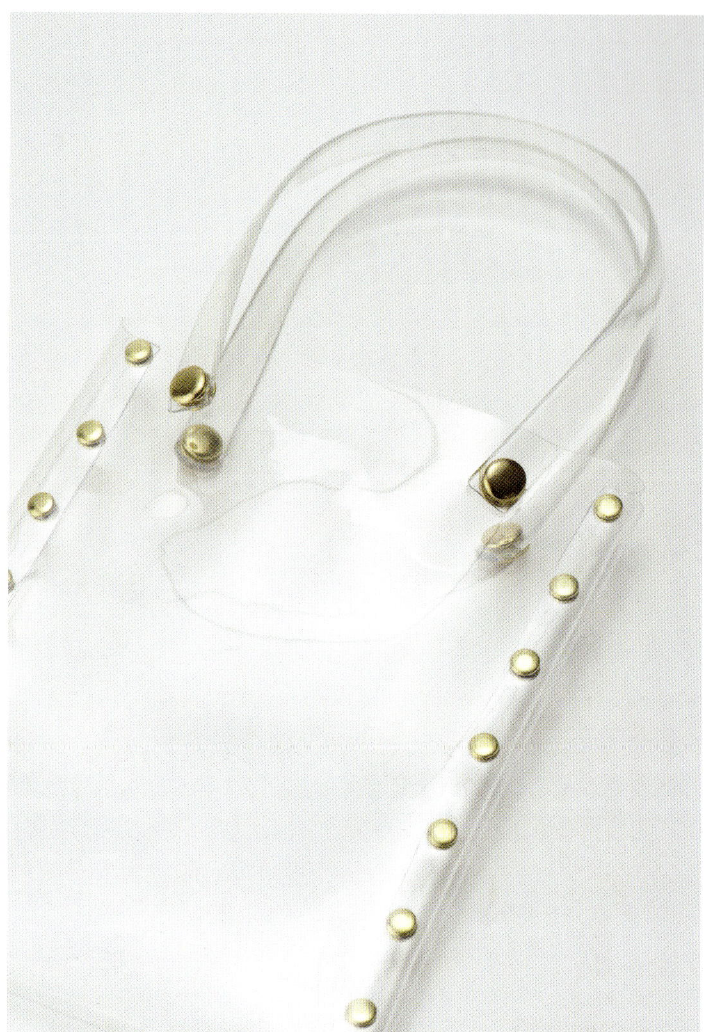
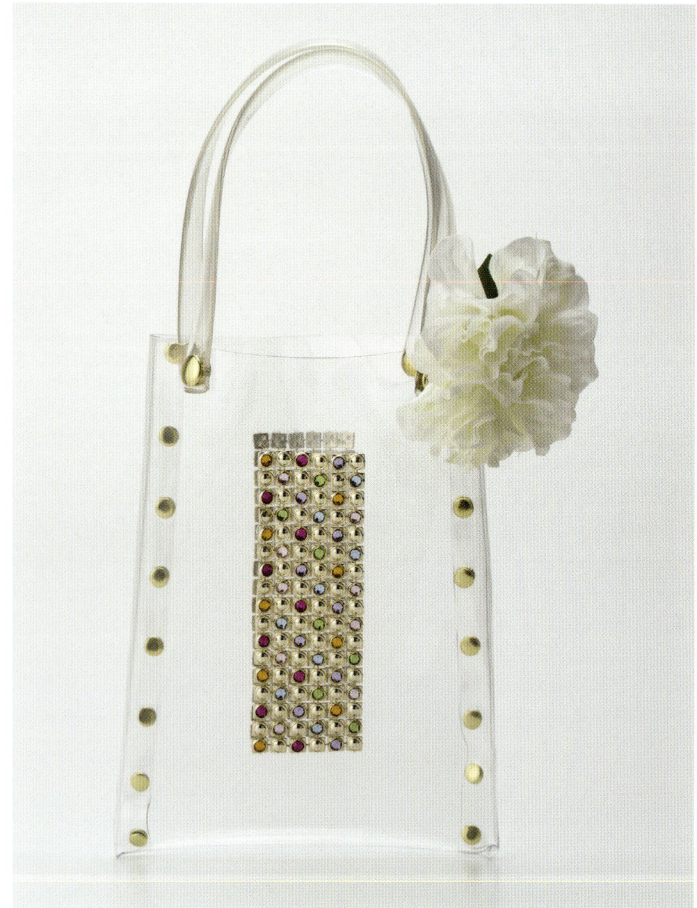
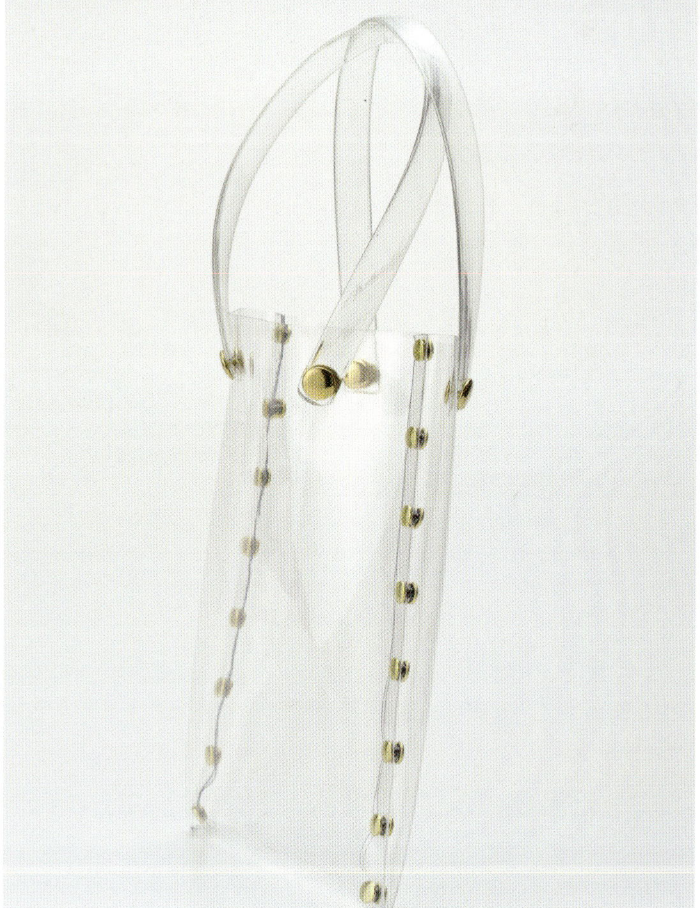

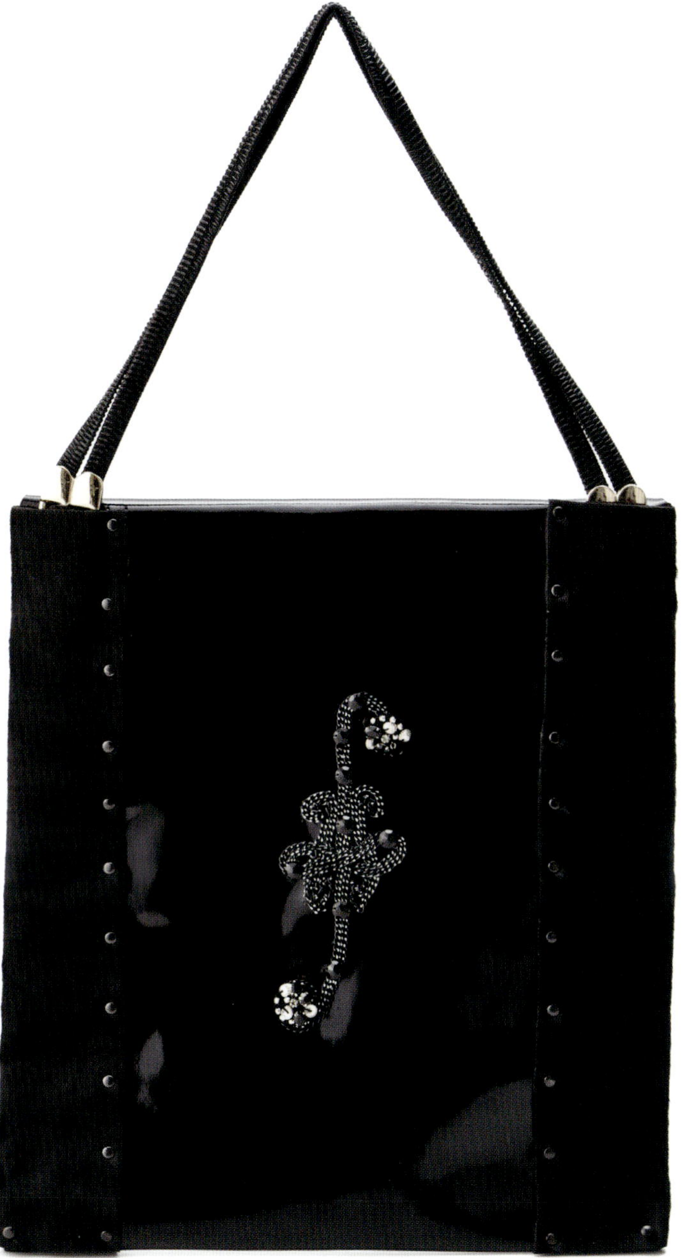

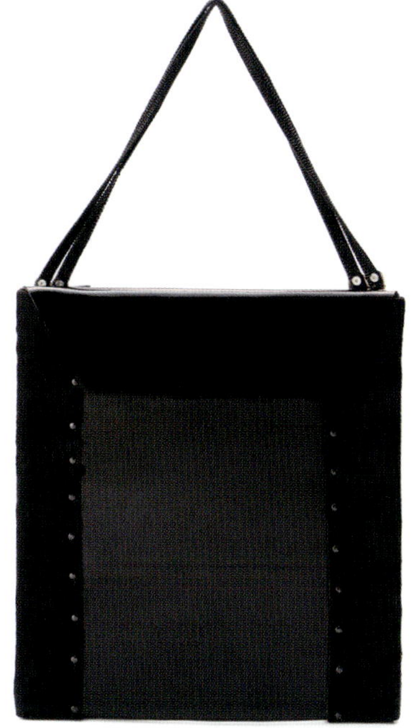

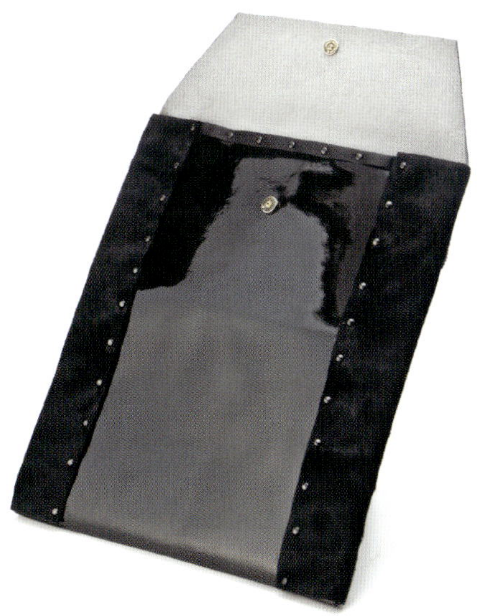

ANY COLOR
DE: Fumie SHOJI

Designed to change appearance as content changes, the bag is transparent, but it is still adorned with ornaments so that it would not appear too plain when emptied.

BLACK QUARTET
DE: Fumie SHOJI

The "BK" skillfully plays with the color black by using different material to present it, via various textures to compose rich visual layers.

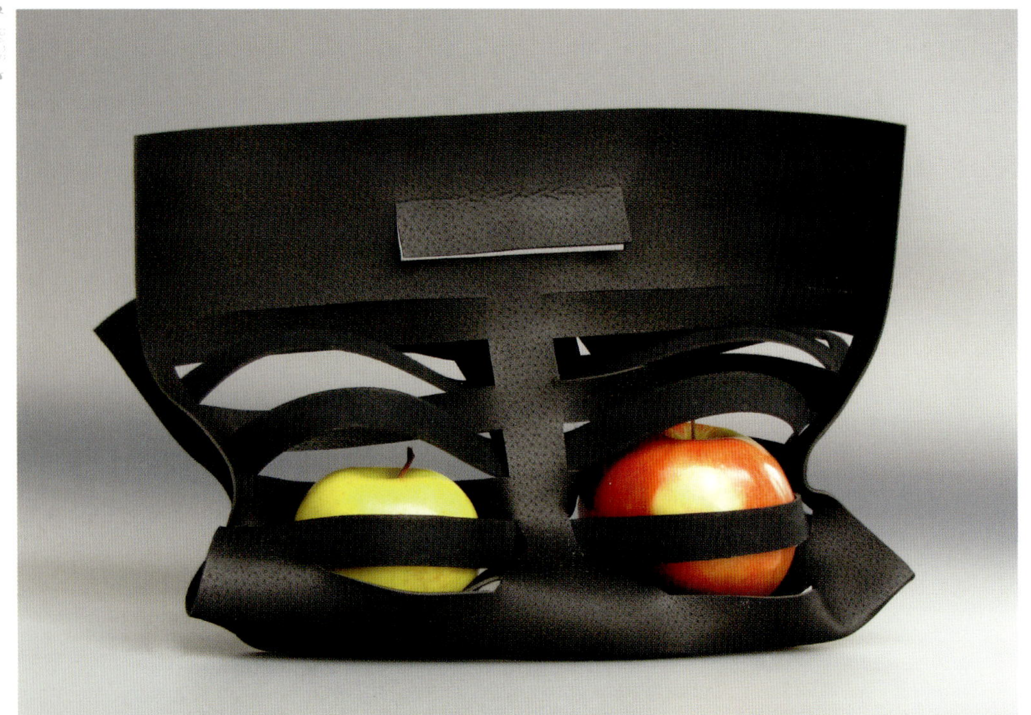

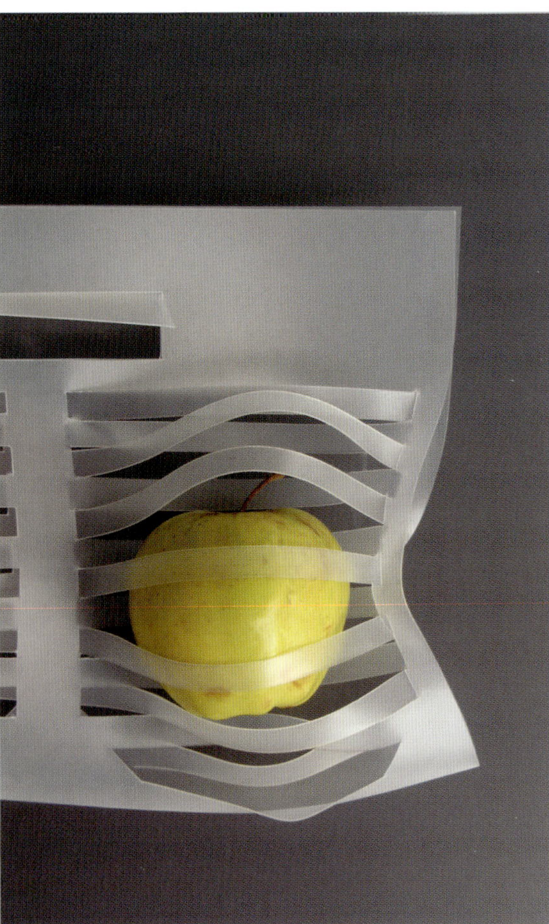

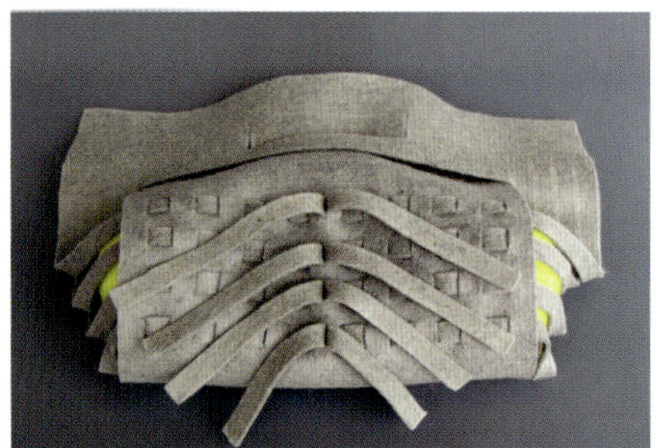

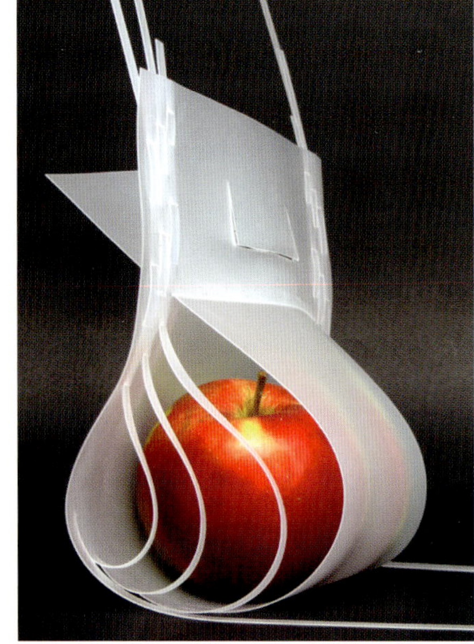

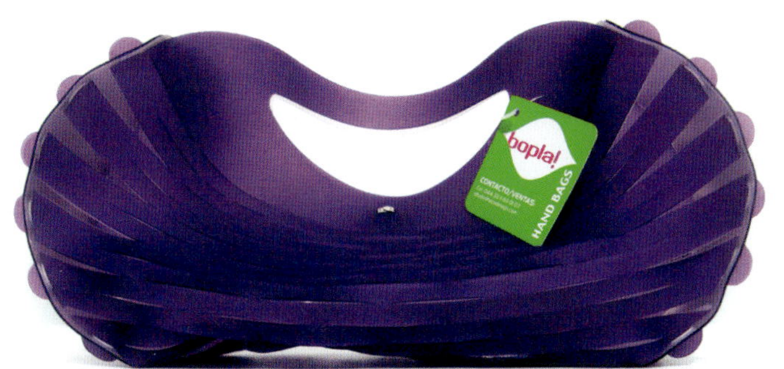

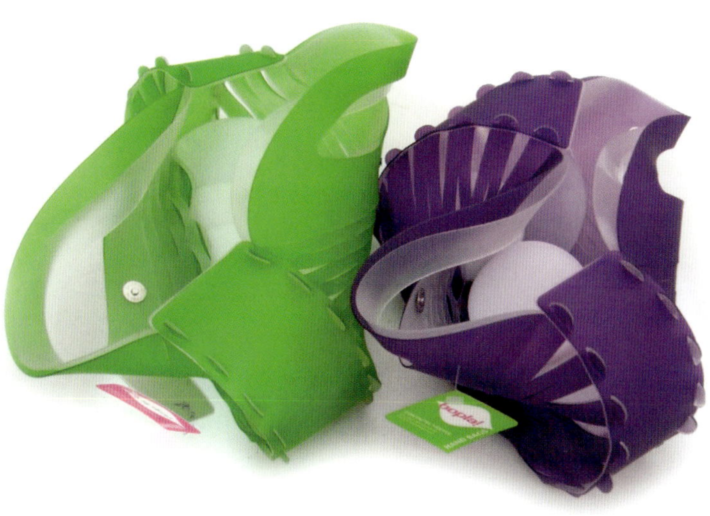

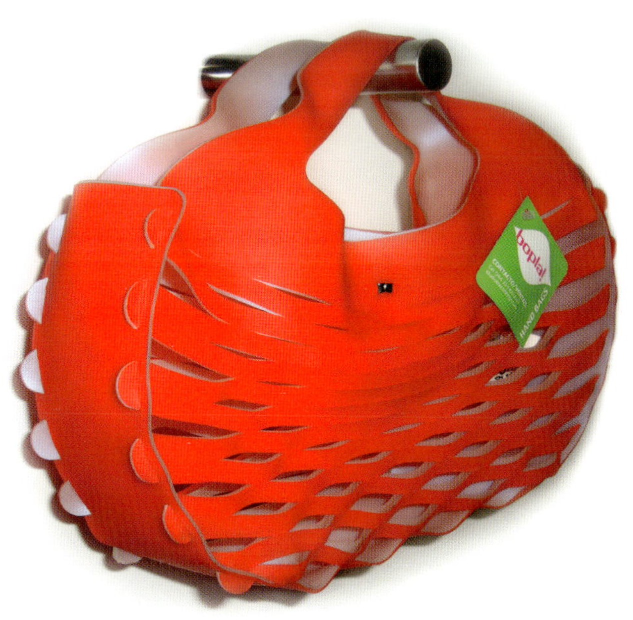

APPLE BAGS
DE: Jikka Ottlik

This series embraces works made of various materials, such as felt, plastic and leather, all in a bag big enough to carry two big apples perfectly.

BOPLA!
DE: Adrian Cervantes (AICO)

"Bopla!" is a series of bags made of flexible material for great functionality, characterized by their unique and peculiar shapes.

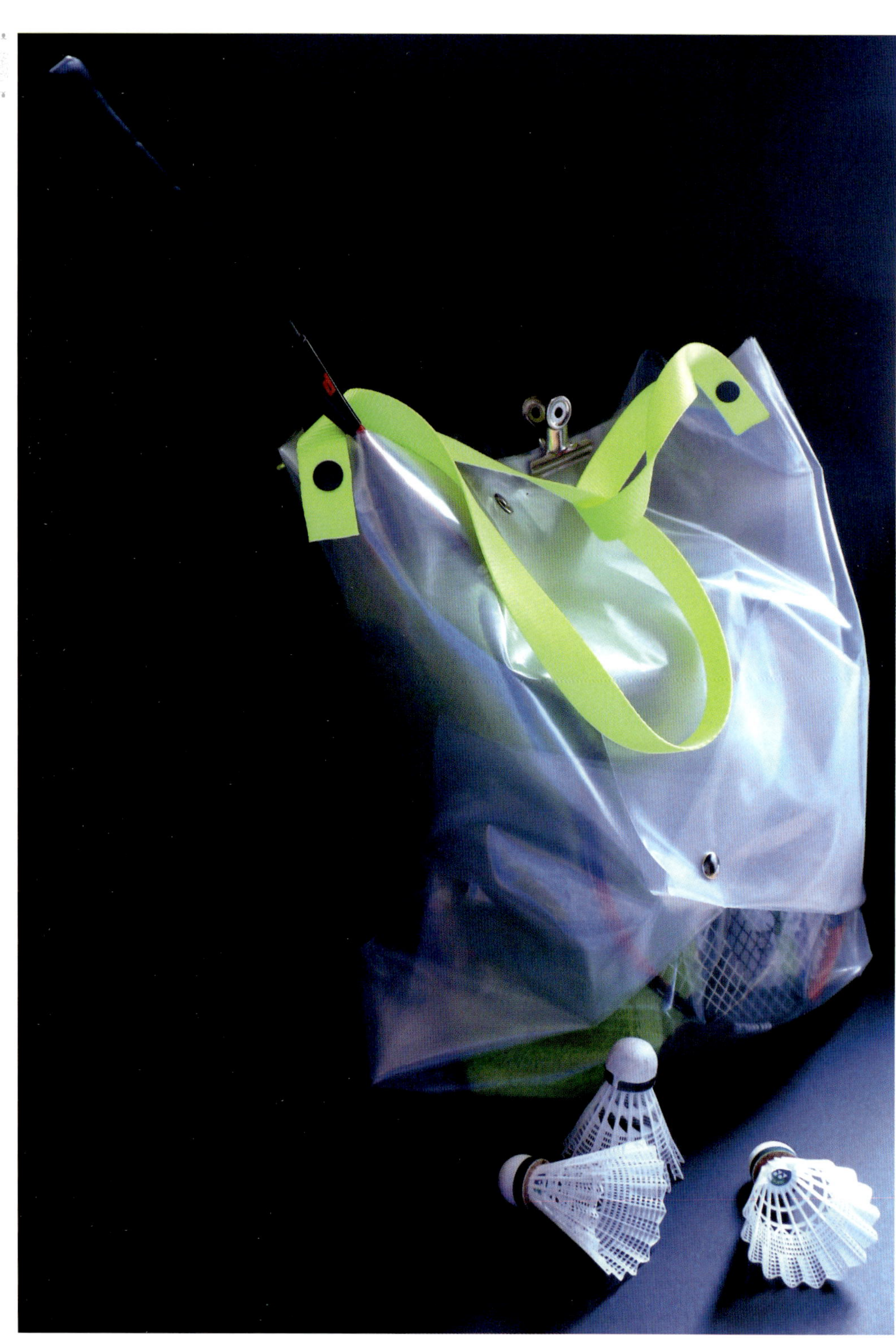

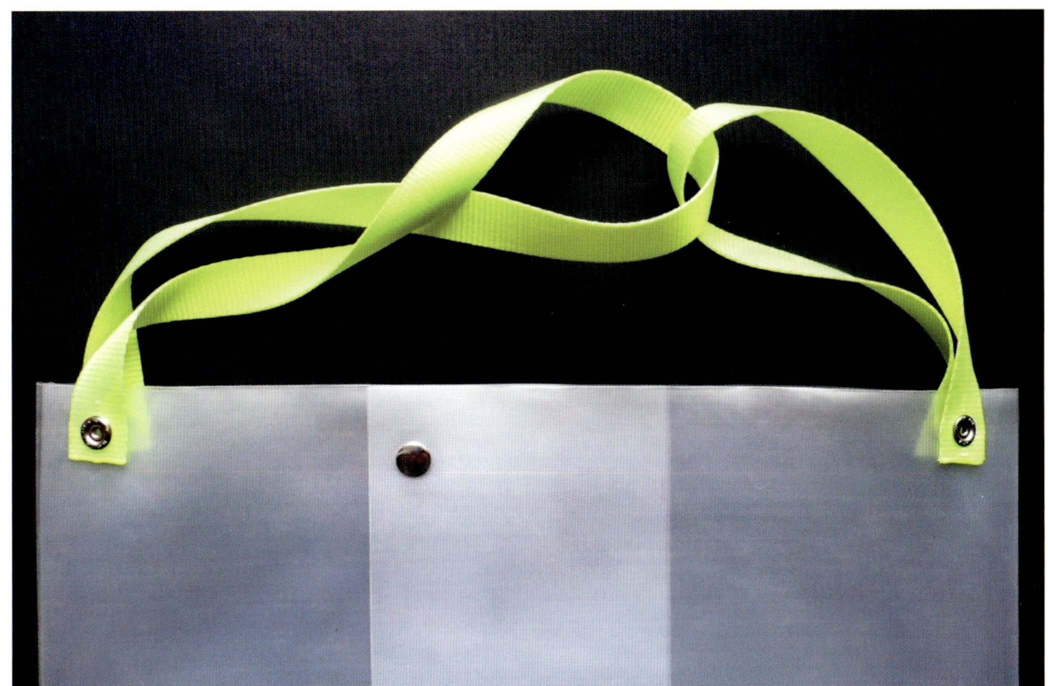

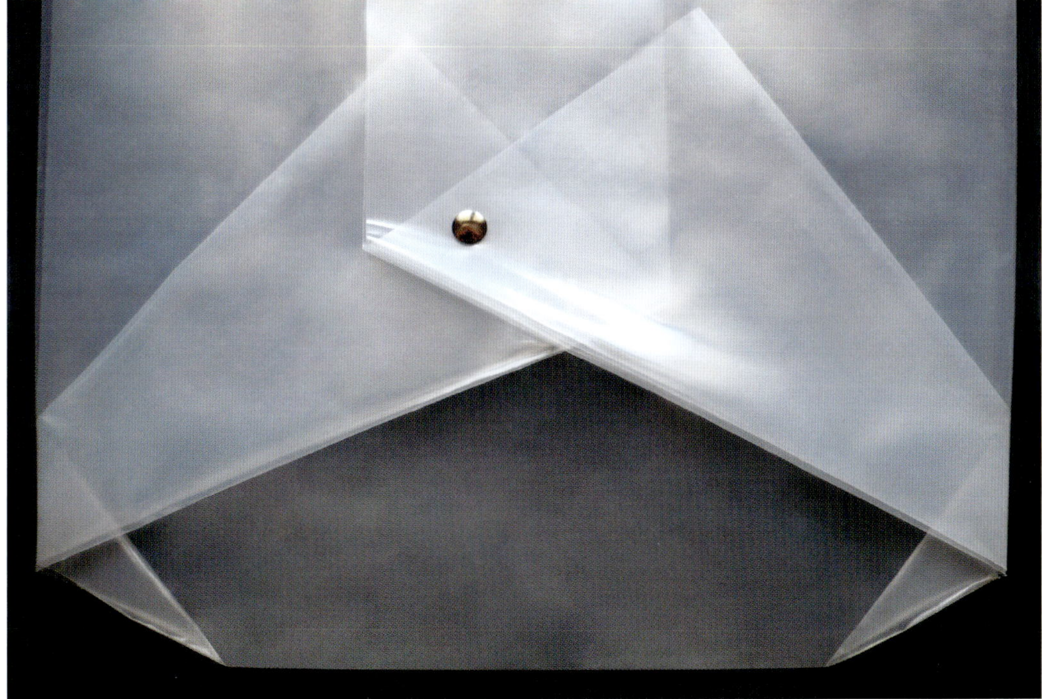

NEON STRAP BAG
DE: Alena Kurfürstova

This design is a simple folded plastic bag, made of a transparent
polyethylene and metallic poppers, completed with a carrying strap in
striking color.

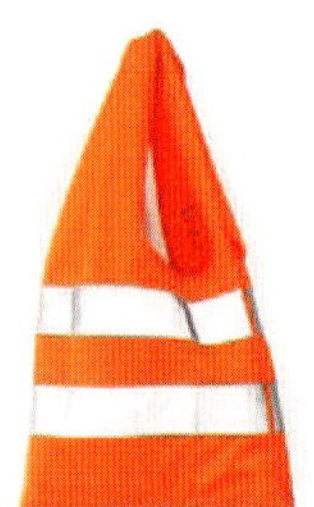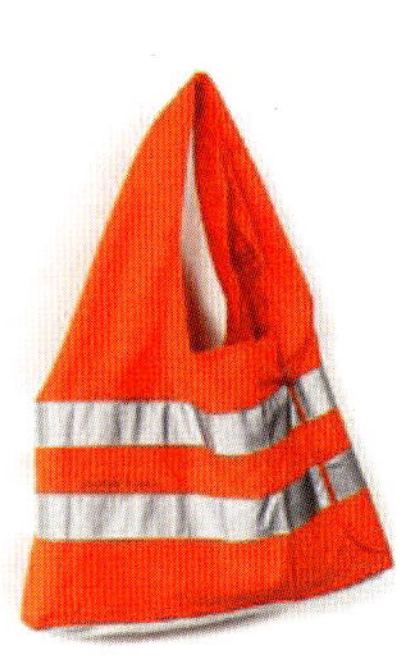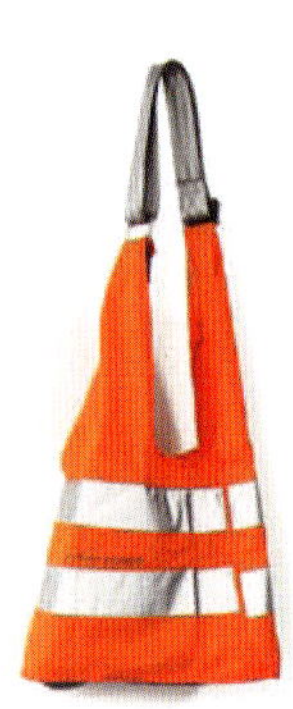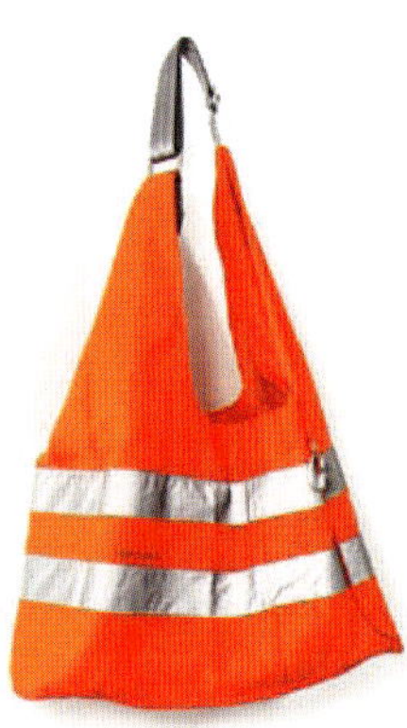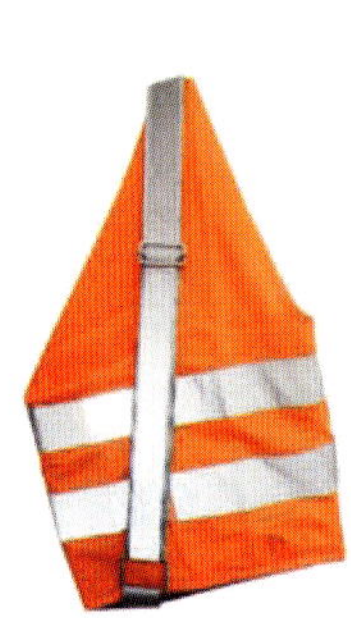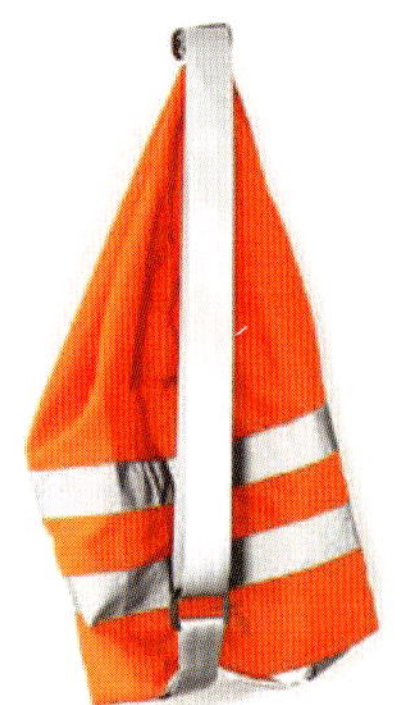

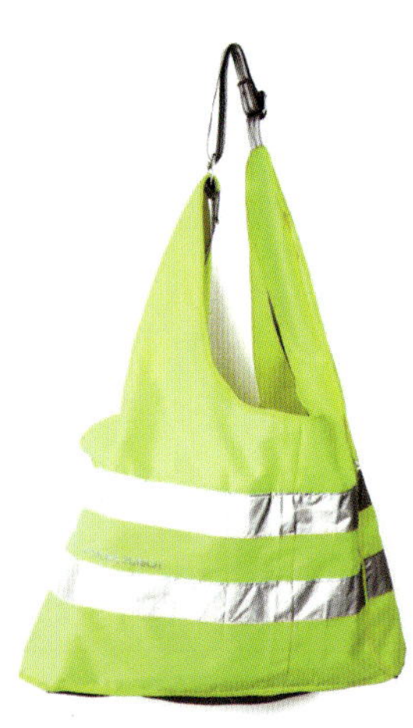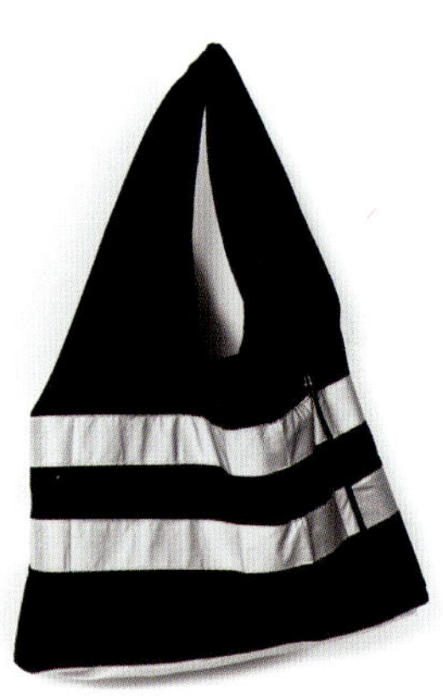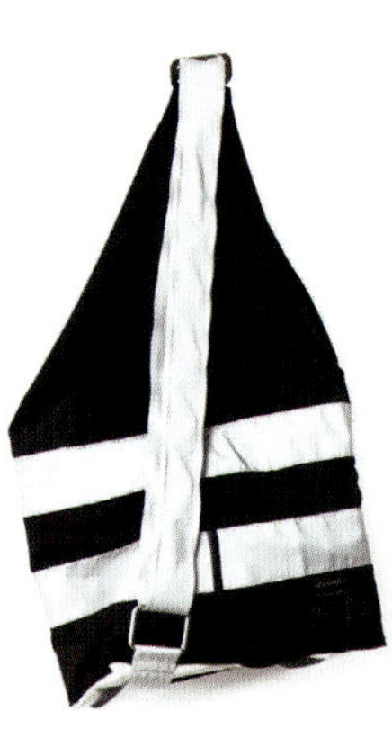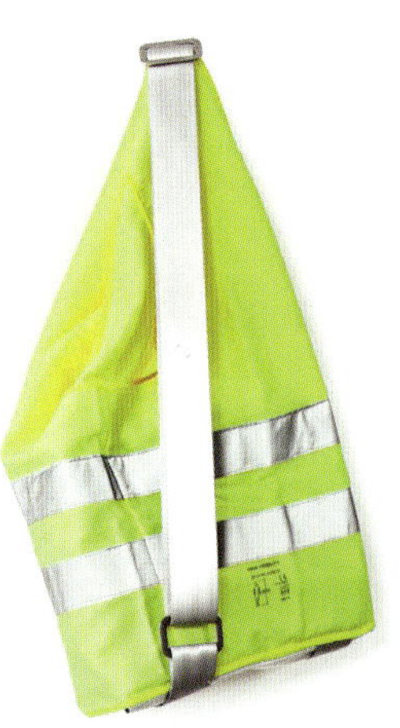

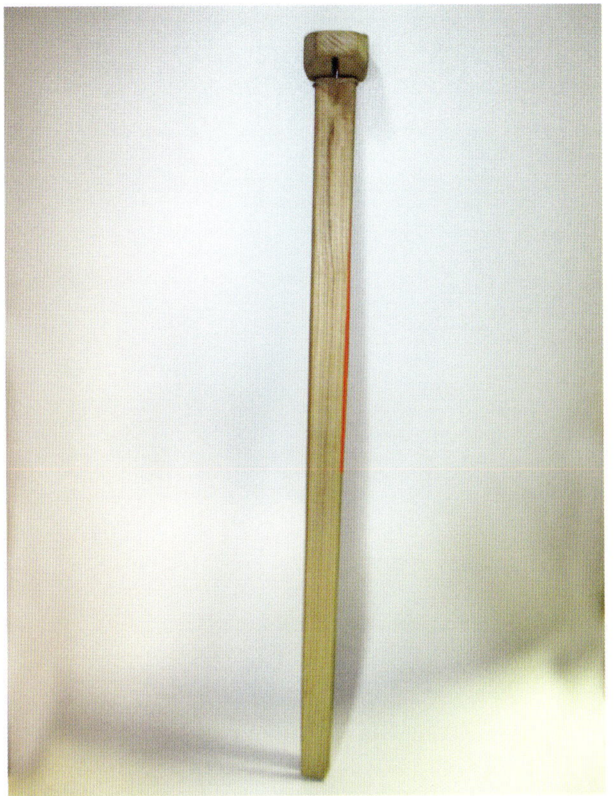 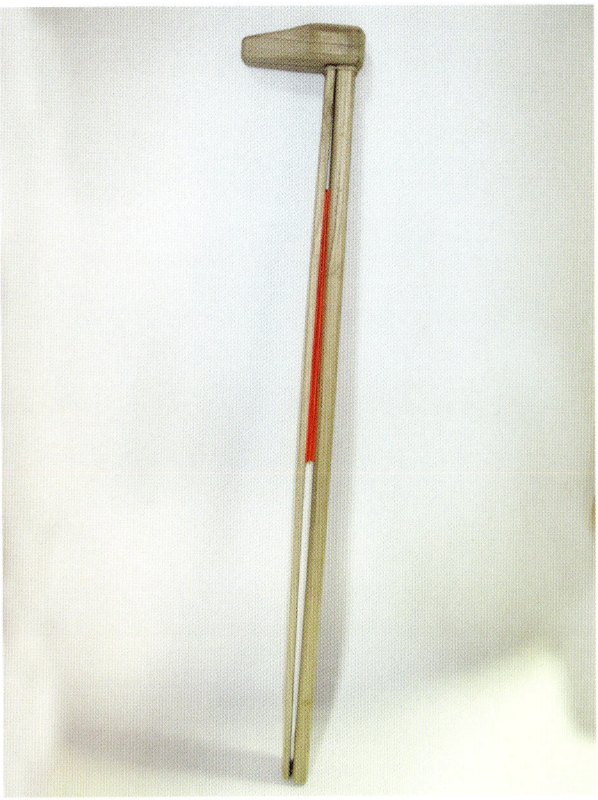

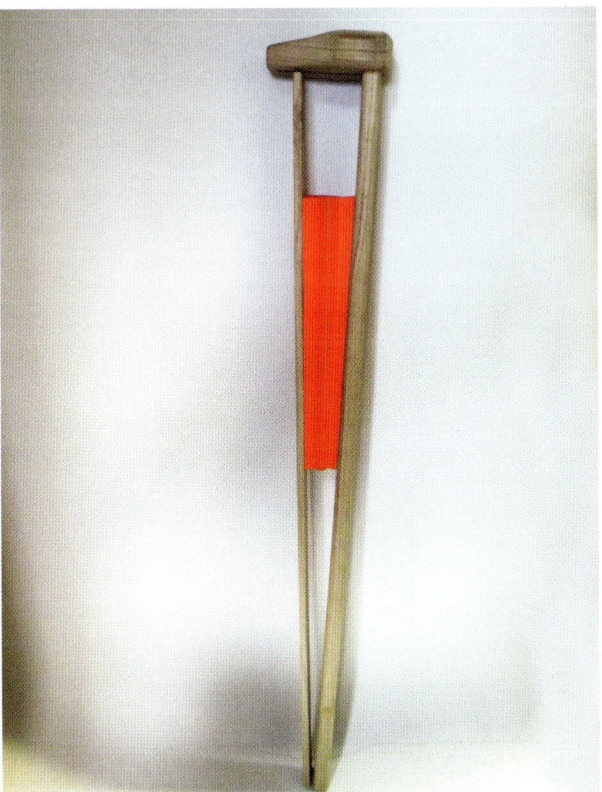 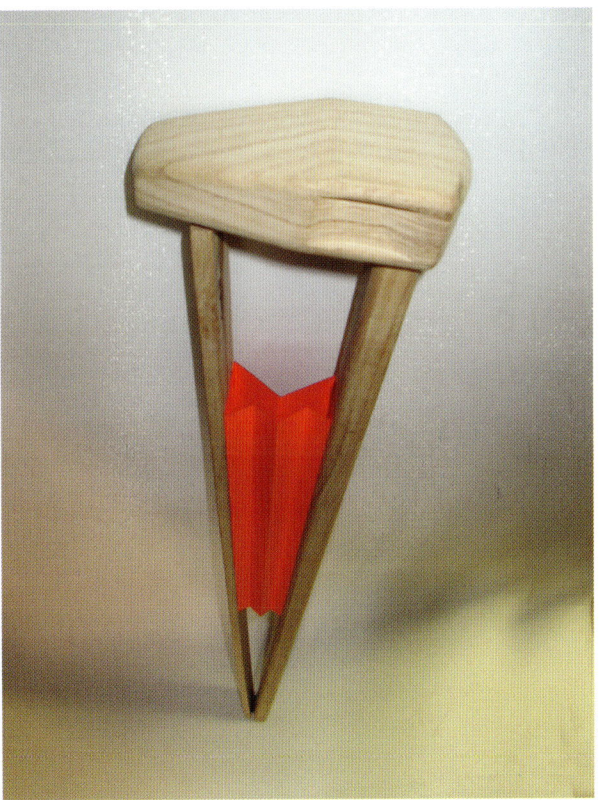

HIGH VISIBILITY BAGS
DA: Sputnik Zurich

Borrowing the striking colors from safety vests, this series is sure to get attention. They come in different models to suit varied preferences.

GHOST BAG
DE: Vittoria Negrin

Aiming to better assist those who need a walking stick, the "Ghost Bag" features a container for odds and ends, which opens with only a flick of the thumb.

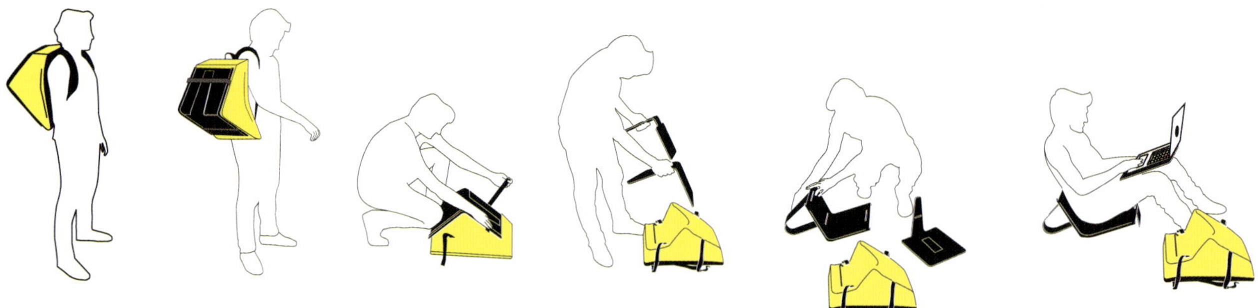

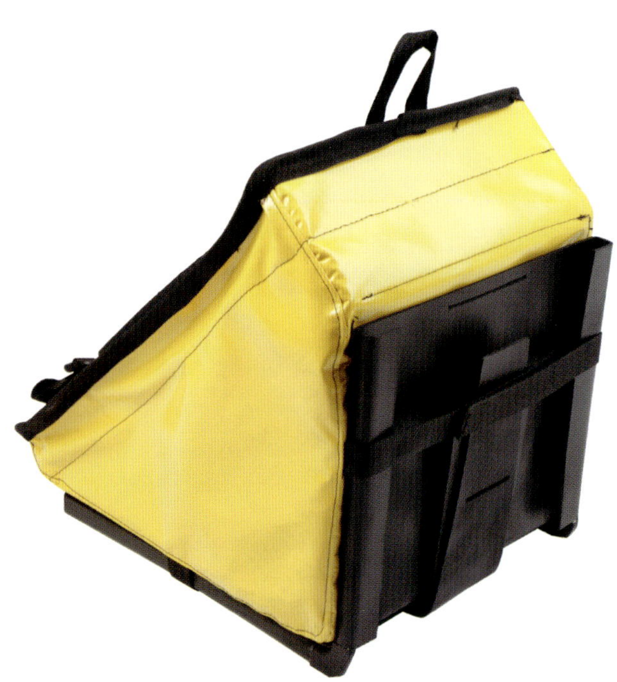

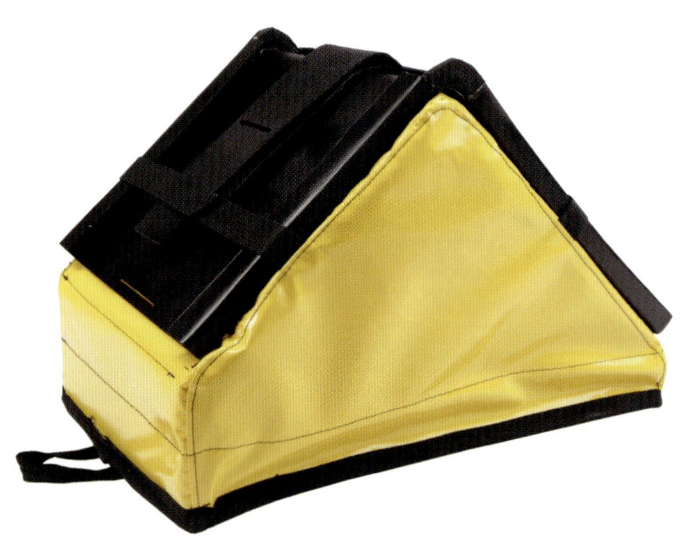

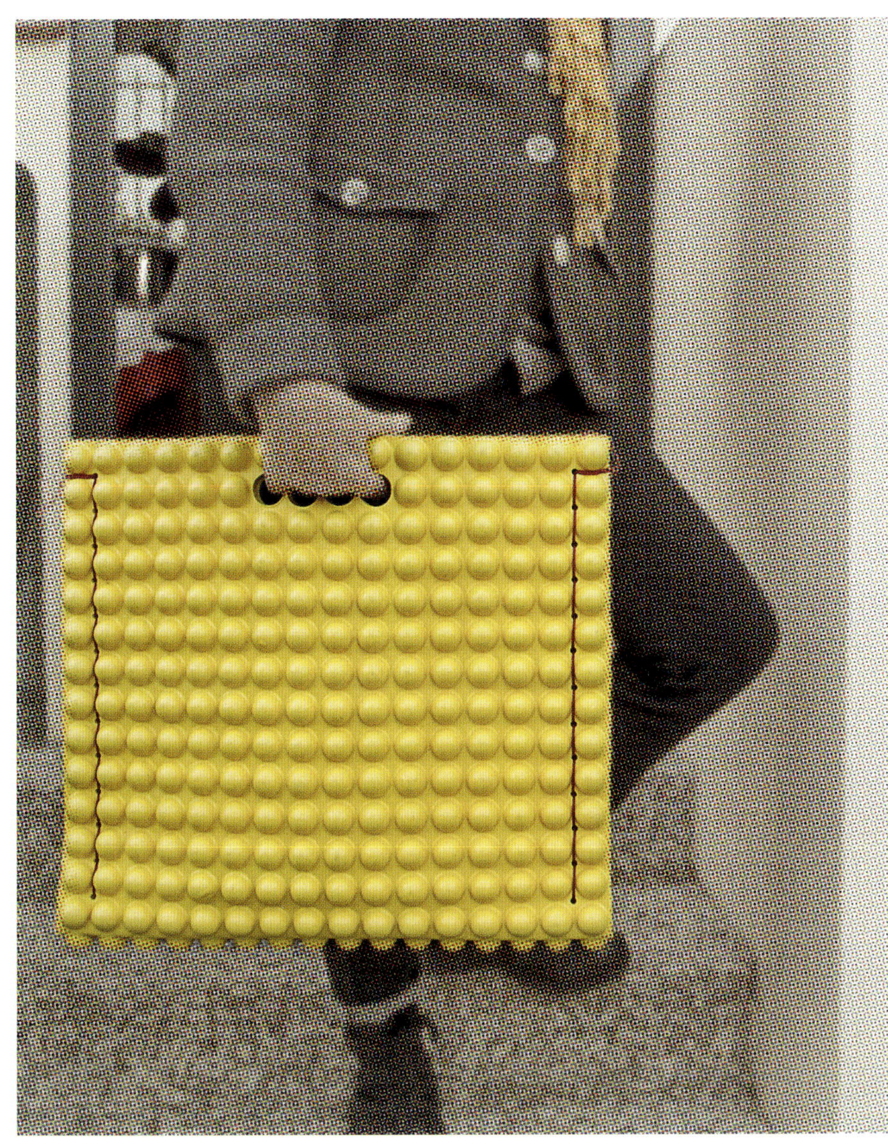

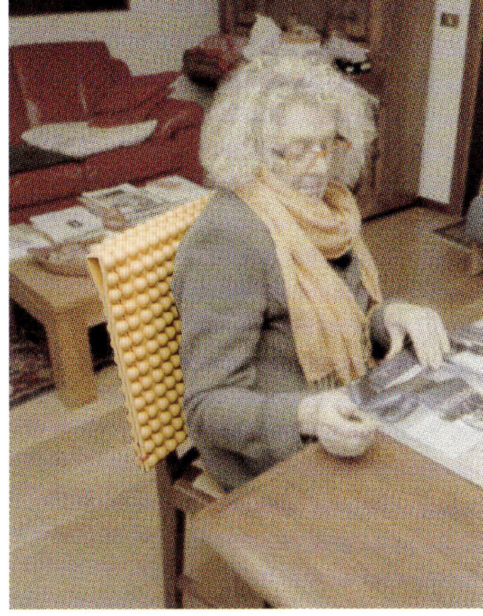

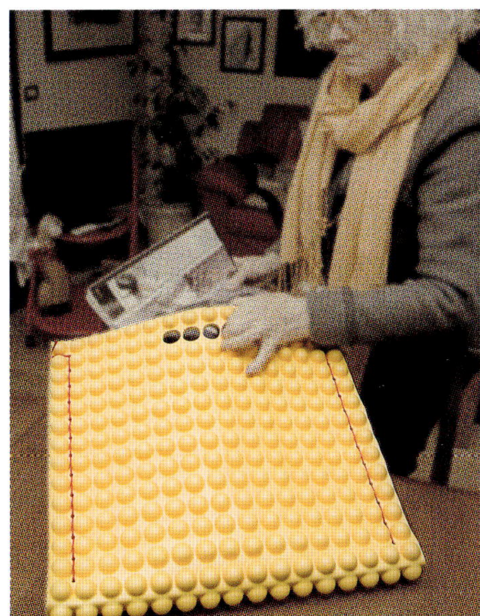

CHAIRBAG

DE: Laura Pison, Elisabetta Costa, Giulio Mazzanti

The "Chairbag" is an authentic backpack designed to turn into a comfortable chair with small table to enjoy the outdoors.

FORMOSA

DE: Giulio Perencin

Made of a sheet of an elastic material, a material that returns to its original shape after being crushed, the bag serves various functions. It can be used to carry things or as a backrest.

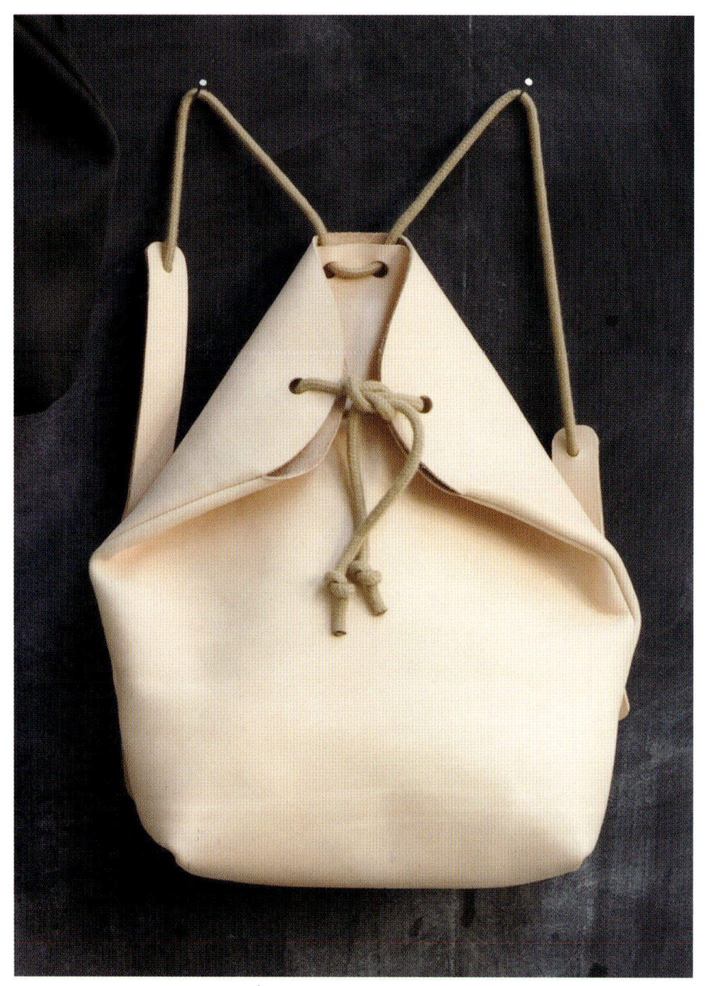
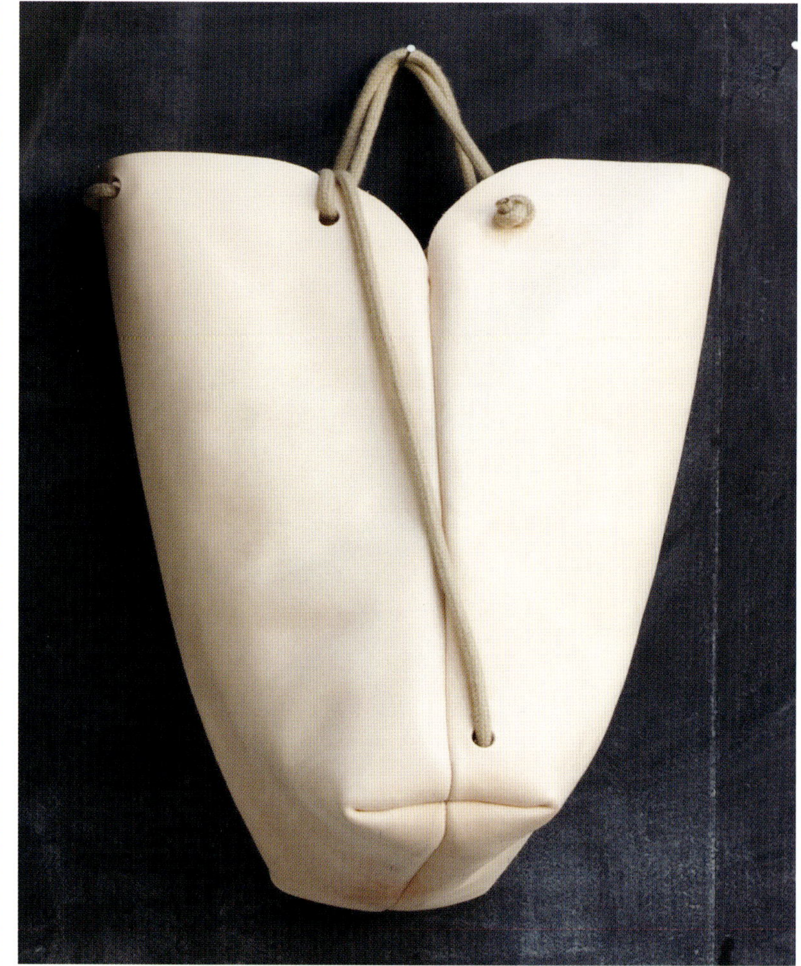

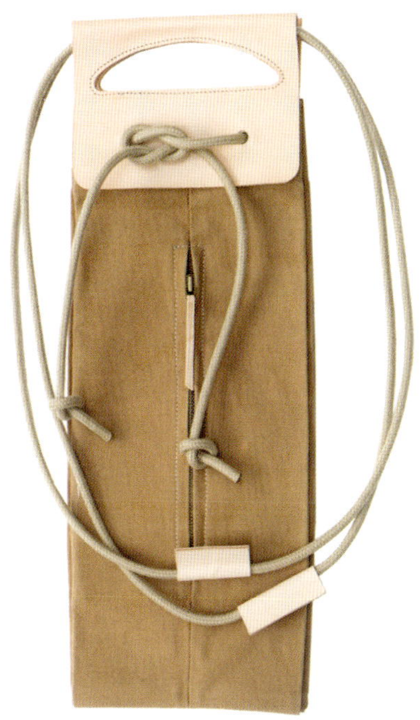

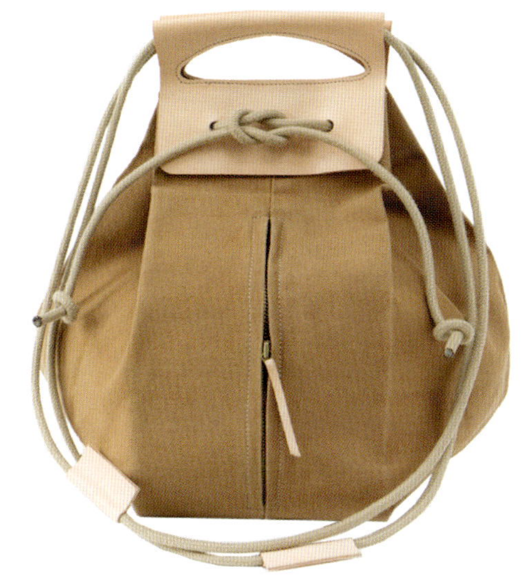

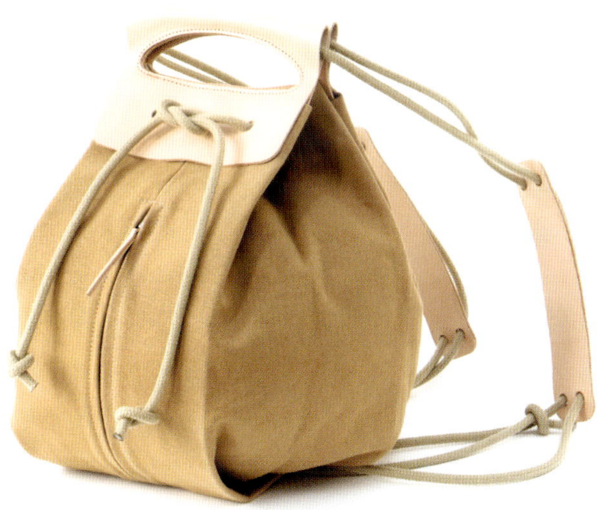

RUCKSACK NUDE
DE: Chris Van Veghel

Designed to be foldable, this design switches from a backpack to a handbag
with simple rope adjustment.

POP-UP BAG BUTTERSCOTCH
DE: Chris Van Veghel

Based on only three folds, this bag becomes entirely flat when emptied and
can be worn differently when the strings are tied in differing manners.

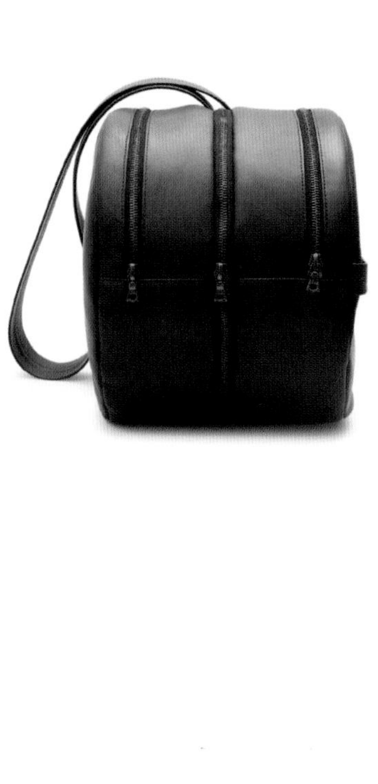
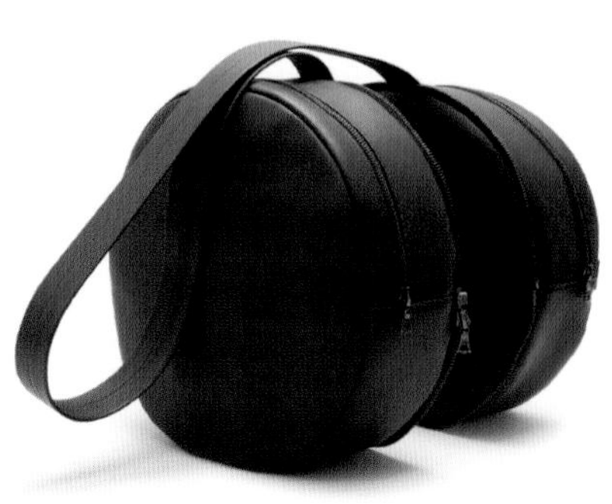
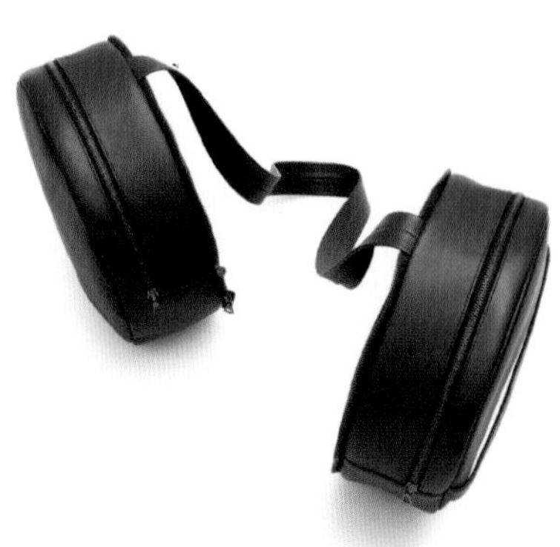
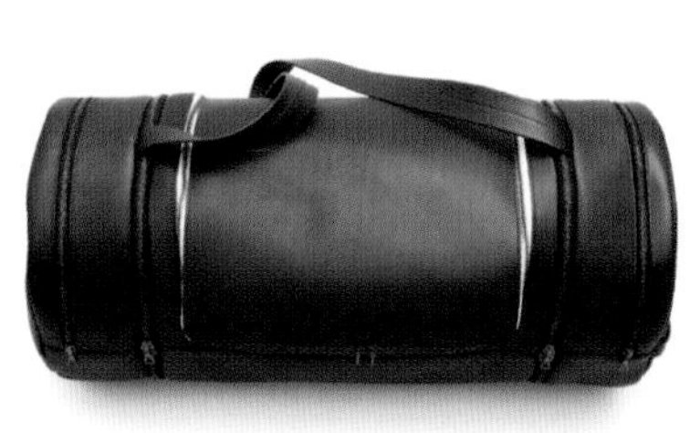
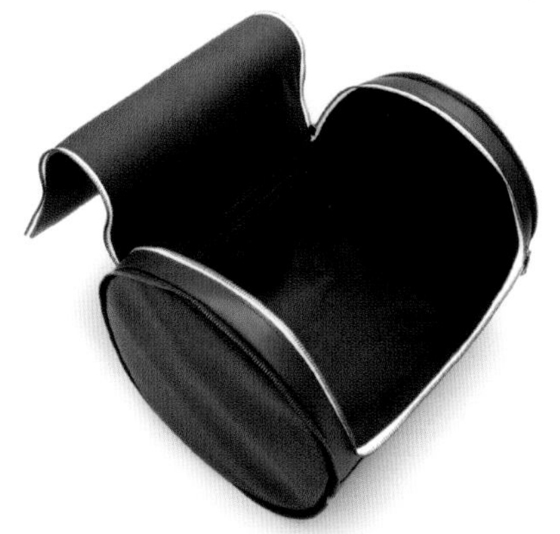
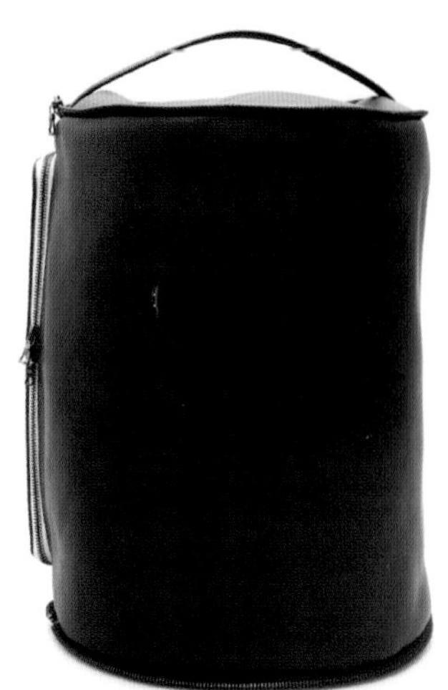
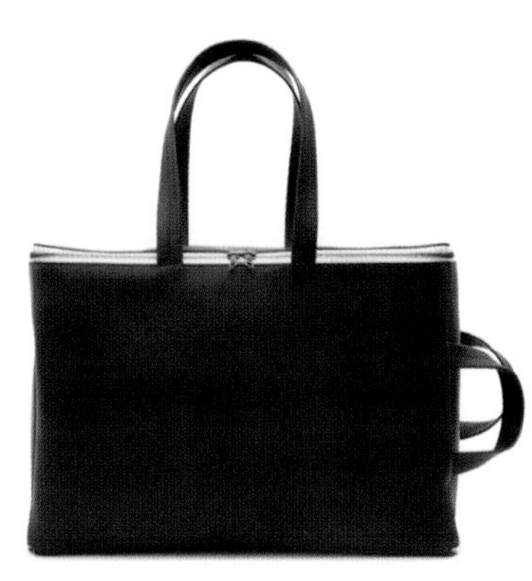
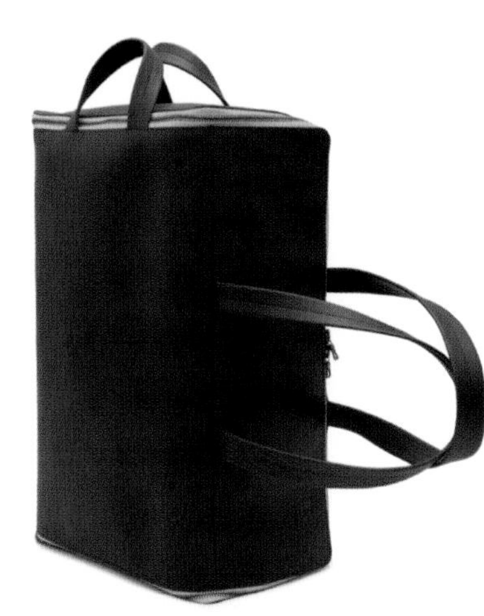
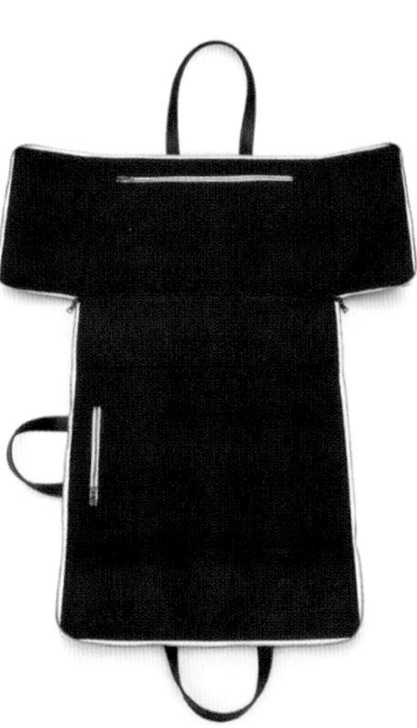

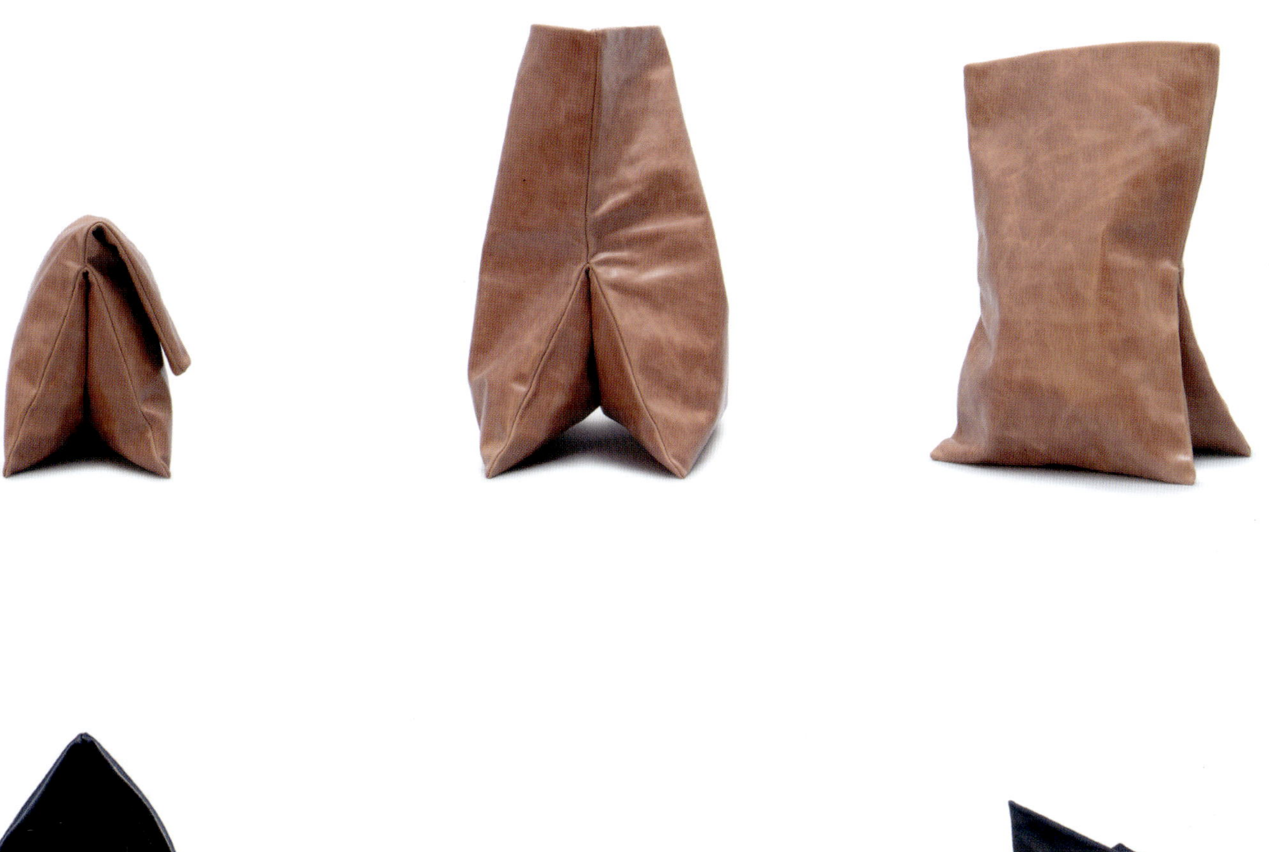

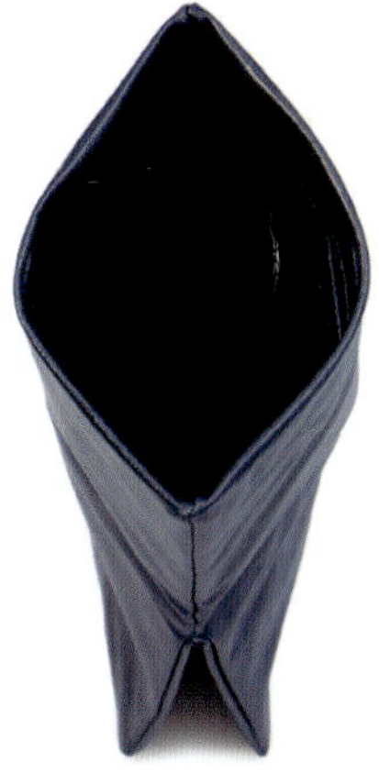

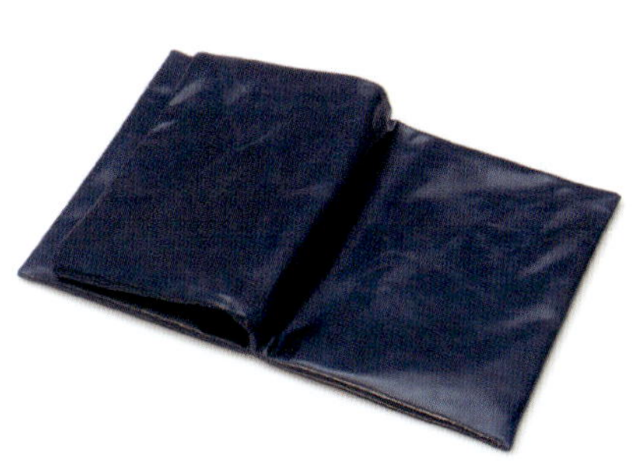

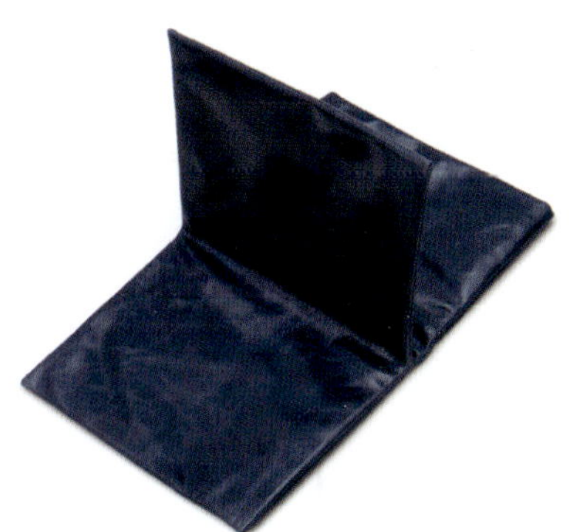

OTAAT
DA: Otaat

The "Otaat" is characterized by monochrome panels, wrap-around zippers,
integral construction and striking shapes.

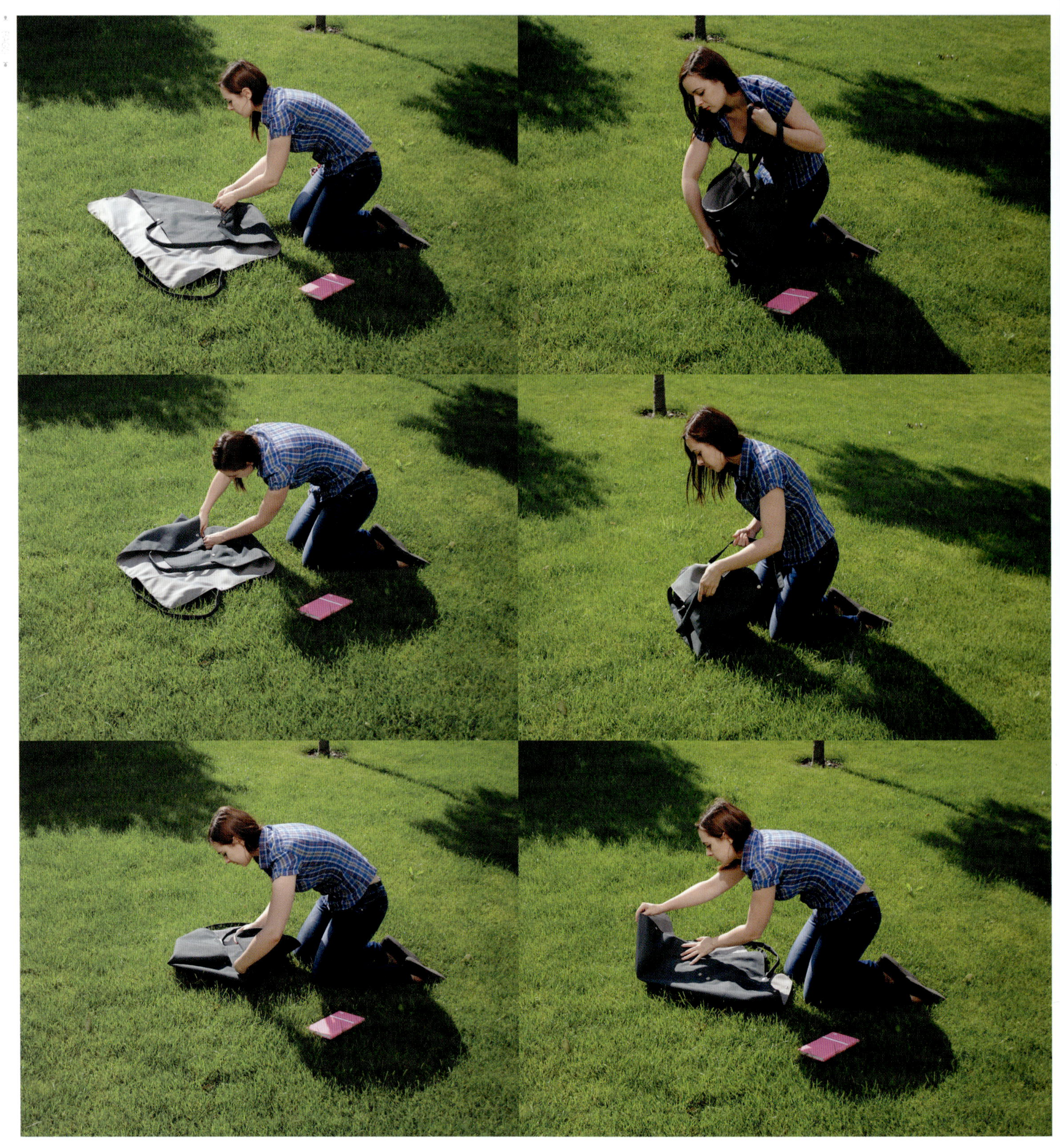

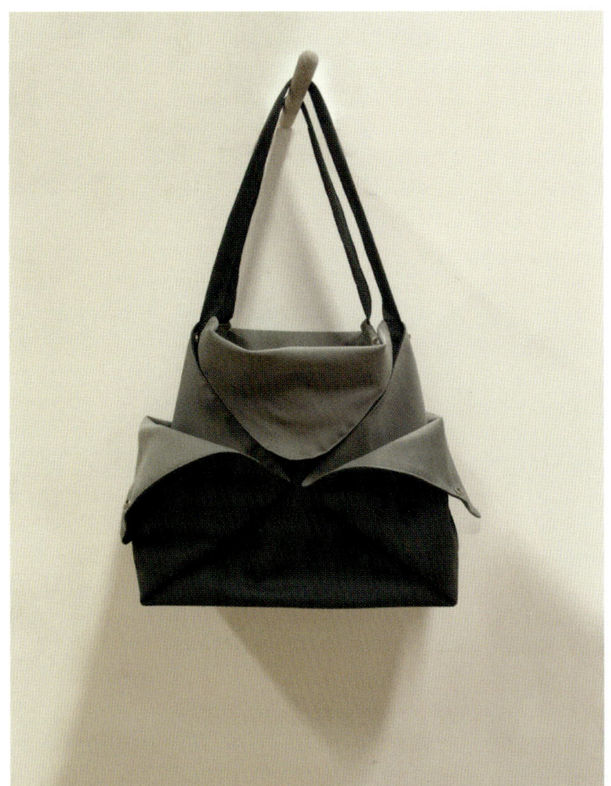

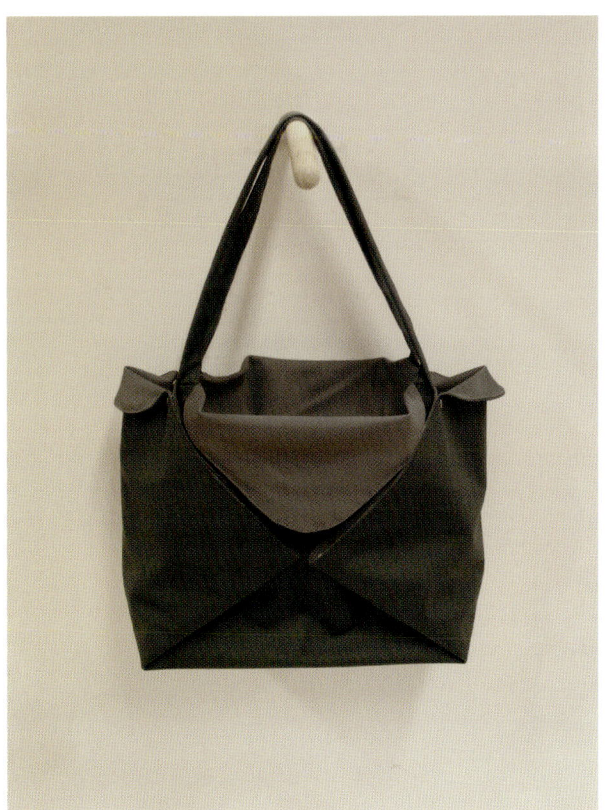

BIG PICNIC BAG
DE: Bc. Aneta Marholdová

Designed with a fastening device, the bag easily unfolds, expanding
enormously to a dimension of 1000x1000mm. When used as a picnic blanket, the
bottom of the bag can support a glass or bowl.

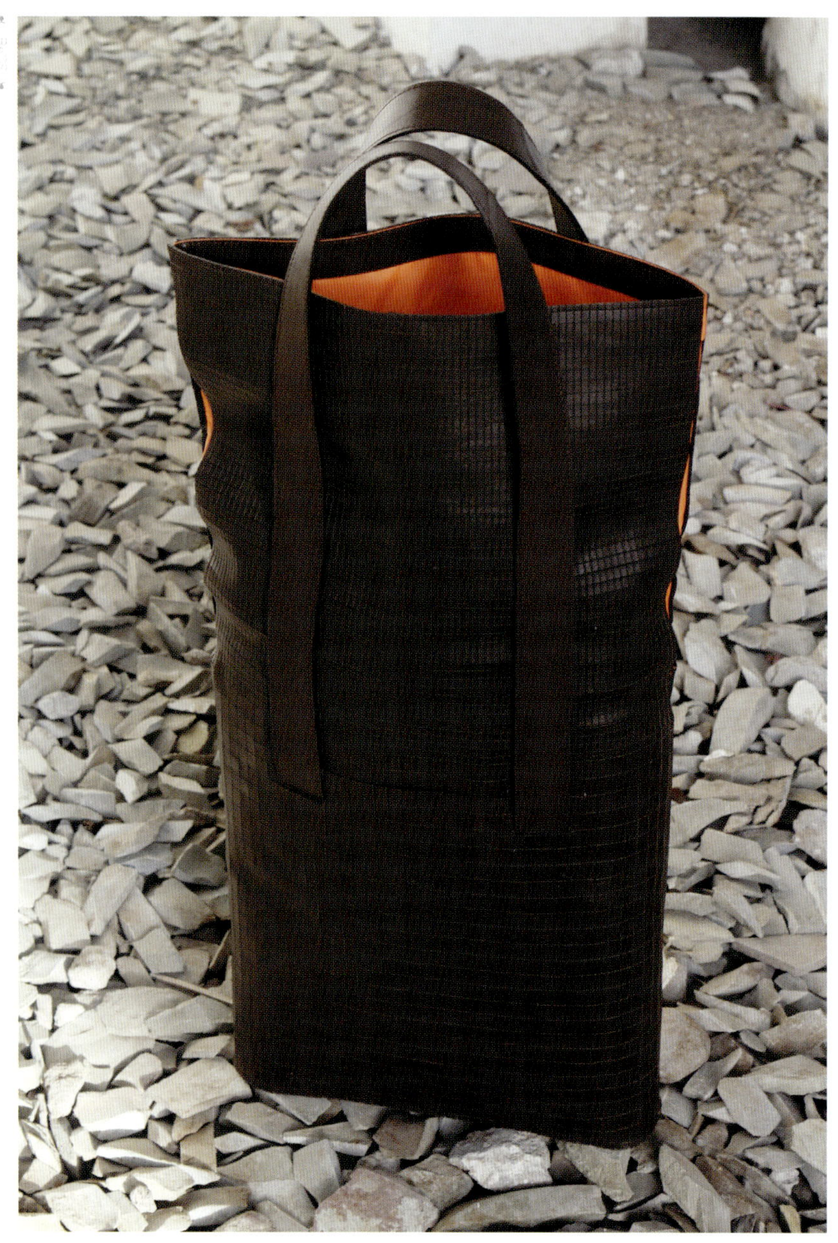
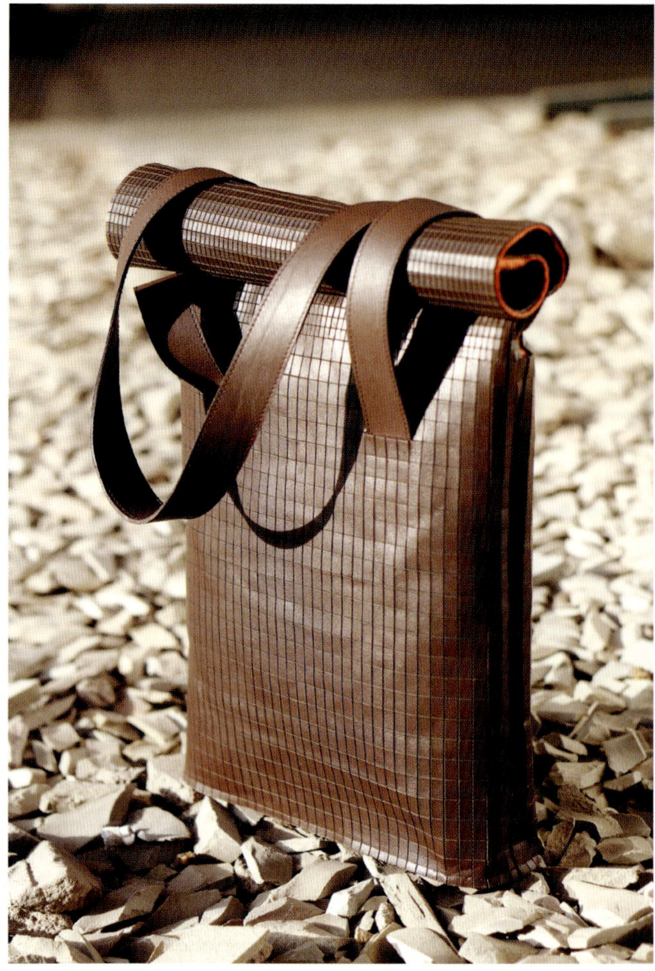

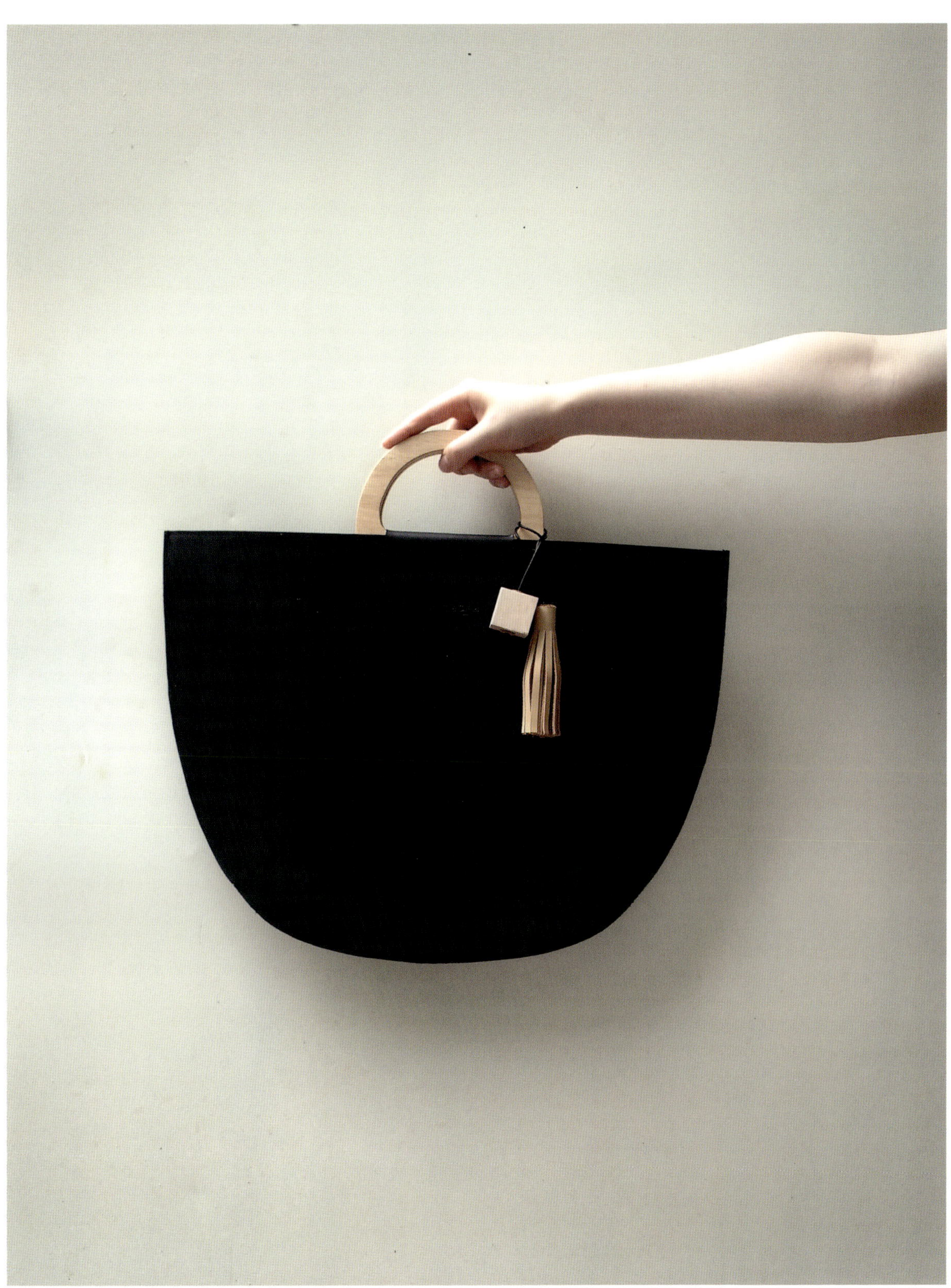

RECHERCHÉ
DE: Abhilasha Jhalani

Aiming to create a leather tote with dramatic proportions and style, this
design has only one storage space, the capacity of which changes with
folding and rolling. It was created entirely in leather, even the stiff body
part.

WOODEN HANDLE BAG
DA: Black Swan

Highlighted by the wooden handle, this design present a harmonic combination
of texture and color.

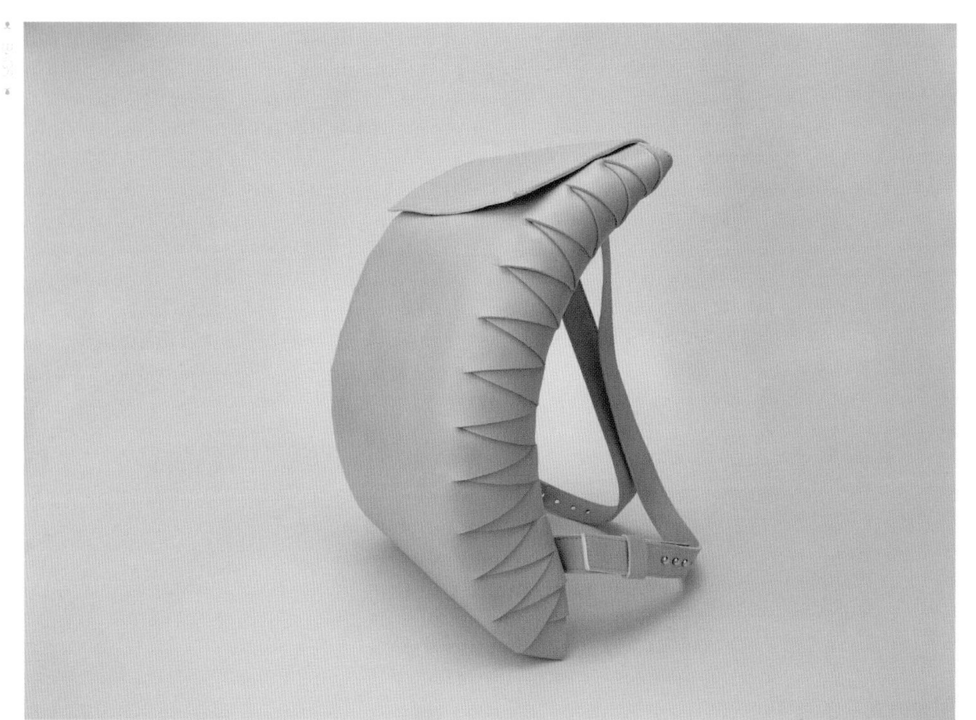

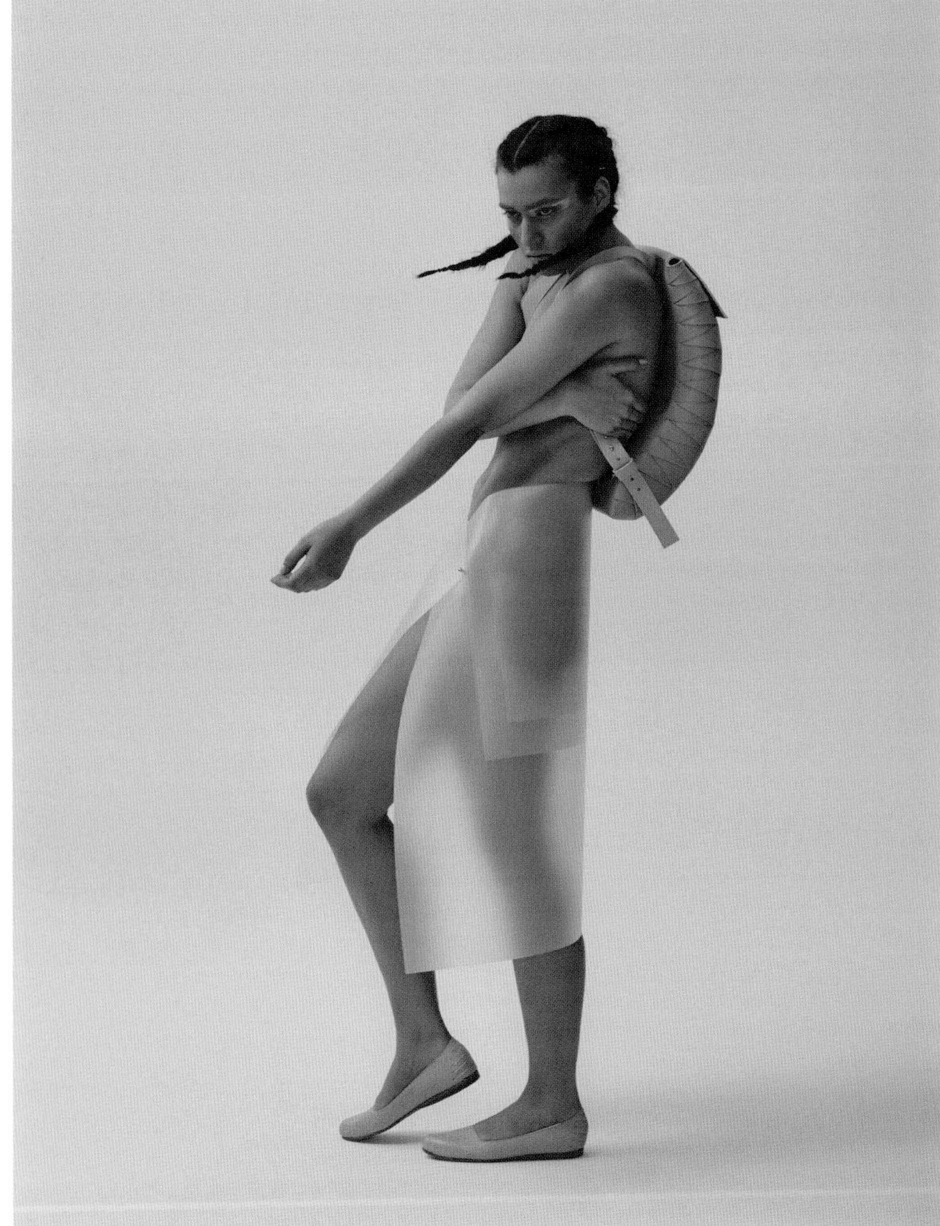

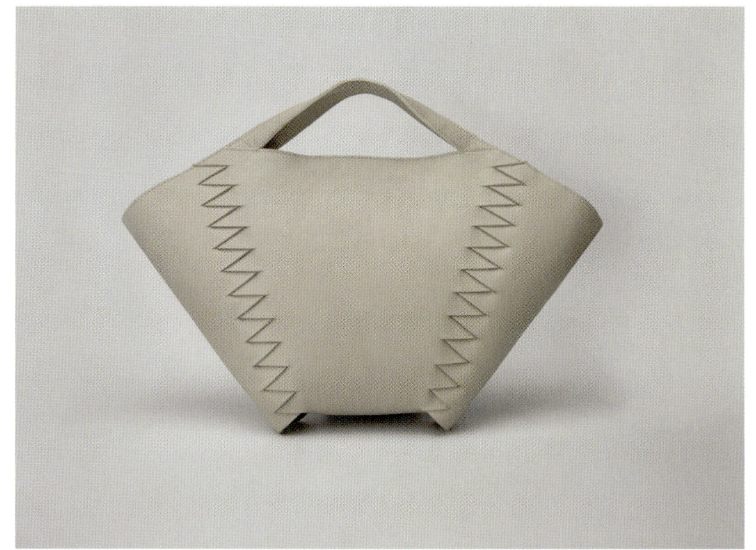
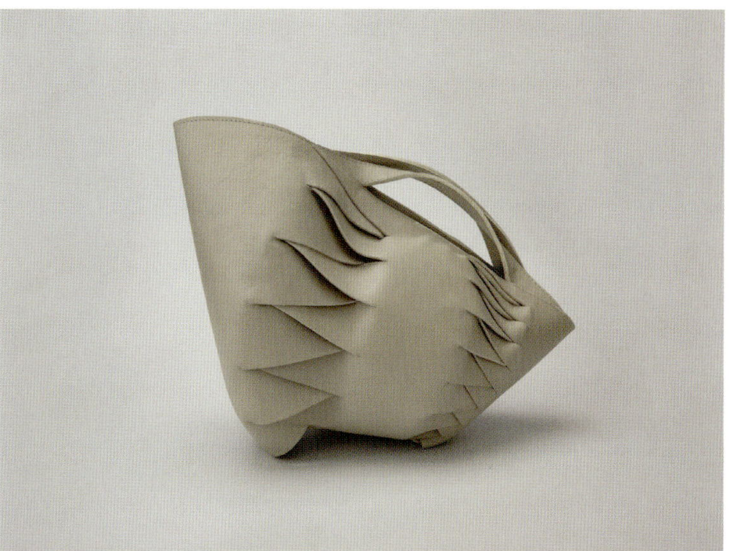
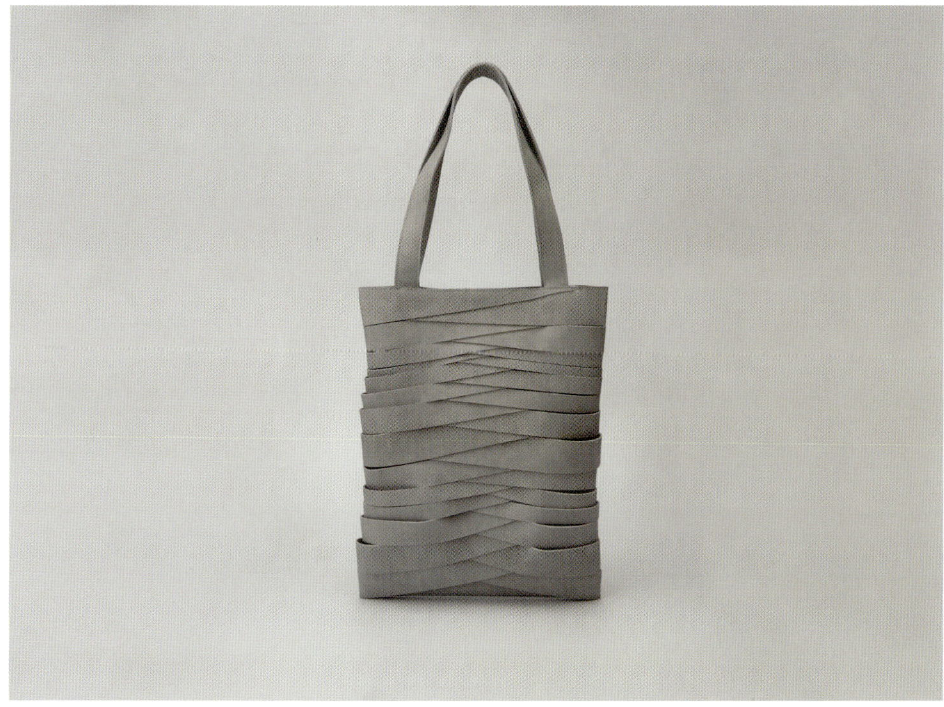
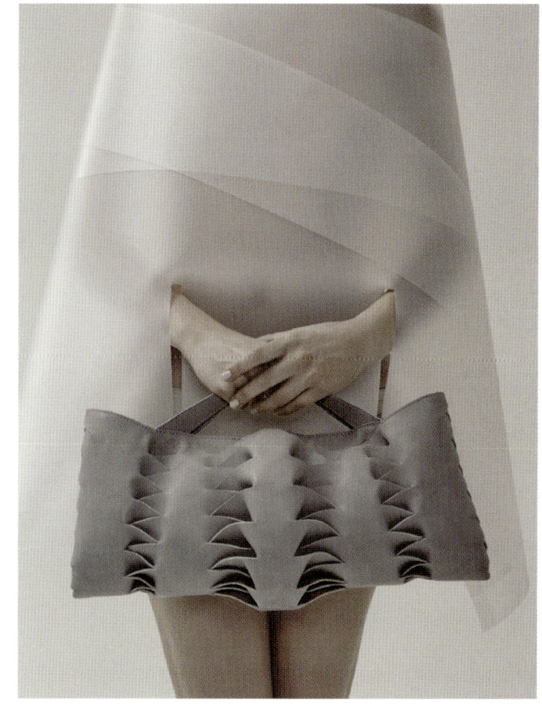

SYSTEM AND FORM
DE: Agnes Kovacs

Combining a hair braiding techique and a one-piece flat surface, the designer used cowhide and pigskin to create this bag in various shapes fixed with studs.

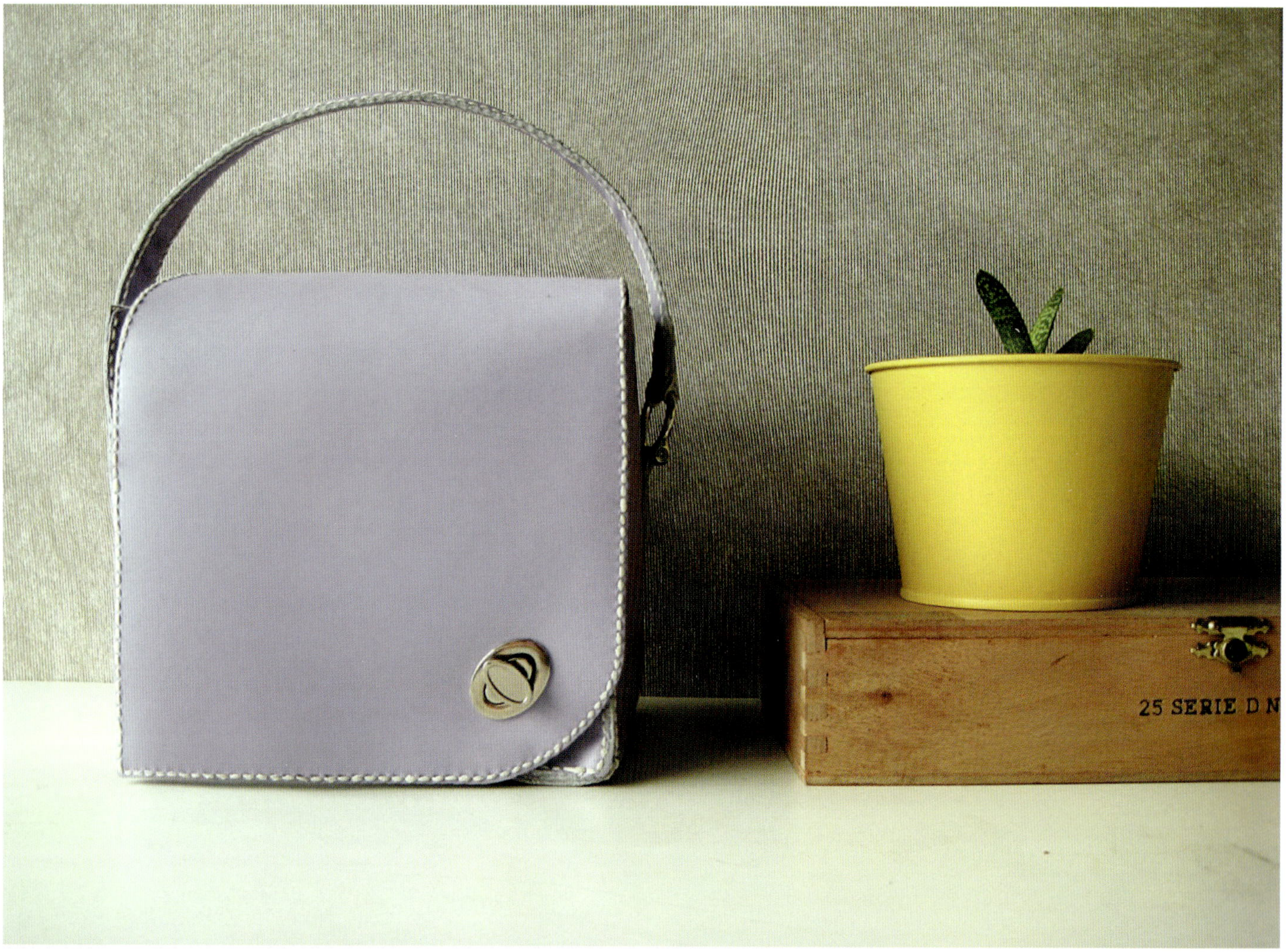

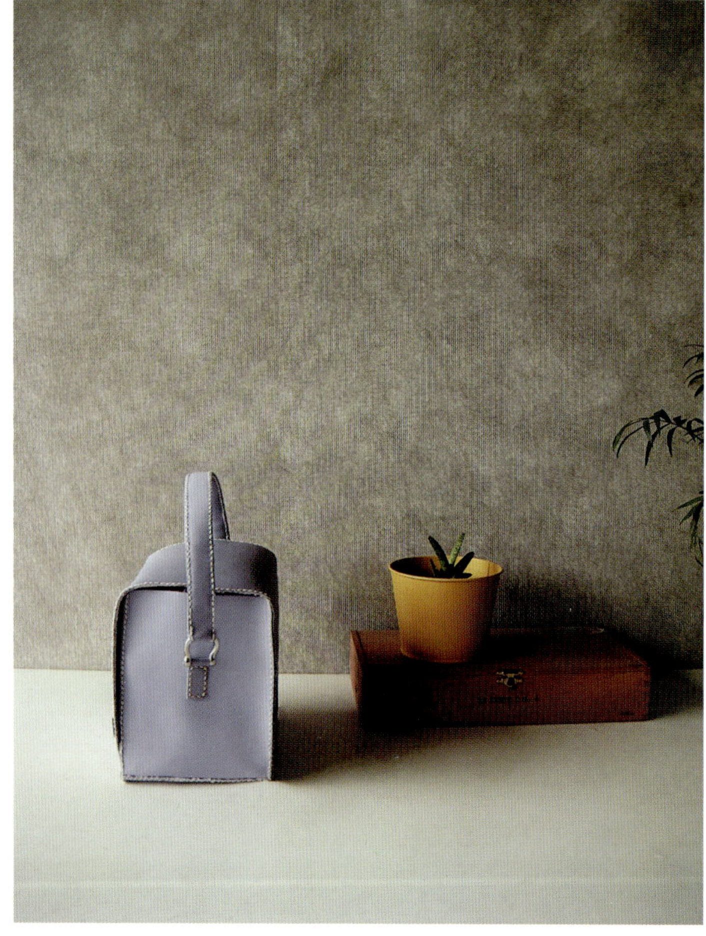
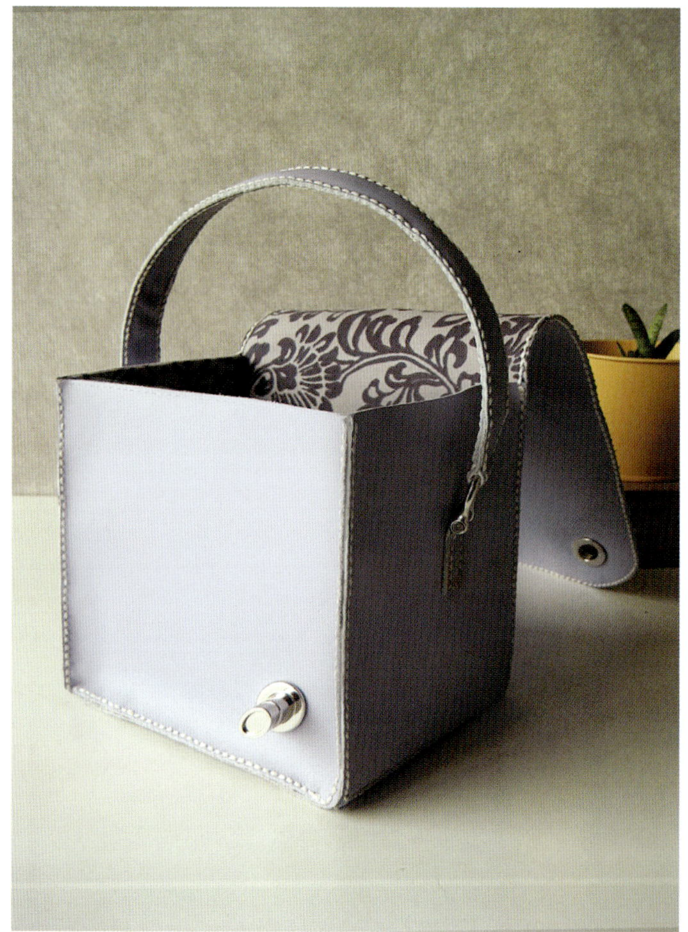

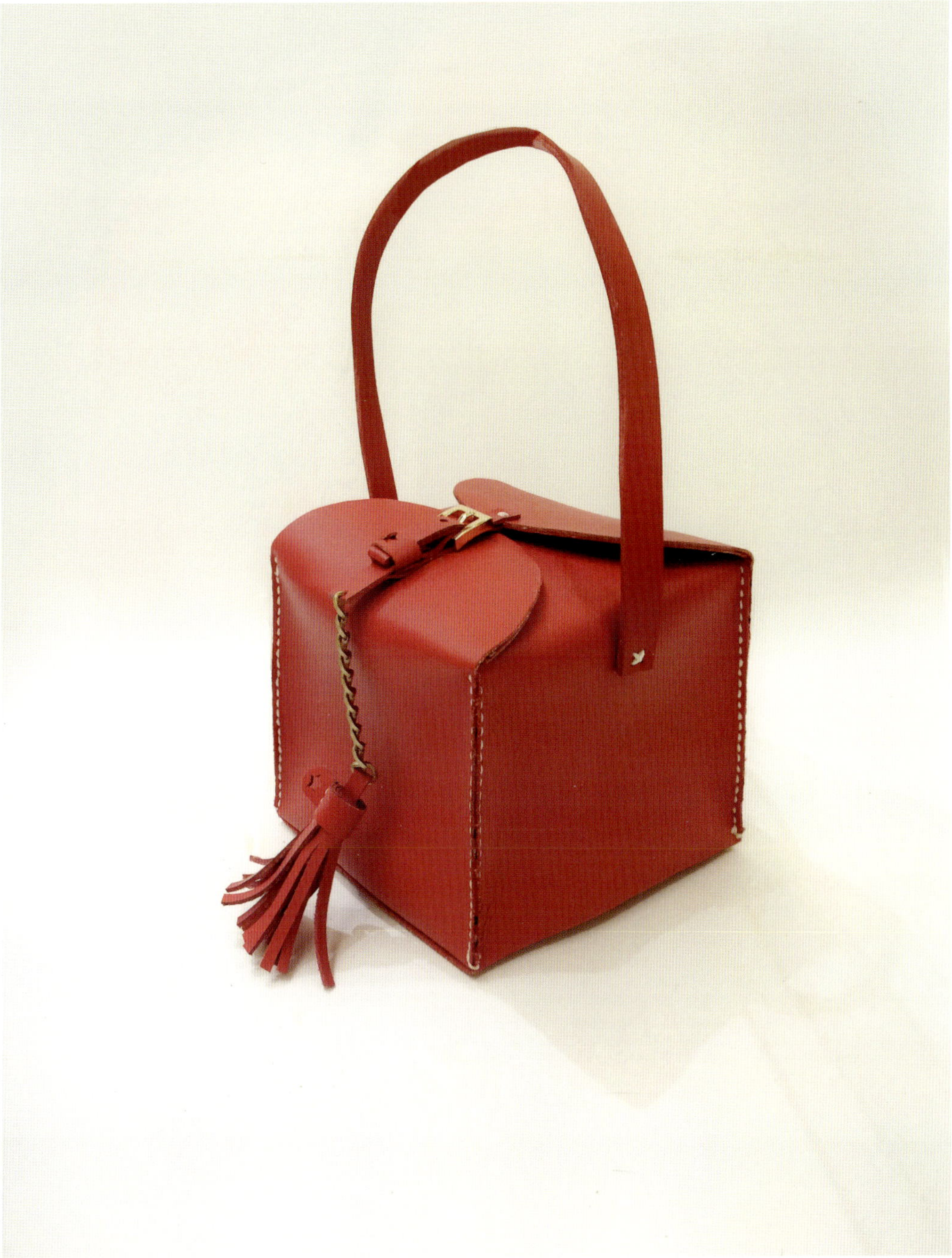

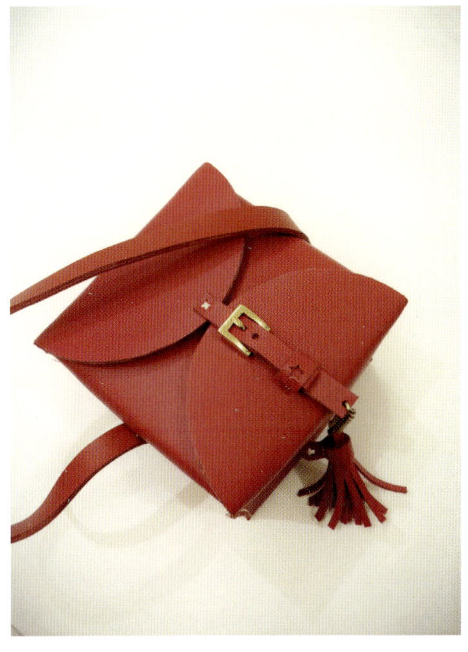

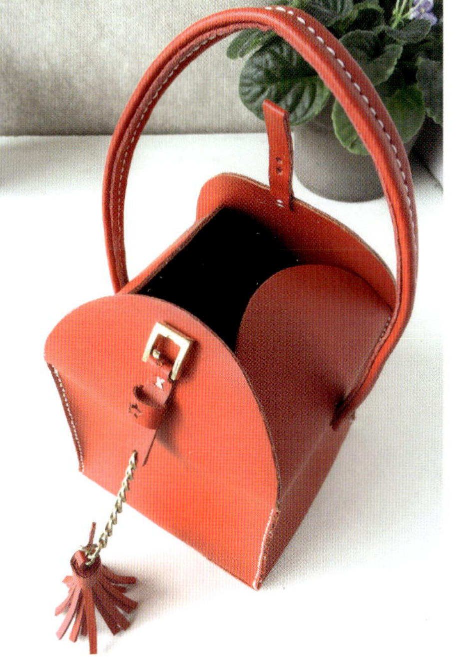

CUBE HANDBAG
DA: Zemoneni

Shaped like a cube, the purple one flips to reveal storage space while the
red model pops open like a Chinese take-out box.

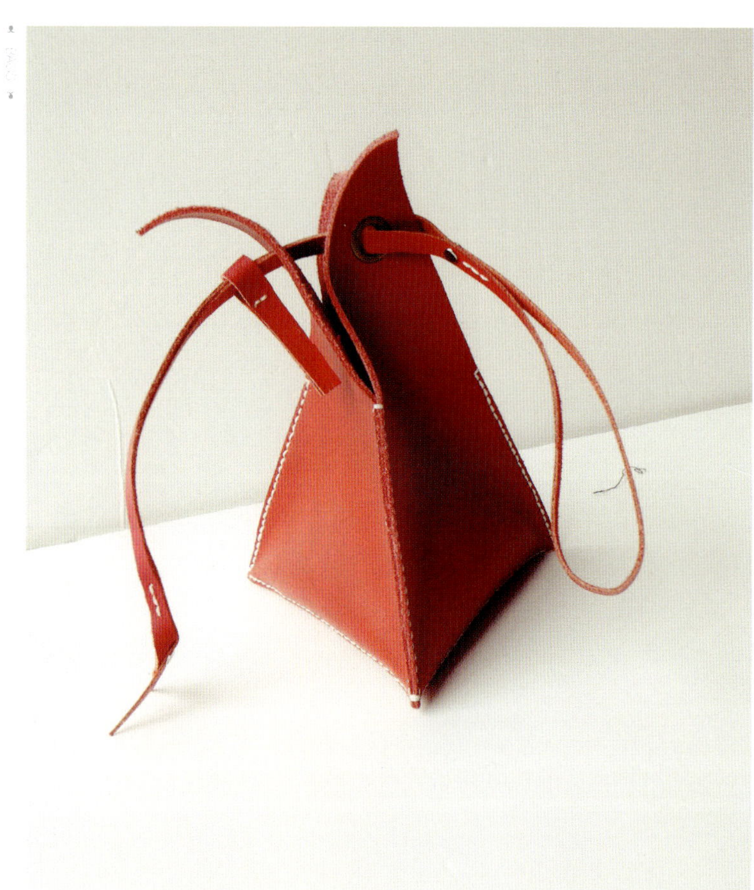
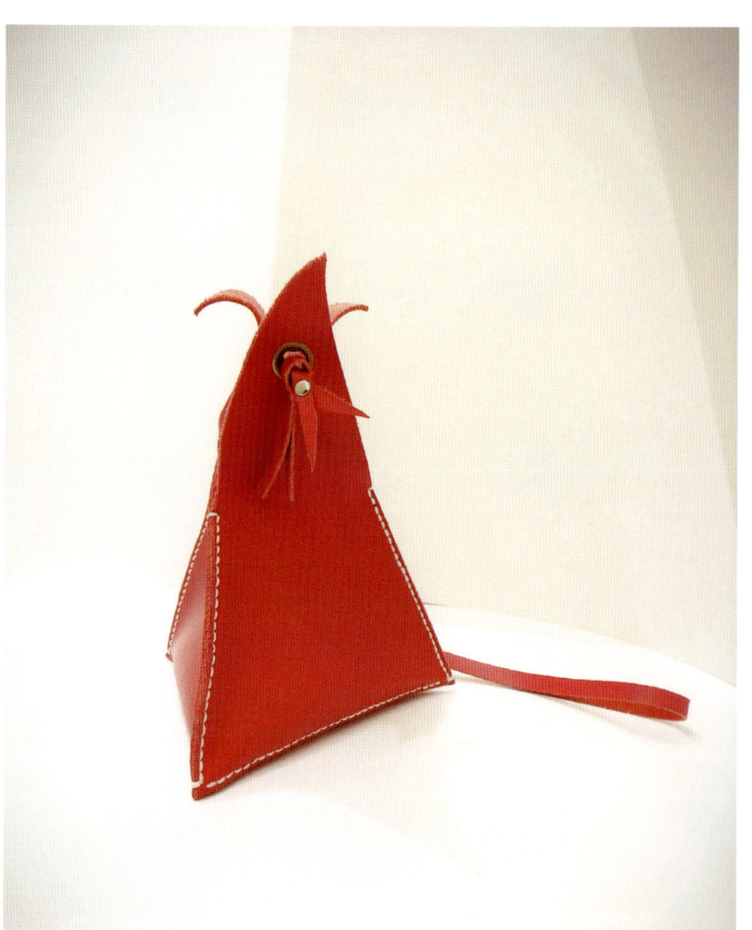
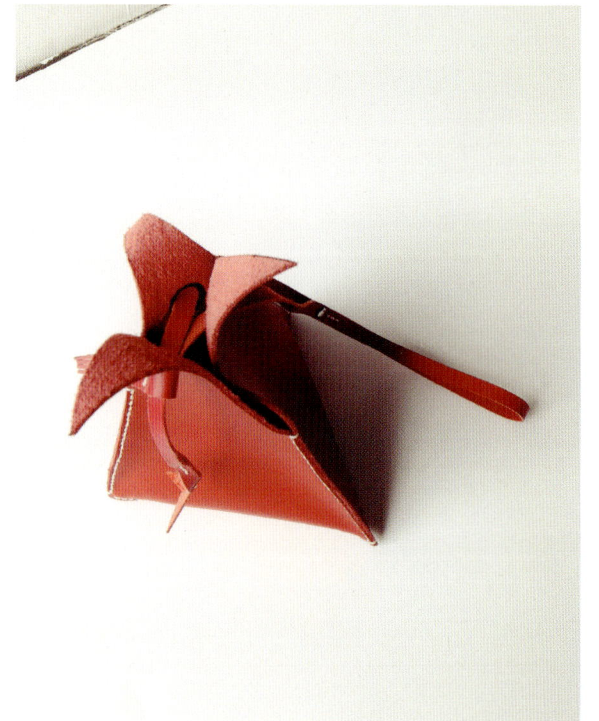
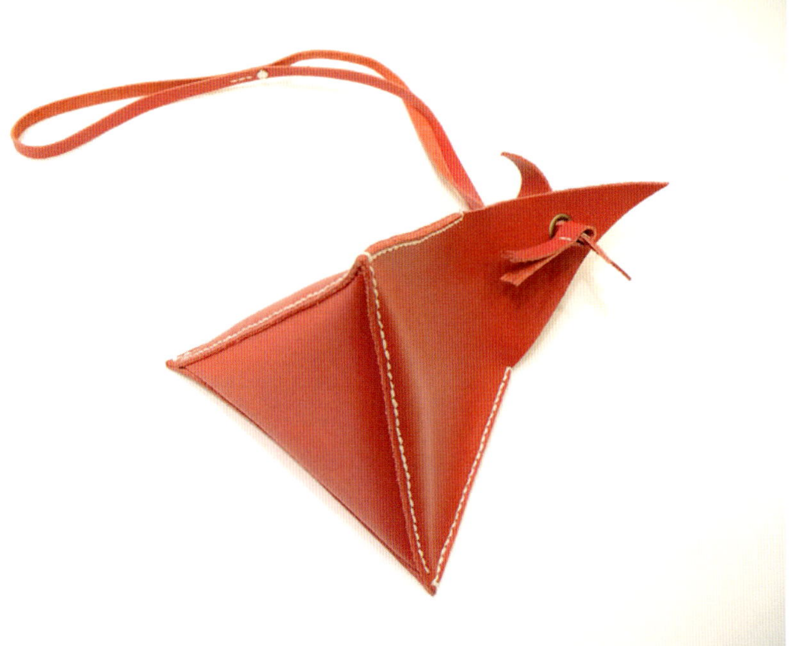

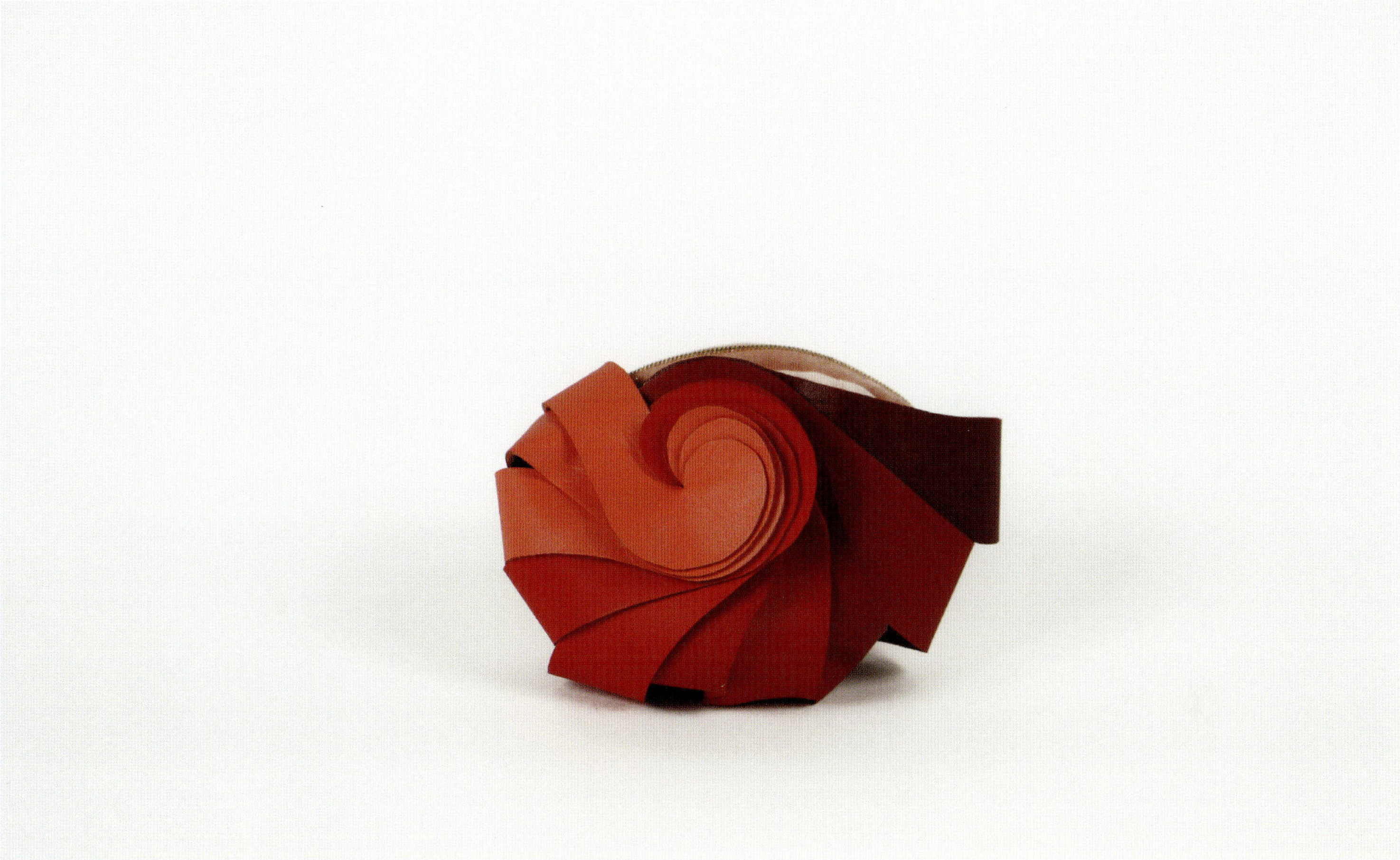

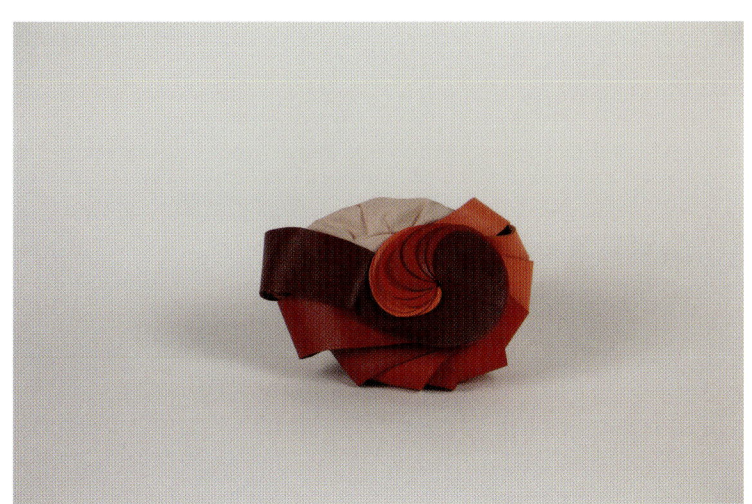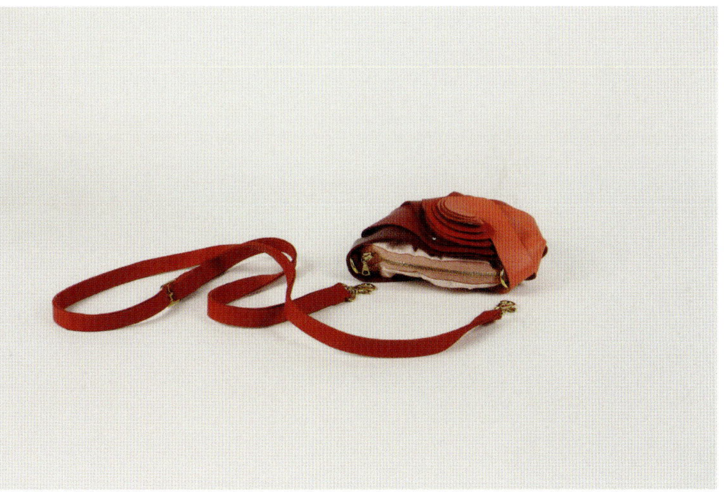

TRIANGLE HANDBAG
DA: Zemoneni

Characterized by its small size, the design is a regular tetrahedron, eye catching and perfect for a party.

FLAMINGO
DE: Zhulin Chanel Shi

Inspired by the movement of a flamingo turning its head and neck to caress its feathers, the design aimed to capture this flexibility and burning red color.

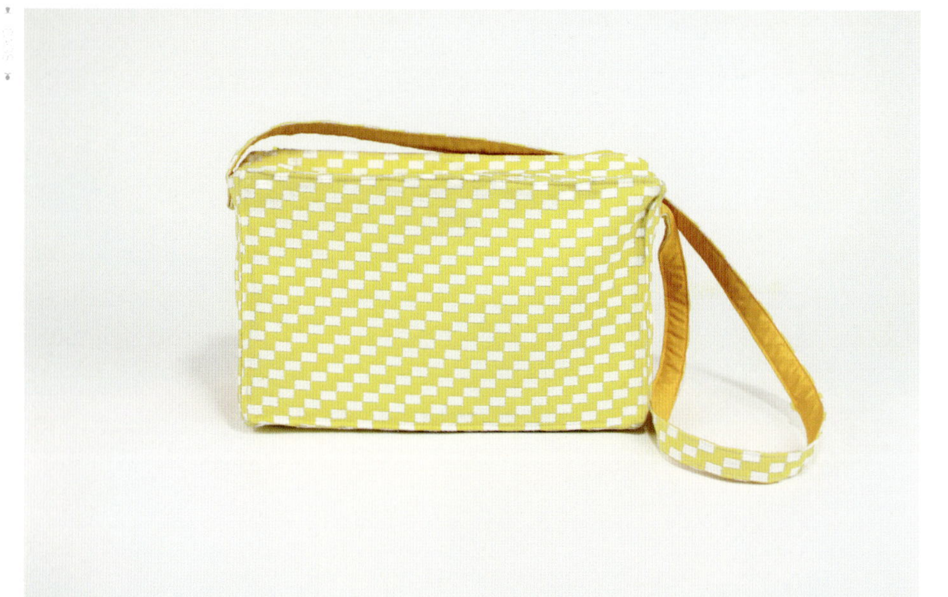

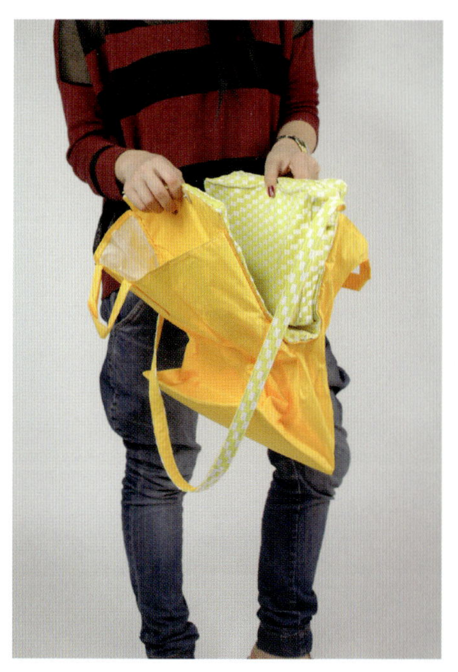

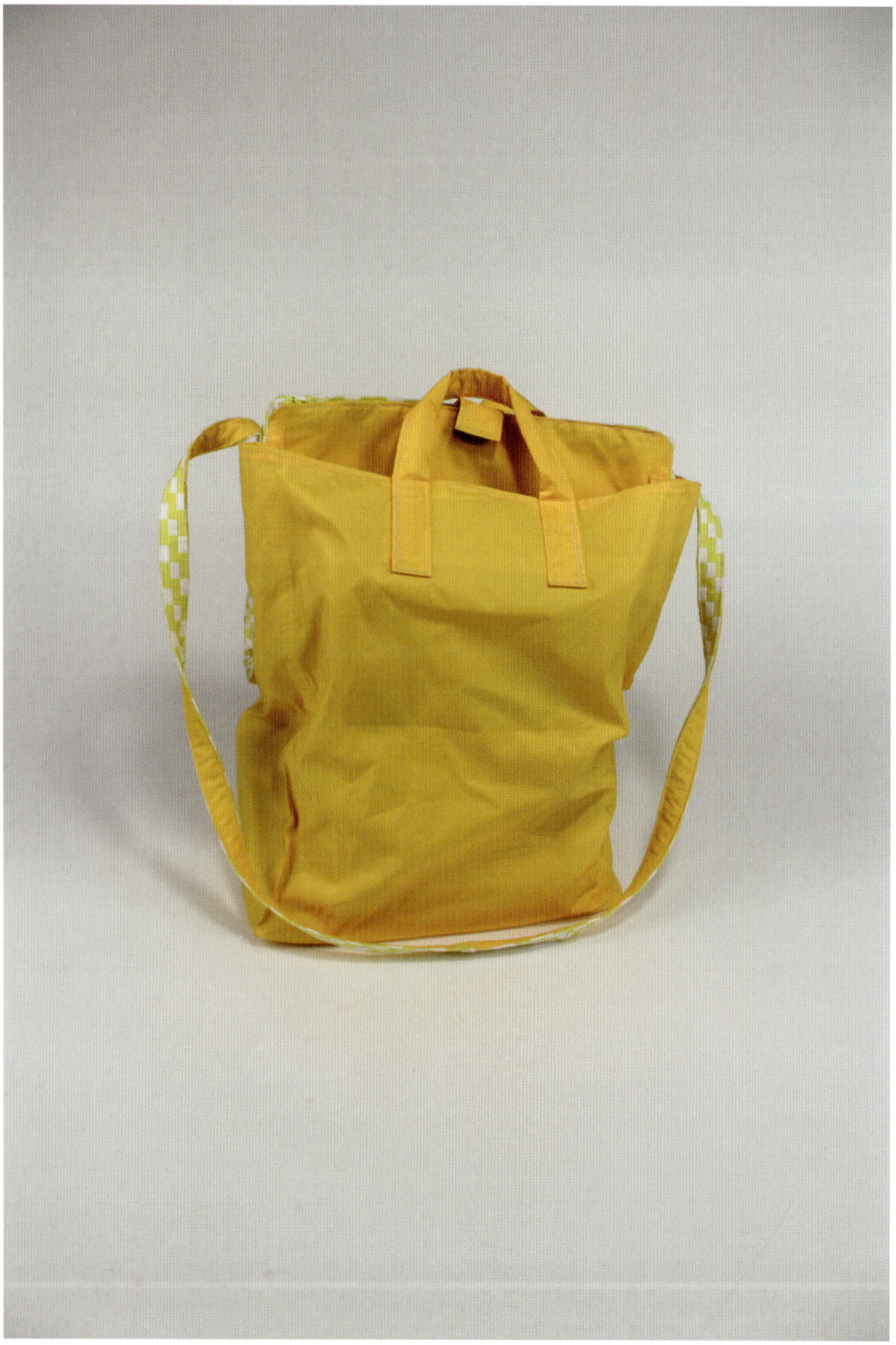

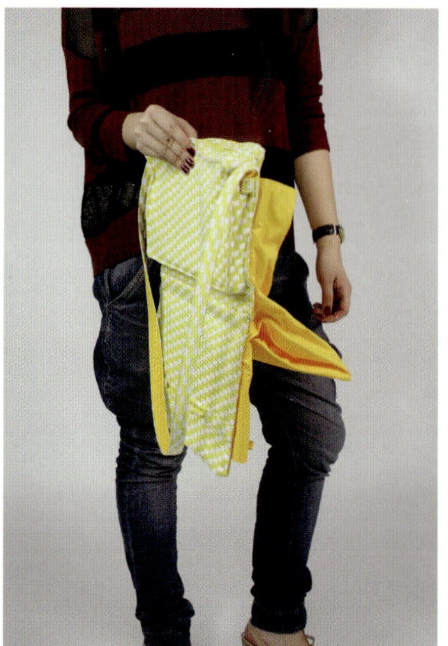

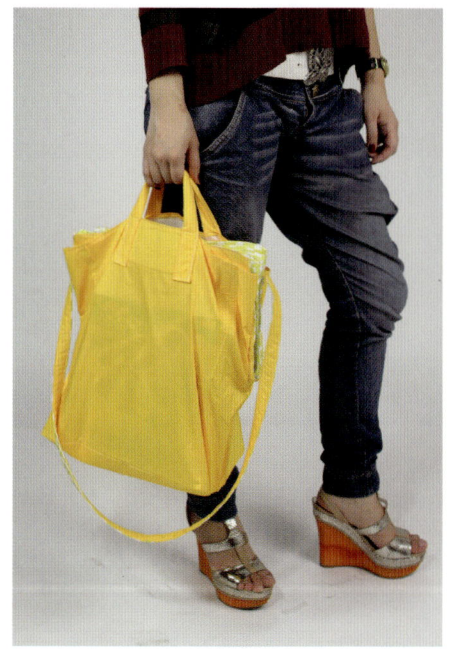

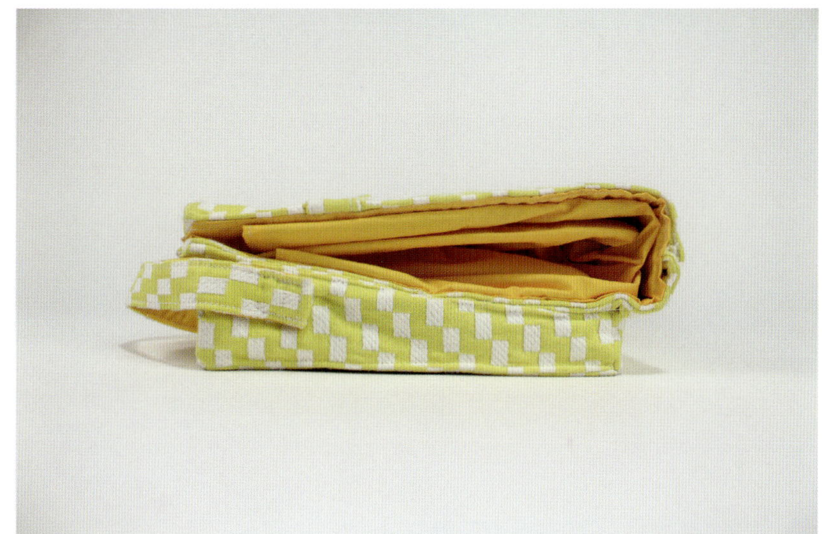

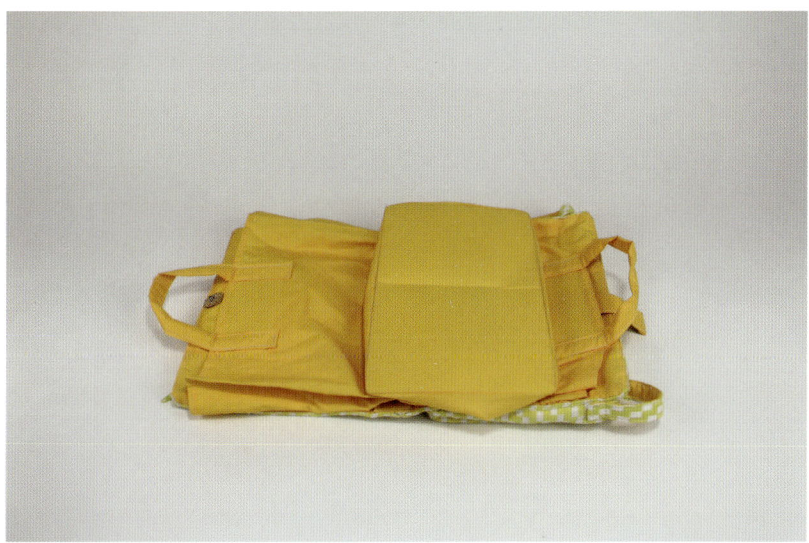

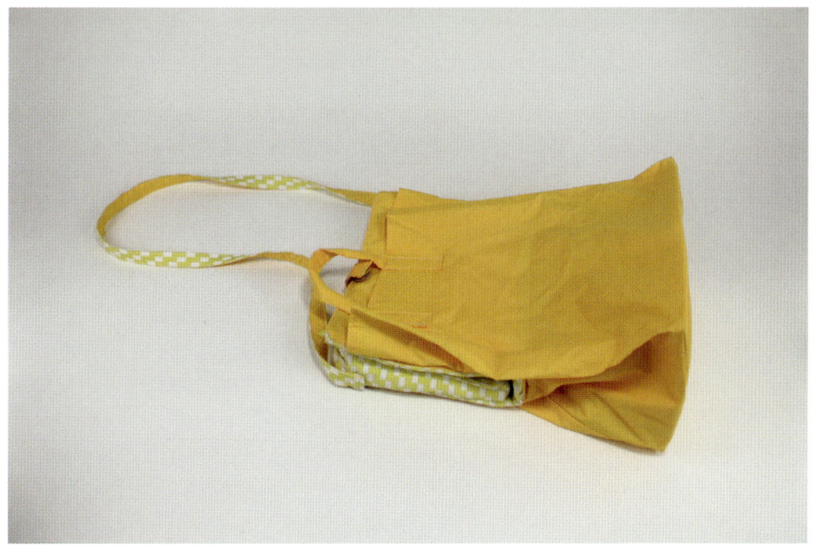

TRANSFORMABLE TOTE
DE: Zhulin Chanel Shi

Designed to meet different needs, this bag can transform from a shoulder bag
into a larger tote.

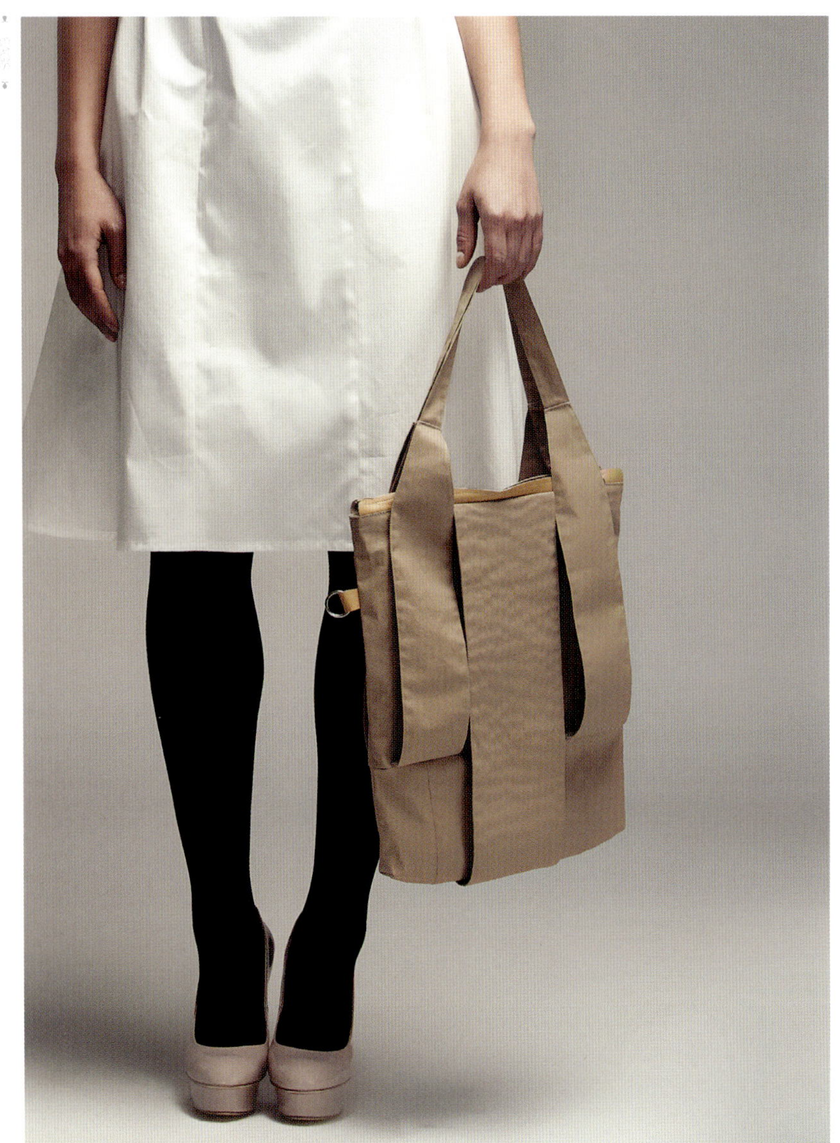

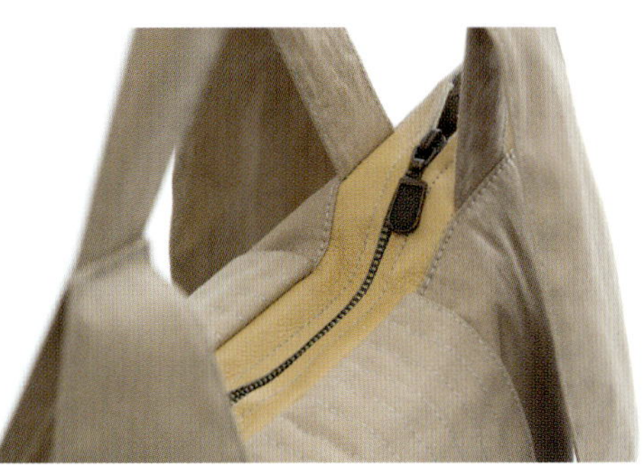

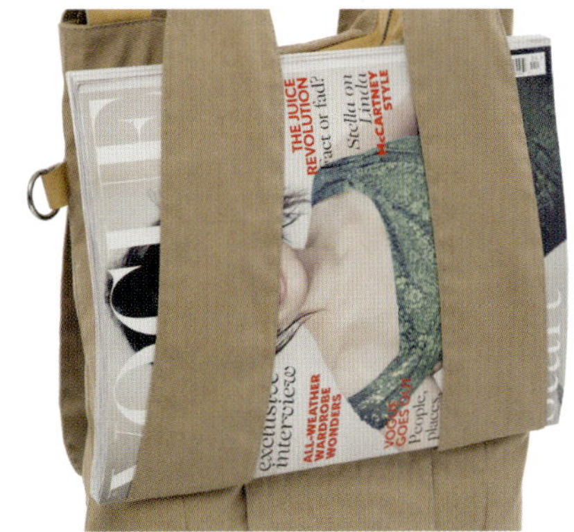

VOGUE
THE JUICE REVOLUTION
Fact or fad?
Stella on Linda McCARTNEY STYLE
ALL-WEATHER WARDROBE WONDERS
extensive interview

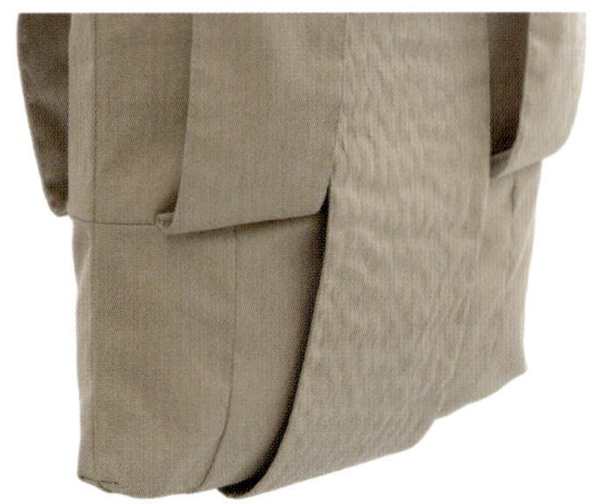

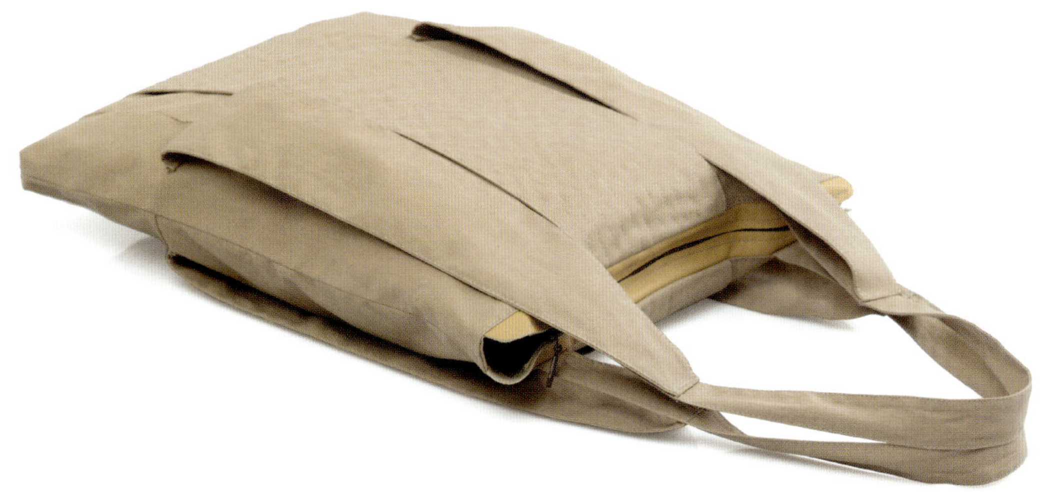

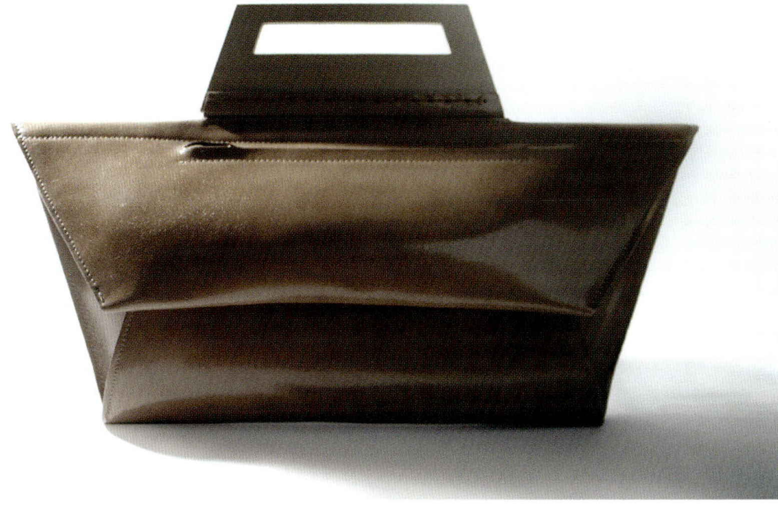

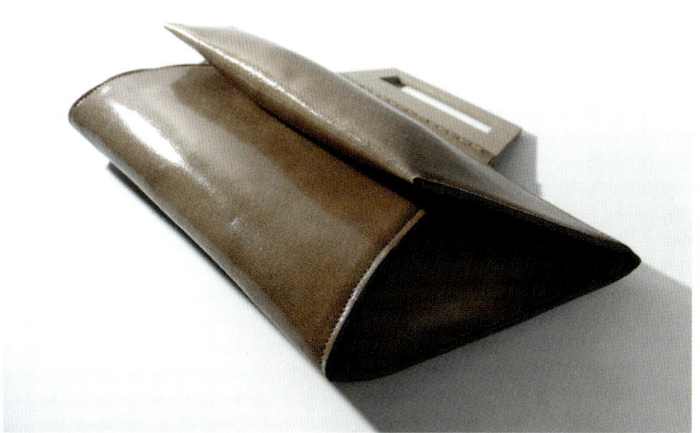

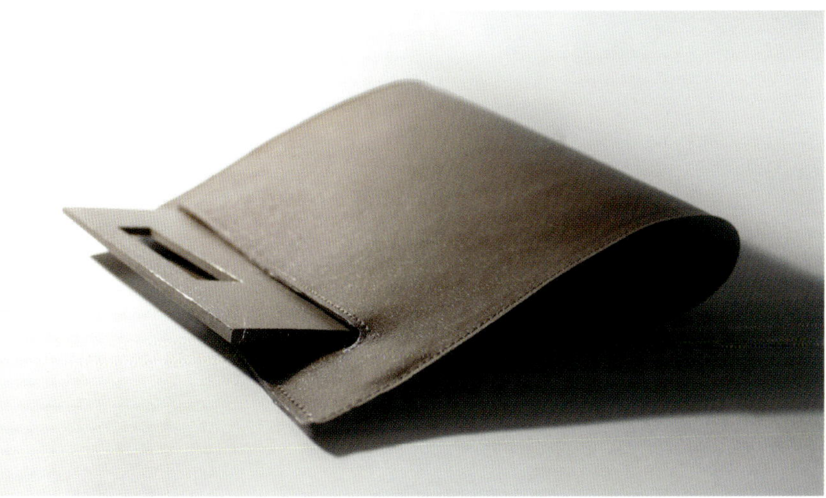

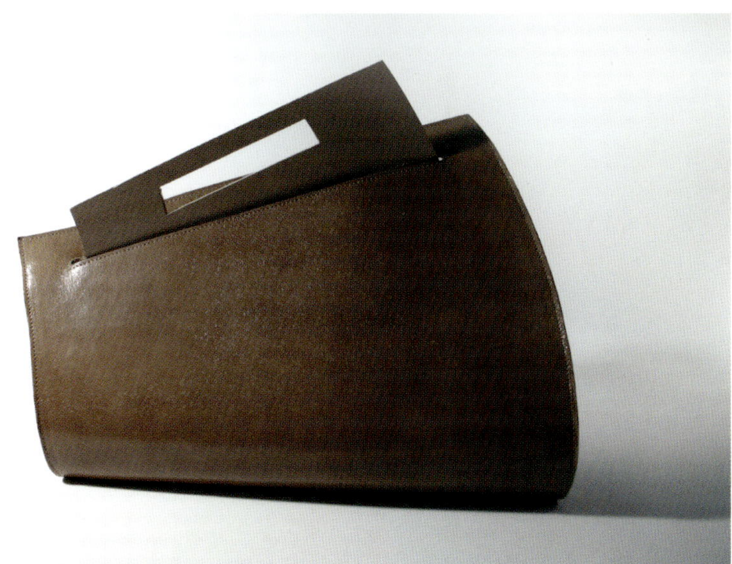

INSERTABLE BAG
DE: František Kubeš

Making adornment practical, this design turned the side straps into a holder
for a magazine or an umbrella.

WOODEN HANDLE BAG
DA: Laura Papp

This designer created two bags, utilizing the idea of folding something into
itself. The first bag has two storage pockets, with a wooden handle shaped in
the same form as the bag, while the second bag is completed as it inserts
slots into the slit.

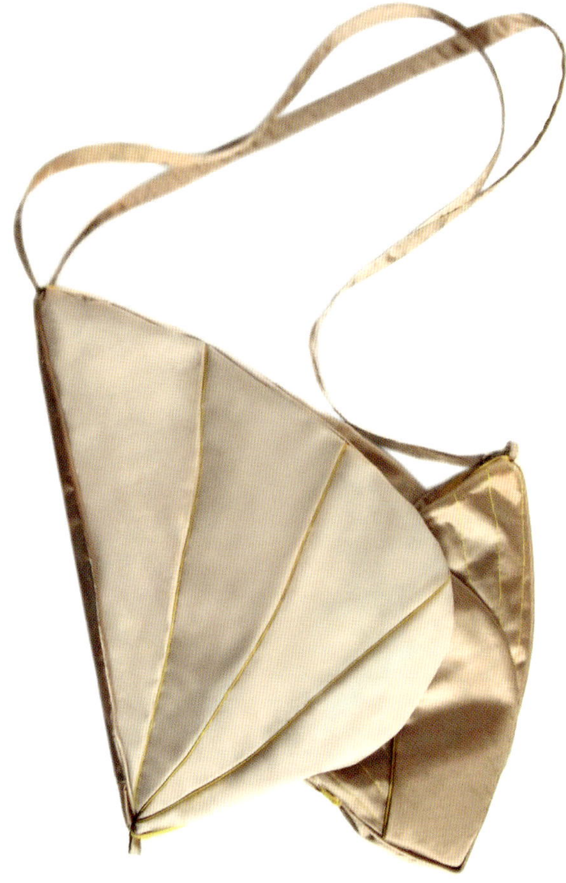

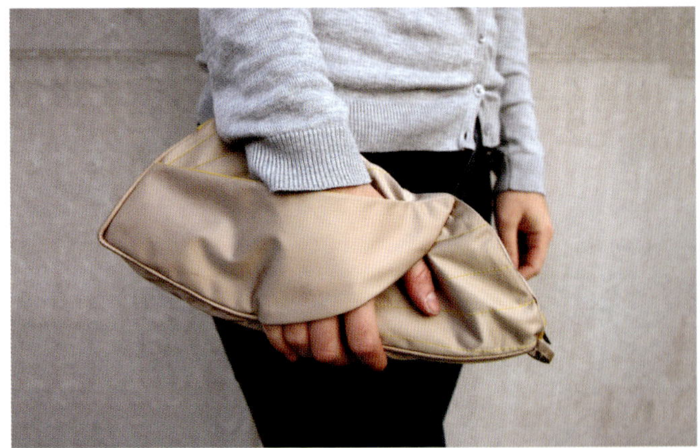

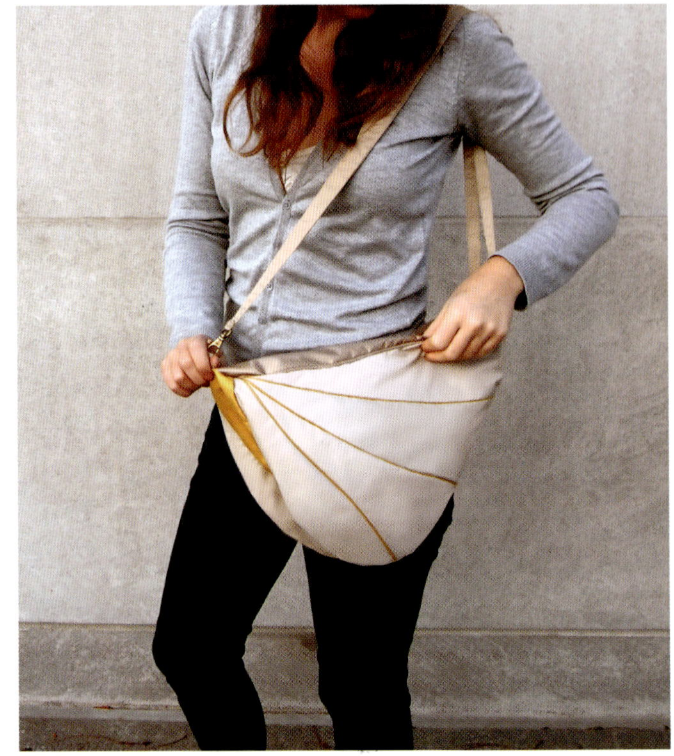

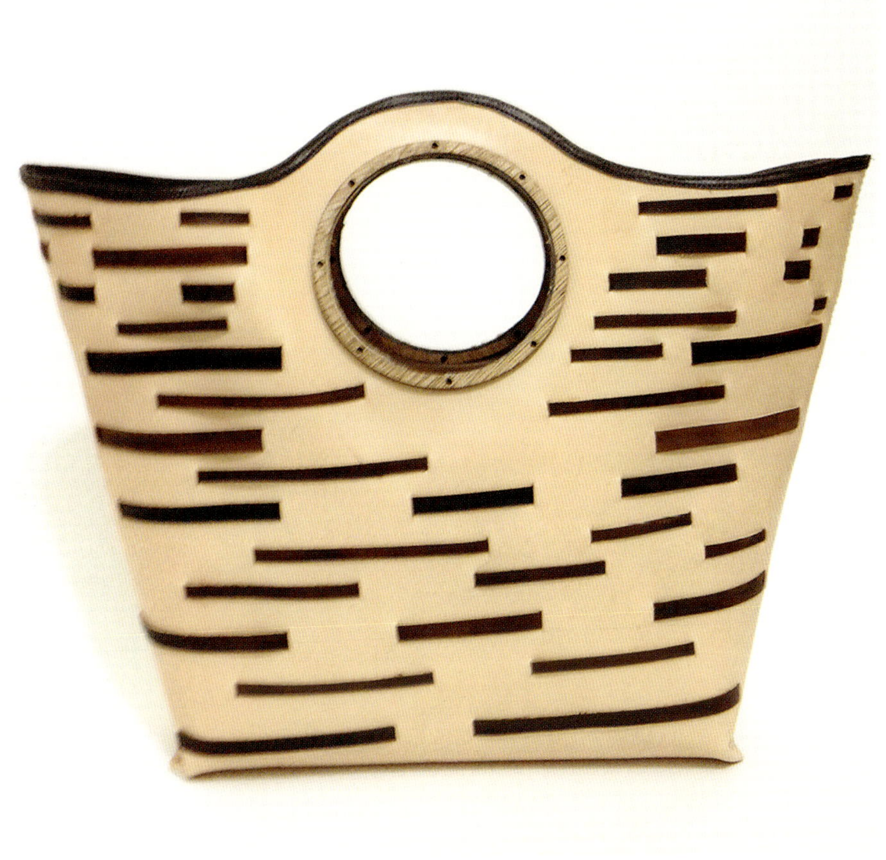

DORÉ
DE: Lisa Dudley

Designed as a transformative bag, the "Dorè" can switch from a clutch to a
shoulder bag as needed, keeping the owner prepared for all occasions.

WEAVING BAG
DE: Minjung Kim

Inspired by Leonardo Drew's sculpture, this bag was made using weaving
techniques with Veg tan leather and a dyed strap.

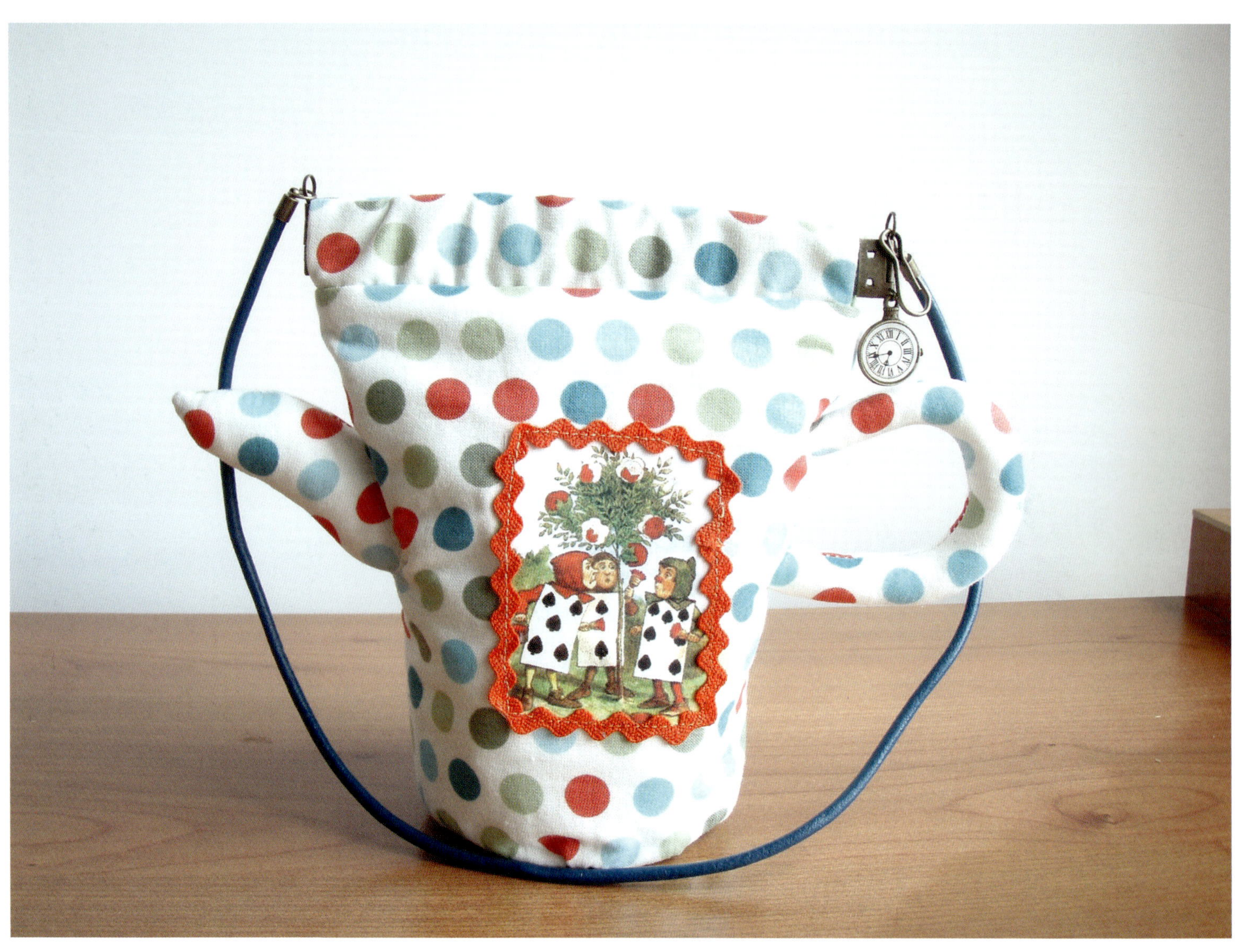

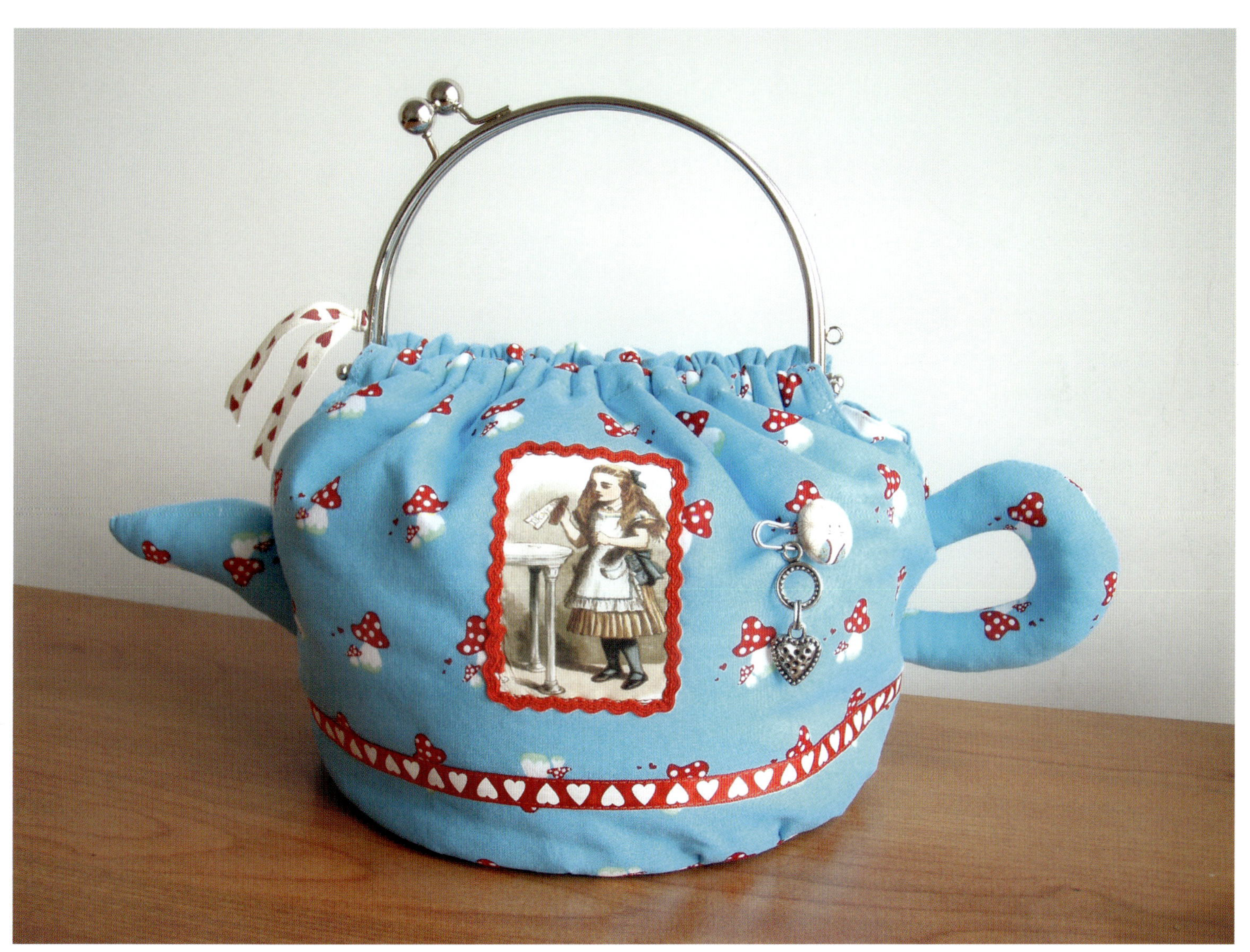

ALICE IN WONDERLAND POUCH
DE: Helena Silva

Inspired by the beloved tale, the designer created two teapot pouches, with
visual elements from the story, like the mushroom, a pocket watch, playing
card soldiers and the painted roses.

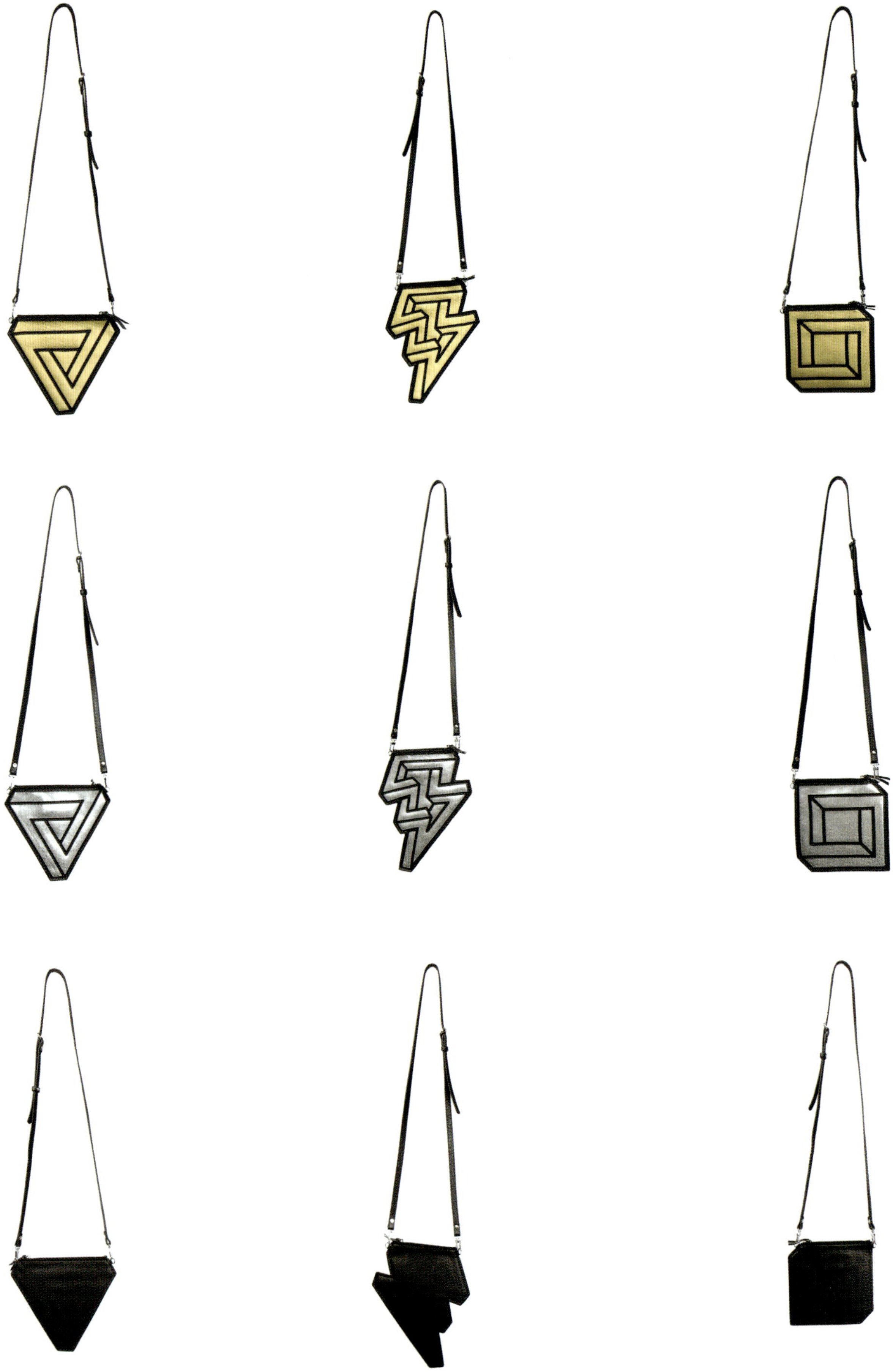

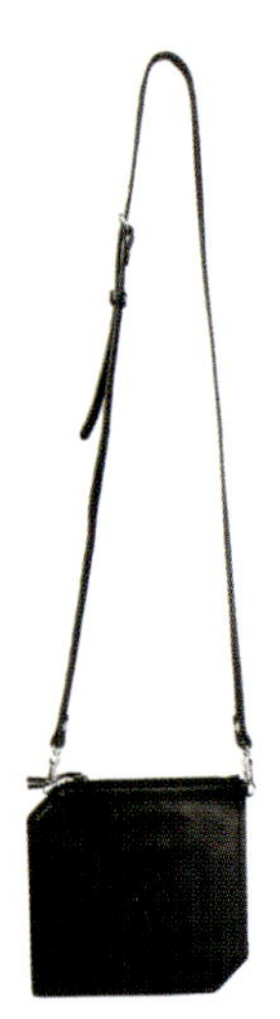

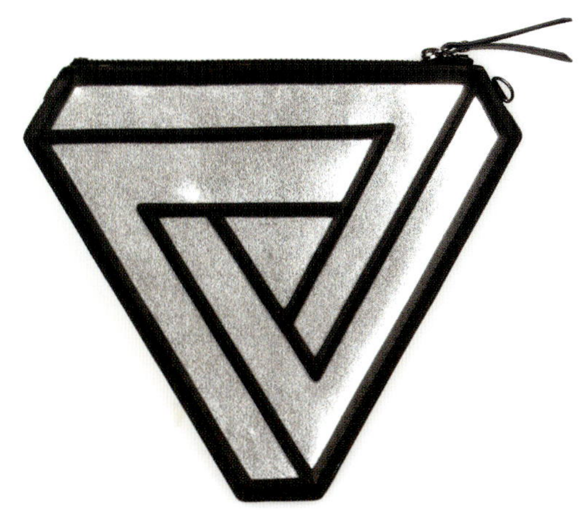

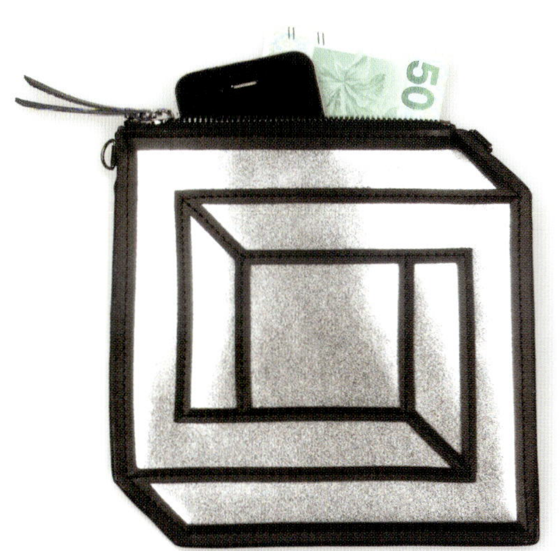

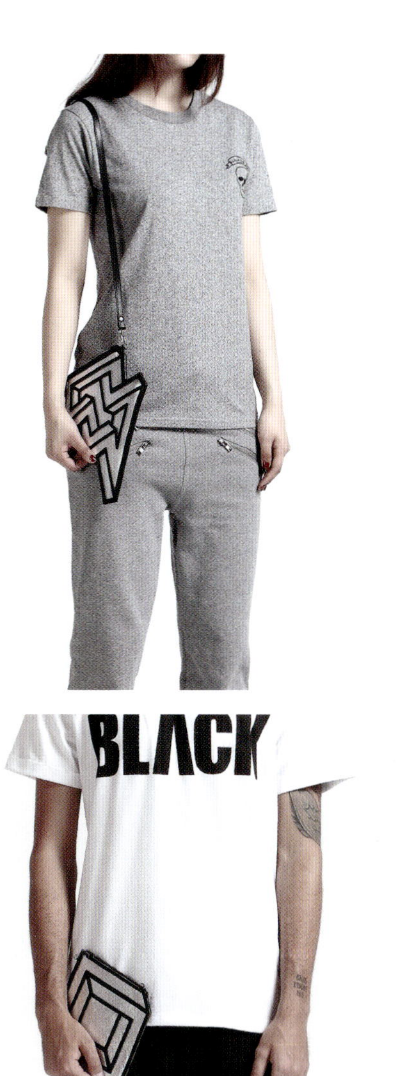

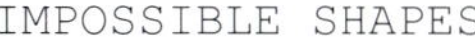

IMPOSSIBLE SHAPES
DA: Black Head

Playing with impossible shapes and 2D effects, Black Head created a series
of clutch/shoulder bags that would look like a sticker on one's body when
worn or clutched.

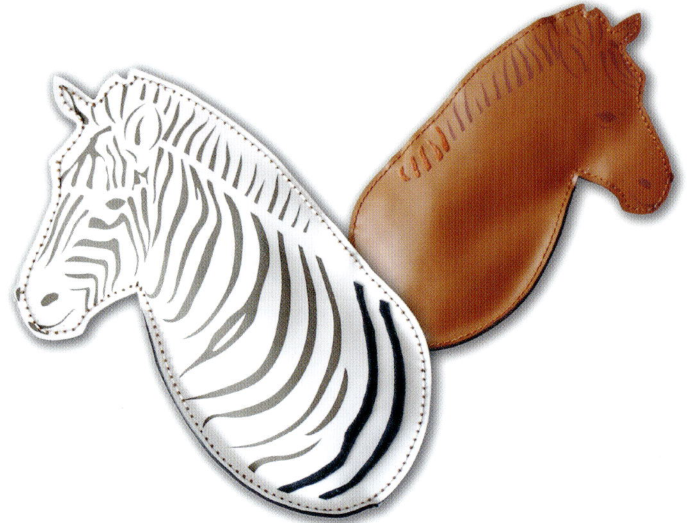

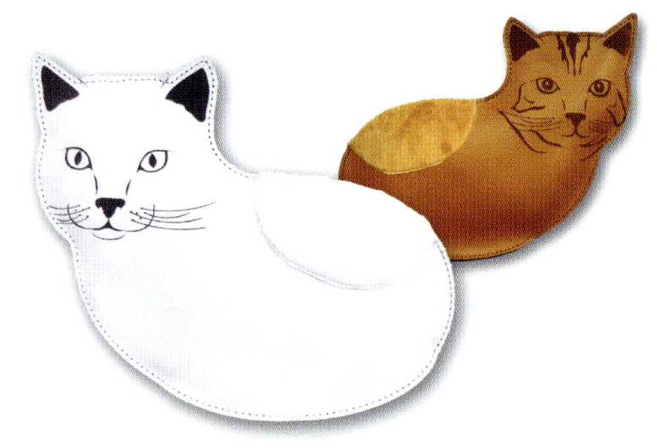

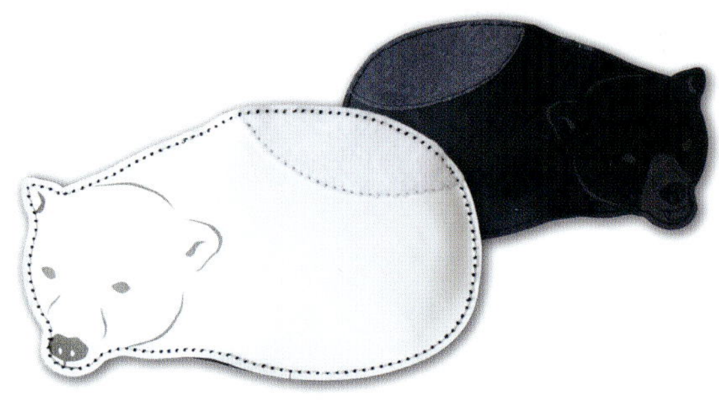

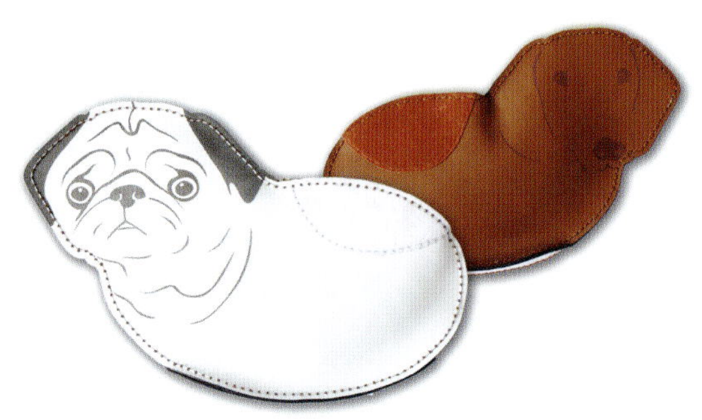

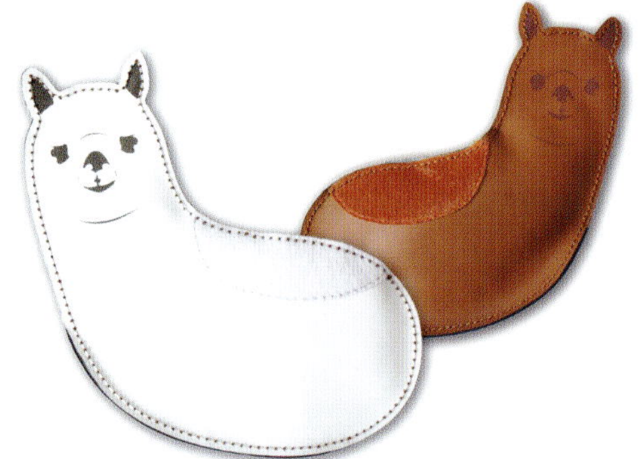

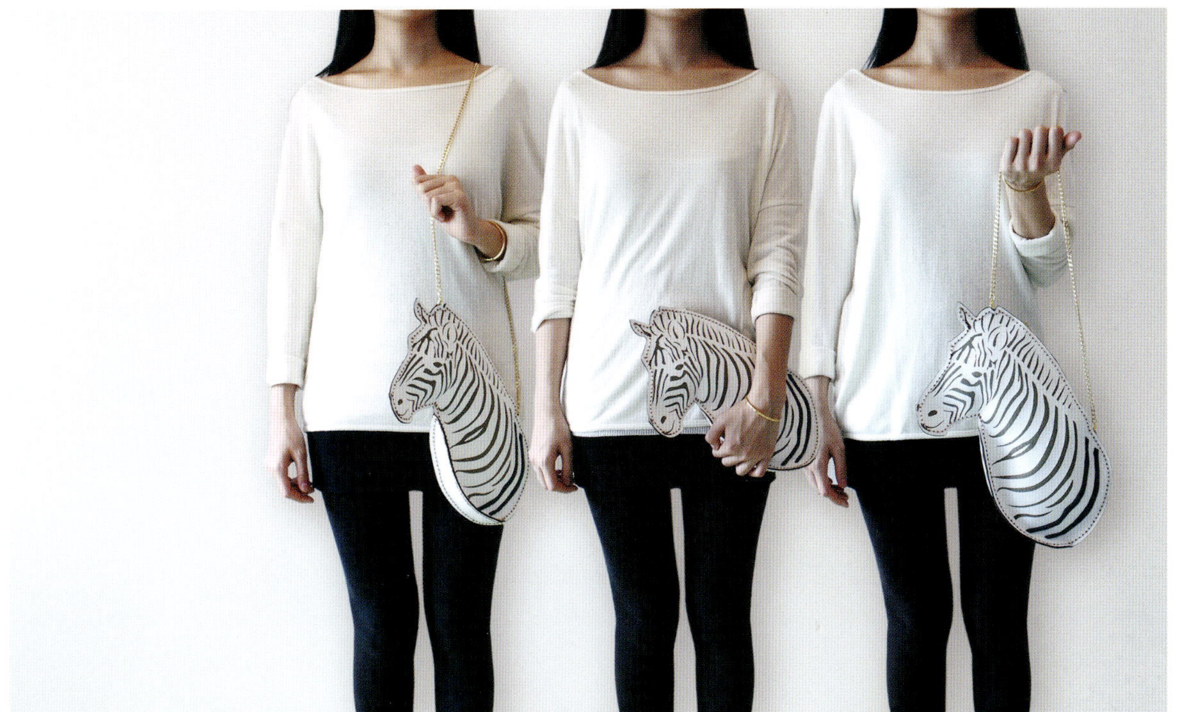

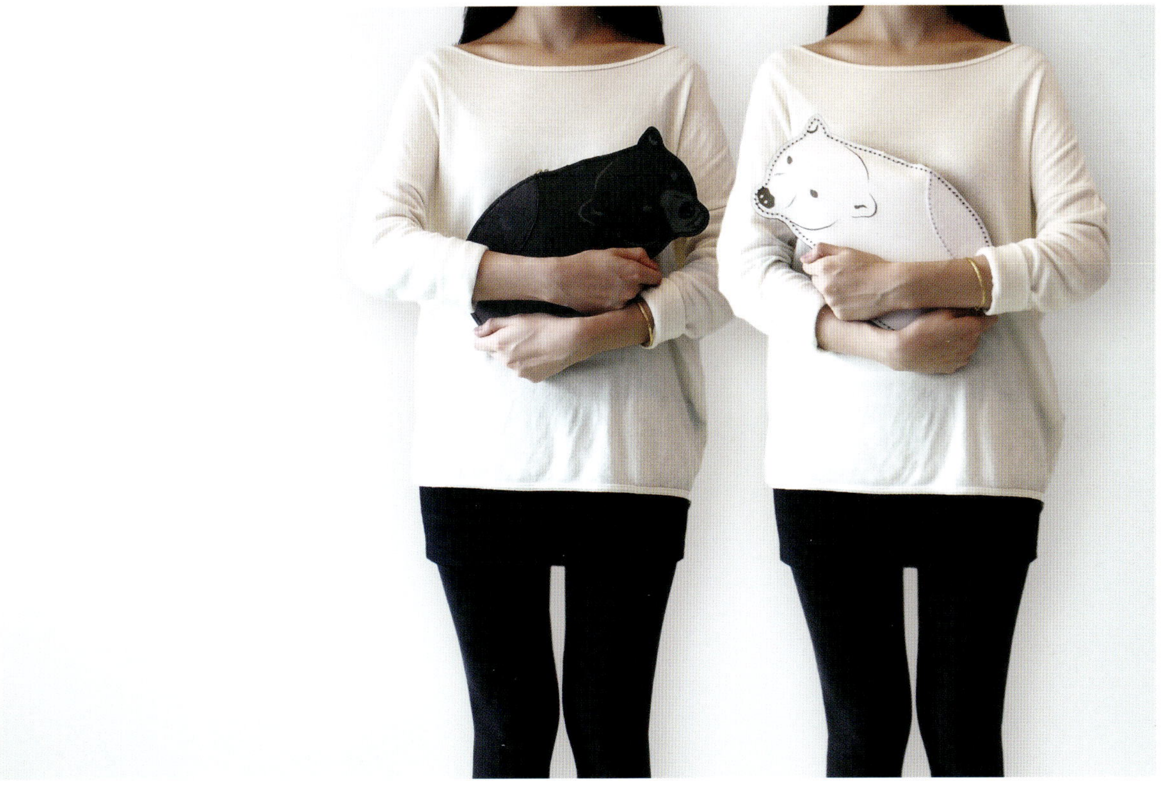

WE ARE FAMILY HAND BAG
DE: UUendy Lau

"We Are Family" is a collection of animal shaped bags, representing different groups of people. Created with double-sided graphics, the design illustrates animals of a similar breed with different skins.

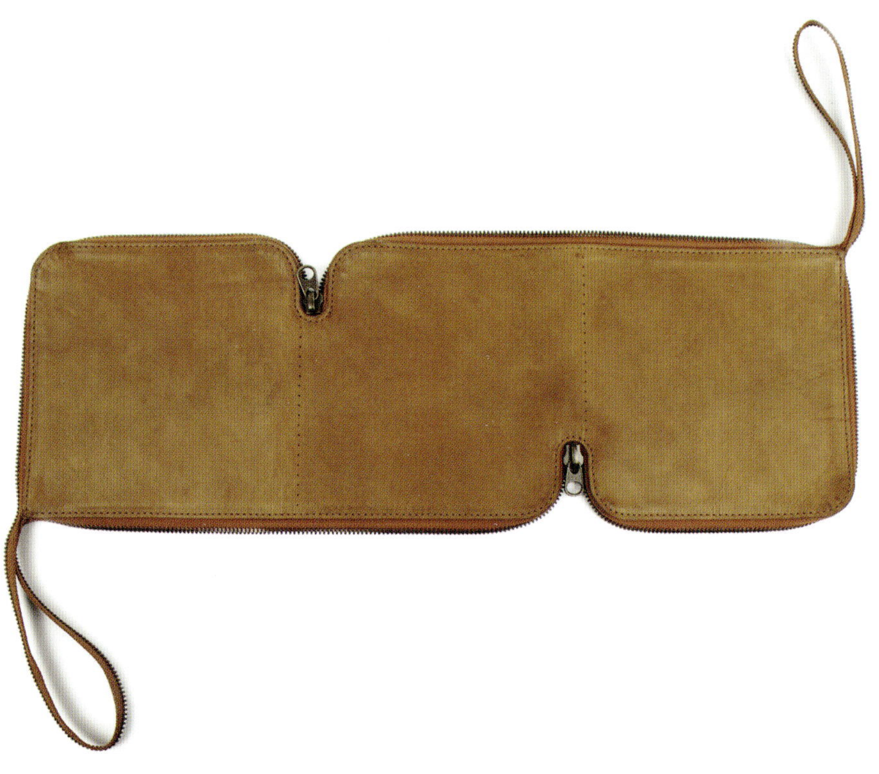
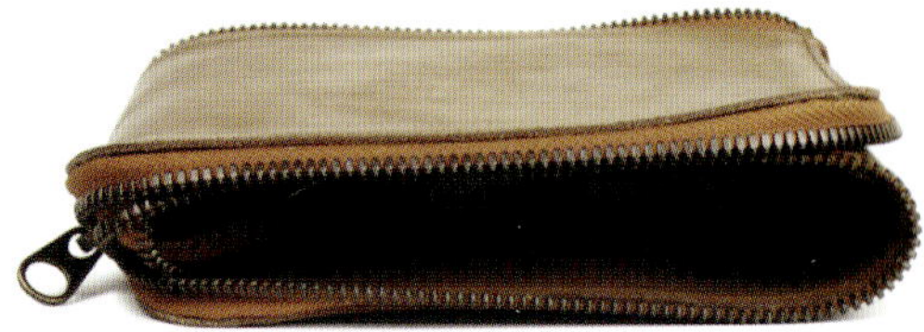
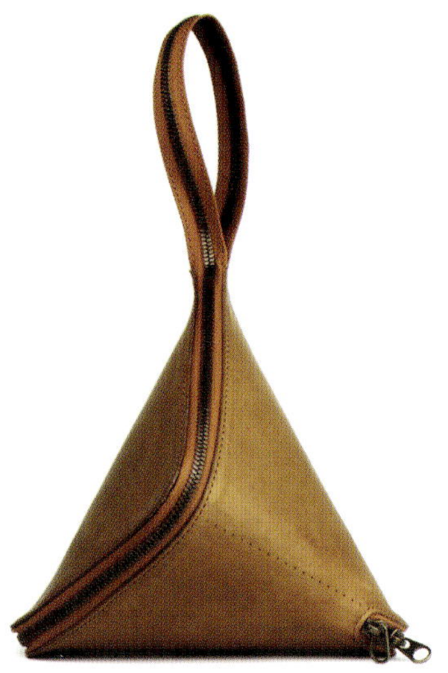
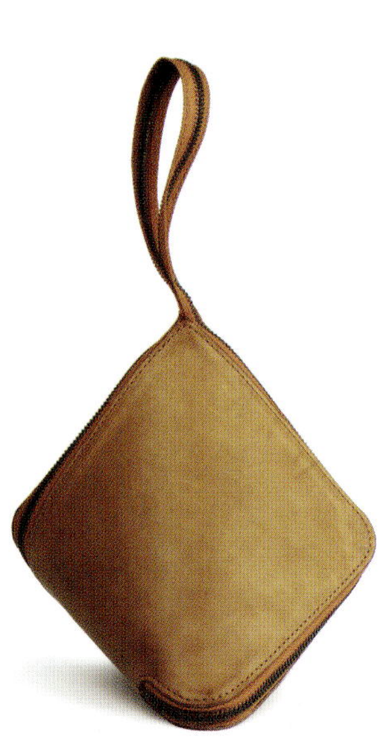

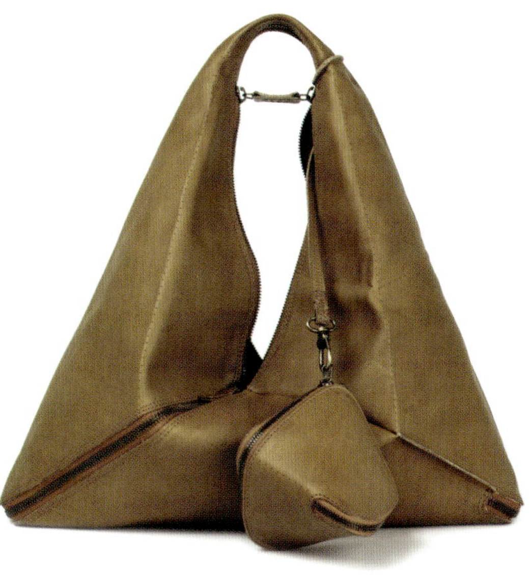

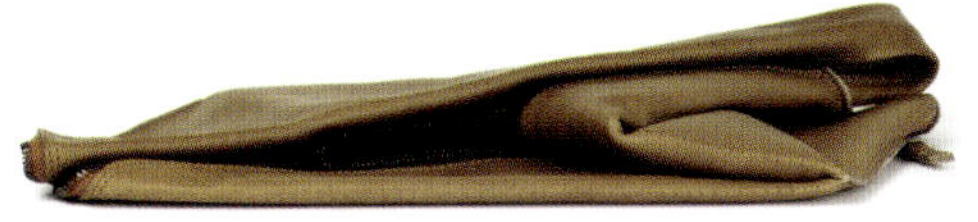

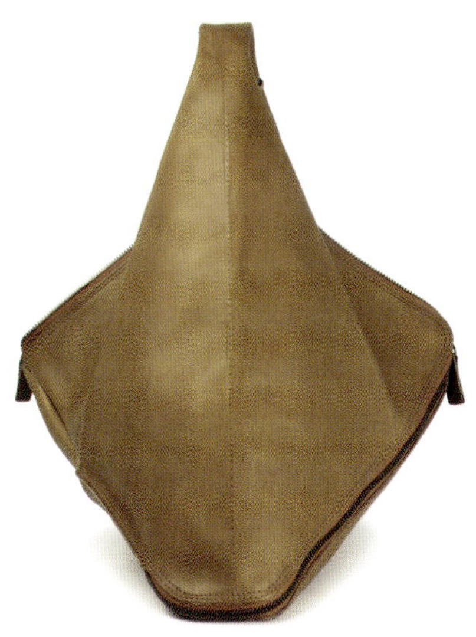

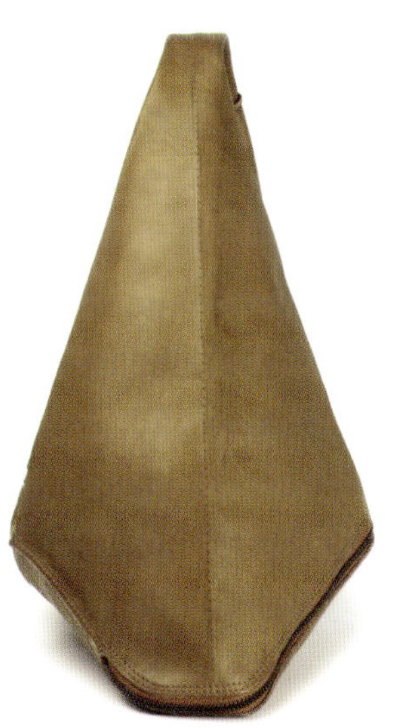

ONE PIECE BAG
DA: Loope

Formed by one rectangular piece of leather and a zipper, "One Piece Bag" is
based on a special system inspired by the traditional Japanese "furoshiki".

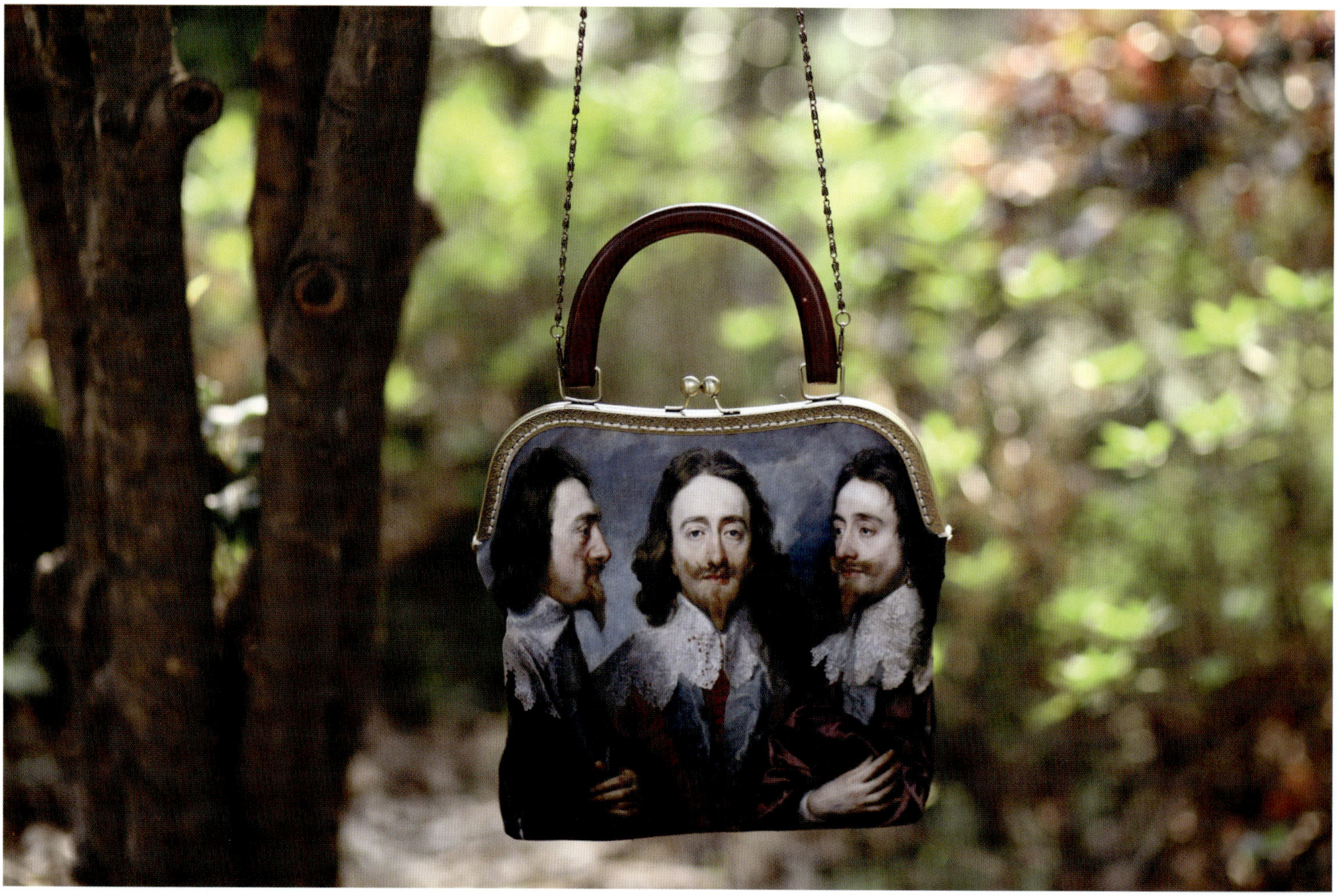

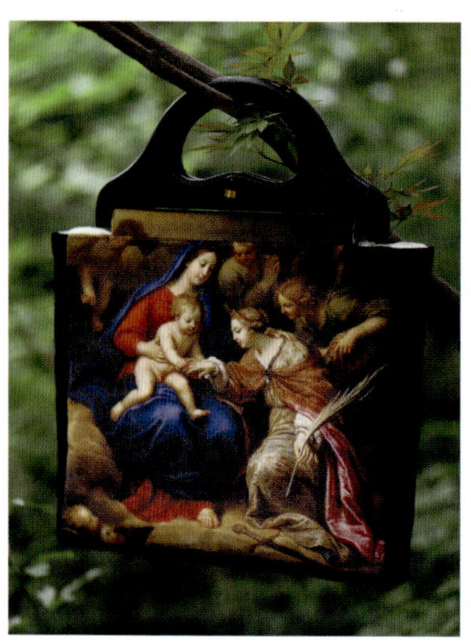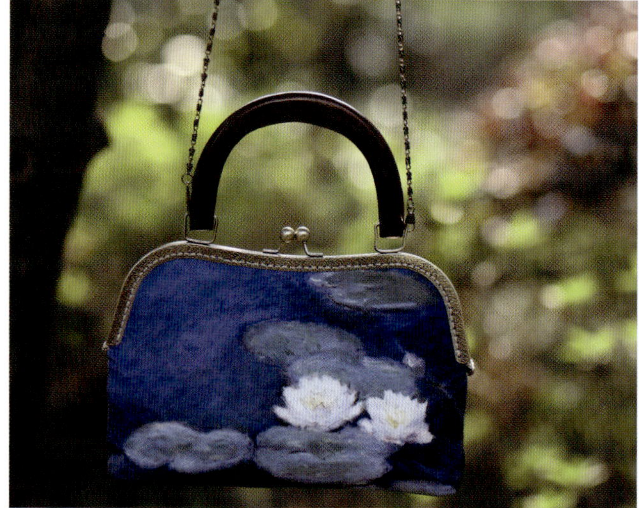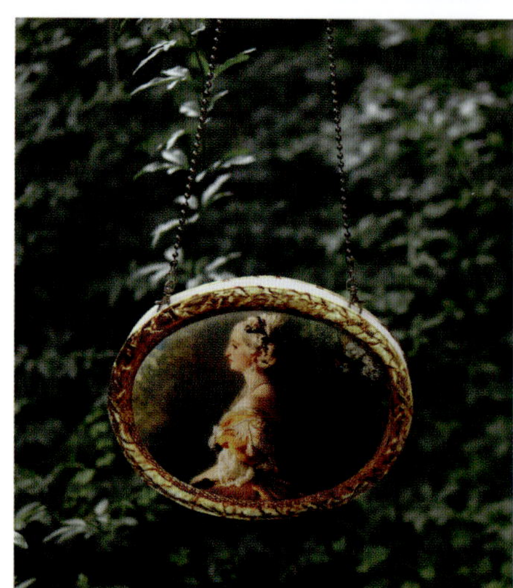

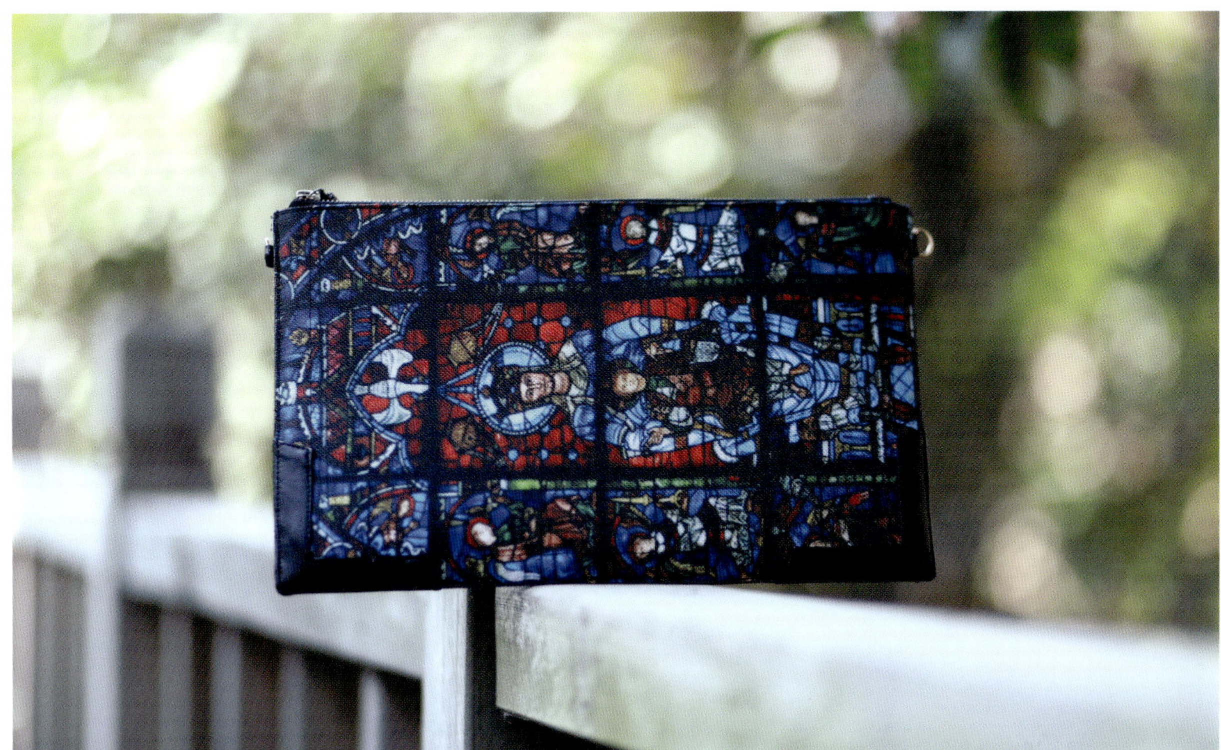

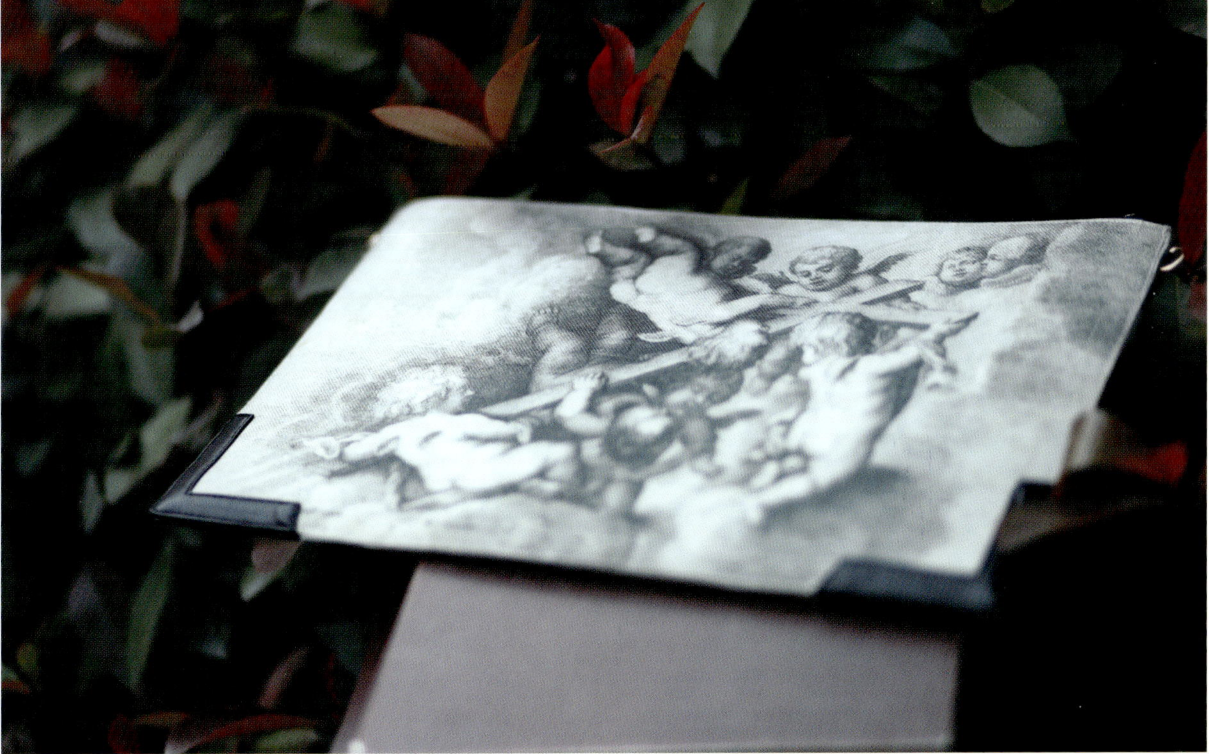

OIL PAITING BAG

DA: Xun Ruo

This series is printed with famous paintings, complemented with vintage bag design and delicate ornamental details to create a luxurious feel.

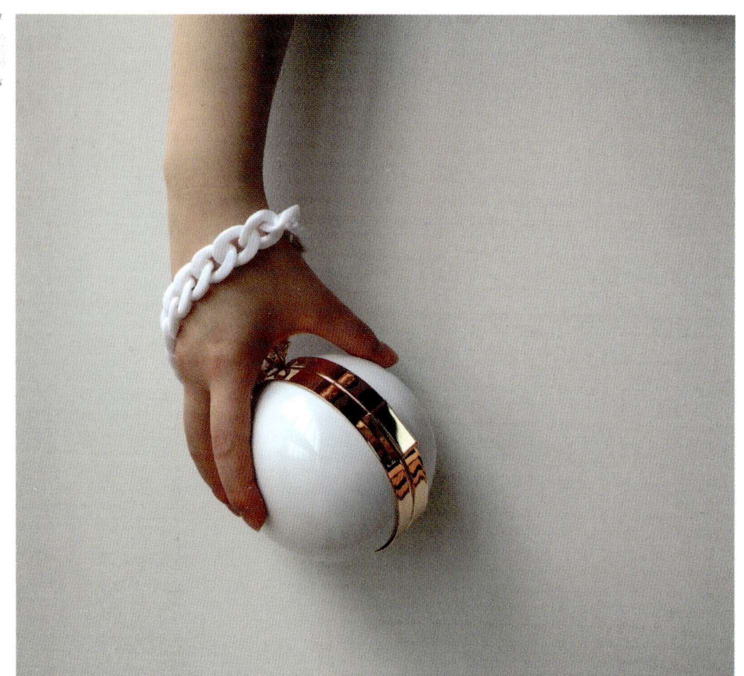

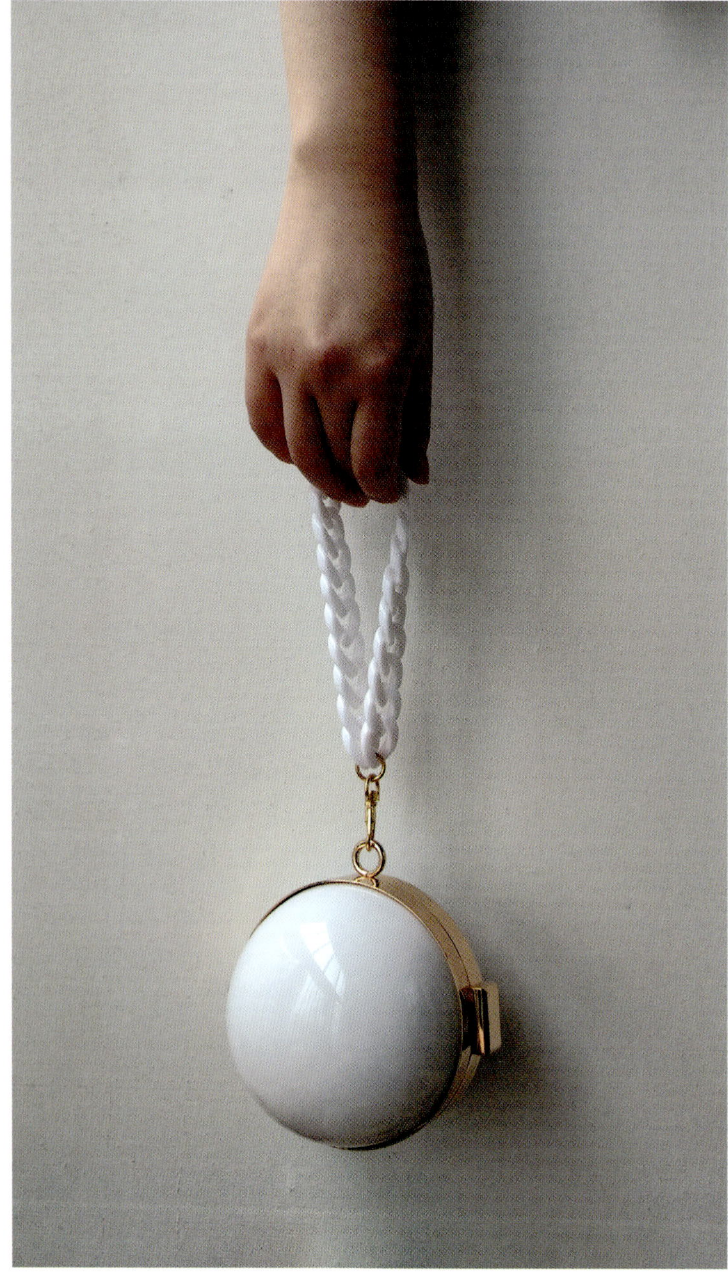

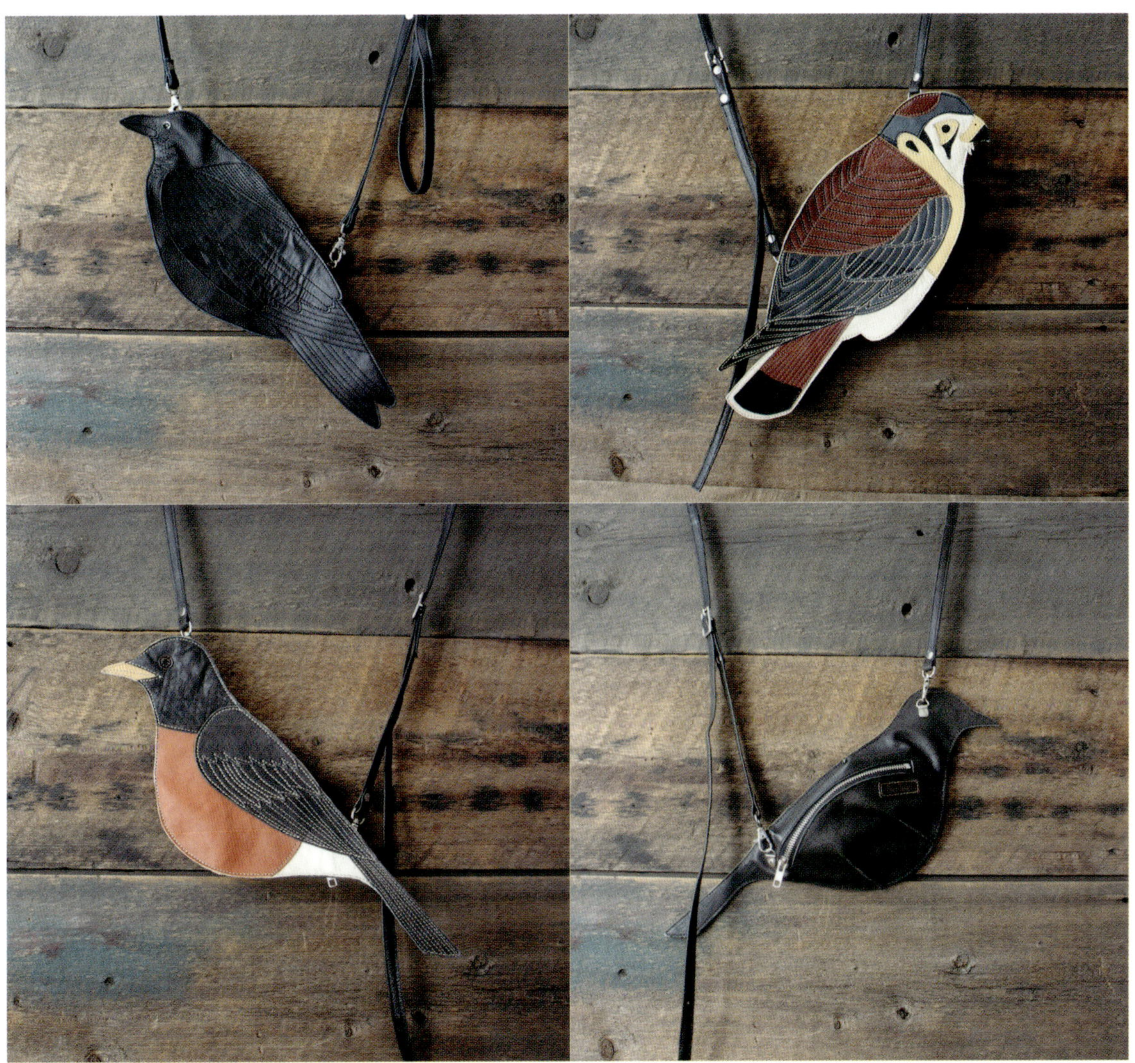

WHITE OVAL
DA: Comme Des Cygnes

Distinctive in shape, the "White Oval" has a comfortable grip and is
lightweight.

BIRD BAG
DE: Marc Simard

Using many colorful threads, designer hope to create a bag to reproduce the
natural beauty of a bird plumage.

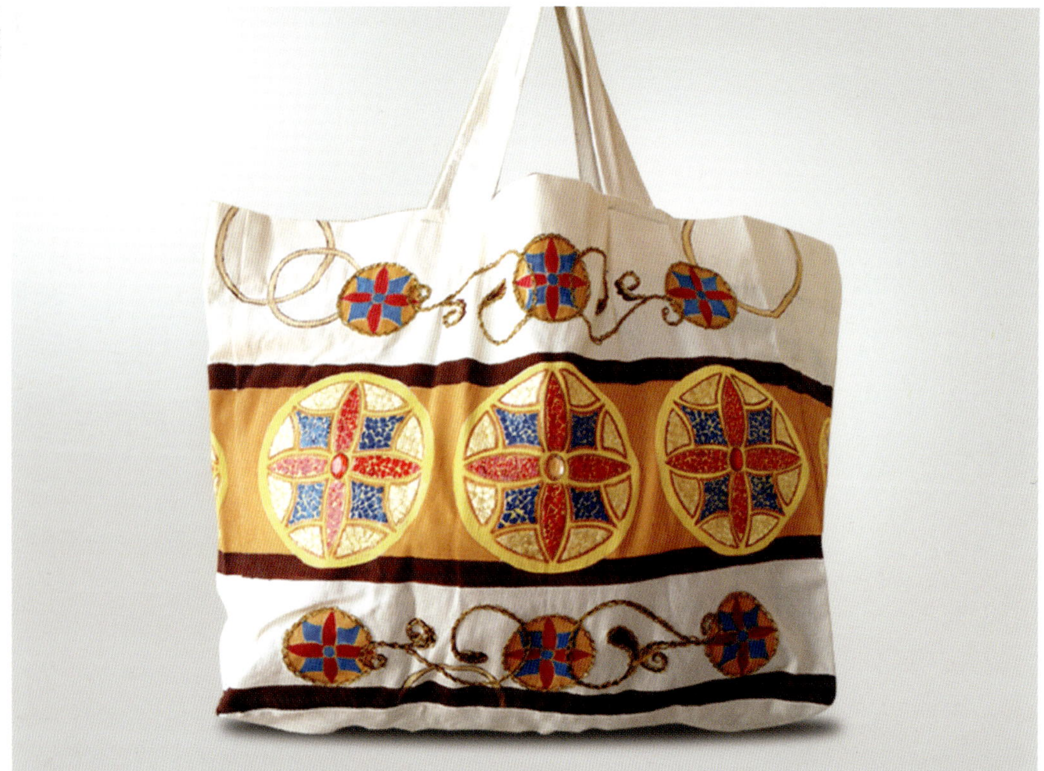
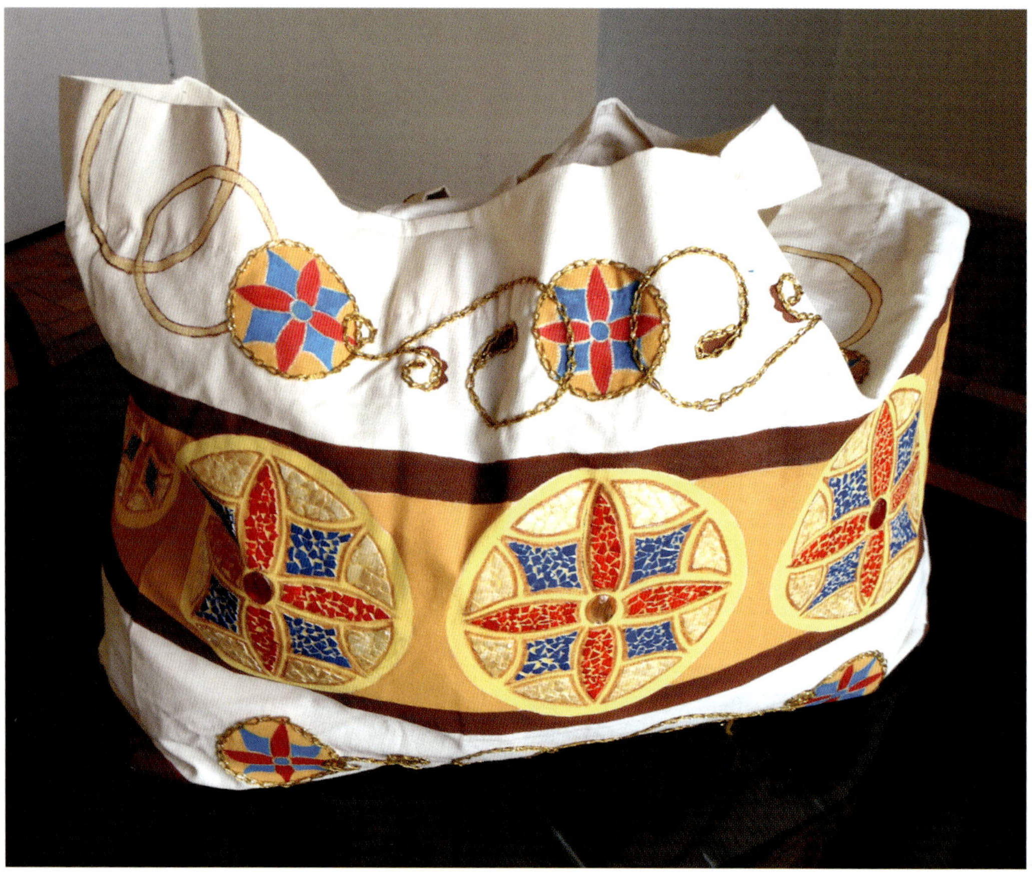

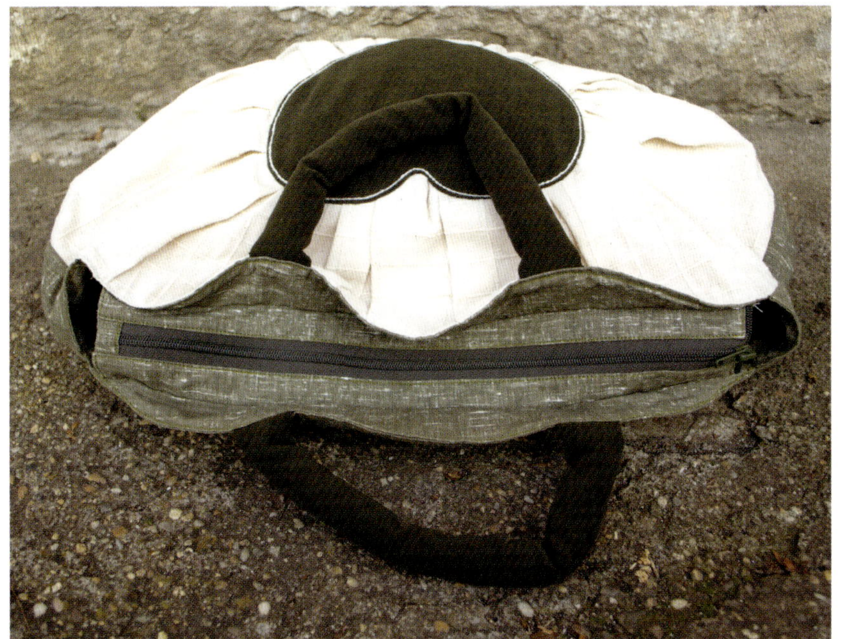

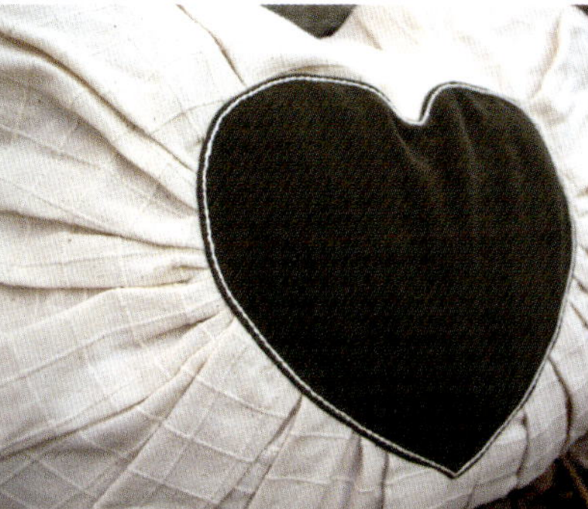

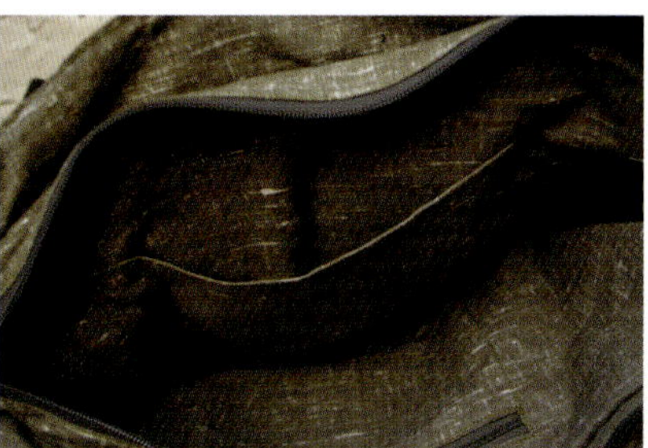

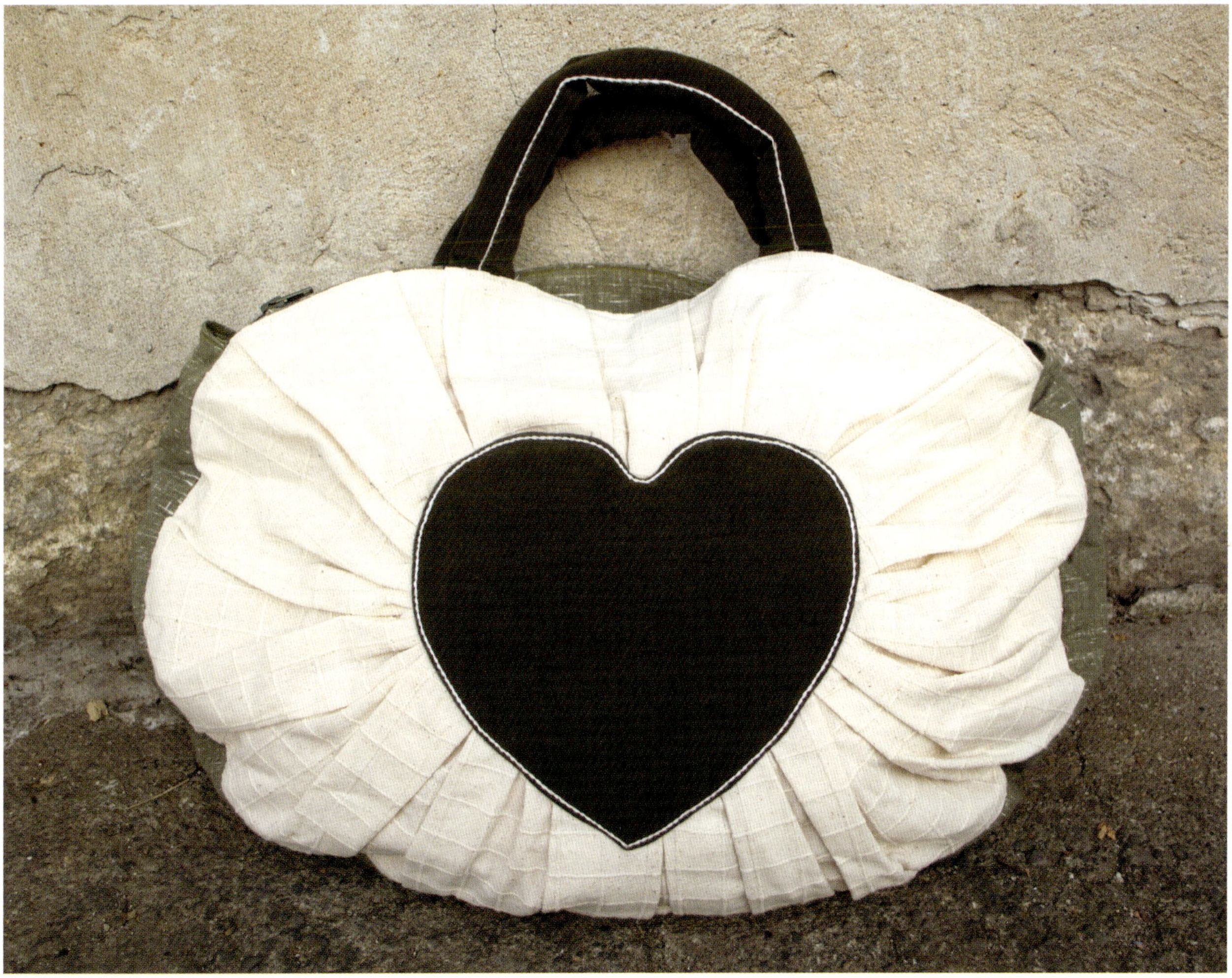

ECO BAG BIZANTYNE
DE: Alessandra Sartori Mattei

Inspired by Byzantine, floral ornaments and halos were used as the principal element. The central drawing, which mimics stained glass art, was made with eggshells, while the rest was created using tissue painting, embroidery, and stones.

CREAM AND ARMY GREEN HEART HANDBAG
DE: Yana Hari Karabelova

This oval-shaped handbag uses army green and the natural cream color of unbleached cotton. The front side of this bag is ruffled, and a large soft plush heart, stuffed with wool, is attached to the body of the bag with stitching. The handles are made in the same way.

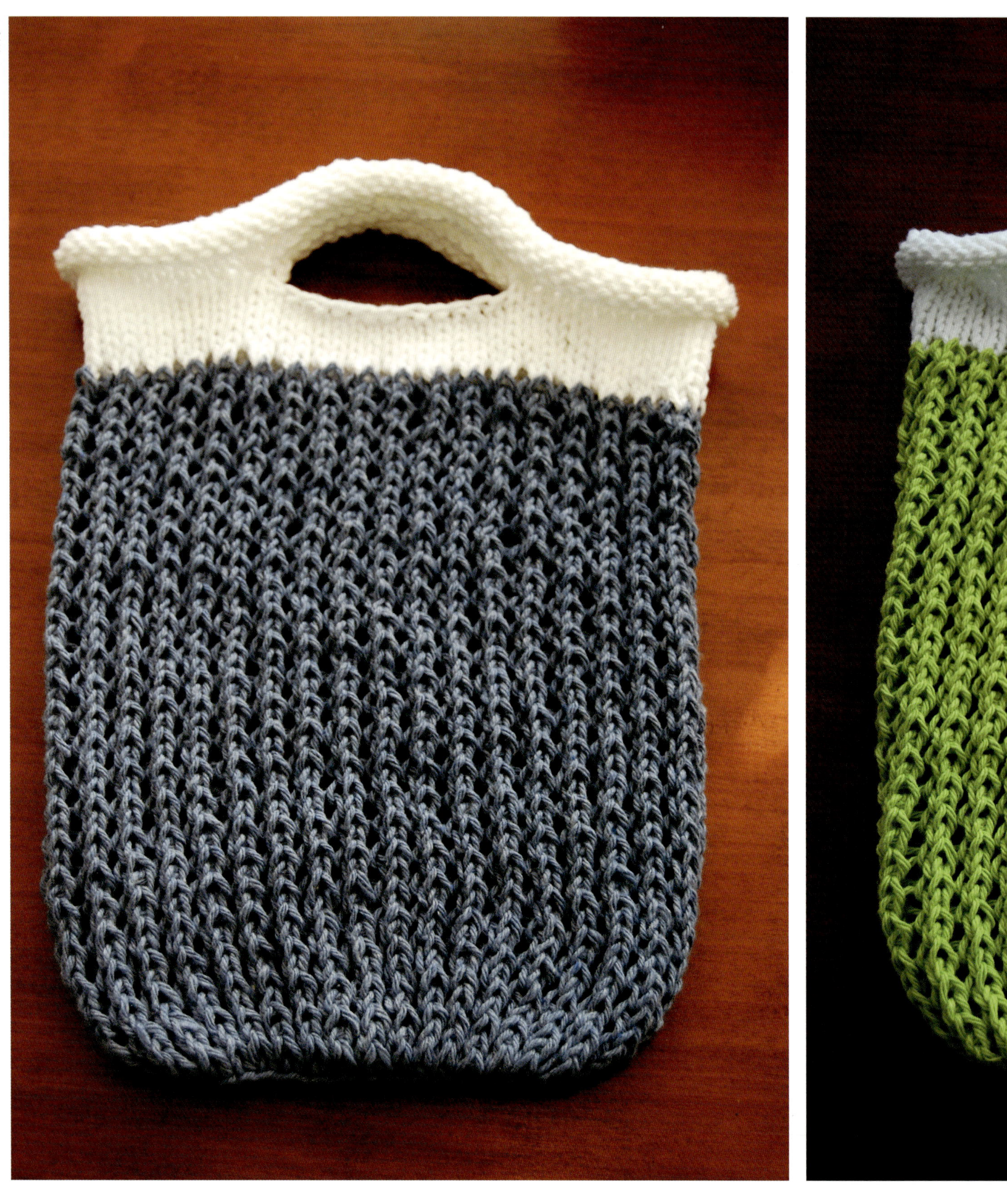

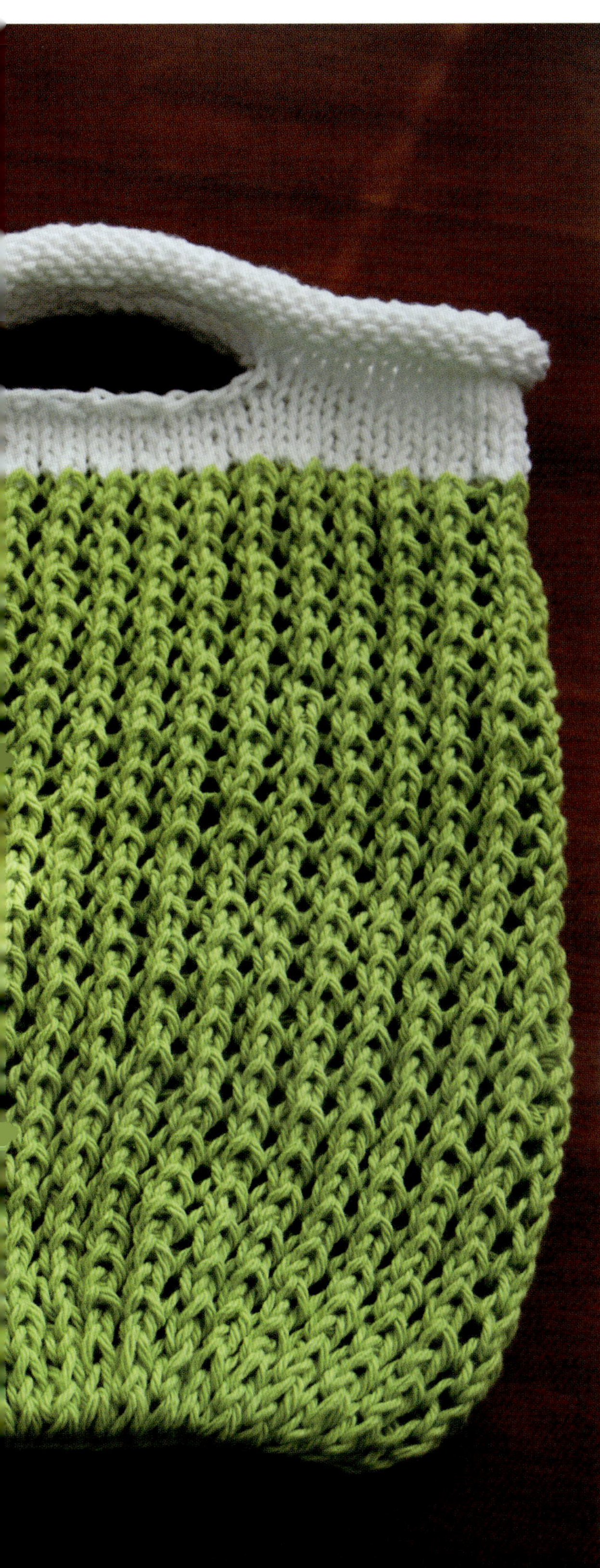
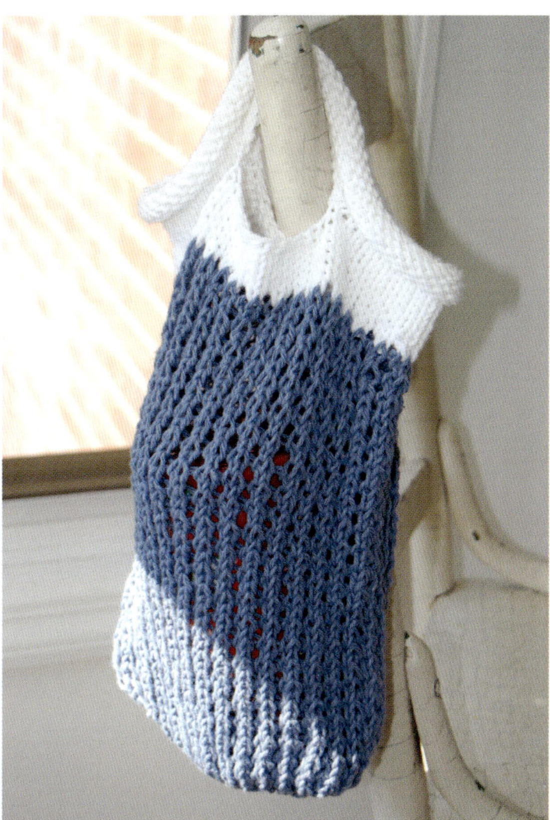
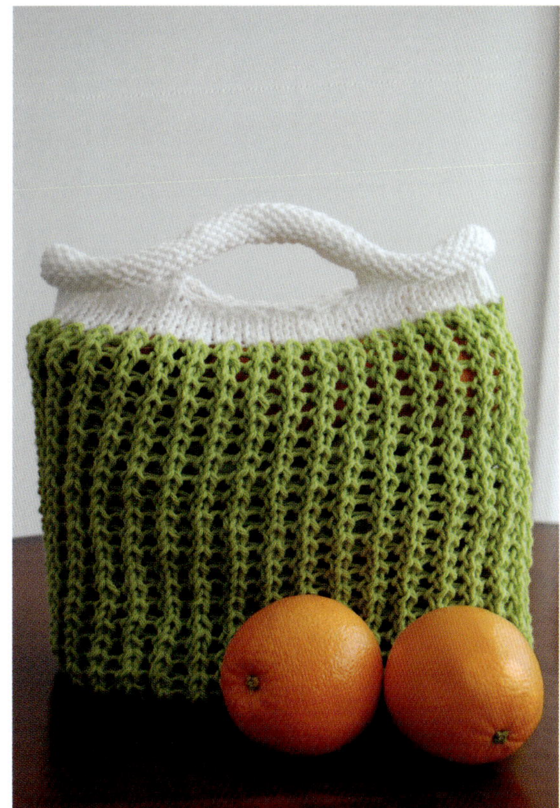

MARKET BAG
DE: Jana Trent

With the handle seamlessly integrated with the body, this bag can stretch to
hold more than a standard plastic grocery bag does. In addition the cotton
material gives it a pleasant, tactile feel.

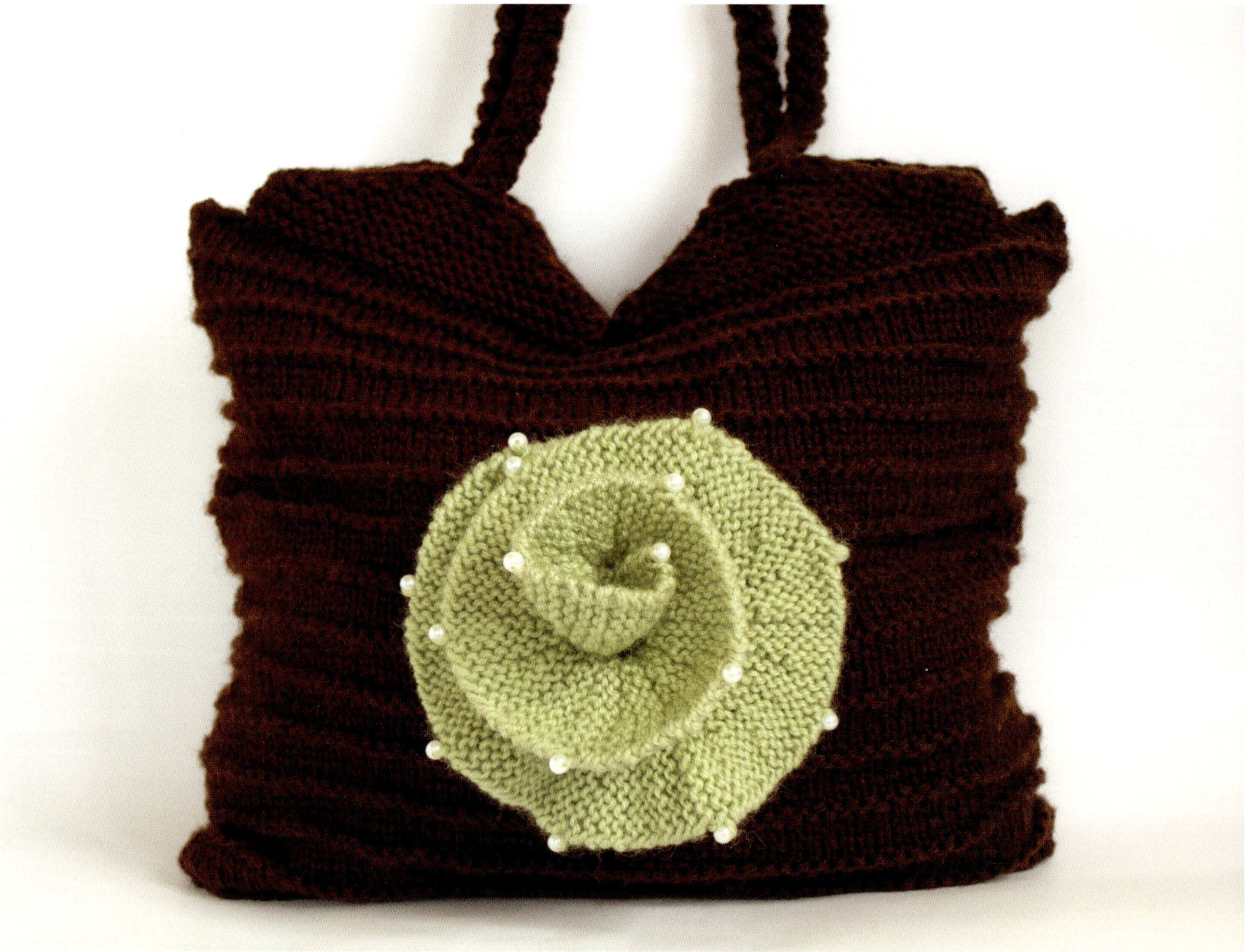

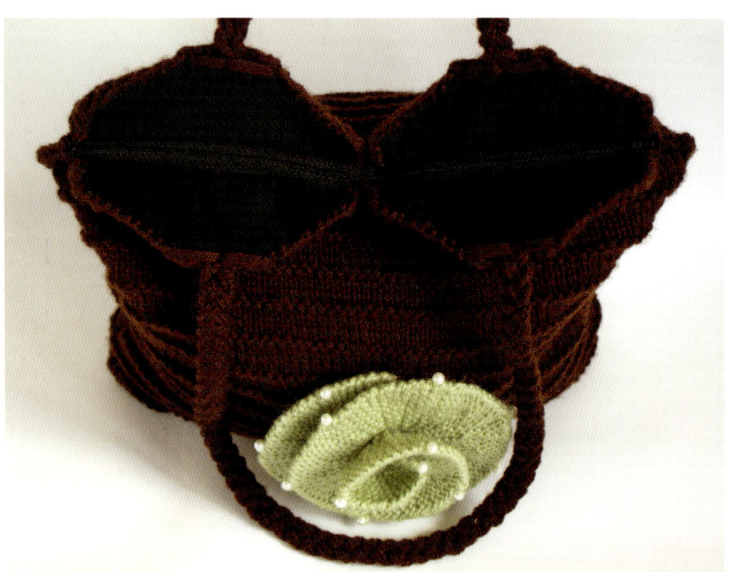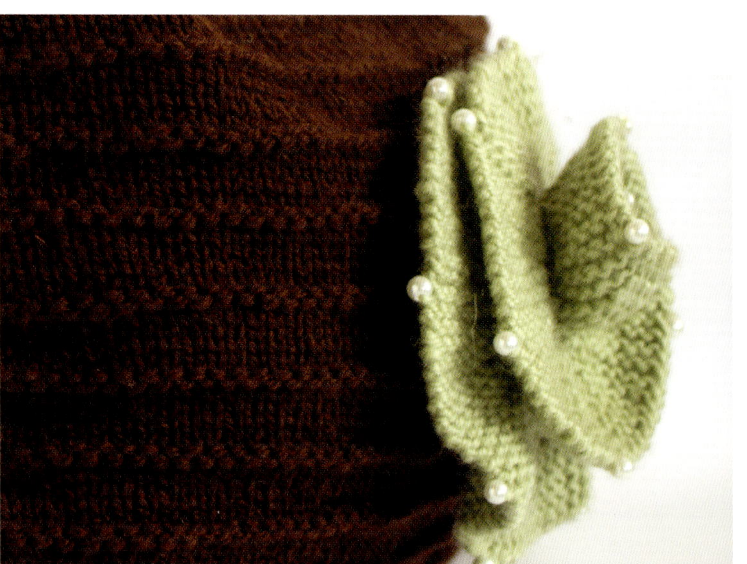

KNIT SHOULDER BAG

DE: Yana Hari Karabelova

In dark chocolate brown and mint green, this bag looks like a yummy petit fours, especially with a large knit flower in front, just like a mint green delicacy fresh out of a pastry bag with creamy white pearls.

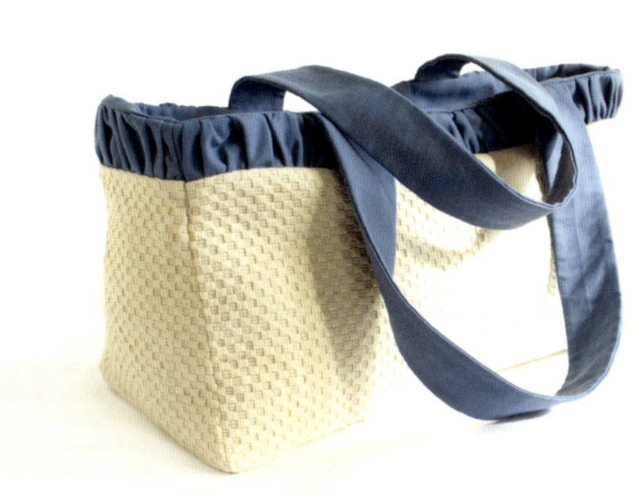 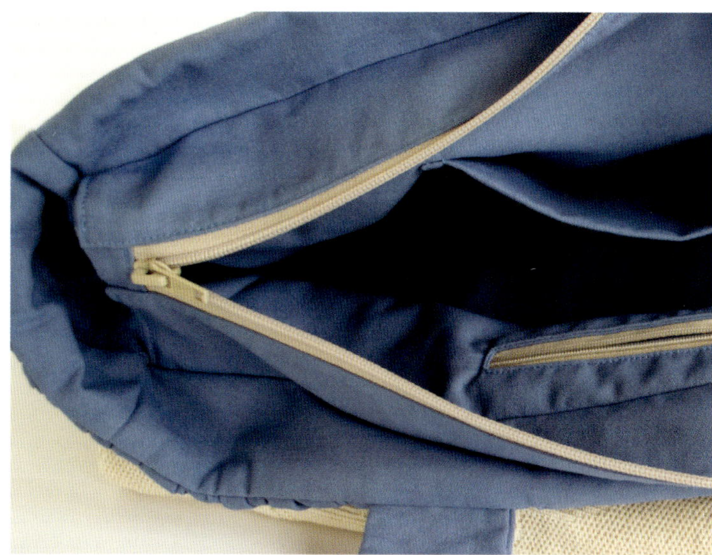

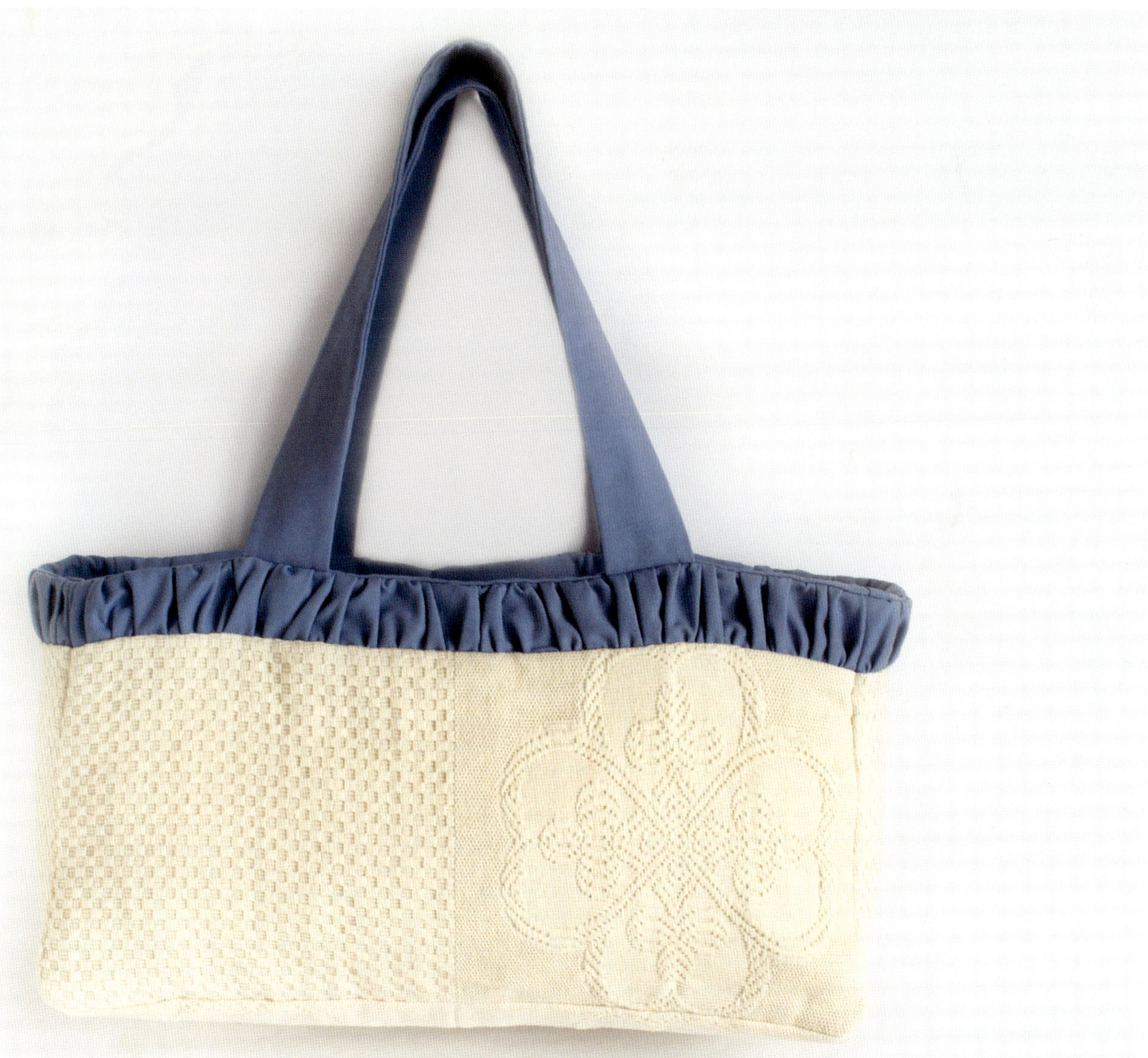

CREAM AND BLUE BAG
DE: Yana Hari Karabelova

In blue and cream, this bag is in tune with long sunny days on the beach.
Upholstery fabric was used for the body and twill cotton for the ruffled part
on top, the handles and the lining.

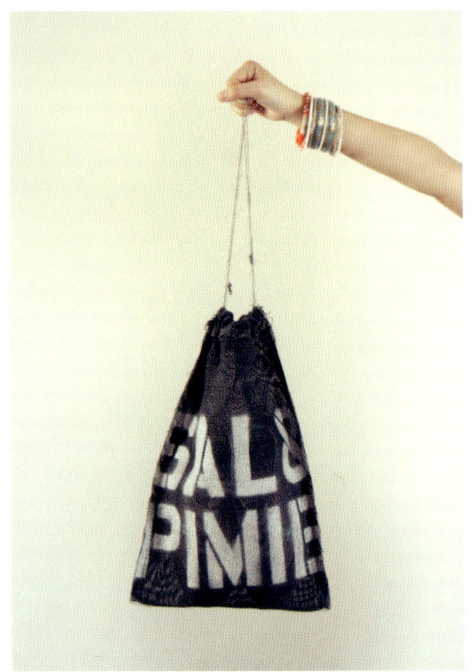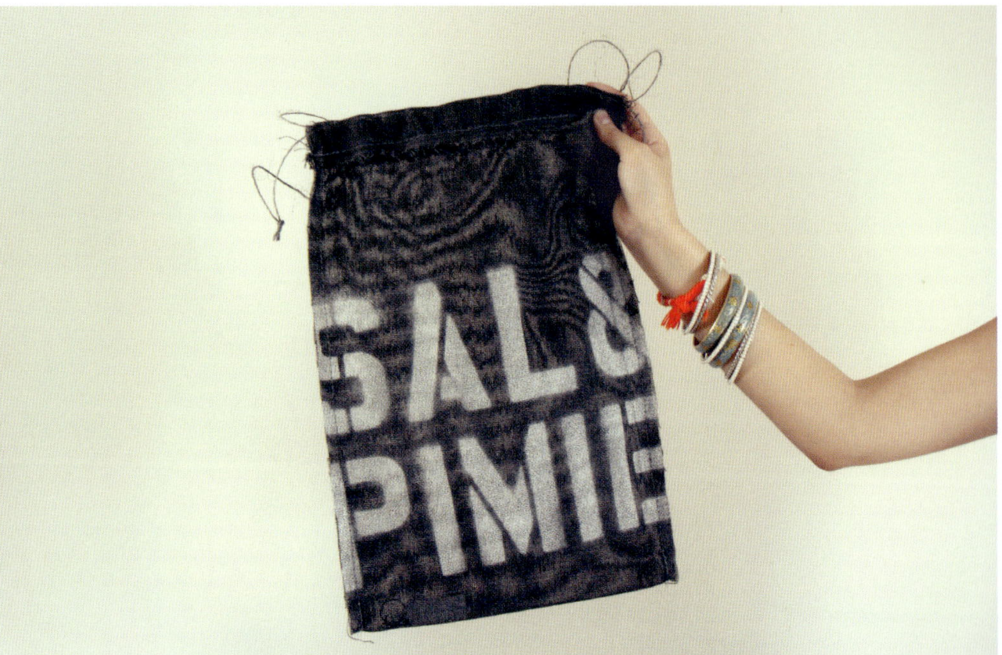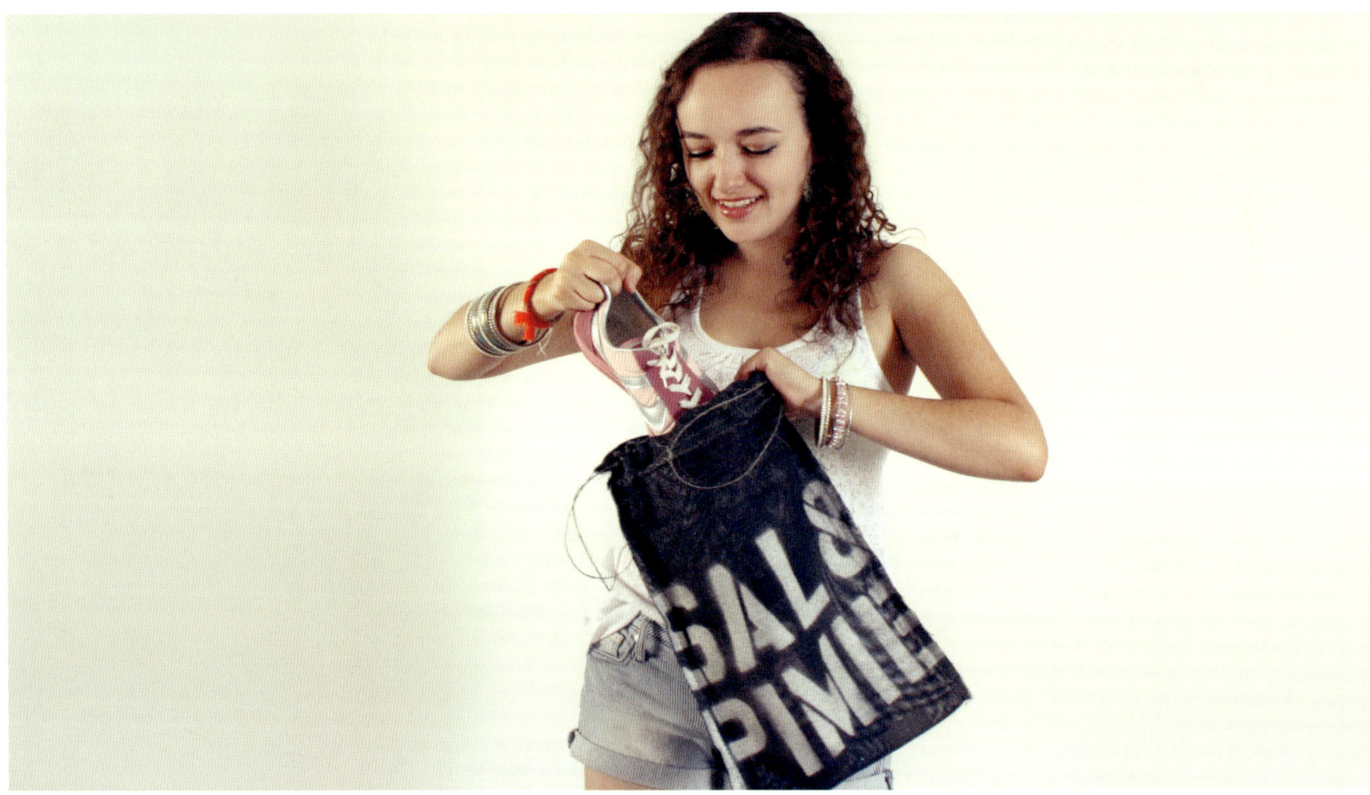

ANNIVERSARY BAG

DA: Ames Studio

Designed as a brand's anniversary gift bag, this bag was made from soft jute and sprayed with silver acrylic using a stencil.

DELICATE MATERIAL

DA: Babich Design and Branding

Designed for a shop featuring handmade soaps, Oleg Babich employed elements of nature - air, water, earth and fire - in a watercolor aesthetic, printed against a white or a pastel color background to convey the refreshing style of the brand.

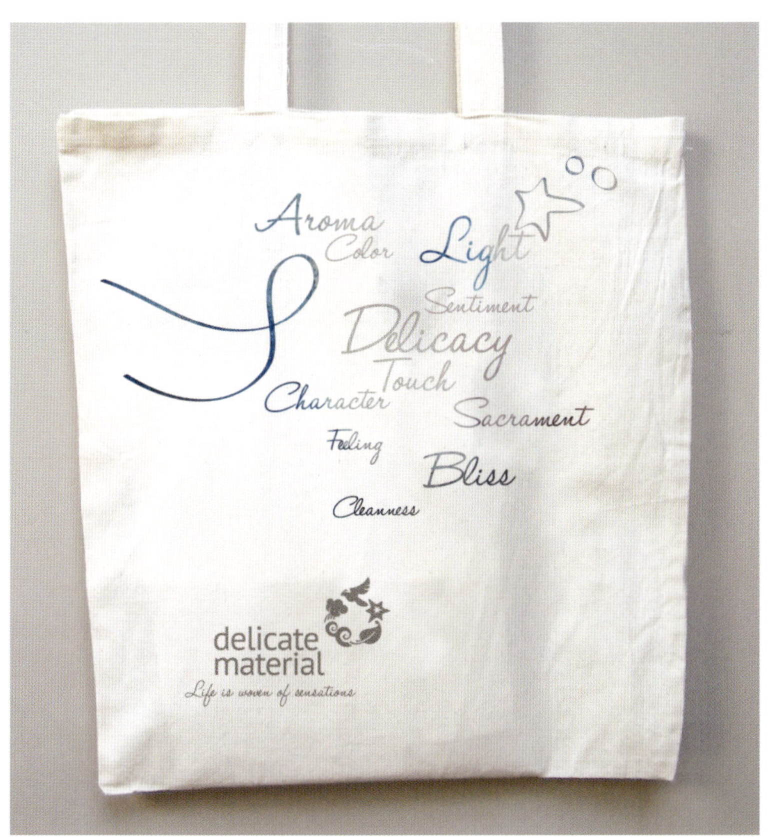

Aroma
Color Light
Sentiment
Delicacy
Touch
Character Sacrament
Feeling
Bliss
Cleanness
delicate
material
Life is woven of sensations

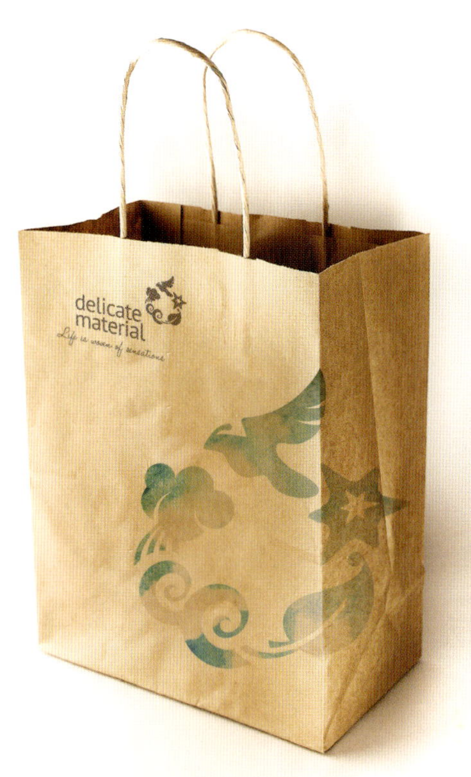

delicate
material
Life is woven of sensations

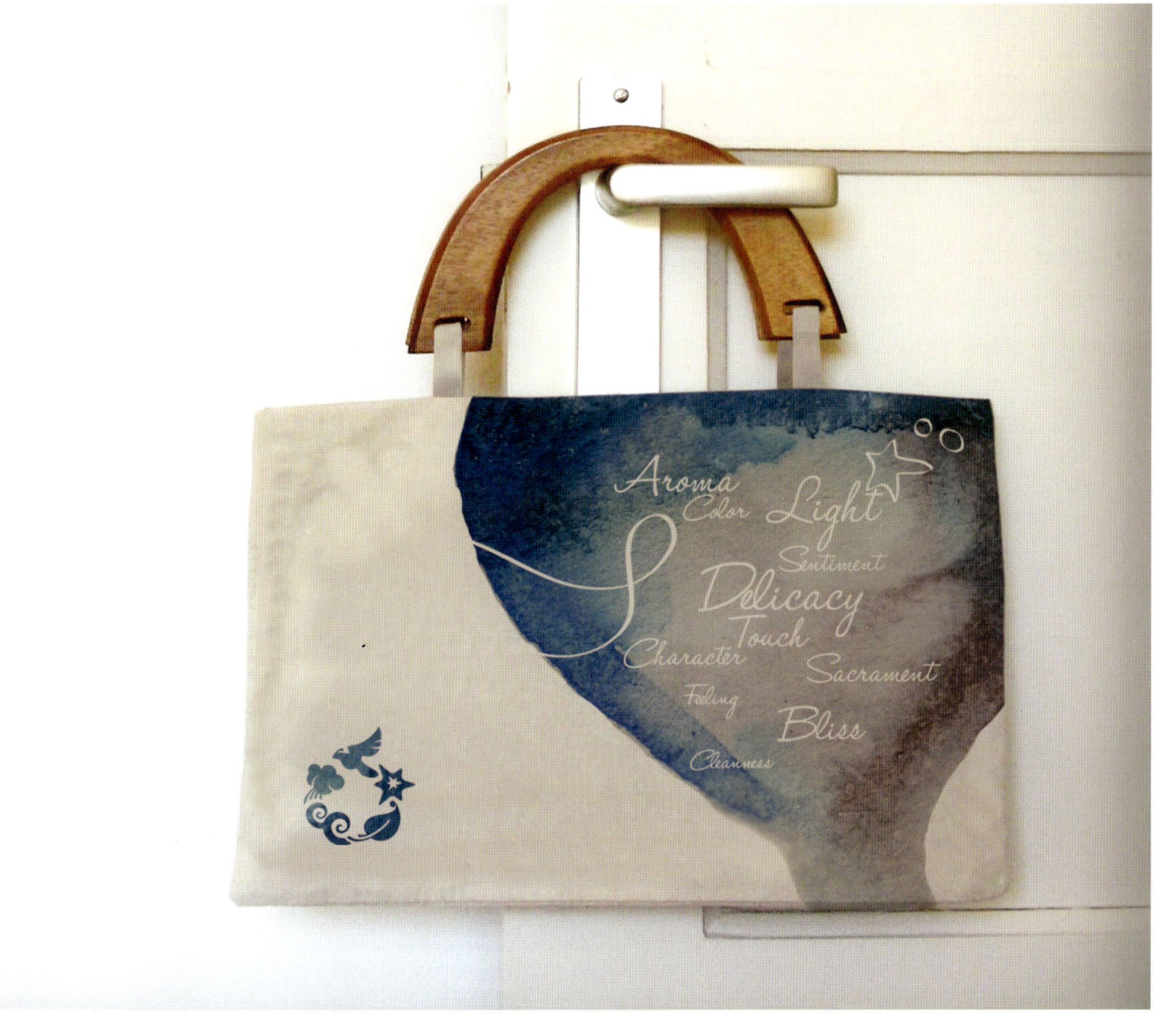

Aroma
Color Light
Sentiment
Delicacy
Touch
Character Sacrament
Feeling
Bliss
Cleanness

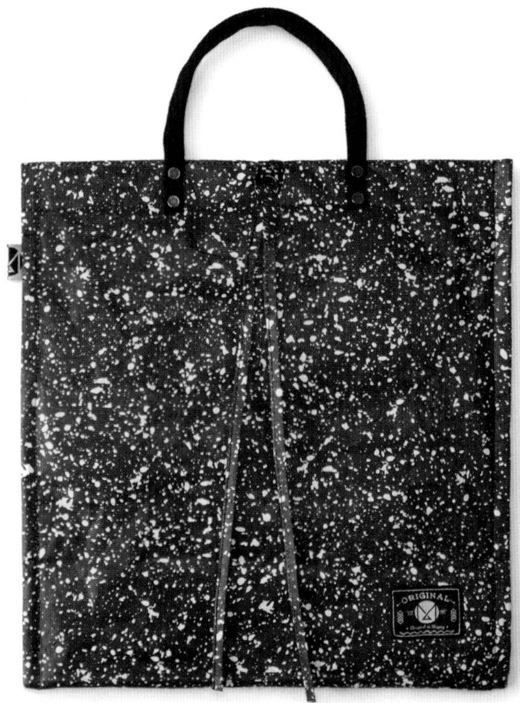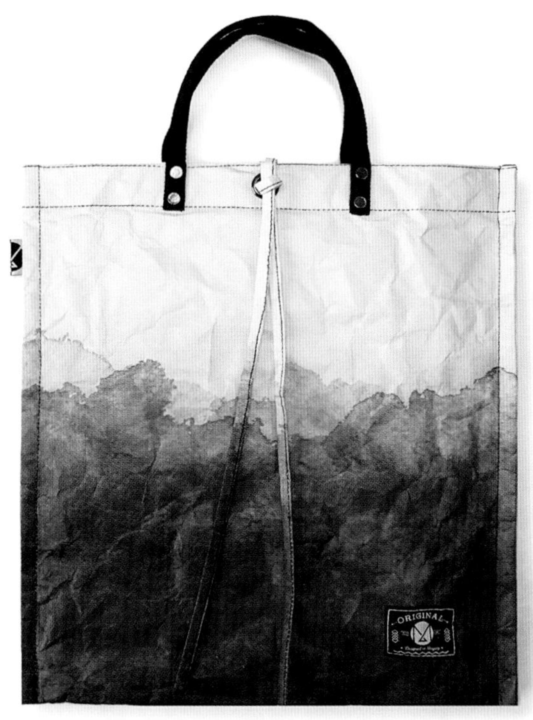

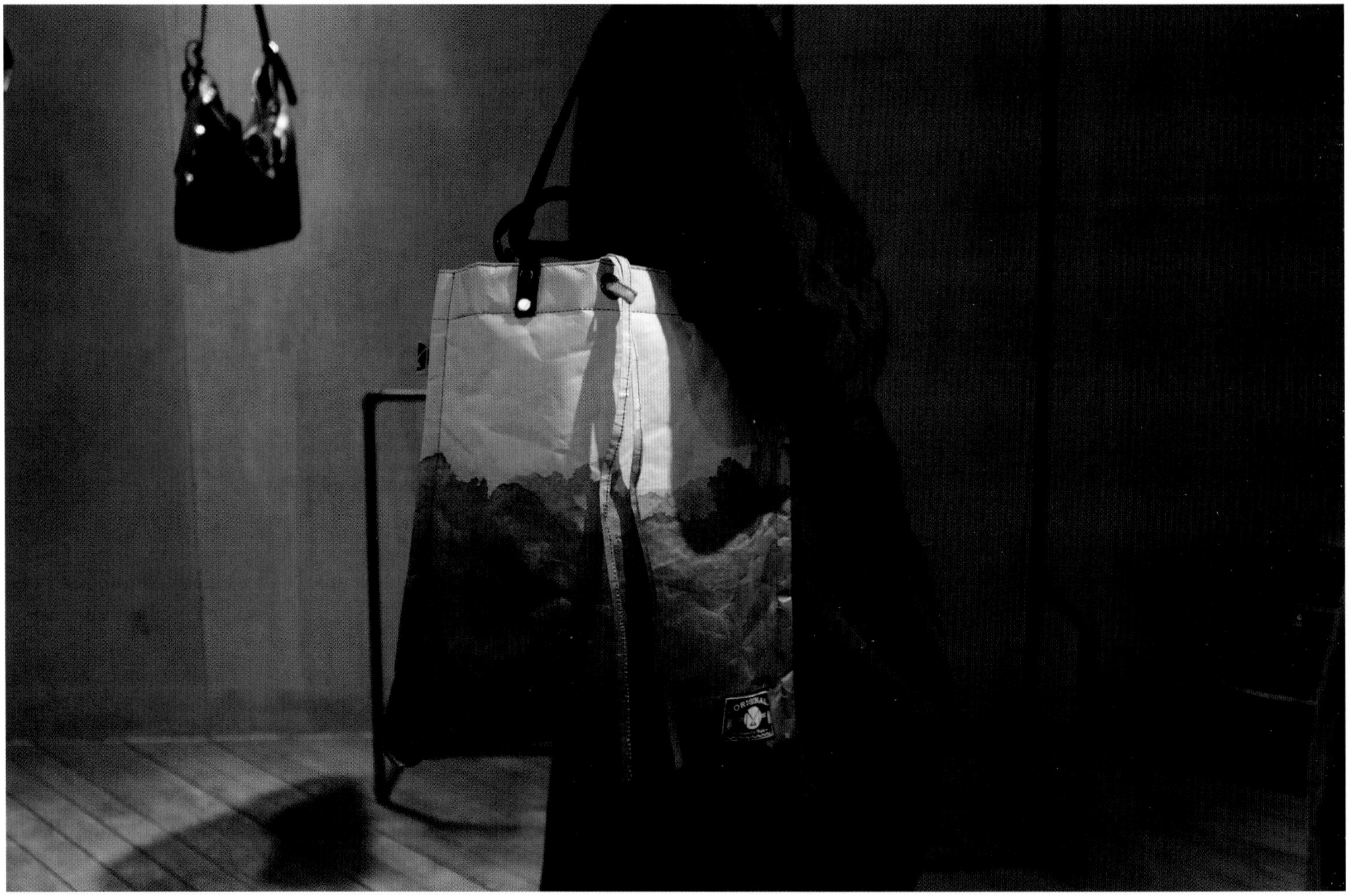

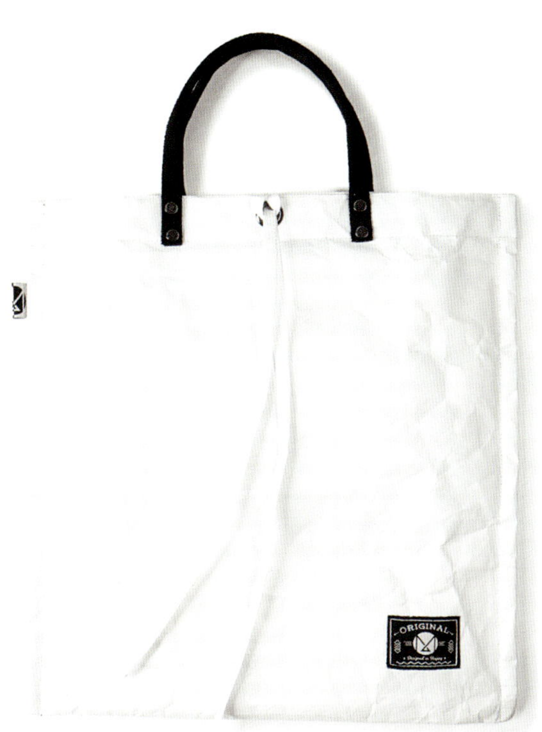

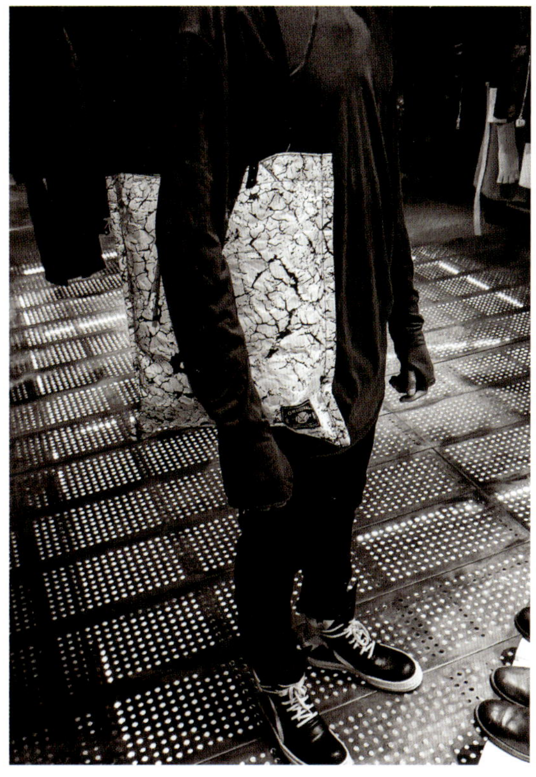

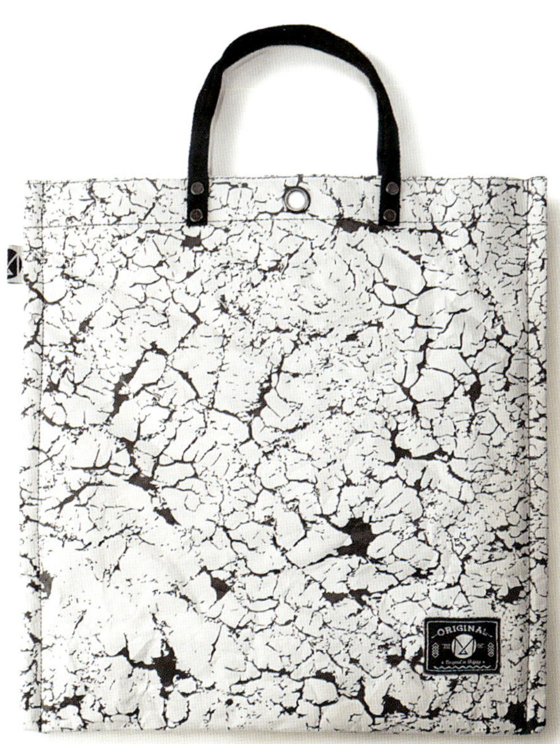

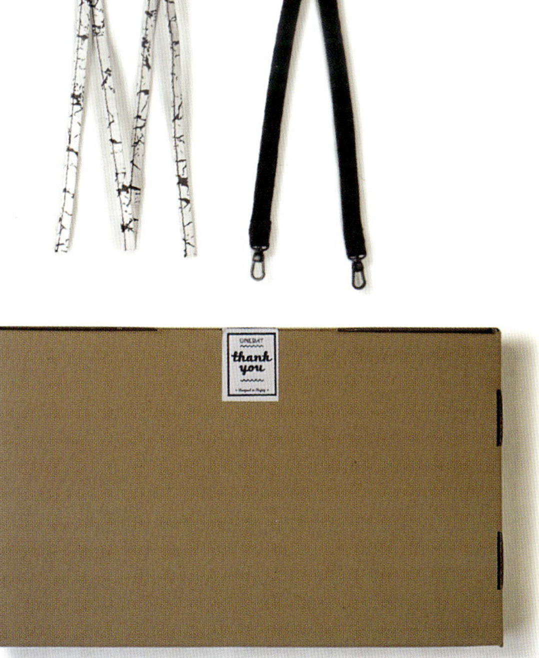

PAPERY BAG
DA: Oneday

Made from Tyvek, the "Papery Bag" series weighs only half as much as
bags made of paper, and is waterproof and durable. The imprint gives
individuality to each bag.

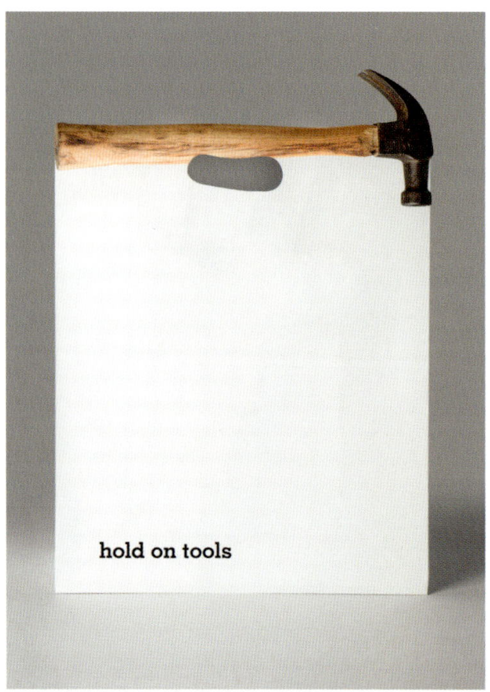
hold on tools

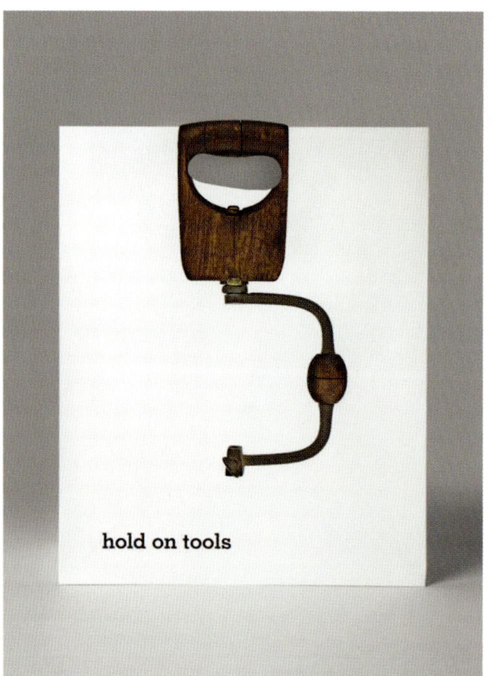
hold on tools

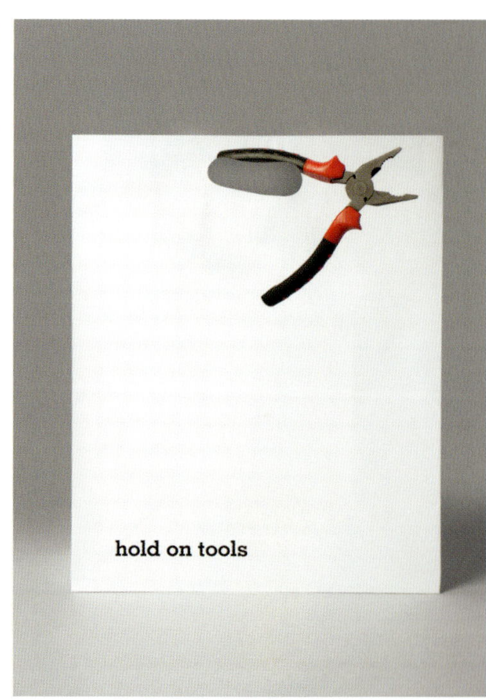
hold on tools

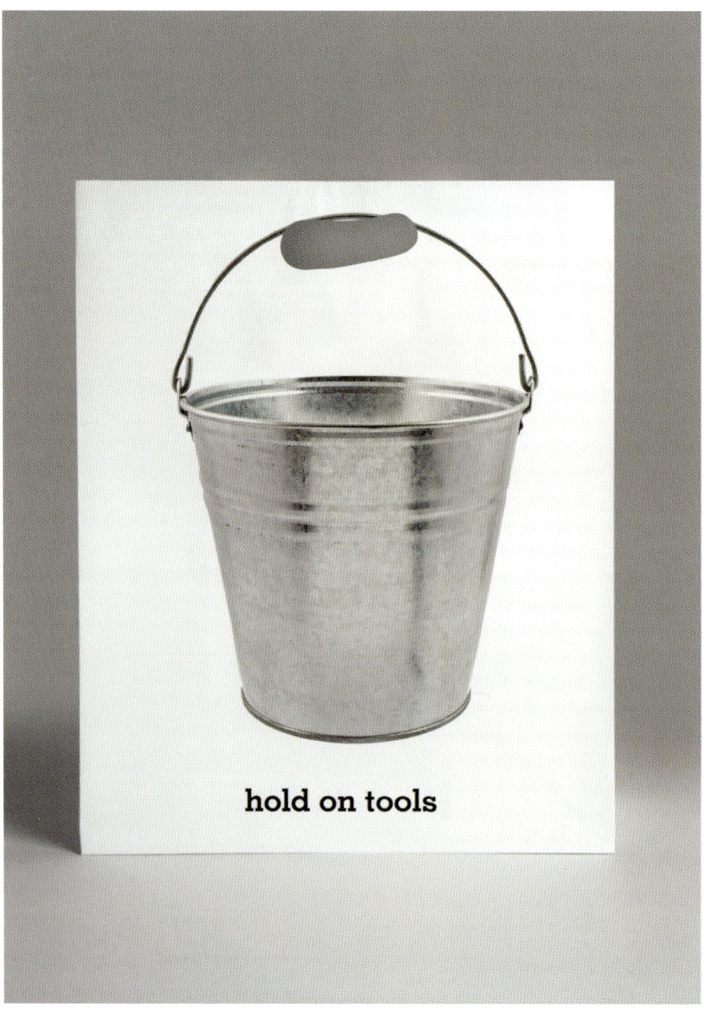
hold on tools

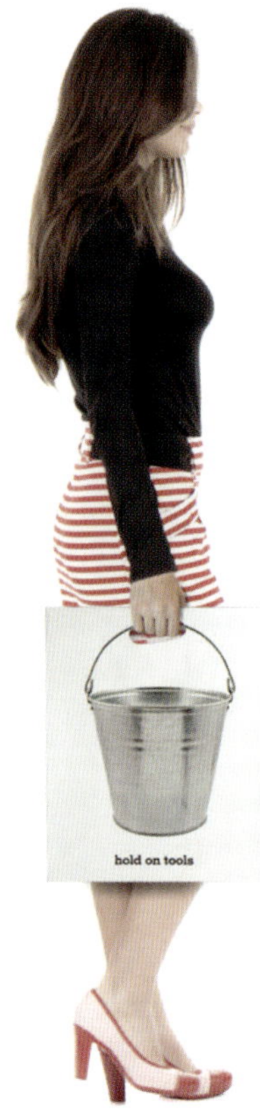
hold on tools

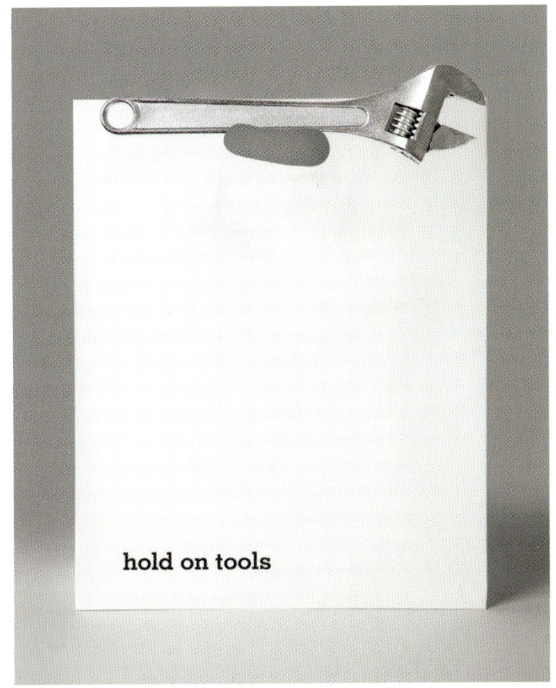

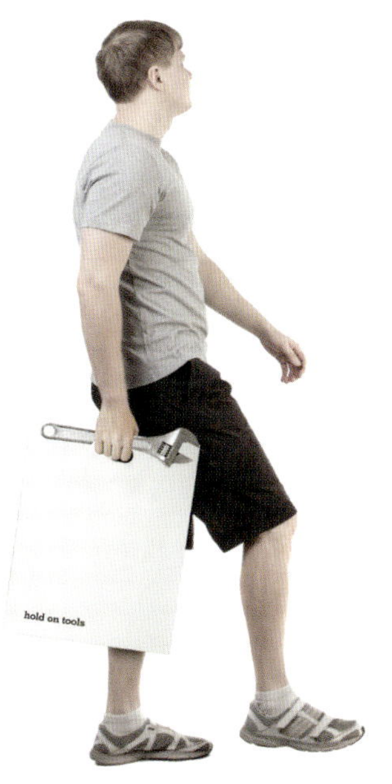

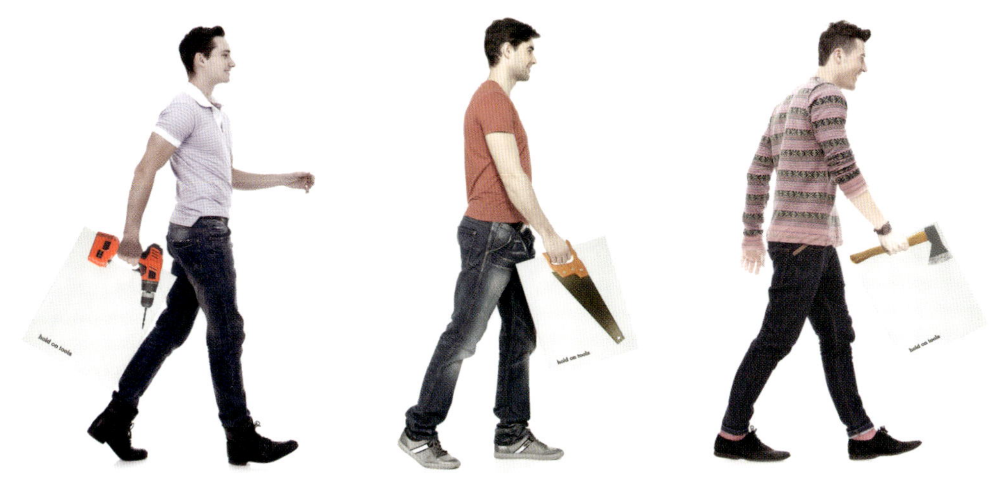

HOLD ON TOOLS
DE: Khudayar Agayarov

"Hold On Tools" are designed to add a sense of playfulness to a tool shop. It is an interesting approach to show that one has just purchased some tools and to attract others to do the same.

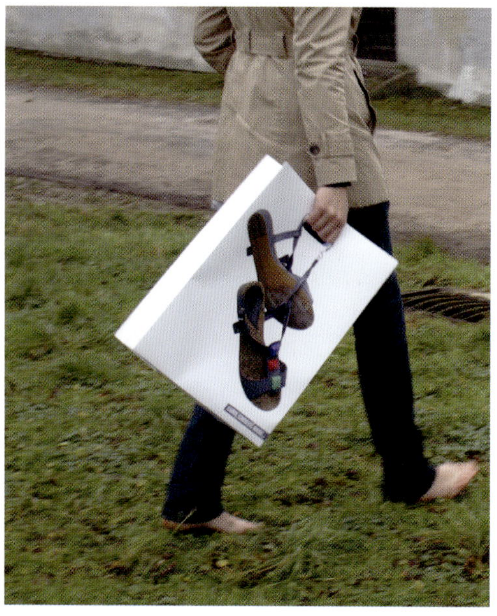
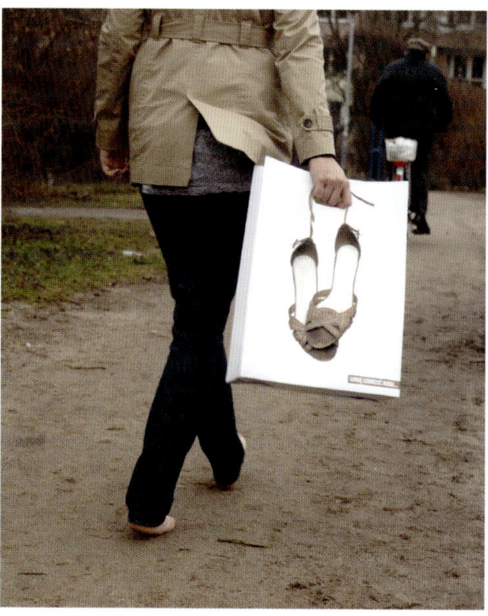
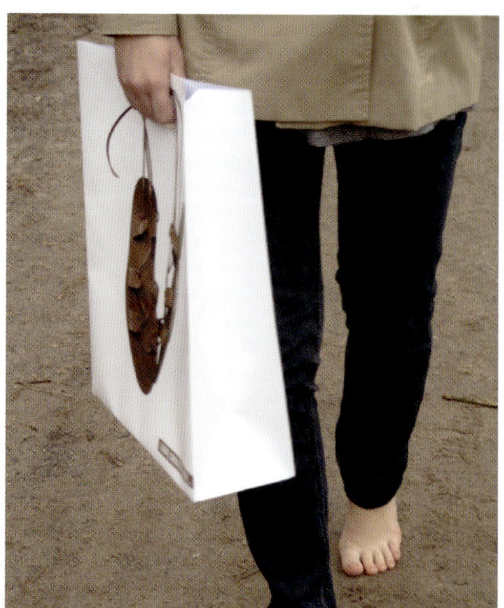

I LIKE WALKING BAREFOOT
DE: Weronika Piatek

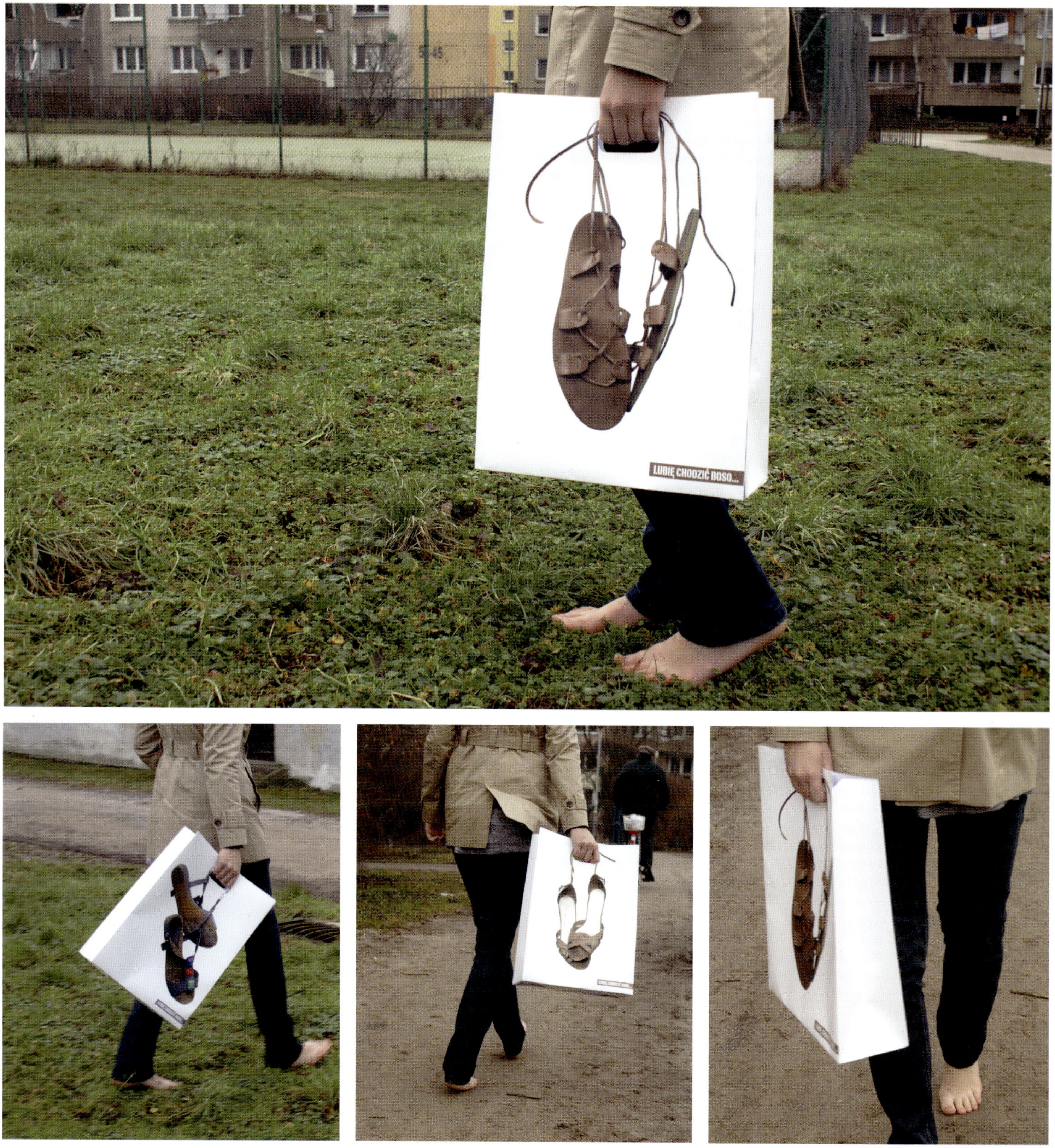

The "Barefoot Bag" urges people to walk barefoot, prompting them to live
a natural and simple life, putting an end to consumerism. Easily confused
with bags for advertisement, as the designer intended, they sell a life
philosophy instead of products.

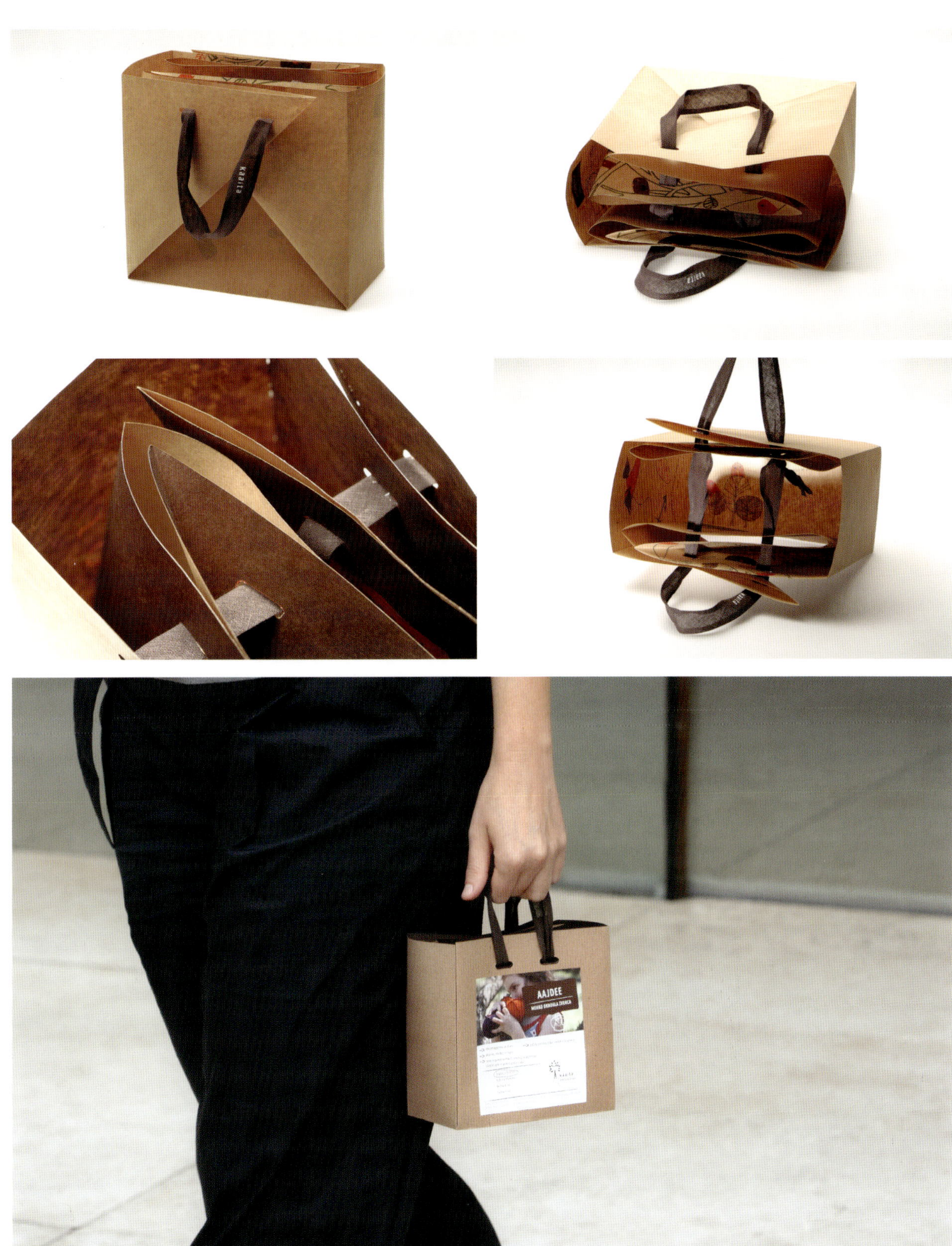

BIGABAGA
DE: Urska Hocevar(Kaaita)

"Bigabaga" is made of a one-piece recycled paper, with instructional folds for users to perform the act of construction before taking advantage of an eco-friendly container.

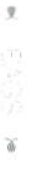

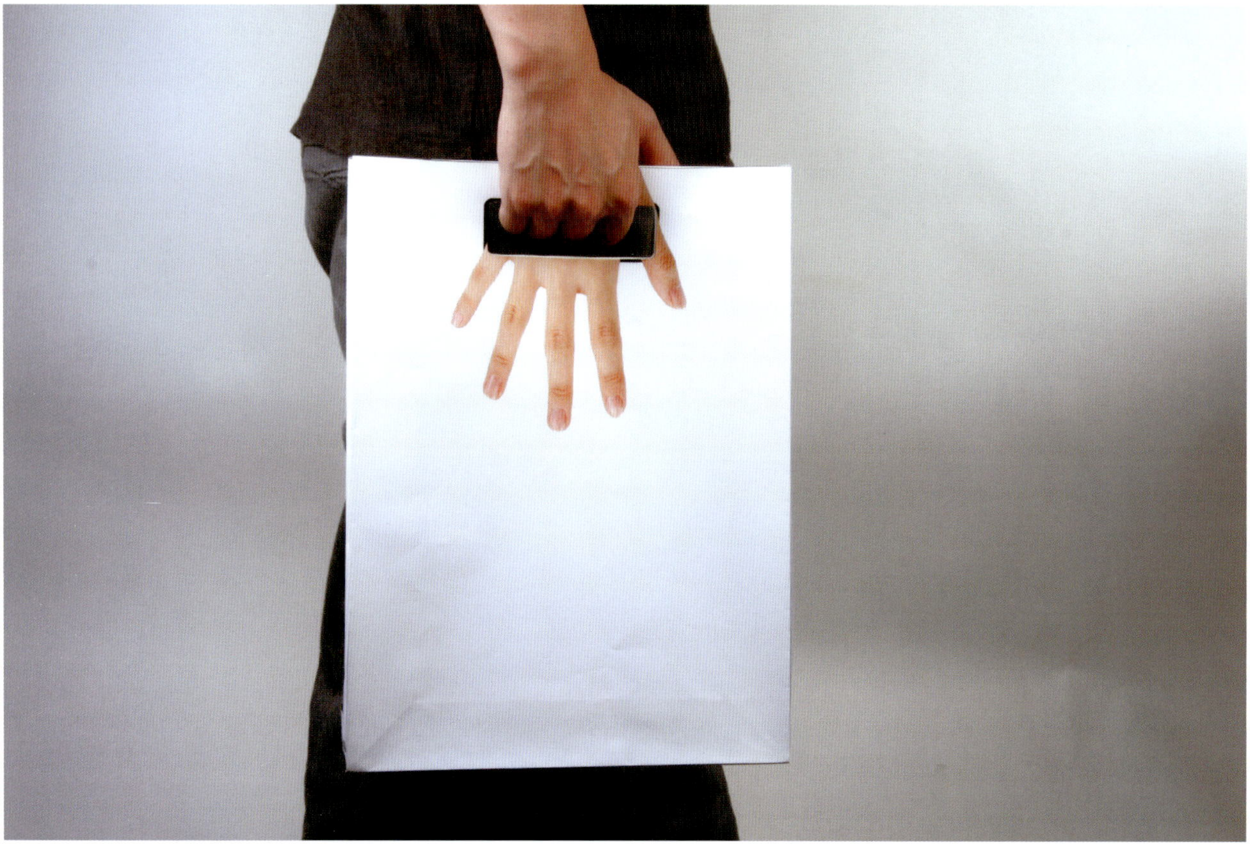

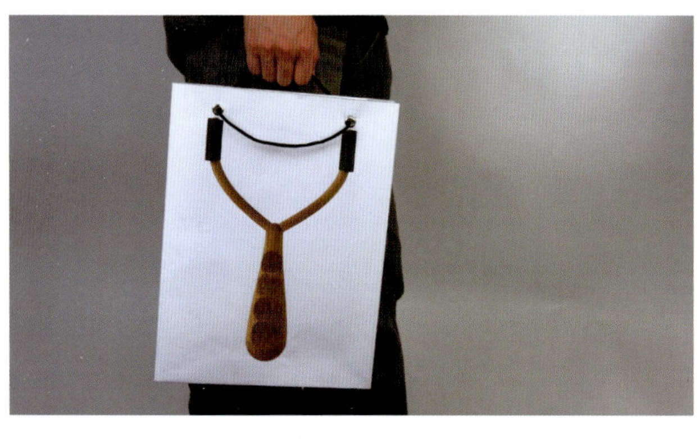

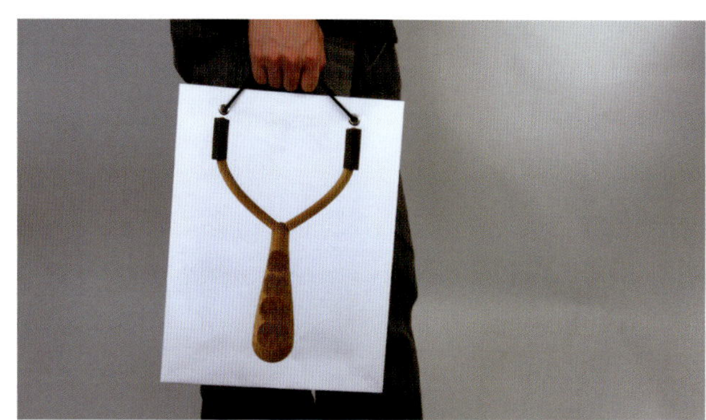

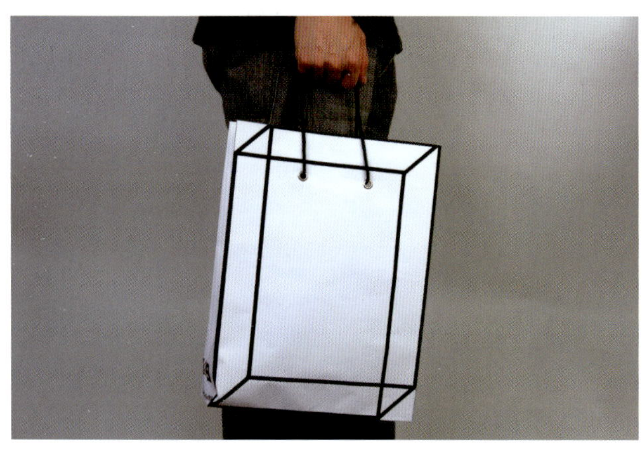

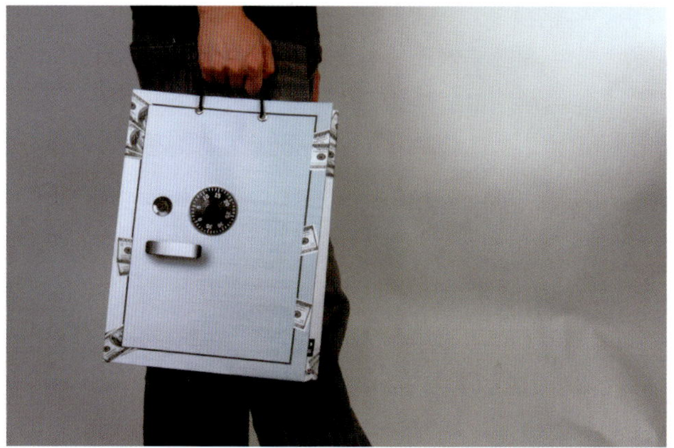

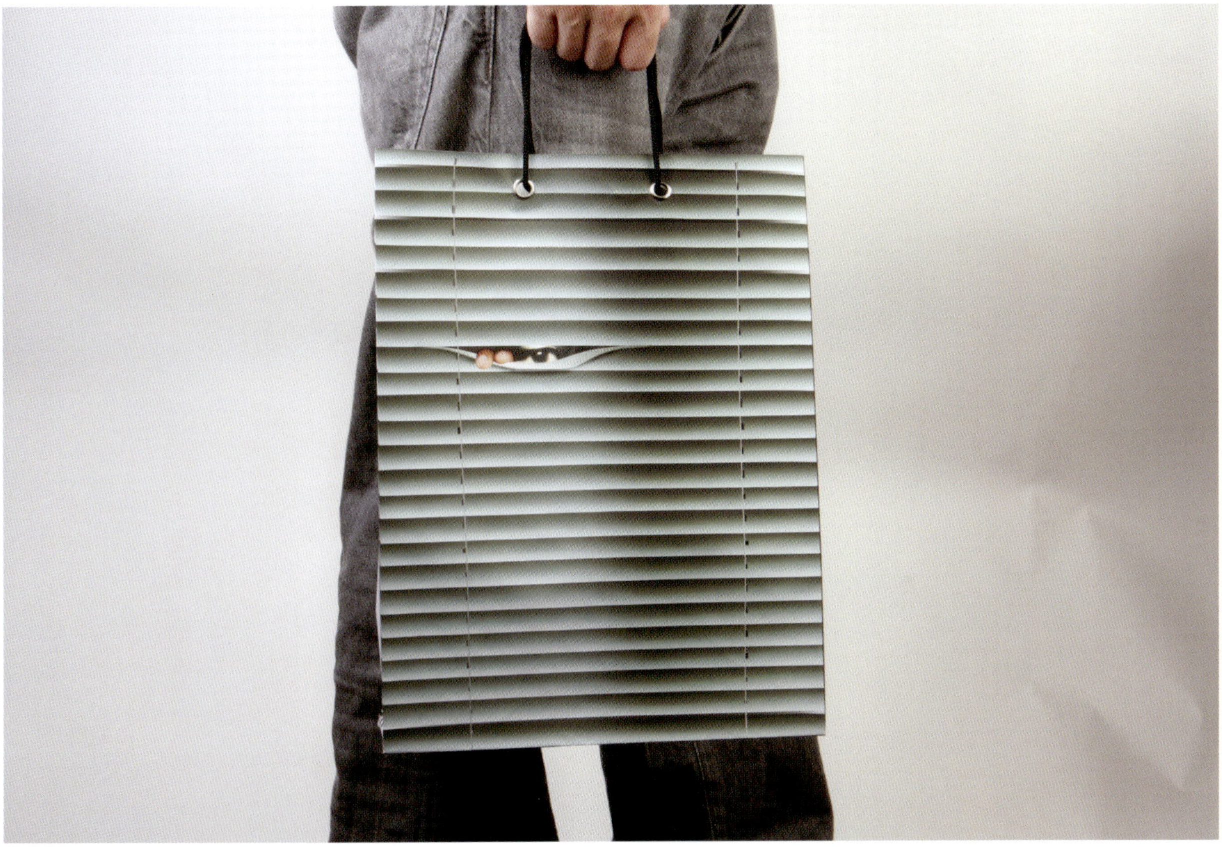

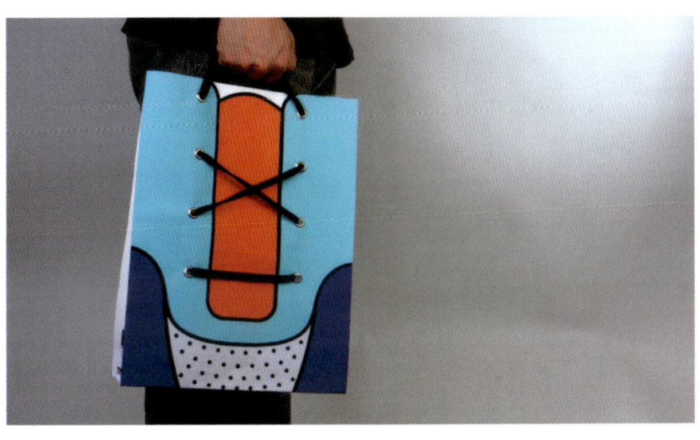

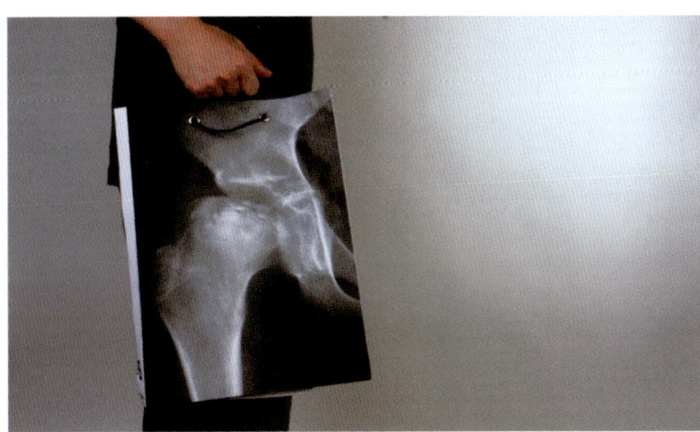

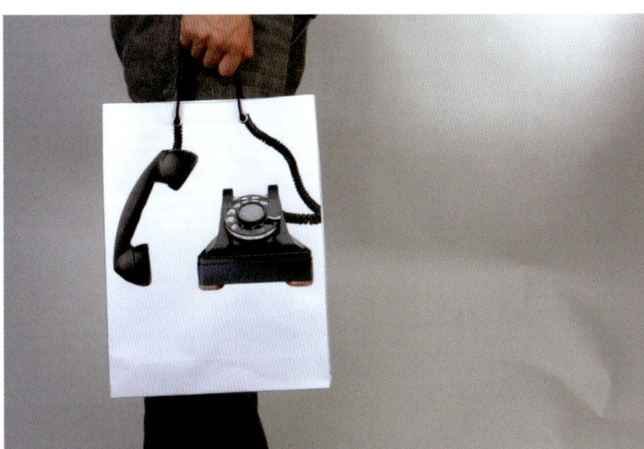

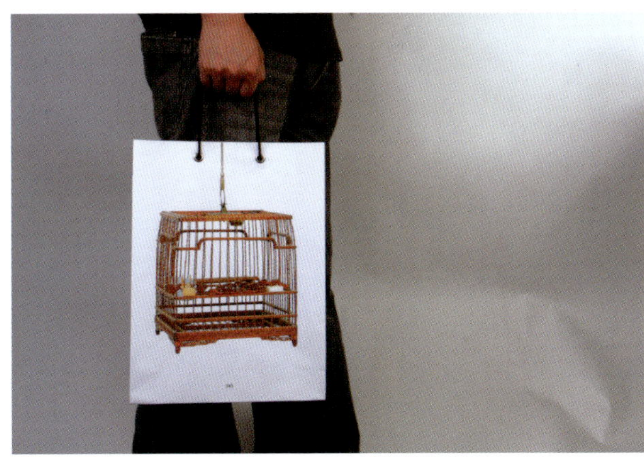

TAOMADESIGN BAGS
DE: Tao Ma

The "Taomadesign Bags," connected with Chinese culture and playfulness, remind
people to carry with them a sense of humor and to relax from time to time.

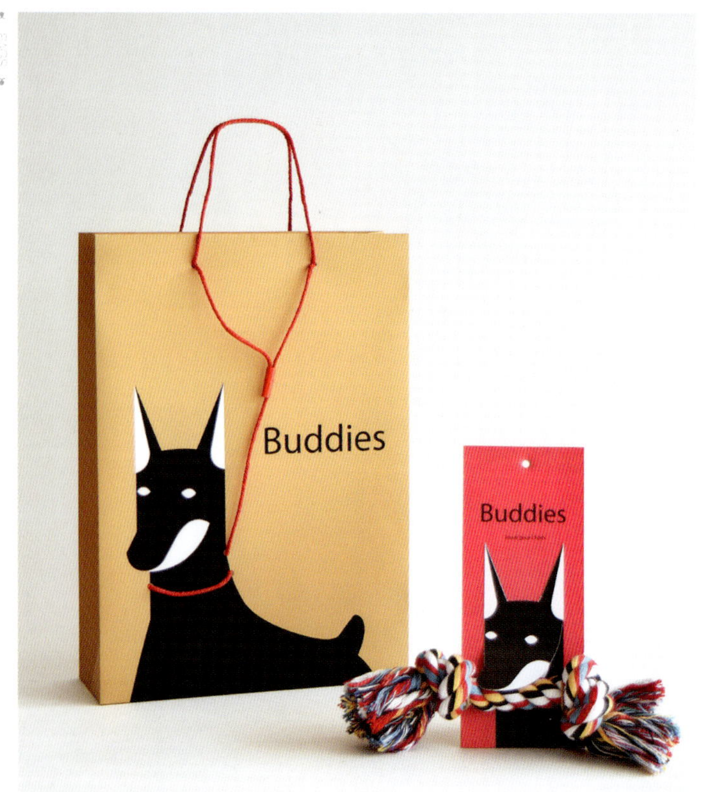

Buddies
Buddies

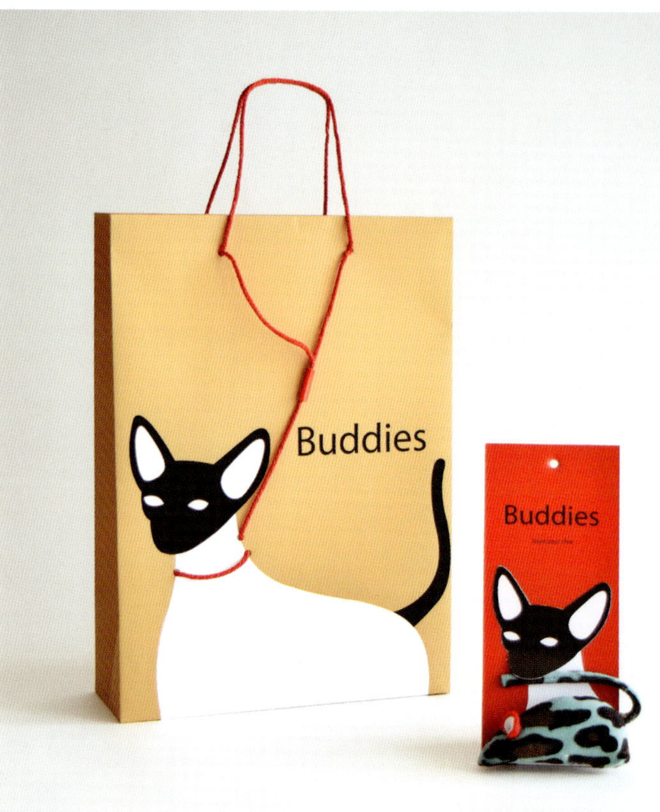

Buddies
Buddies

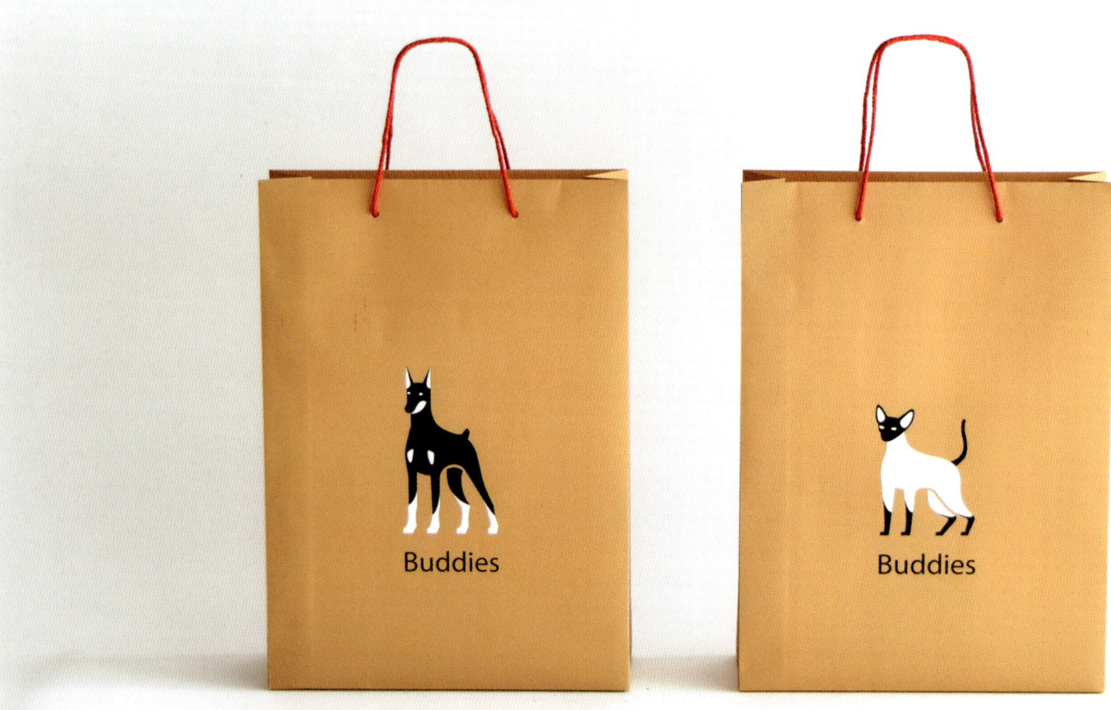

Buddies
Buddies

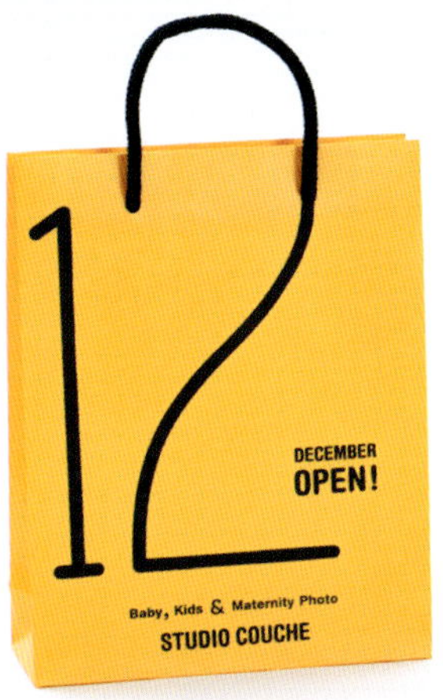

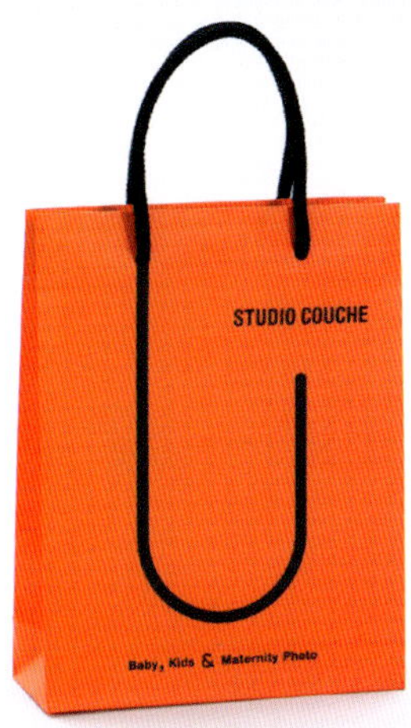

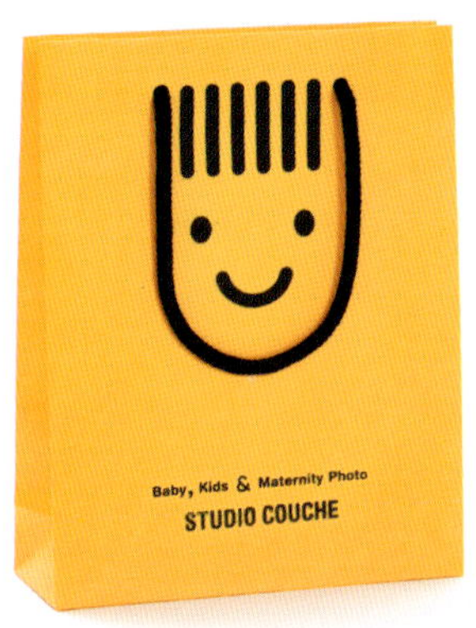

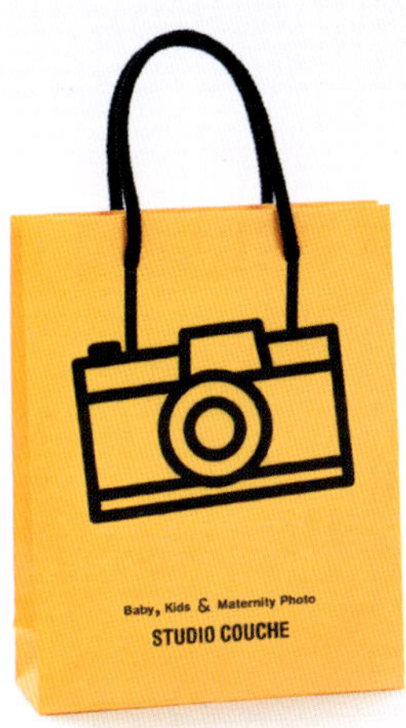

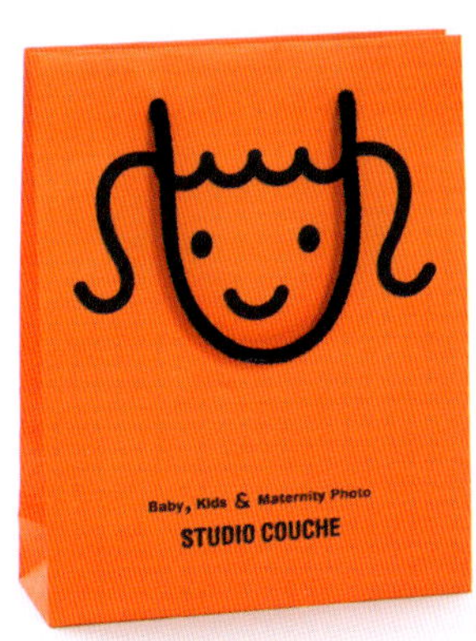

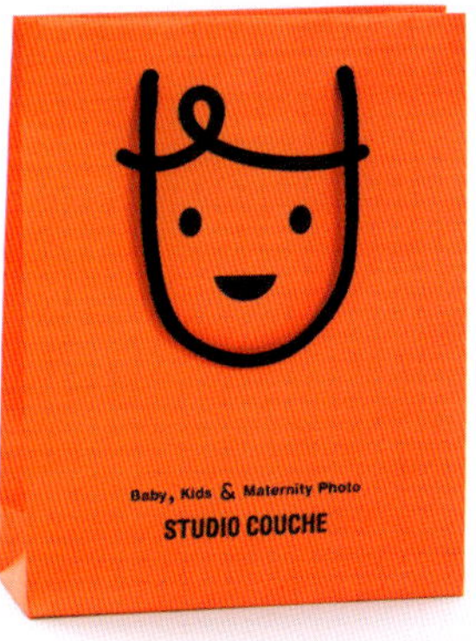

BUDDIES
DE: Yuelan Liu

Intended for a pet toy shop, these bags were printed with pictograms. The handles are like a part of the leash, so that when users carry the bag, it is as if they are walking a pet.

STUDIO COUCHE
DA: Coton Design

Designed for a photo studio for kids, this series was printed with icons of smiling faces, letters and numbers completed with handles.

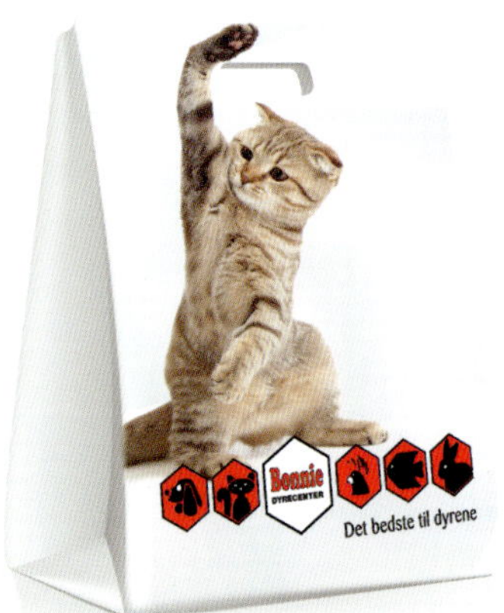
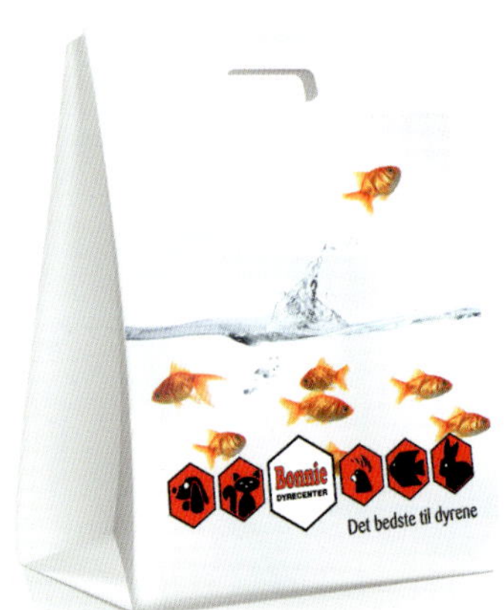
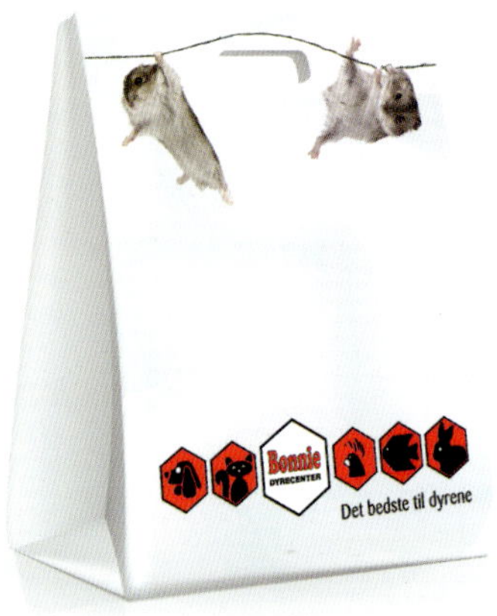
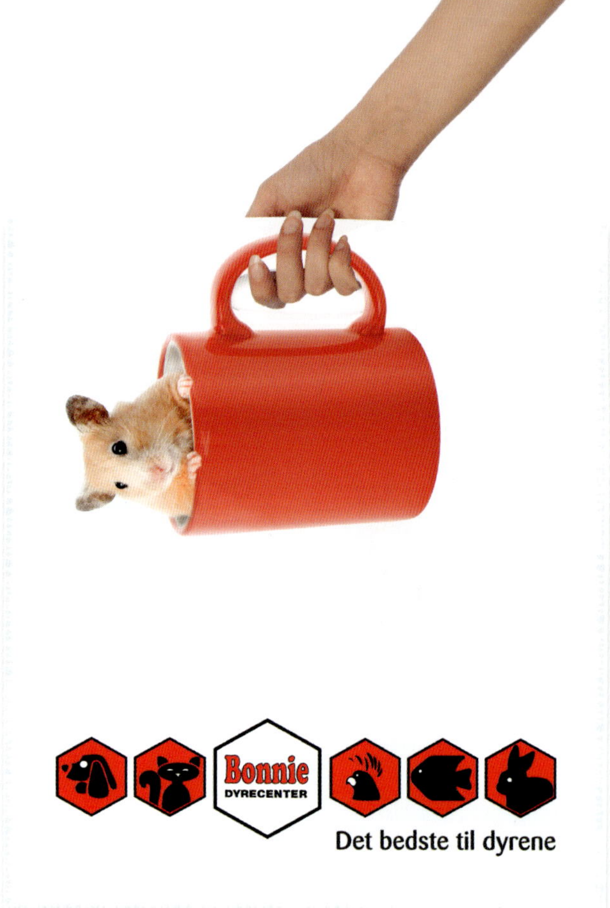

BONNIE BAGS

DE: Björgvin Guðjónsson

A Denmark pet shop wants to give customers a playful impression with interactive bags printed with happy animals, sending the message that they provide: "the very best for your pets."

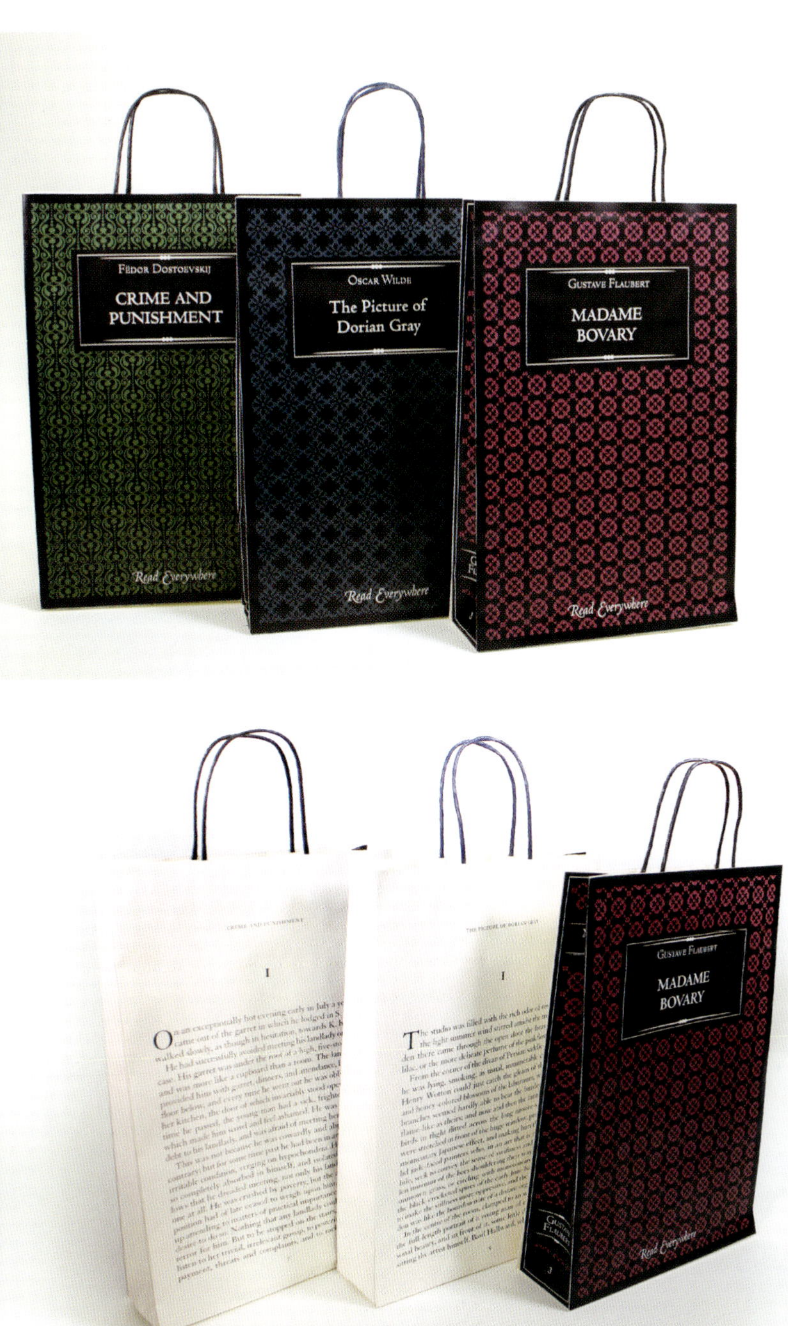

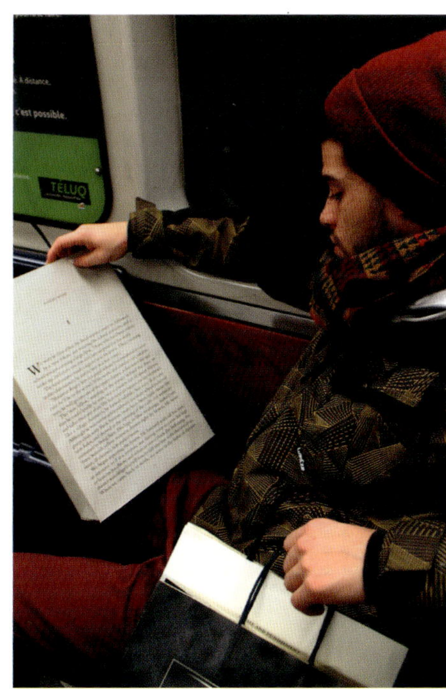

READ EVERYWHERE
DE: Sofia Girelli

Aiming to demonstrate the beauty of reading, this series shows the cover and the first page of some of the best books in the world. They interact with pedestrians who encounter them, acting as an invitation to read.

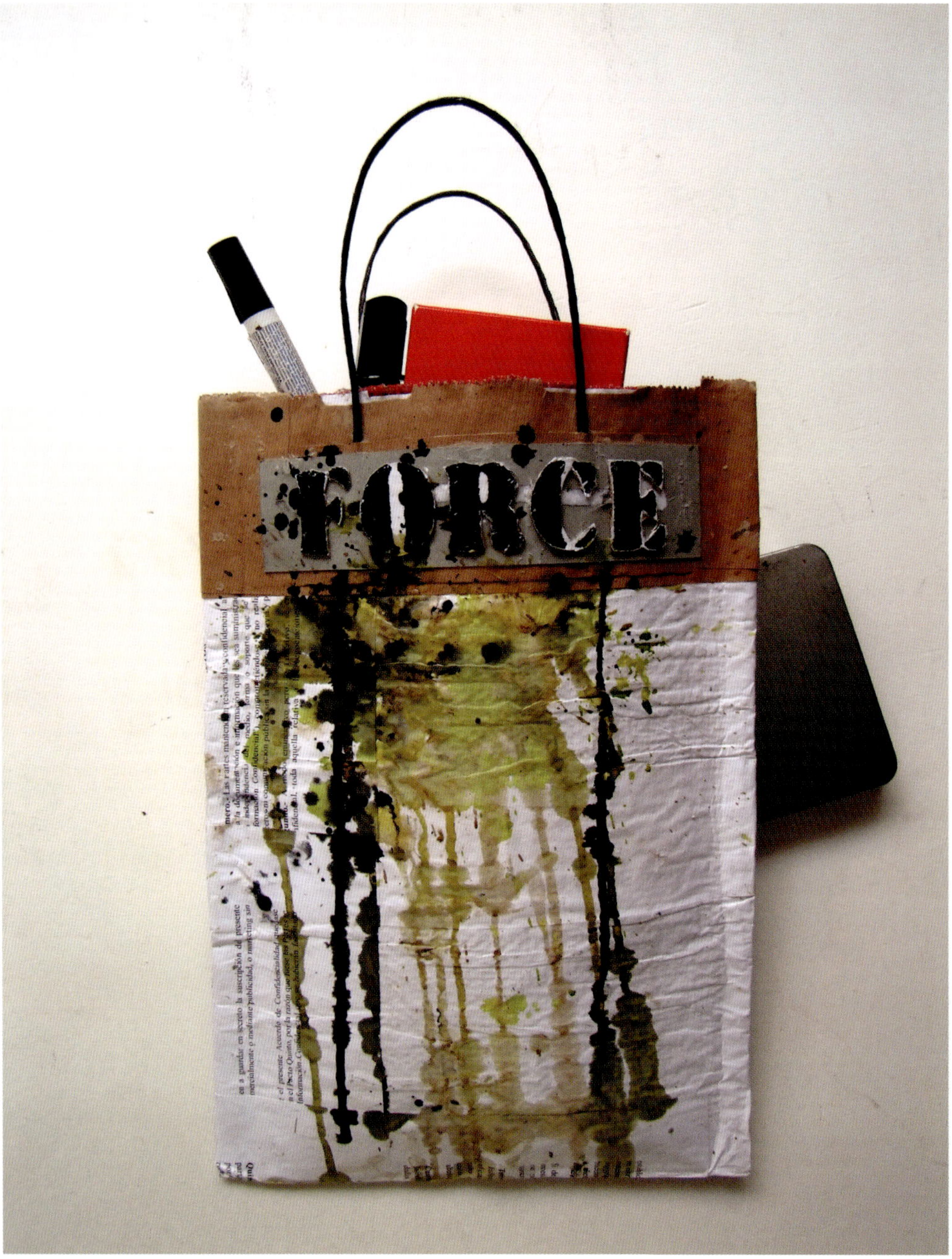

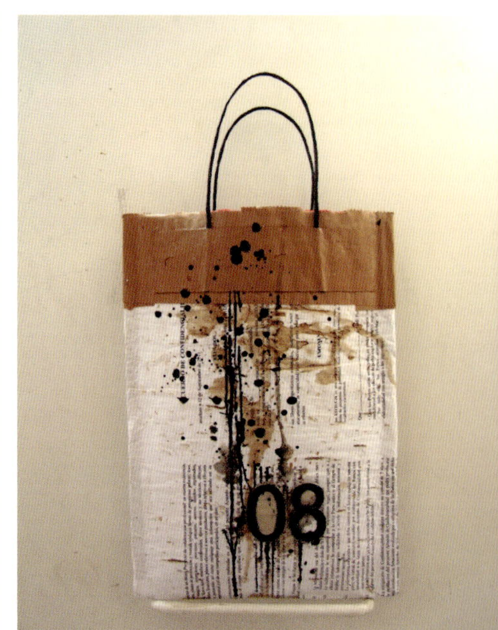

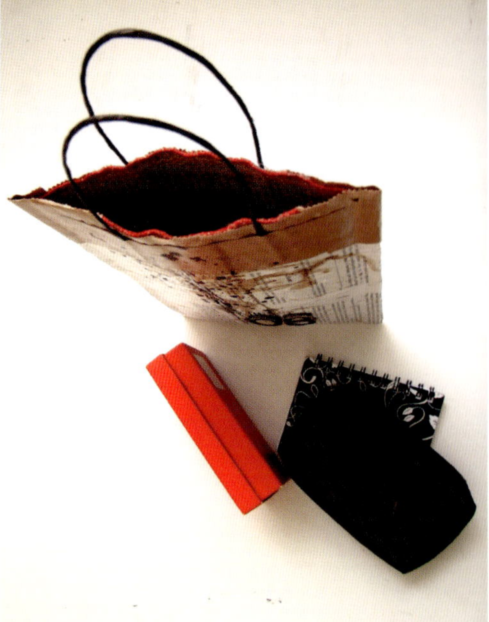

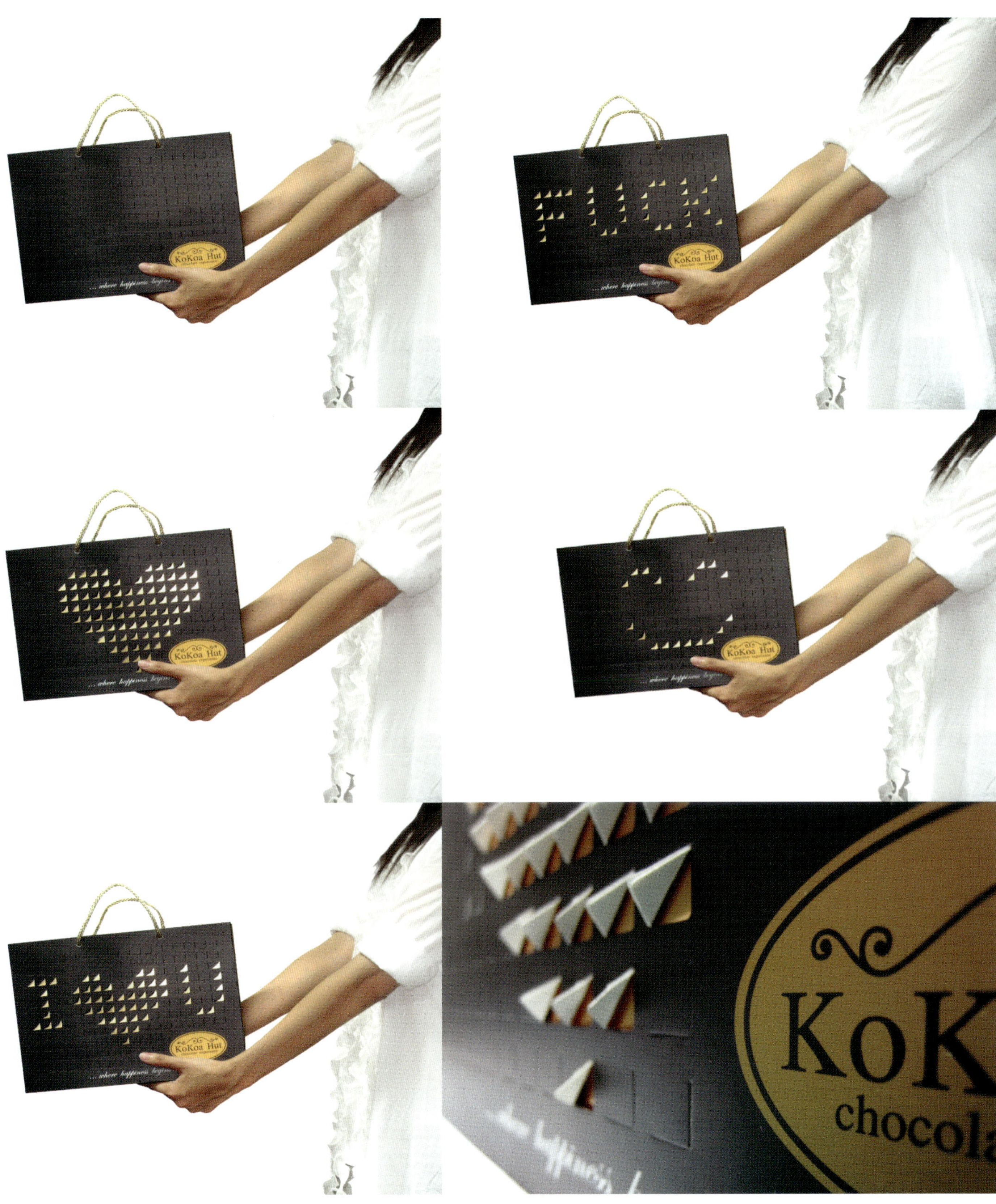

RE-BAG

DE: Paulo Humberto Reis de Almeida e Silva

The name "Re-bag" bears two meanings. First, it was made with recycled jute.
Second, users can participate in the design of the bag by using stickers,
paint, or a piece of paper on the surface.

KOKOA HUT SHOPPING BAG

DE: Passorn Subcharoenpun

Desiged for a chocolate shop, this bag enables consumers to express
their feeling to the gift receivers or just everyone. Through the little
squareboxes, shoppers can flip up the boxes to create images or words.

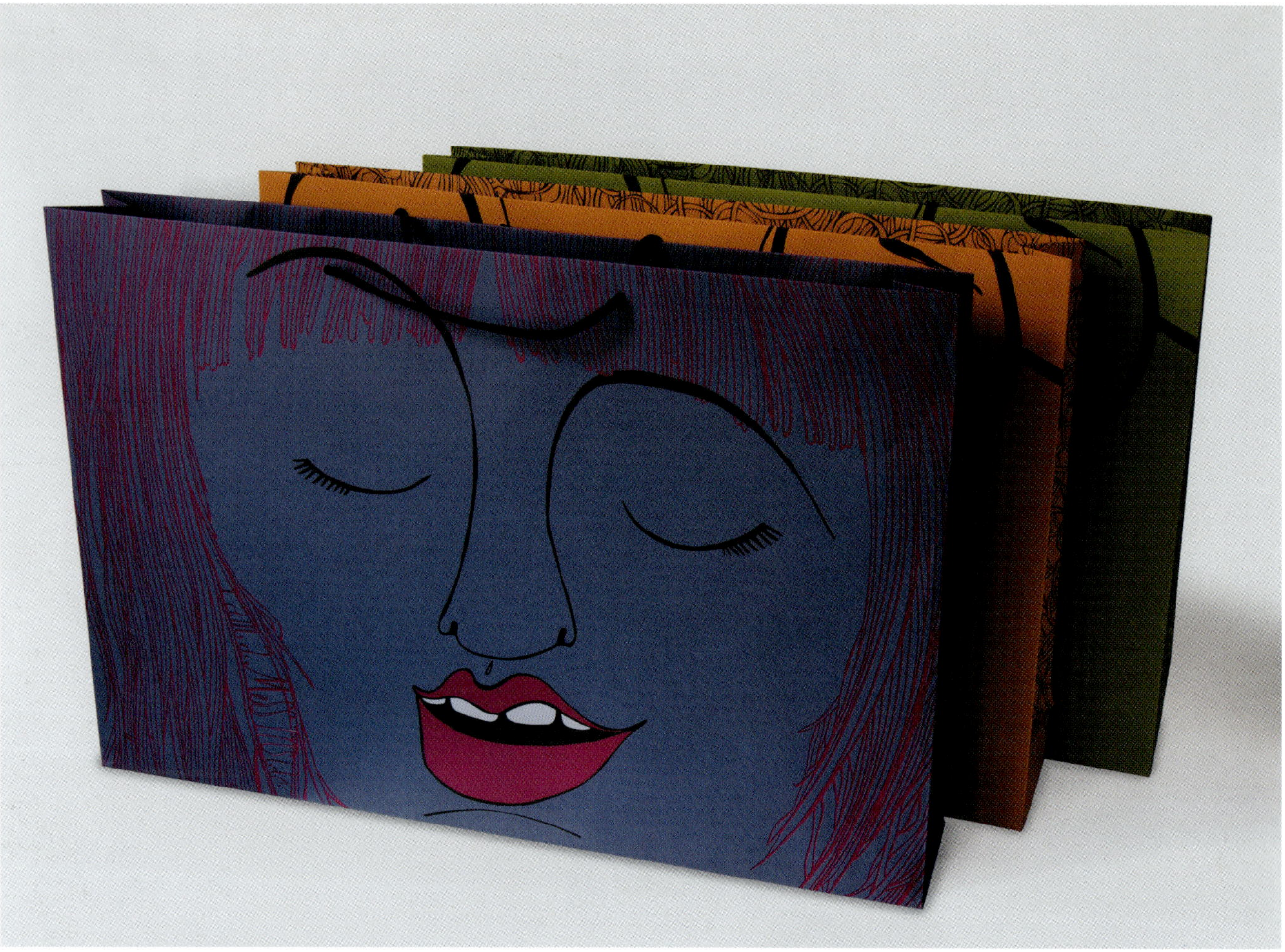

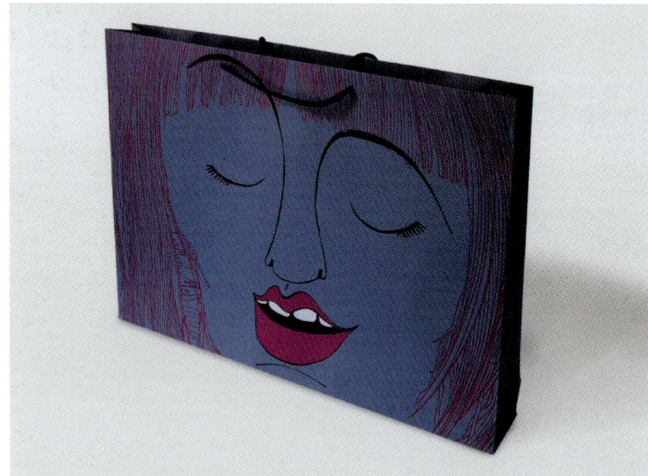

Everybody loves me.

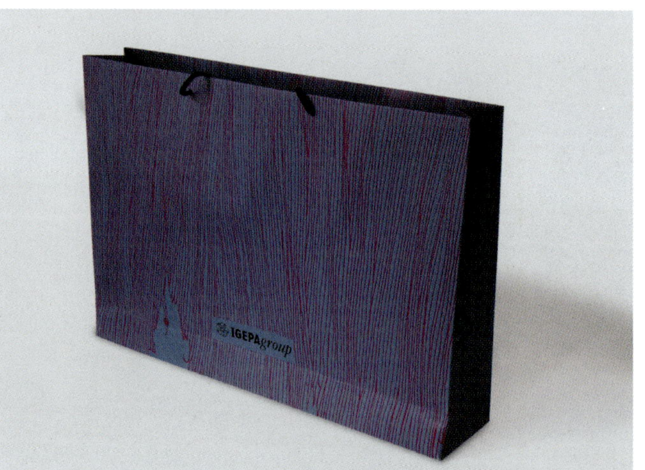

IGEPAgroup

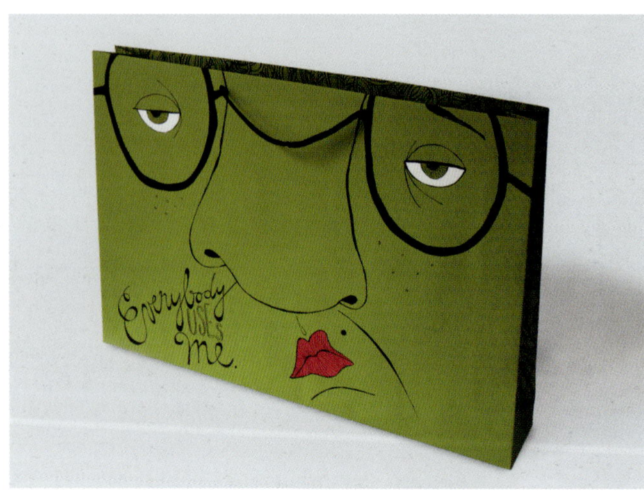

Everybody loves me.

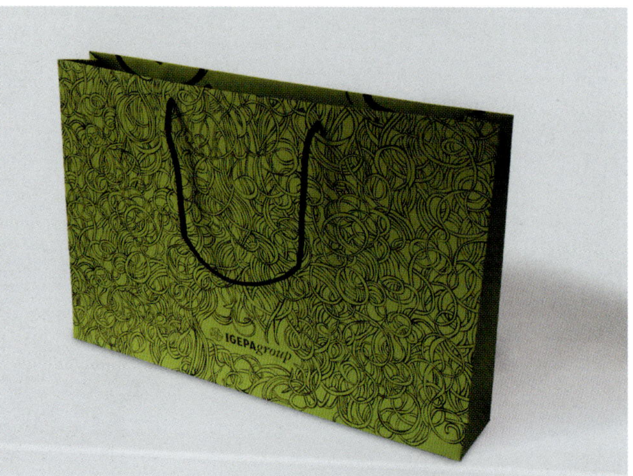

IGEPAgroup

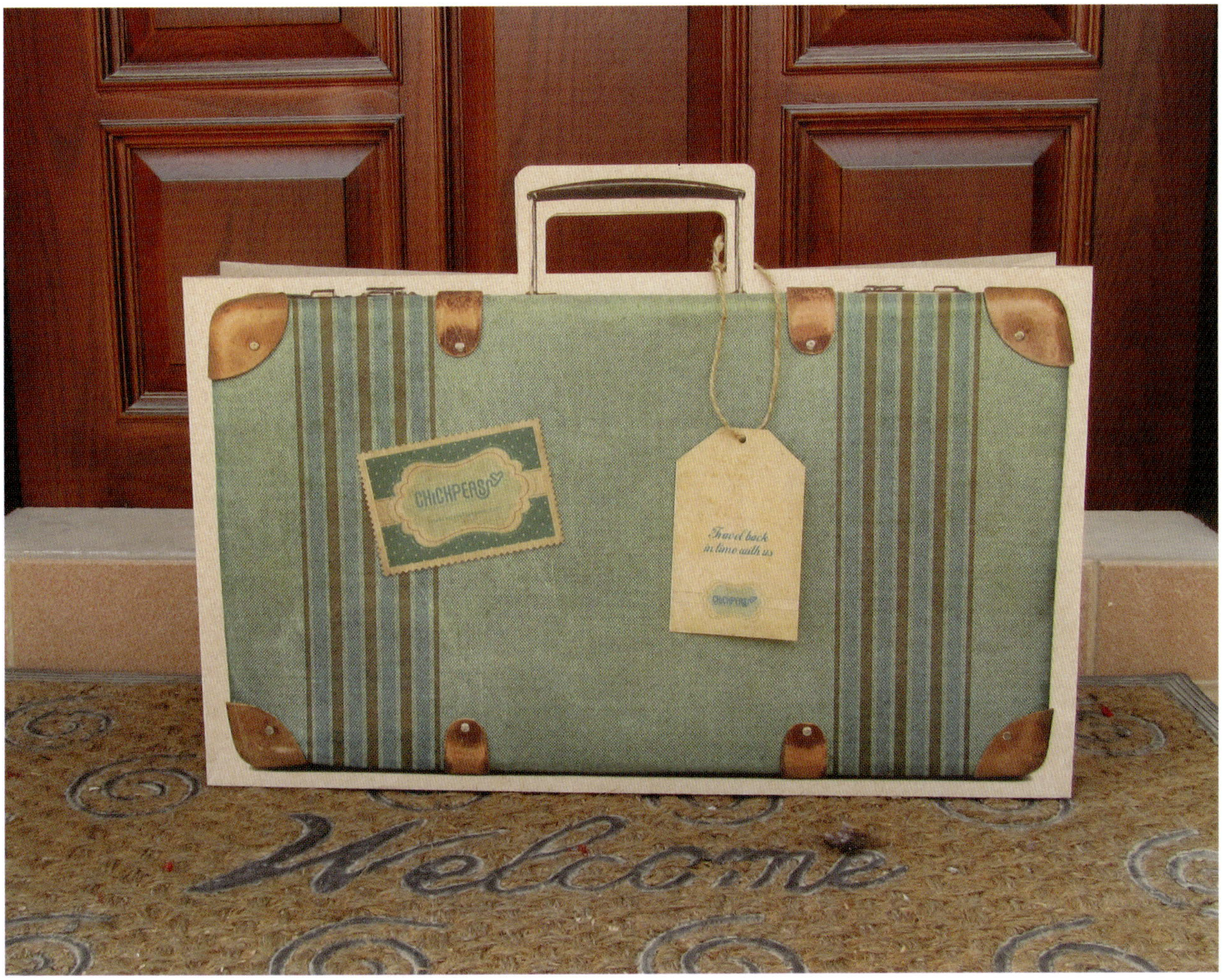

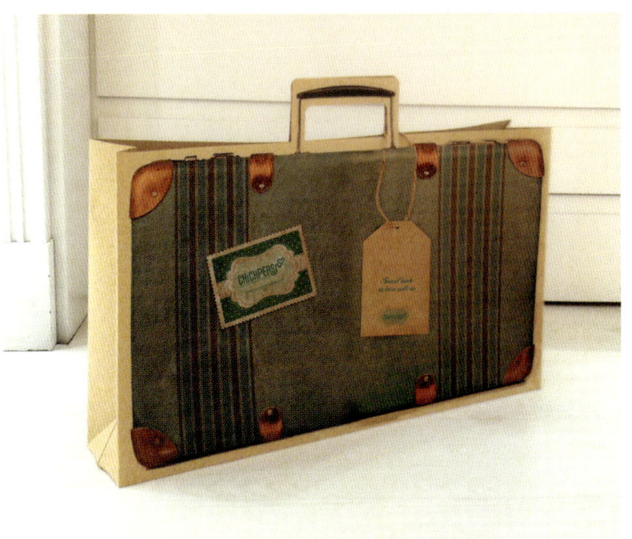

BIG HEAD PAPER BAG
DE: BooBoo Tannenbaum

Depicting giant faces, this series presents facial expressions in various moods, with whimsical quotes like: "Everybody uses me", "I am a mess inside" and "My head is full of things I don't understand."

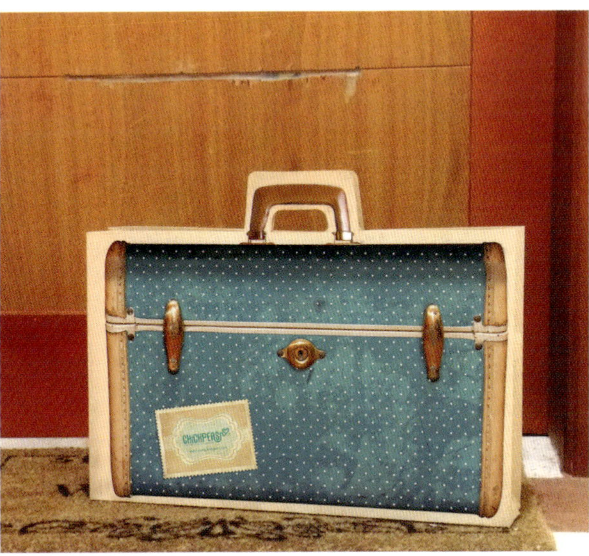

THE TIME TRAVEL BAG
DE: Amira Hassan, Suha Hamid(Wunderman Dubai)

To complement a pop-up, vintage store, this series of shopping bags was printed with vintage travel cases in yellowed paper to complete the antique experience.

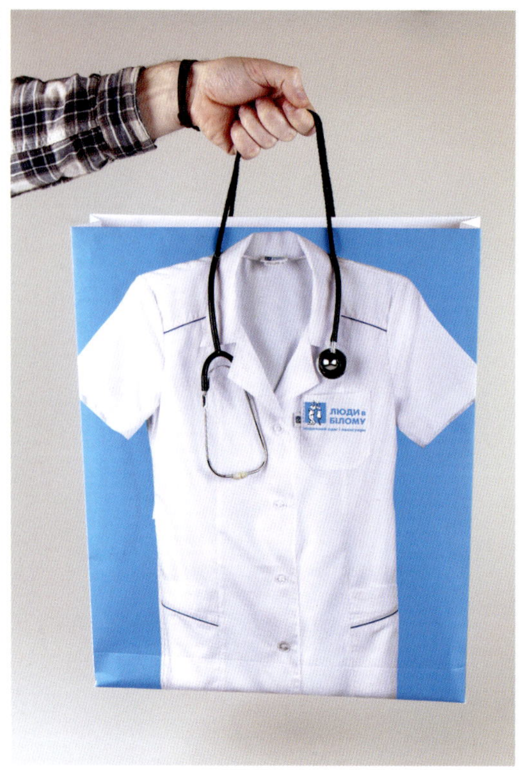
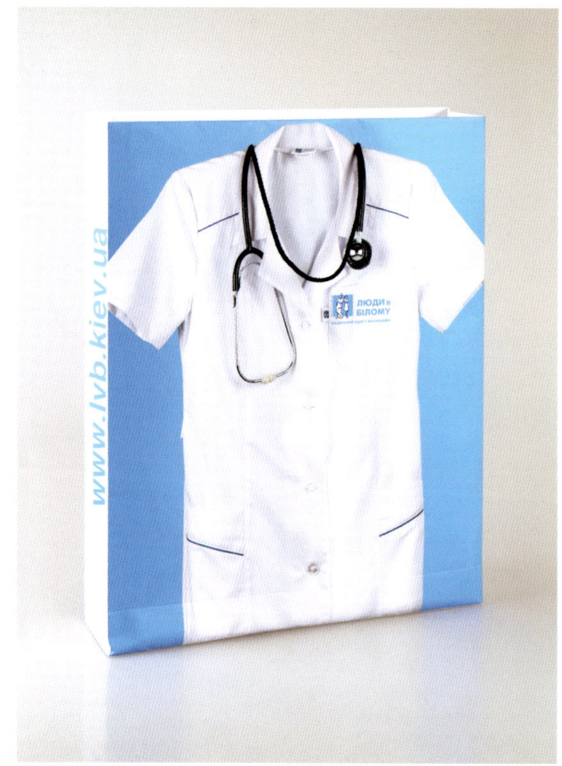

MAN IN WHITE
DA: >STRELA creative agency

This bag is printed with a doctor's white robe, the handle part of the stethoscope hung around the collar.

MOOMAH
DA: Apartment One

Apartment One developed a curious series of illustration for Moomah, based on everyday objects and animals, encapsulating the whimsical wonder of the brand.

BAO
DE: Alessandra Conti

Dedicated to connecting Chinese and Italian cultures with creation upcycled from Chinese manufacturers' waste, this designer created "Bao," a series of reused sacks printed with images of masks from Italian Commedia dell'Arte and Chinese Opera.

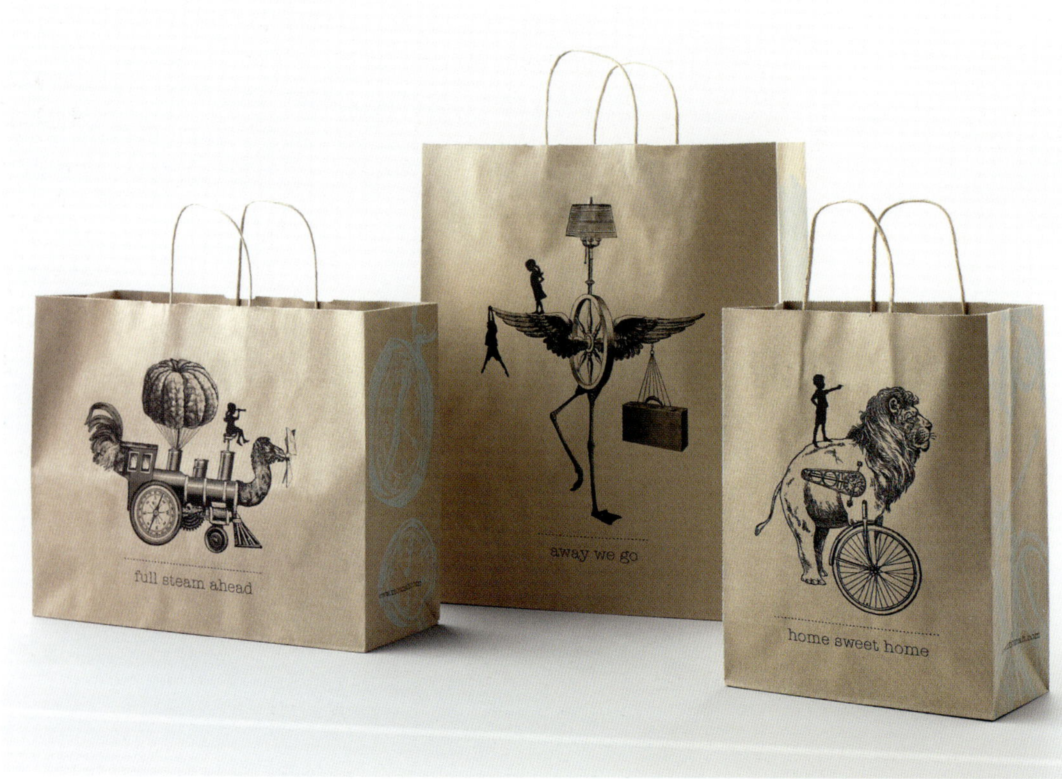

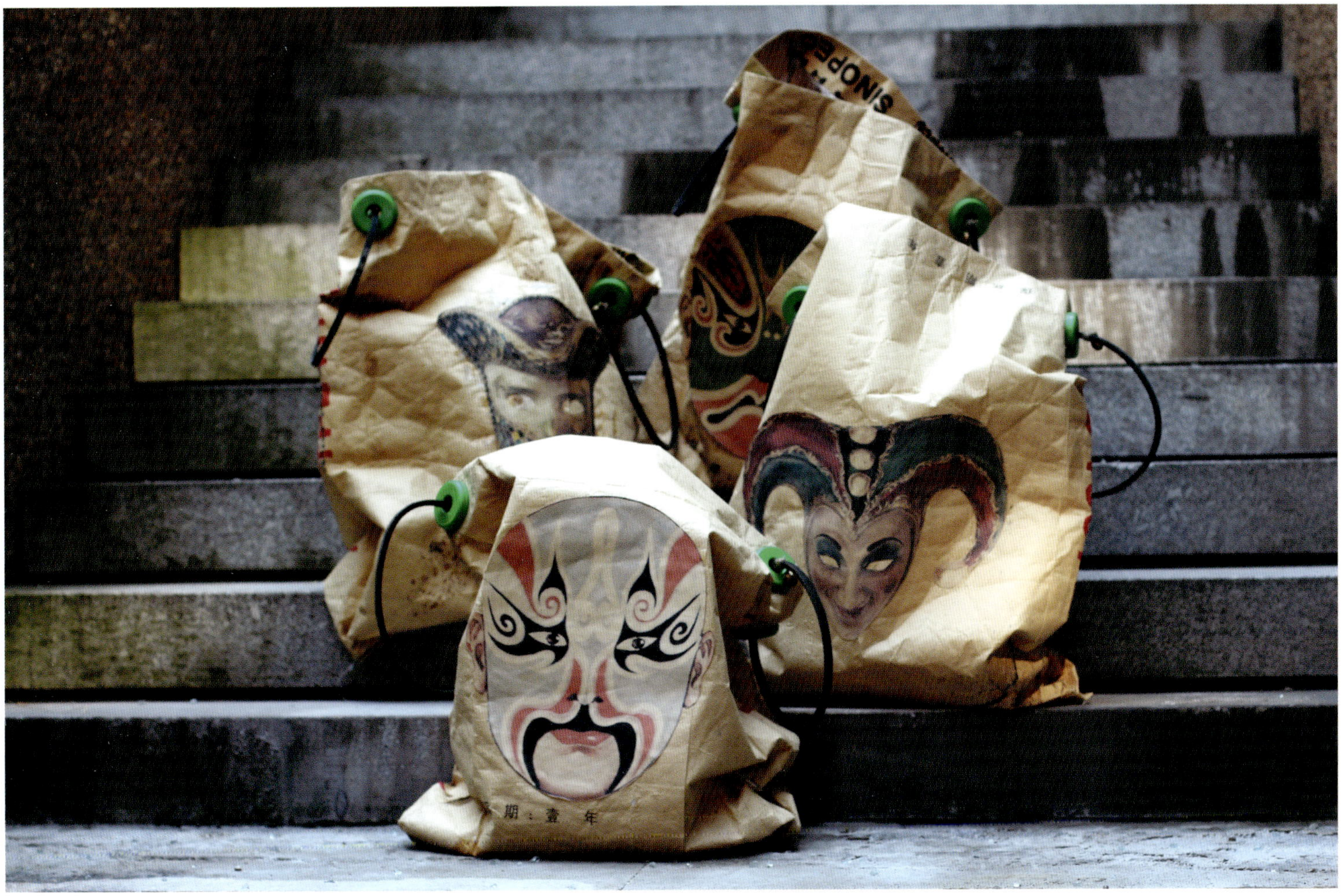

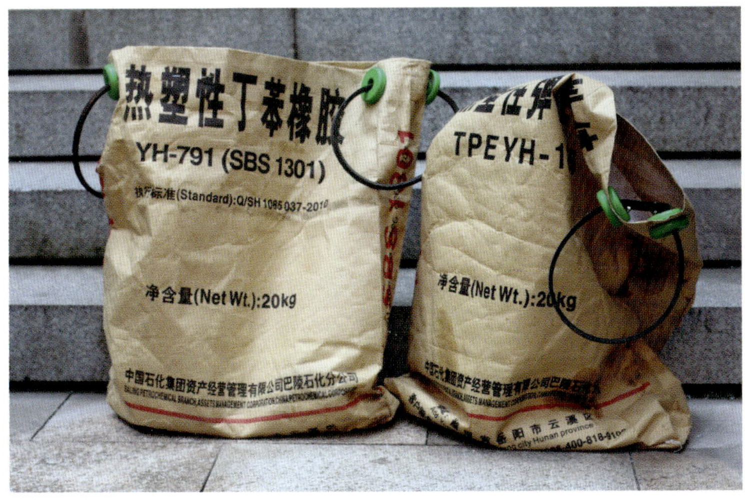

热塑性丁苯橡胶
YH-791 (SBS 1301)
执行标准(Standard):Q/SH 1065 037-2010
净含量(Net Wt.):20kg
中国石化集团资产经营管理有限公司巴陵石化分公司
TPEYH-1
净含量(Net Wt.):20kg

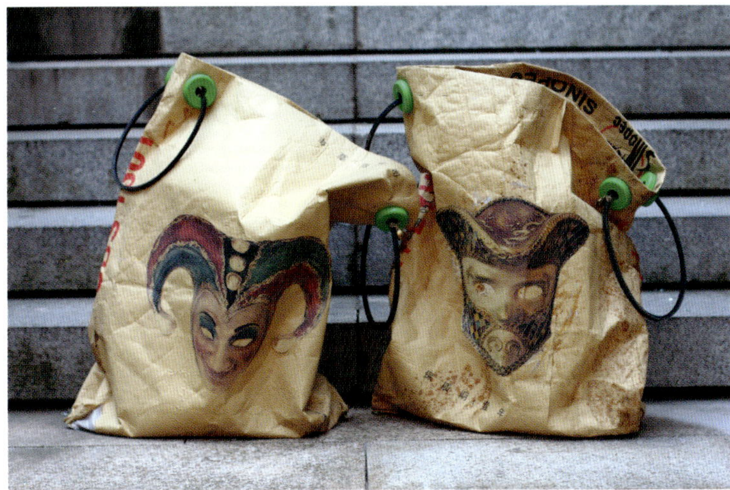

SINOPEC

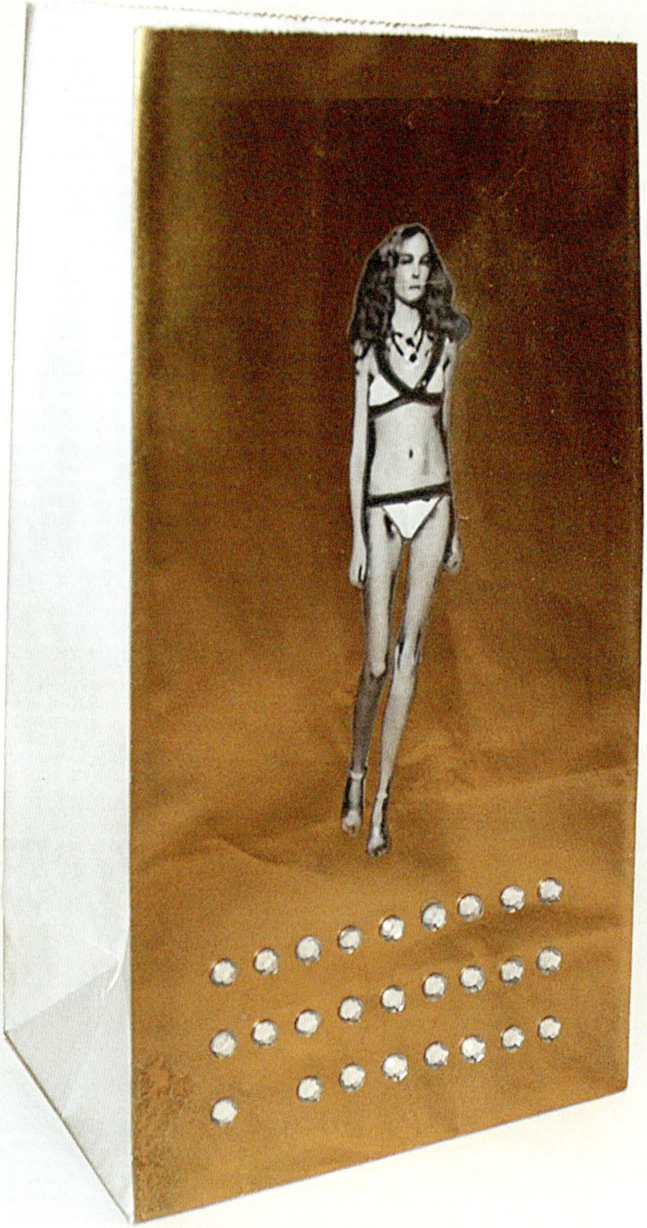

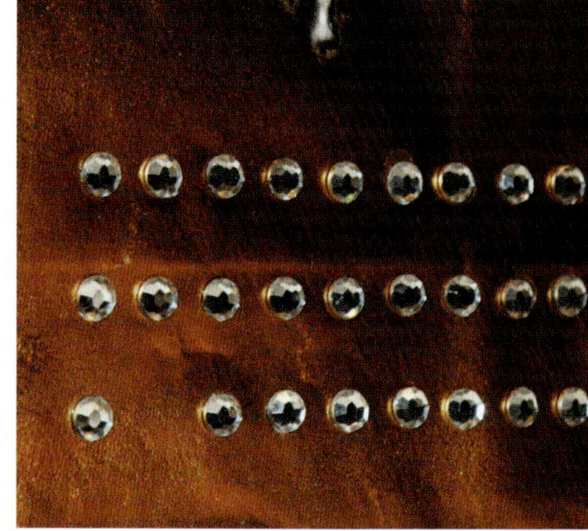

ANOREXIC BAGS
DE: Stab

This design is a golden bag with the picture of an anorexic-like model and shining fake diamonds, a interpretation of the prevalent practice in which already skinny girls vomit to look more like what they see in the magazine.

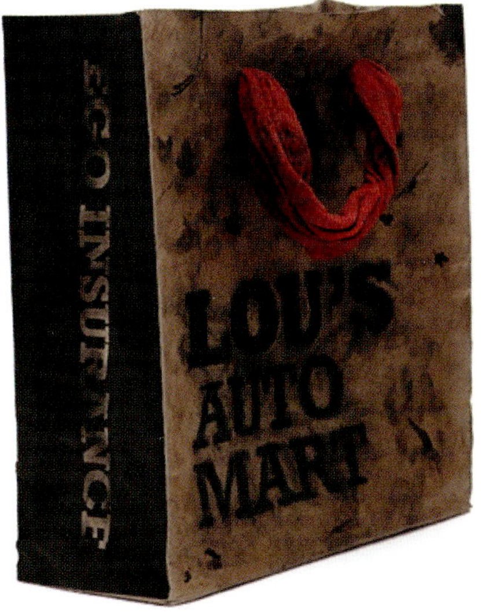

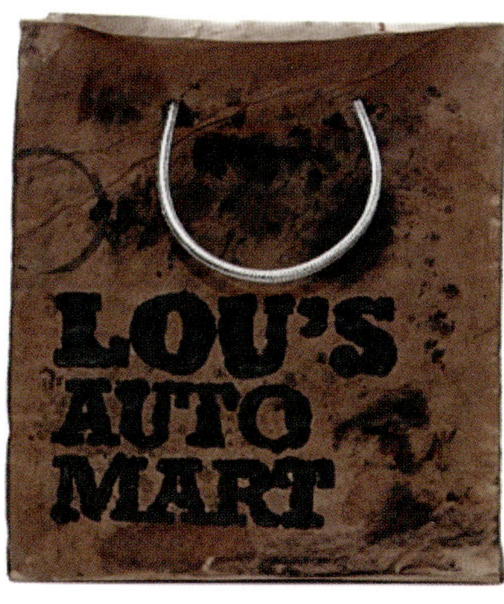

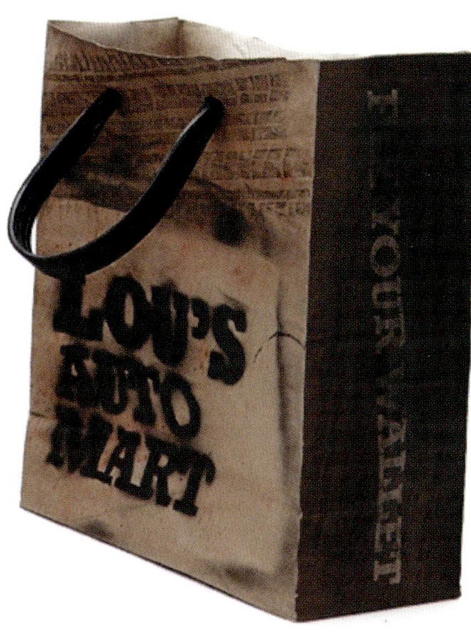

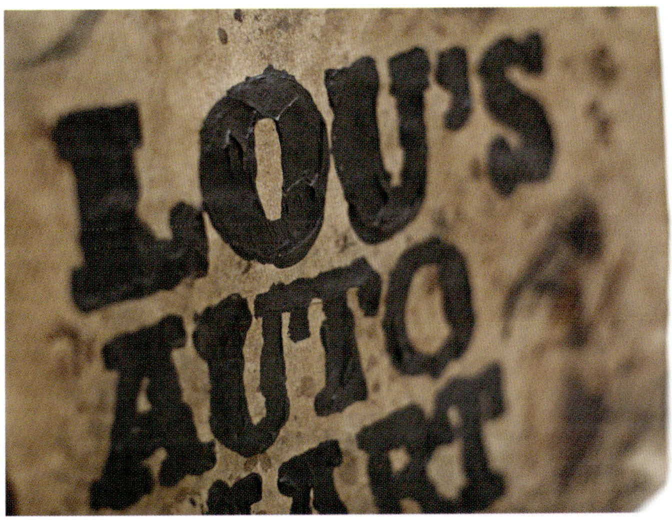

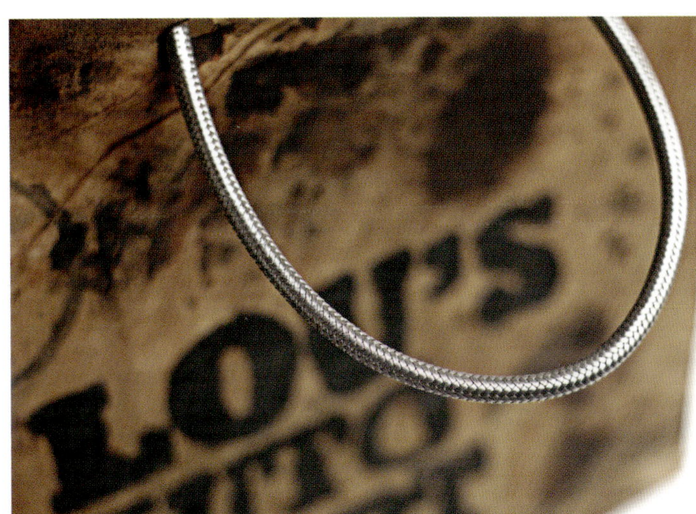

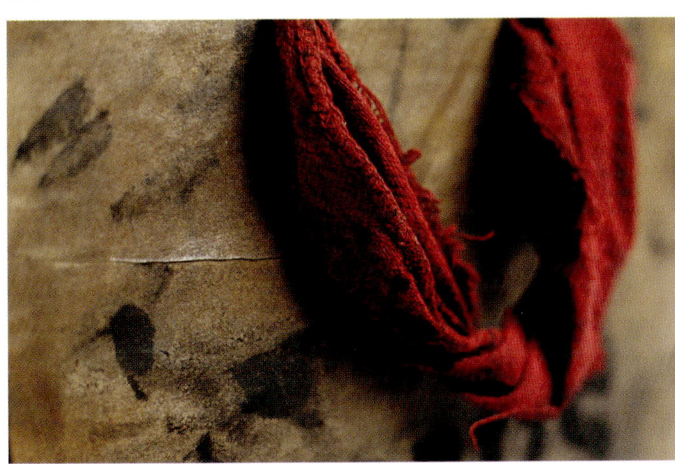

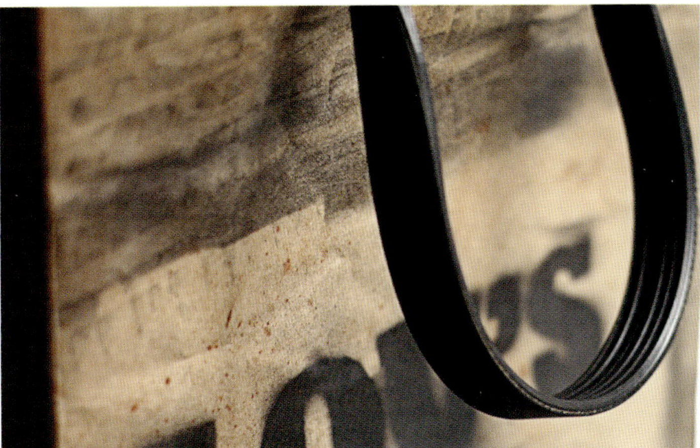

LOU'S AUTO MART SHOPPING BAGS
DE: Michael Gauthier

Designed for a car parts store for DIYer, this bag was created to generate a familiar feel. The bold font was gas-smeared while the handles are made of essentials from the garage - shop rags, engine belts, and braided hoses.

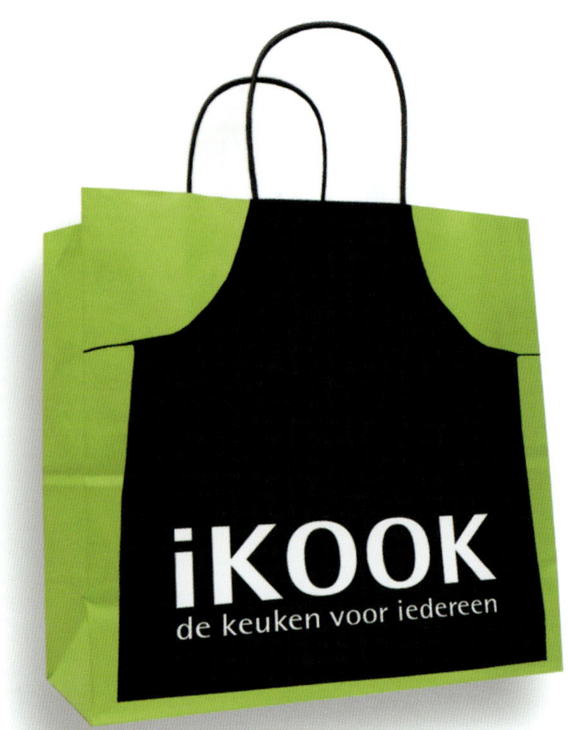

iKOOK
de keuken voor iedereen

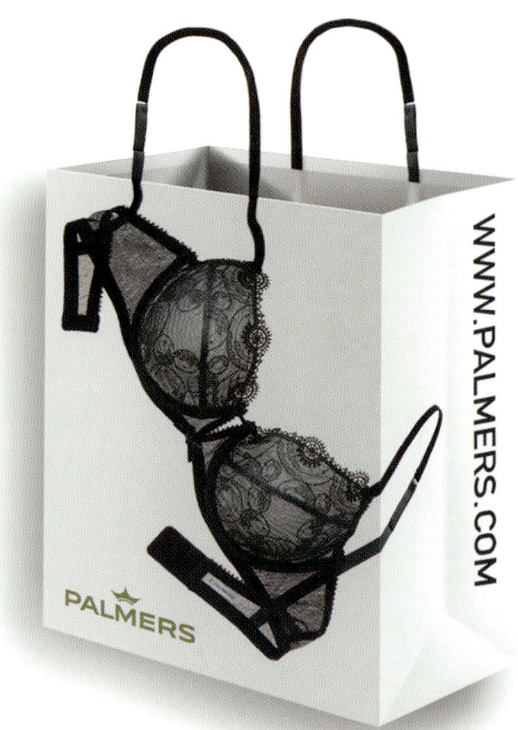

PALMERS
WWW.PALMERS.COM

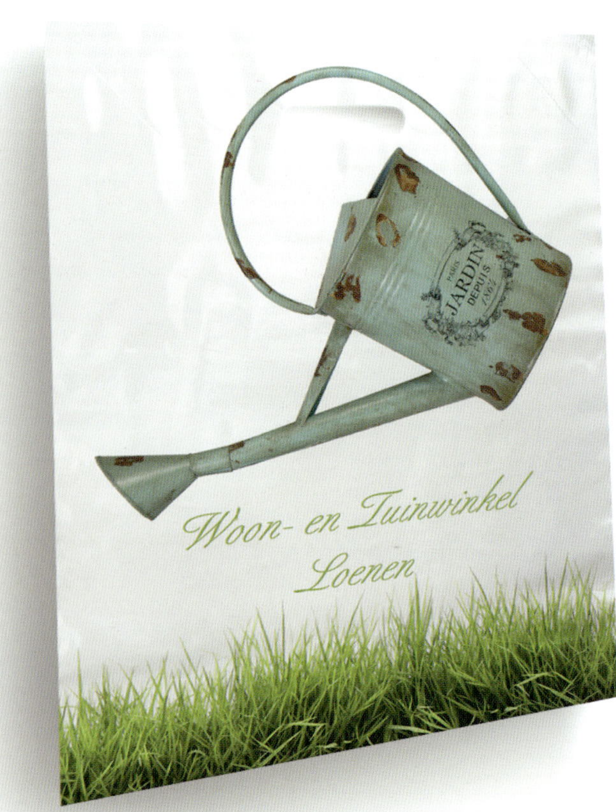

JARDIN
DEPUIS
Woon- en Tuinwinkel
Loenen

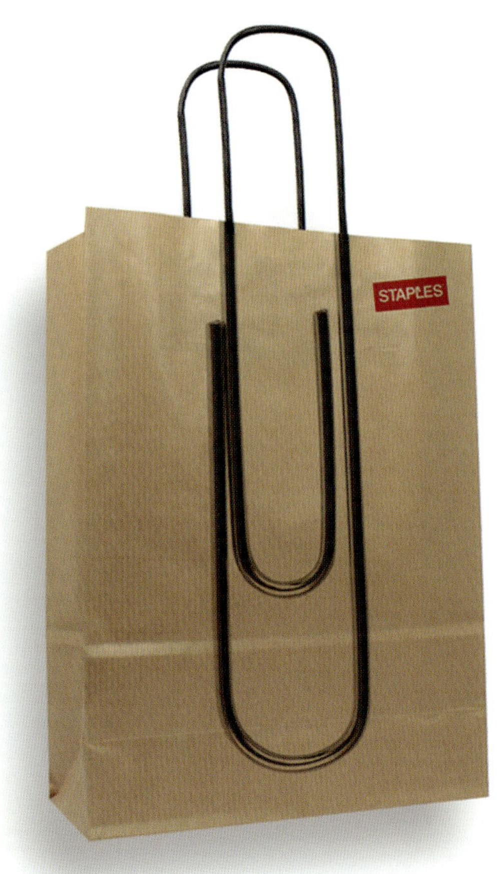

STAPLES

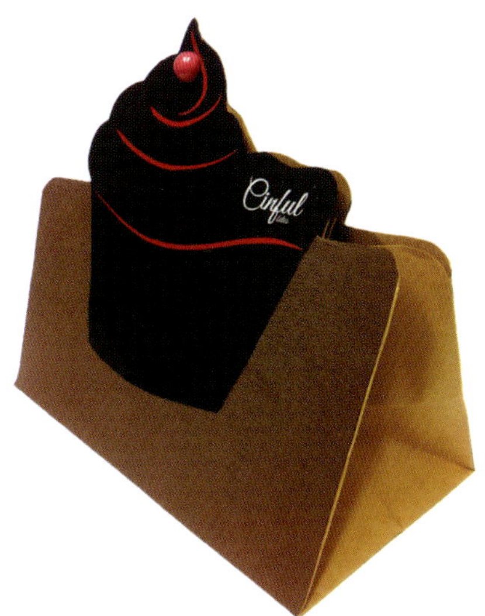
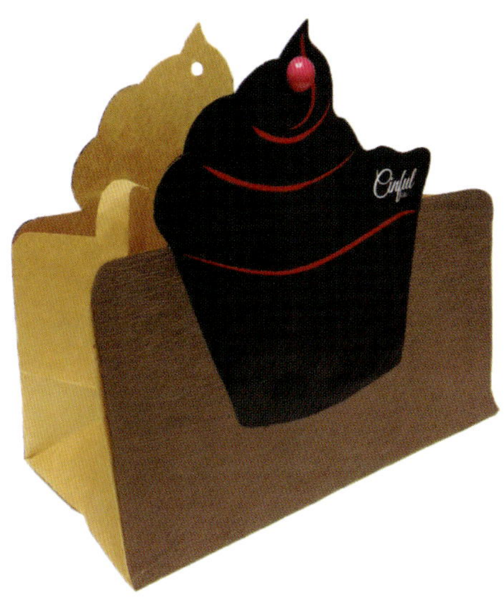

SHOPPING BAG DESIGN CONCEPT
DE: Rob Gros(Twaalfdozijn)

The designer created this series to display
the visual connection between the hand that
customers used to carry this bag and the product
they actually purchase.

CINFUL BITES
DE: Cindy Yambao

This bag's bite-mark impression, textured
material and clutch bag appearance, secured
with a candy-like button, definitely resonate the
sweet, fun and unique style of "Cinful Bites".

HAPPY BAGS
DE: Raphael Mahon

Playing with the holes alongside the handle,
Raphael Mahon simply added a straight line or
a downward curve to compose a smiling face or
other expression, making clever simple and
simple clever.

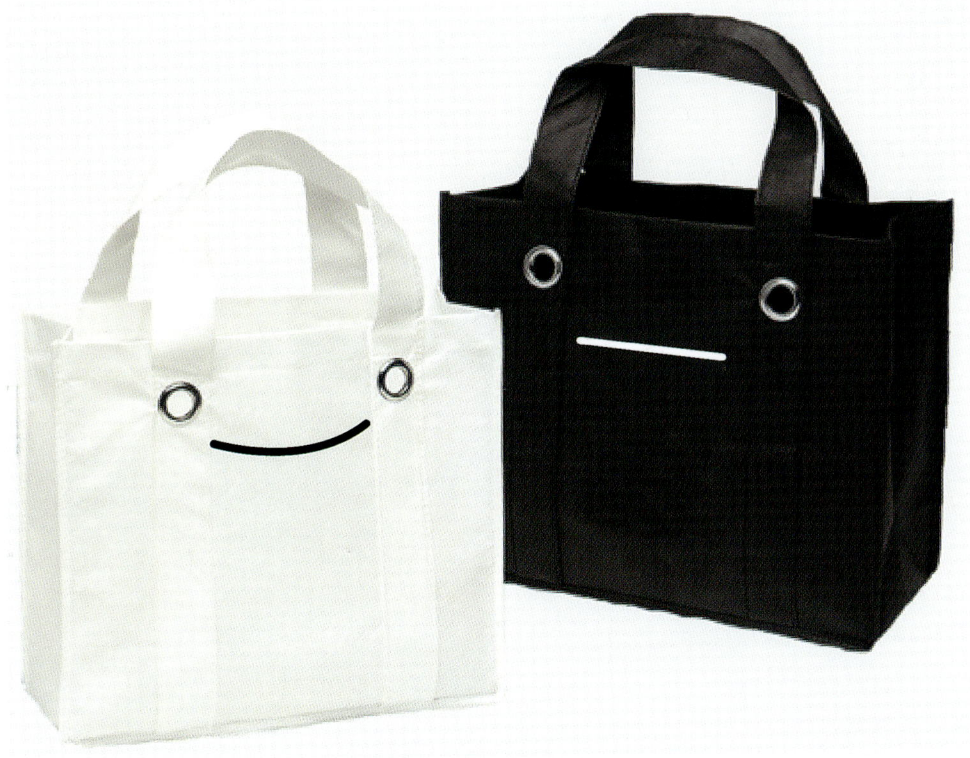

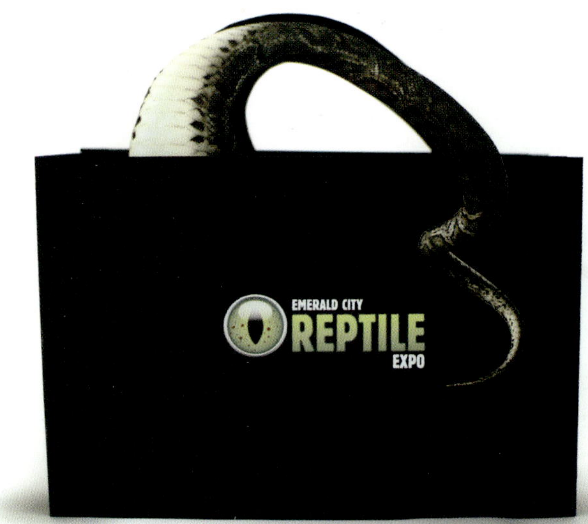

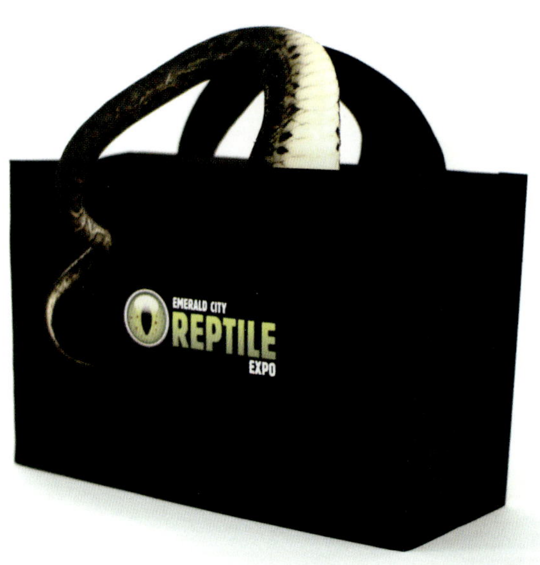

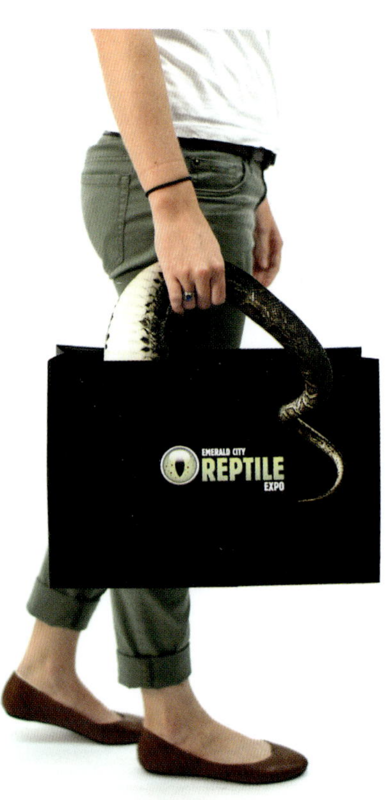

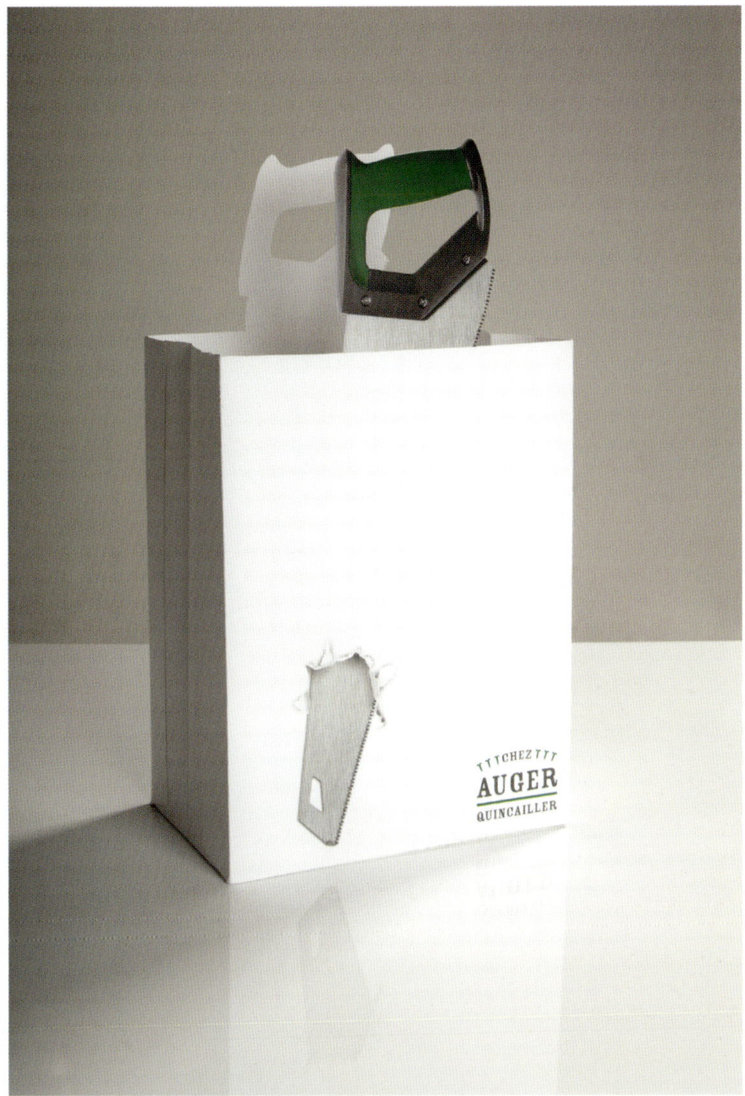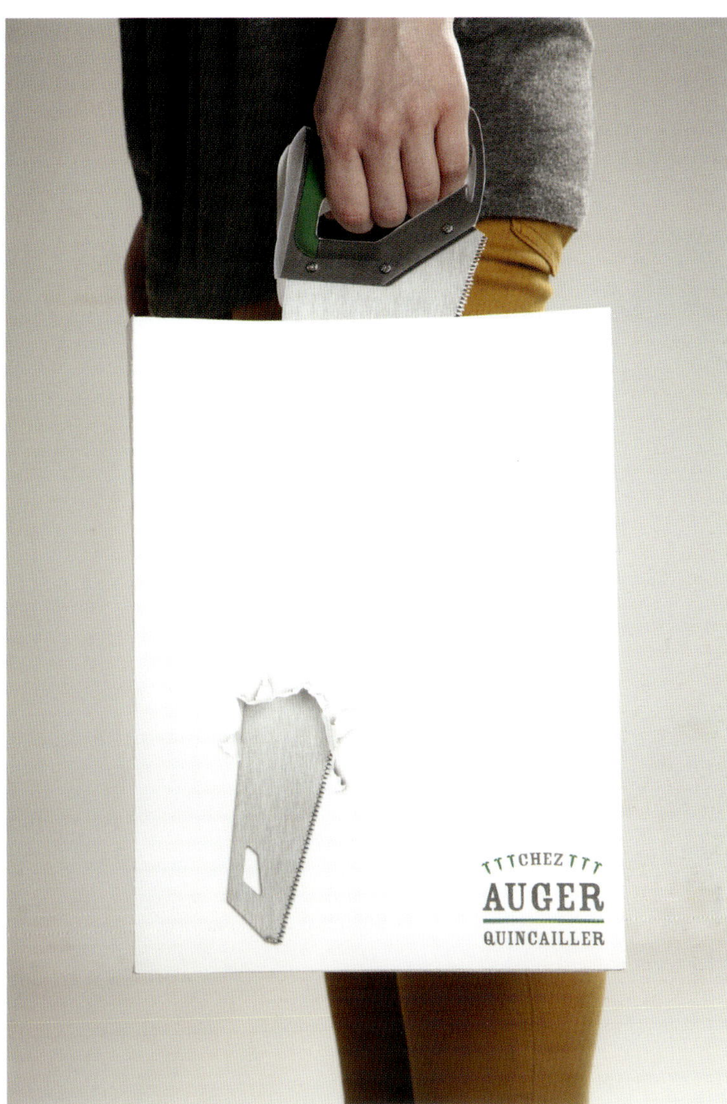

REPTILE EXPO BAG
DE: Cheryl Smith

Designed for Emerald City's annual Reptile Expo, this bag creates an illusion in which the holder is holding a snake coming out of the bag.

CHEZ AUGER QUINCAILLER
DE: France Auger

In this design, the handle of the bag is also the end of the saw.

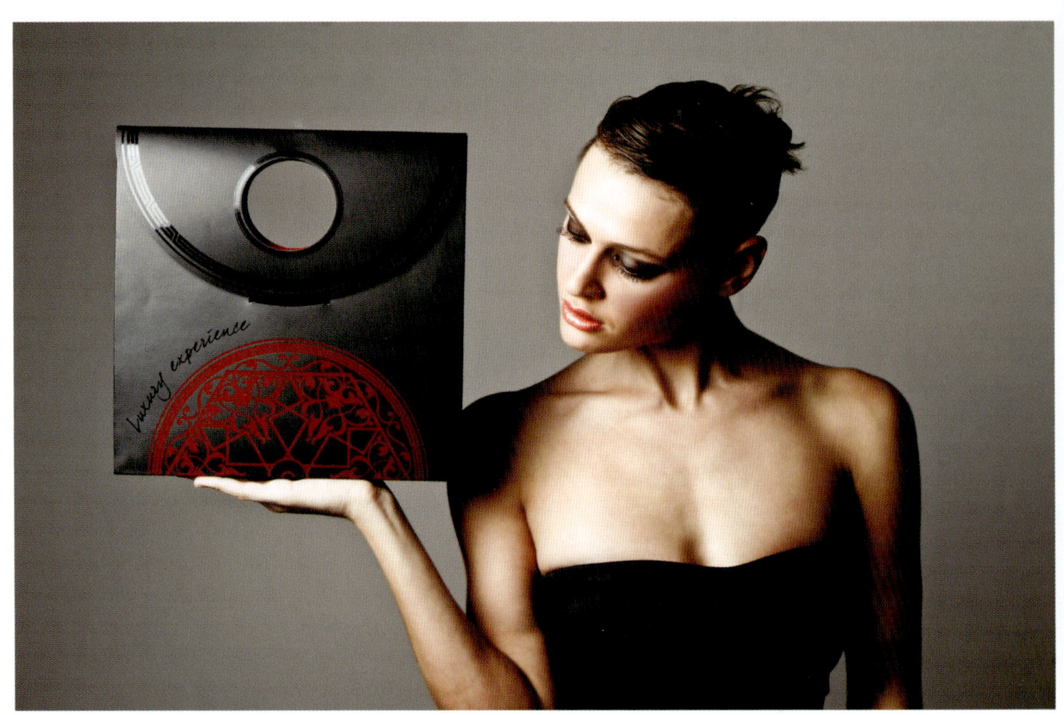
luxury experience

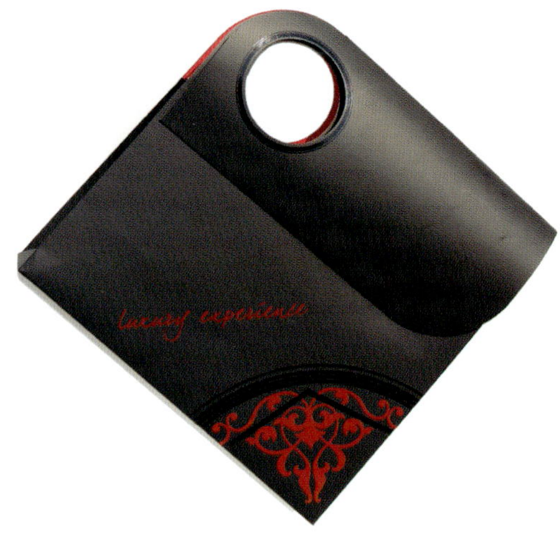
luxury experience

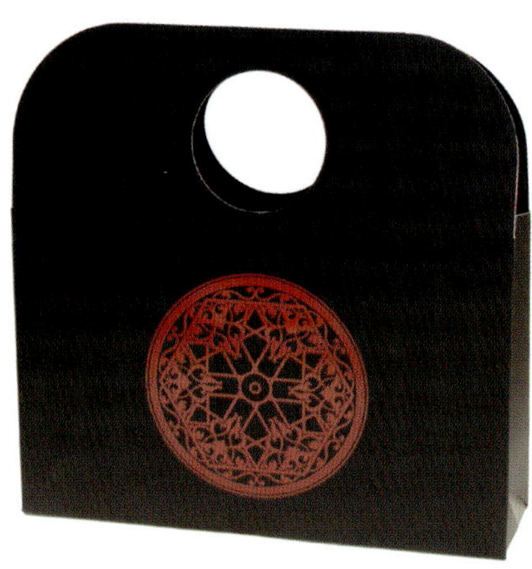

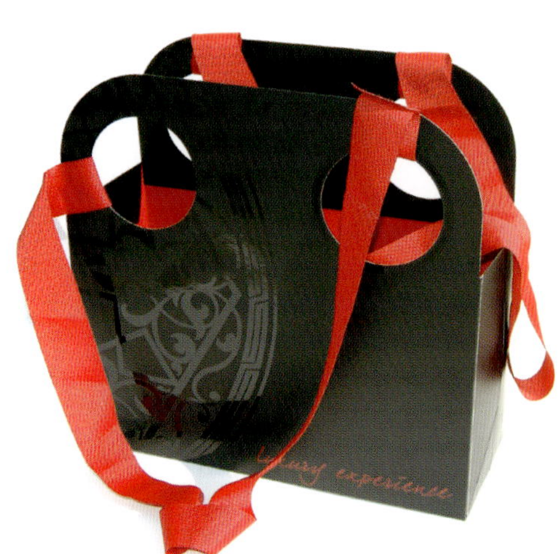
luxury experience

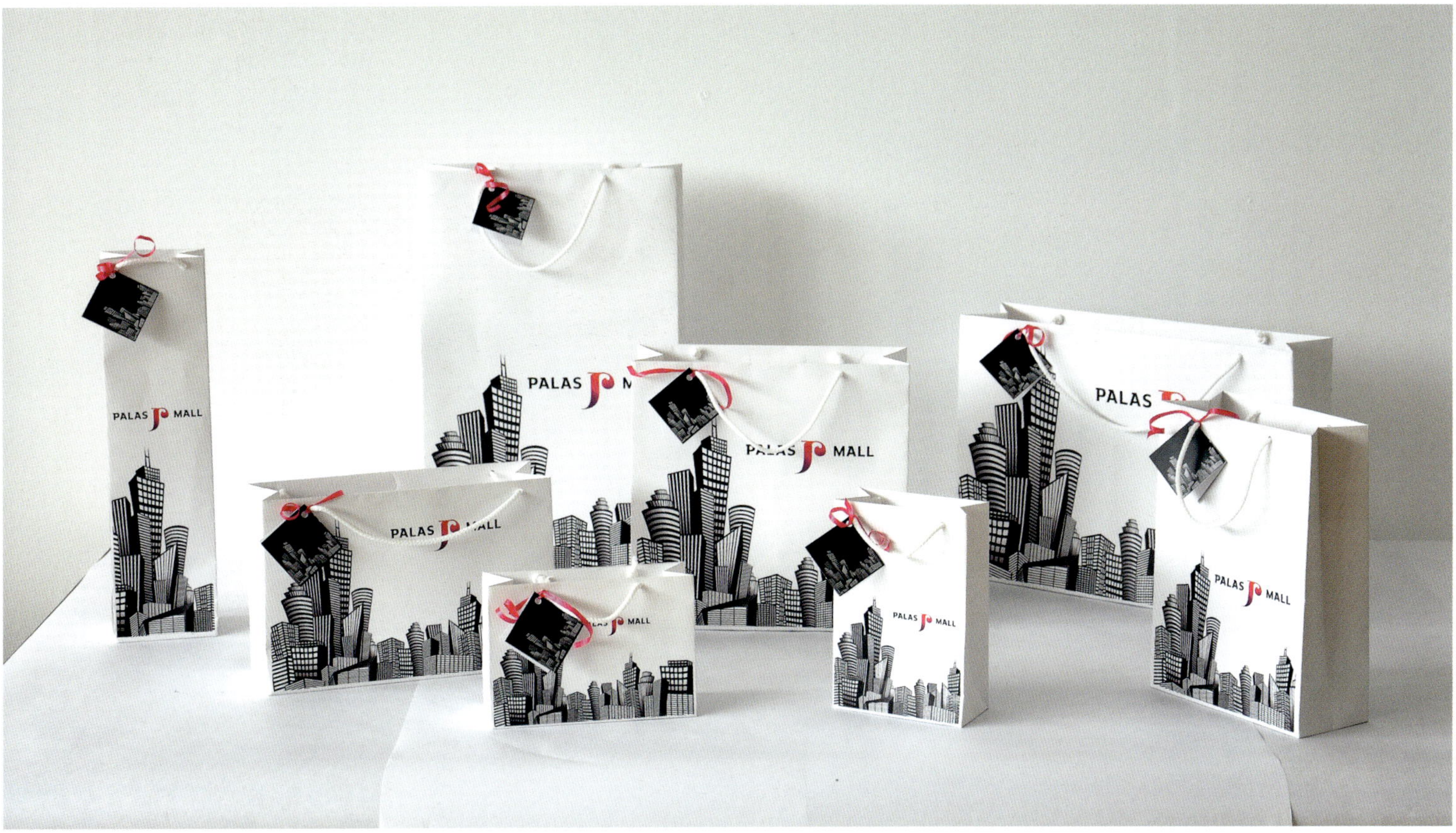

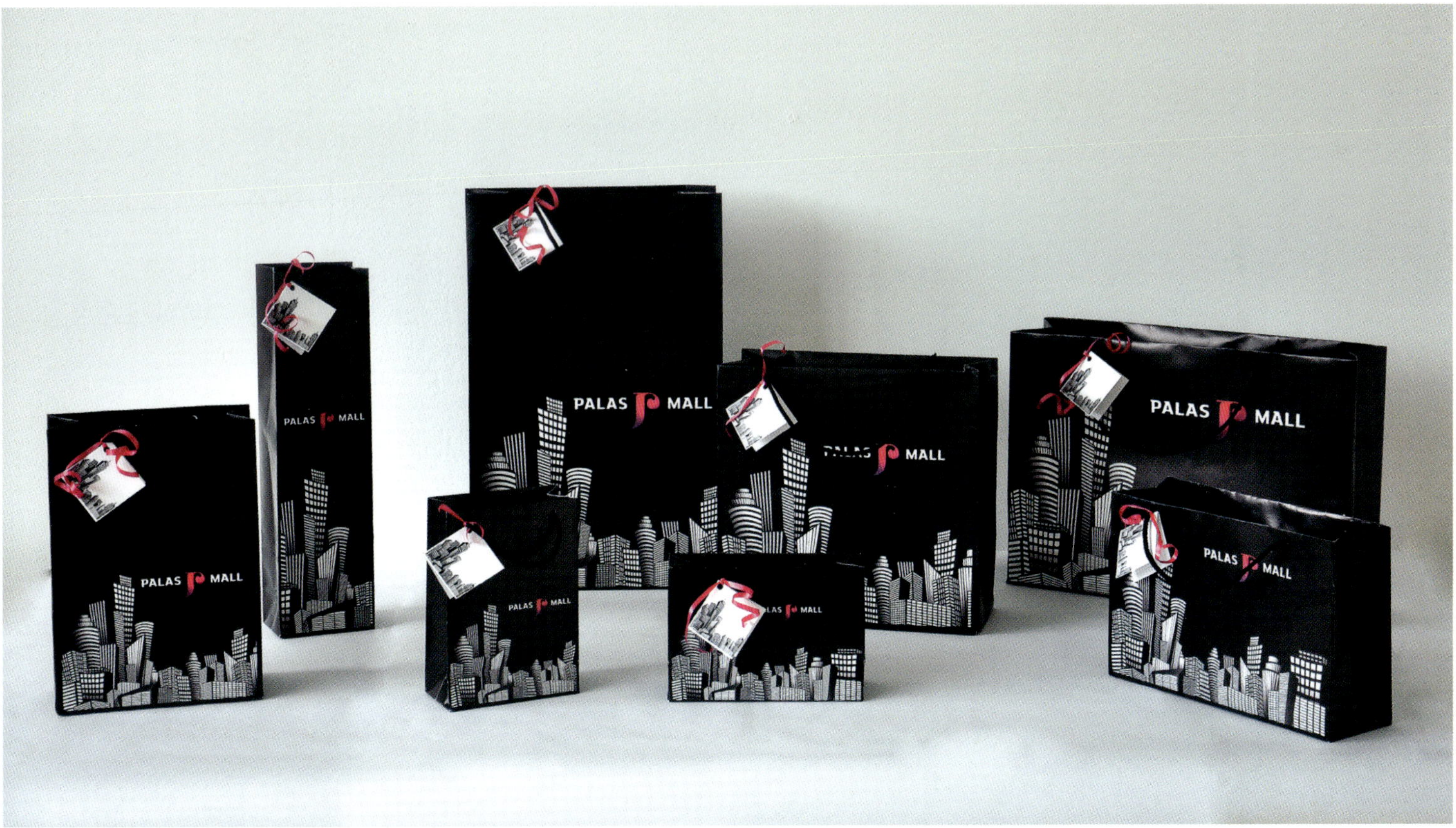

ELITE
DE: Greta D'Angelo

This series was created for an Italian spa company. Black mat ink is used as the background of the outer part while glossy black or red ink was used for the graphic. The interior is in bold red.

PALAS MALL SHOPPING BAG
DE: Gabriela C. Ungur

Highlighting the concept of community, the illustration depicts a series of buildings in different shapes and heights - reflecting the demographic and cultural diversity of the city - fitting perfectly together to convey the idea of a harmonious community.

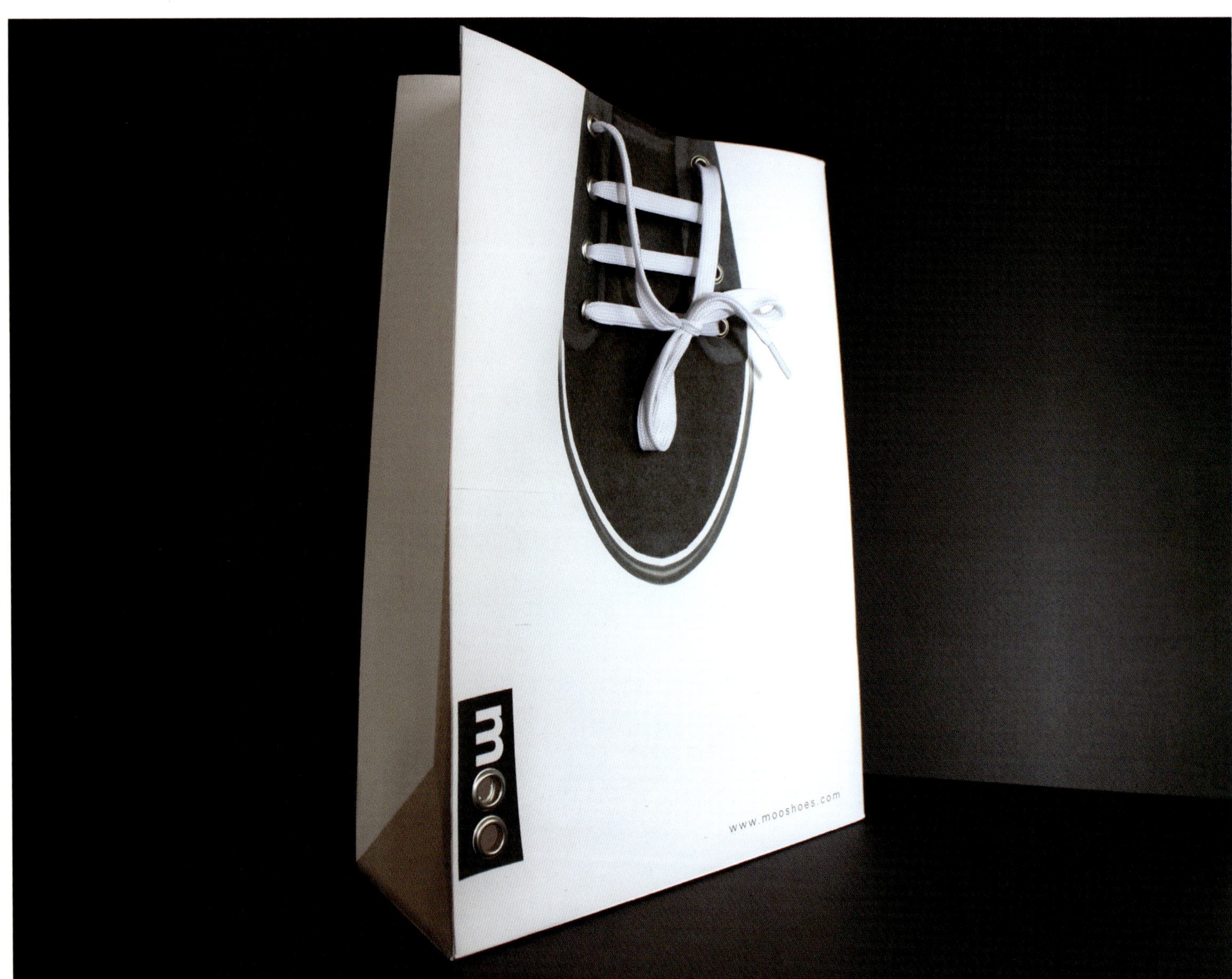

MOO
DE: Alistair Marshall

Created for a footwear company, this bag's handles are actual shoelaces,
which can be taken out as a spare pair of shoelaces.

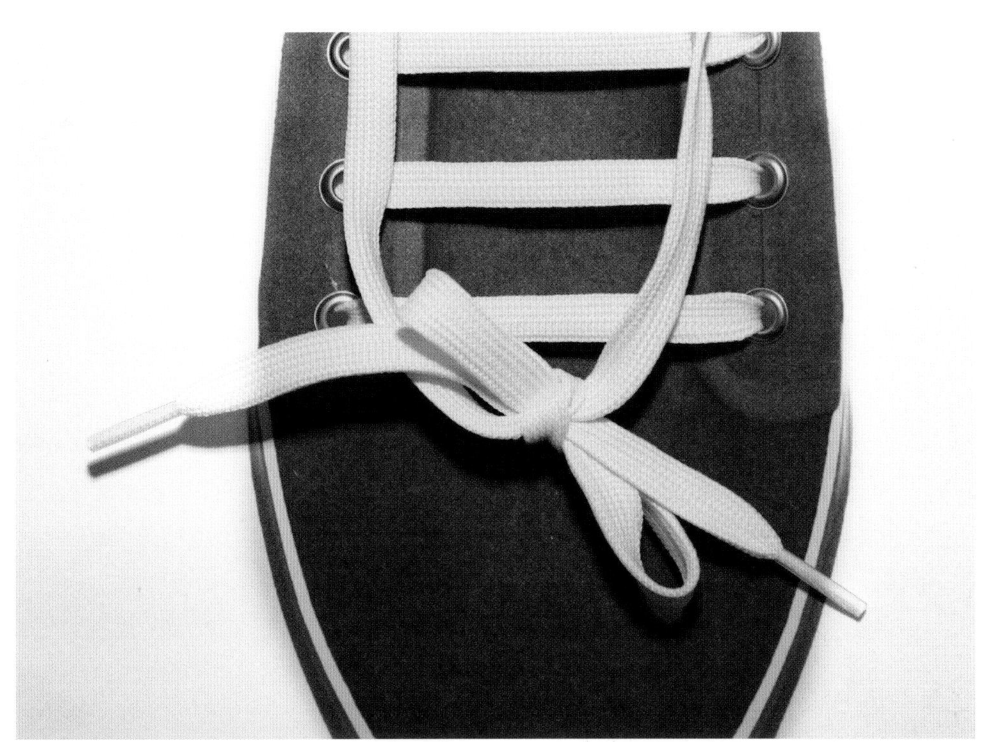

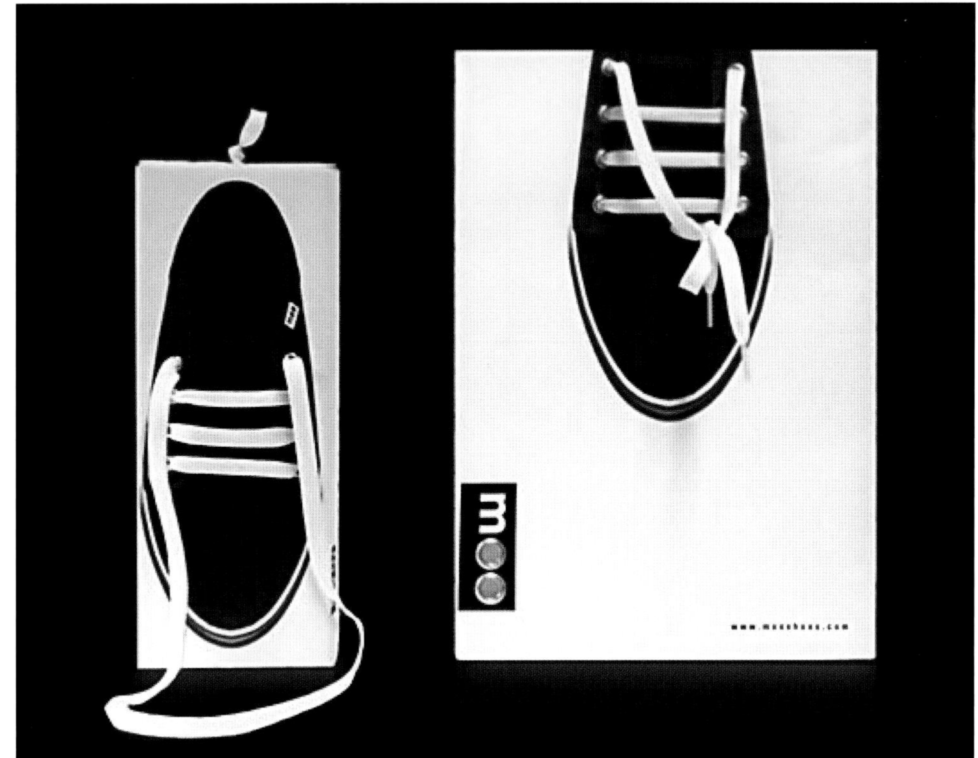
www.mooshoes.com

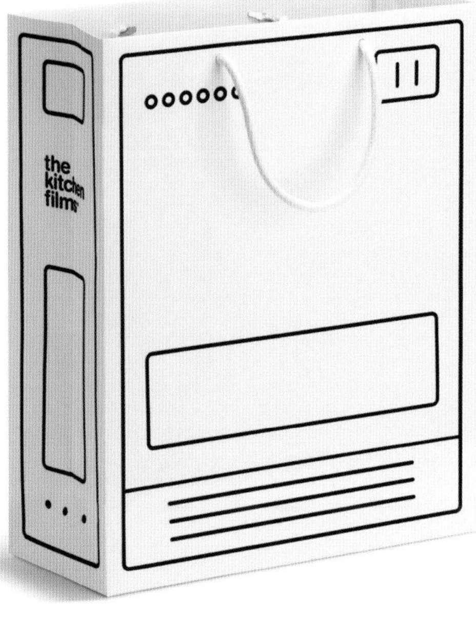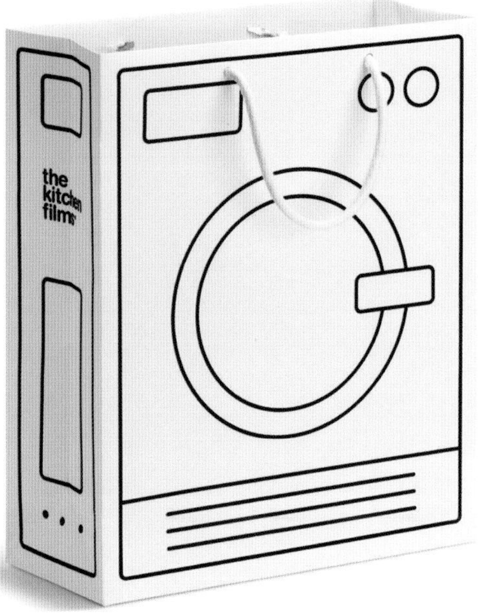

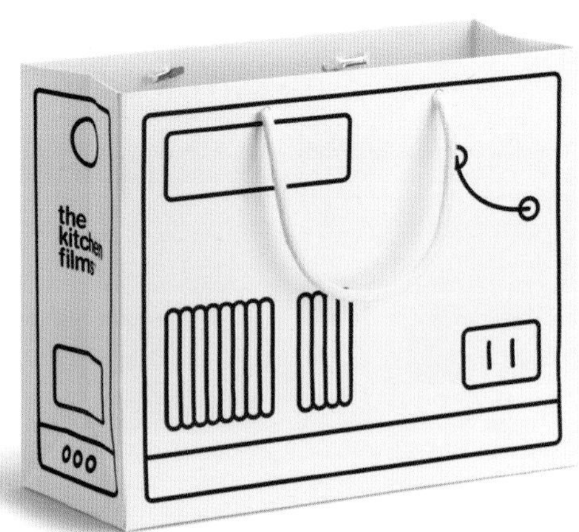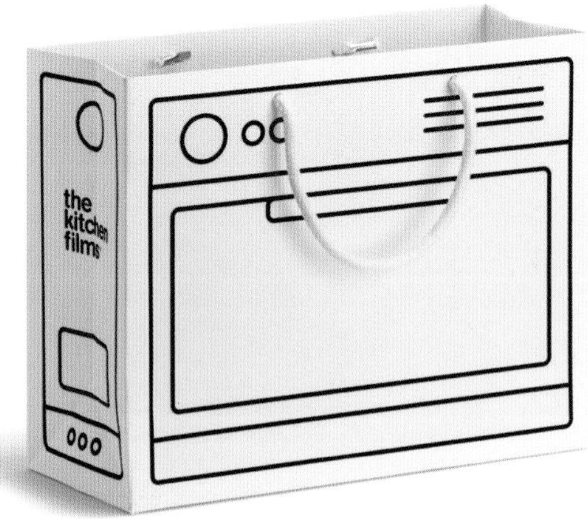

THE KITCHEN
DA:ruiz + company

To visualize the name "The Kitchen Films," paper bags printed with an abstracted microwave oven icon were designed to interact with the business card printed with food, mimicking the cooking process.

HAJDU ANETT
DE: Miklos Kiss

Designed for a fashion brand, this bag uses meat industry wrappings and hunting accessories to correspond with the theme of the season - revealing the hidden animal in all of us.

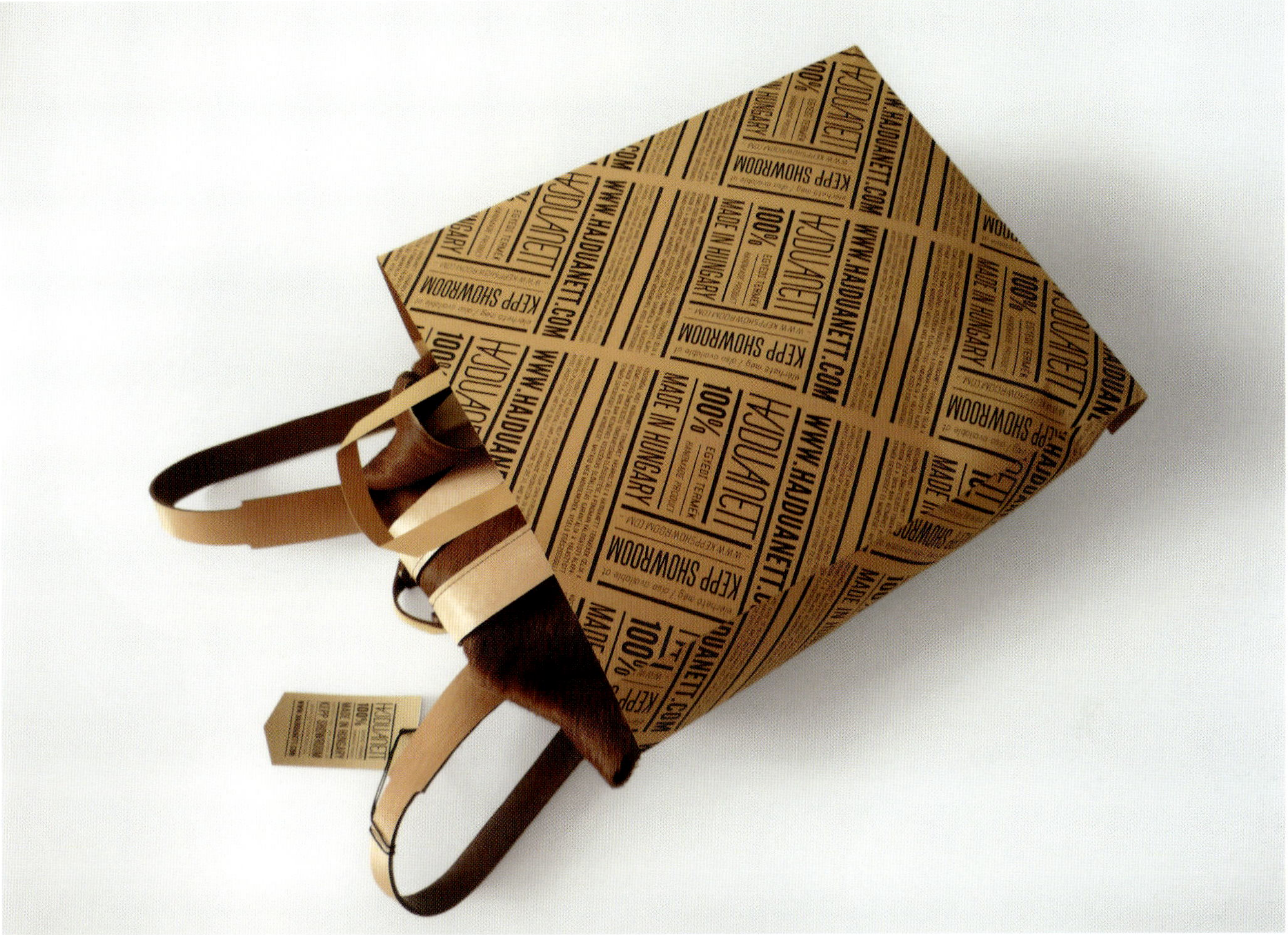

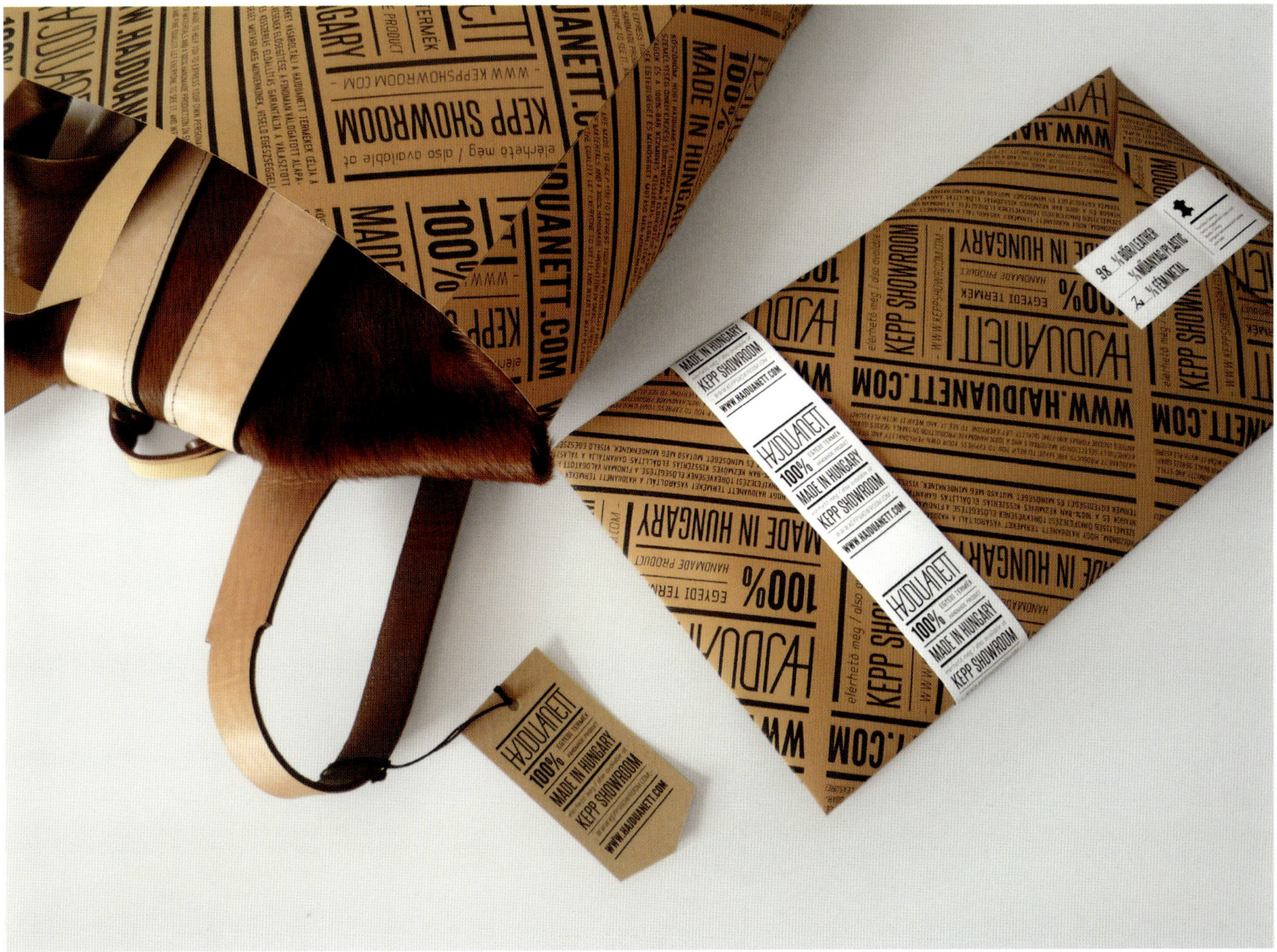

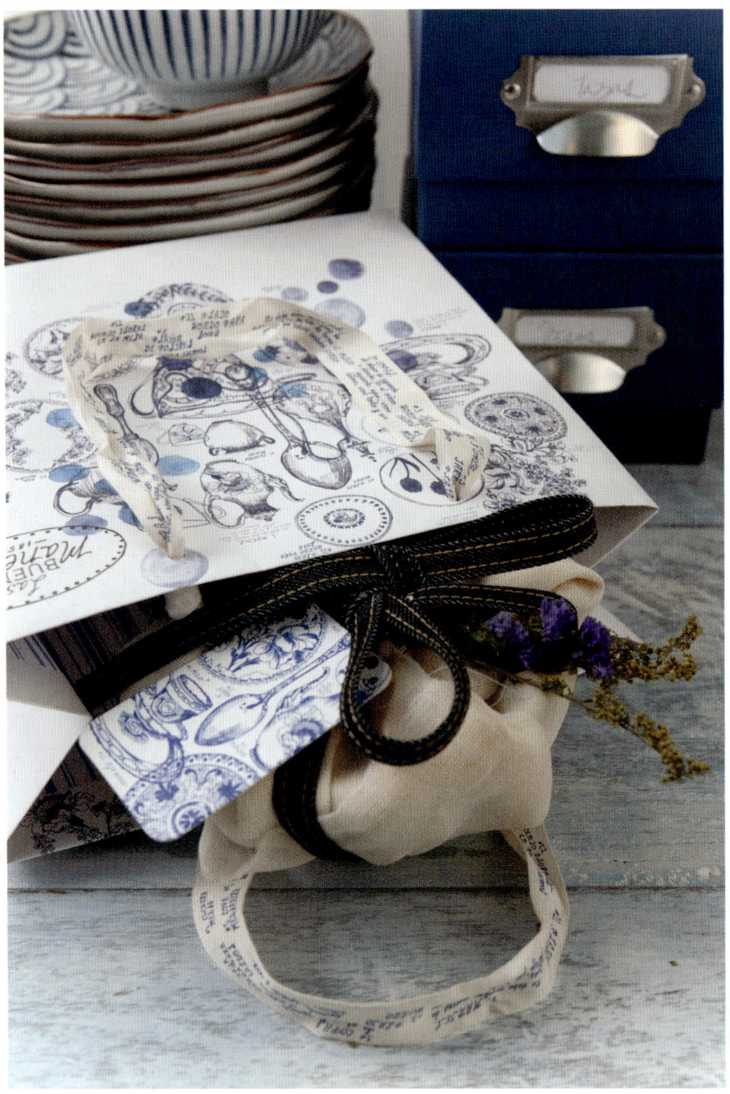

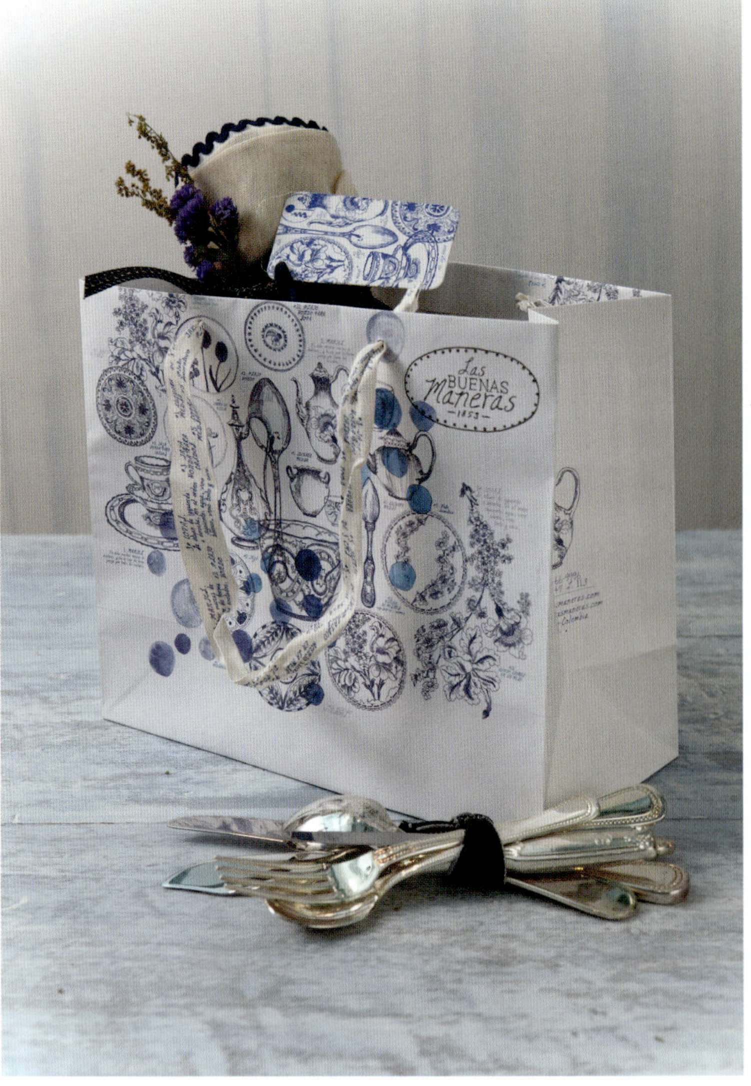

LAS BUENAS MANERAS

DE: Cristina Londoño(Wallnut Studio)

The image running through this bag is created using a blue rollerball pen
and some watercolors, depicting the good old days when table etiquette was
valued.

SEXY MAMA

DE: Carla Hanson

Designed for a lingerie store, these bags are in very feminine pink, purple
and blue in combination with the mysterious black to live up to the name
"SexyMama." The sides mimic those of the corset.

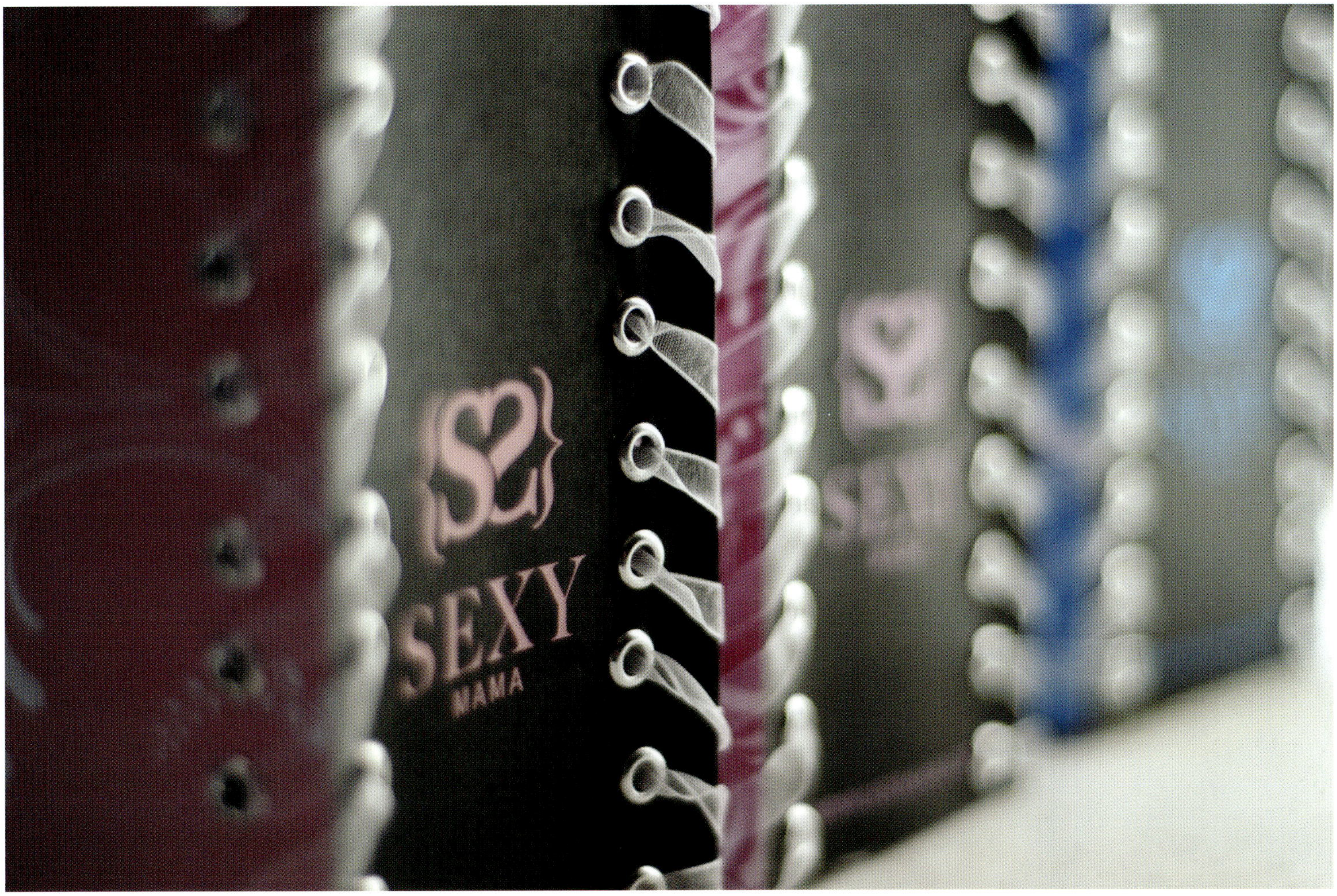

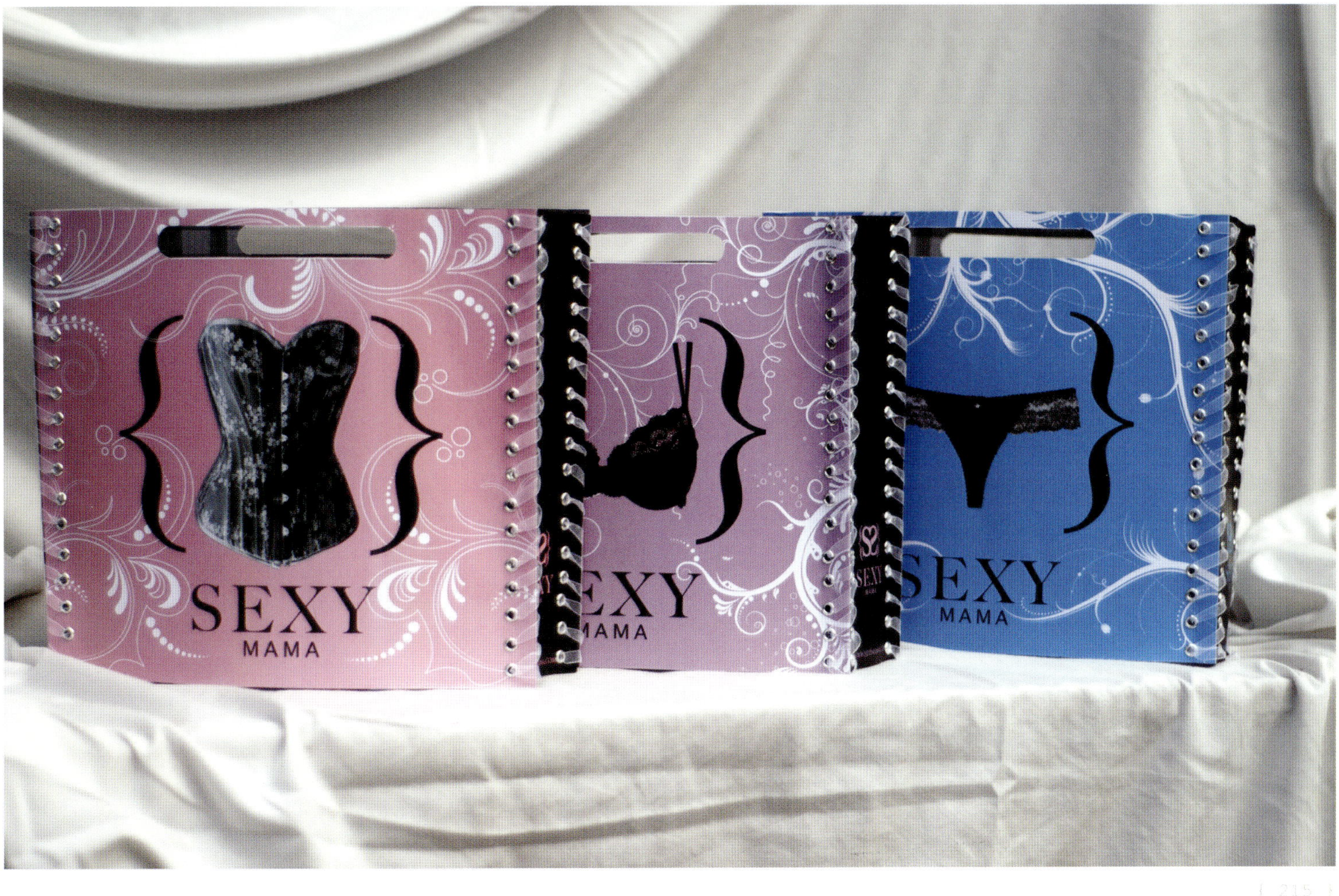

SEXY
MAMA

SEXY
MAMA
SEXY
MAMA

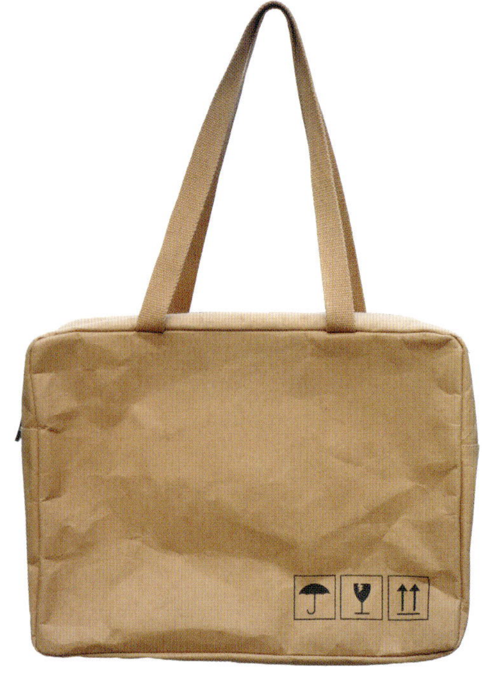

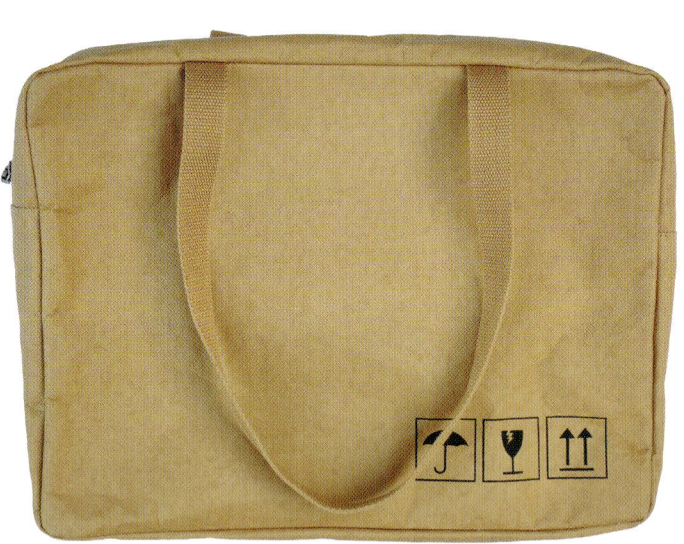

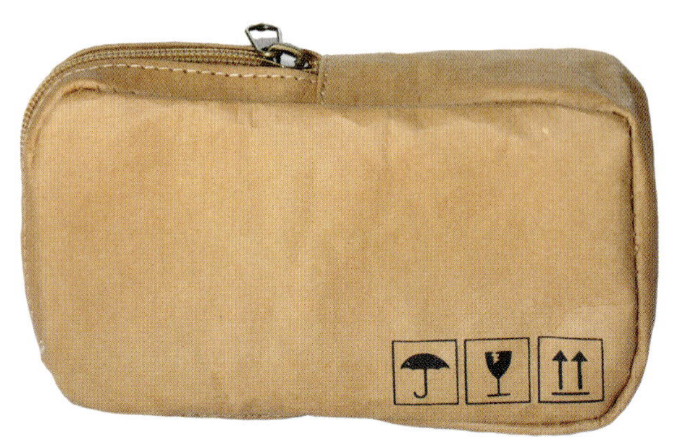

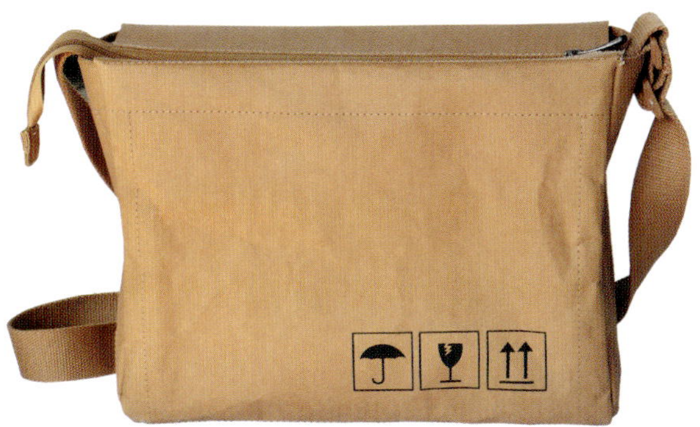

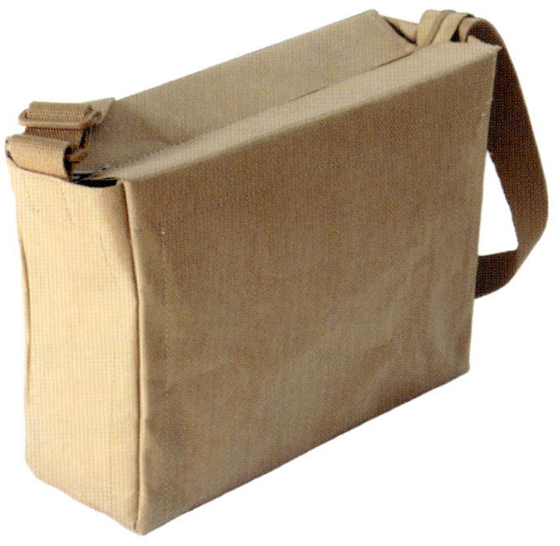

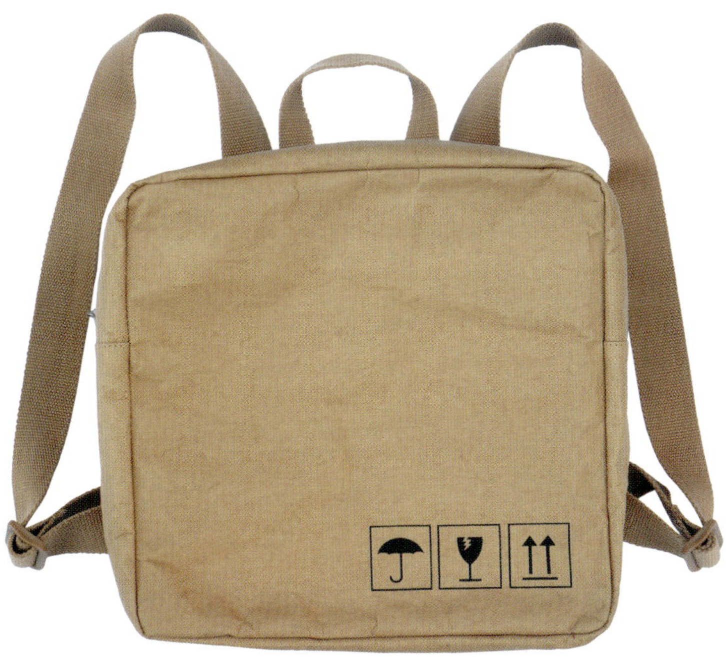

INDUSTRIAL STYLE WATERPROOF PAPER BAG
DA: Off Pop Studio

Made from rinsed Kraft paper, the design has the texture of thick Kraft but is waterproof. They are highlighted with the packing case signs and will crease with usage to become a unique creation of the owner.

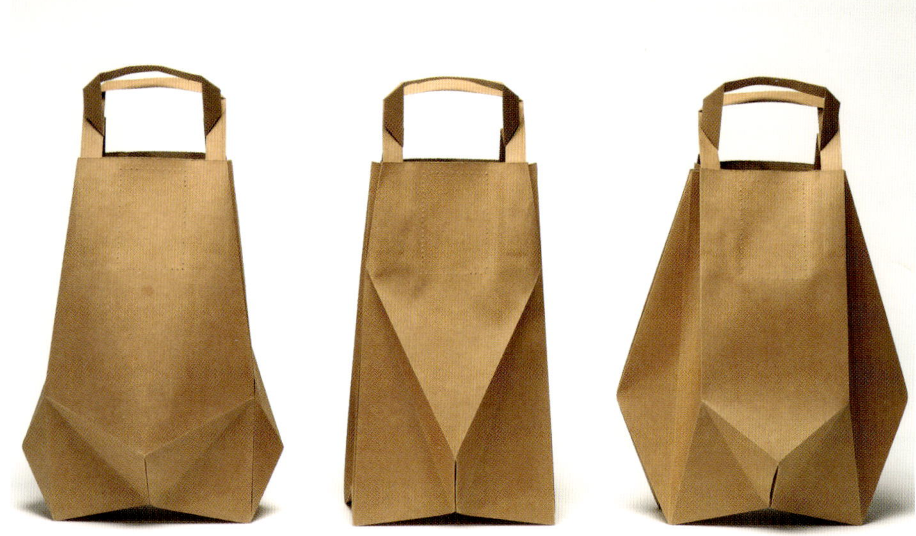

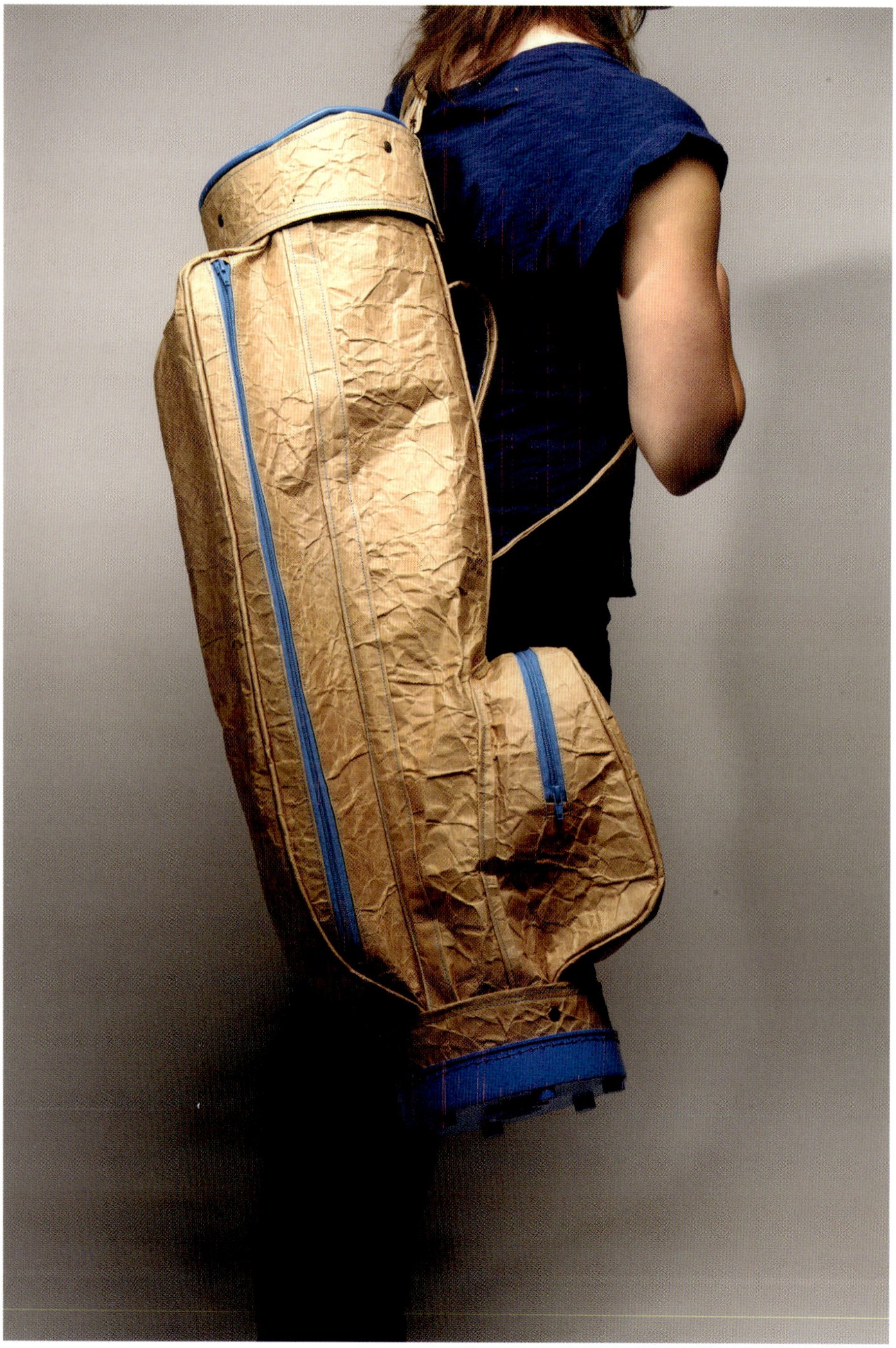

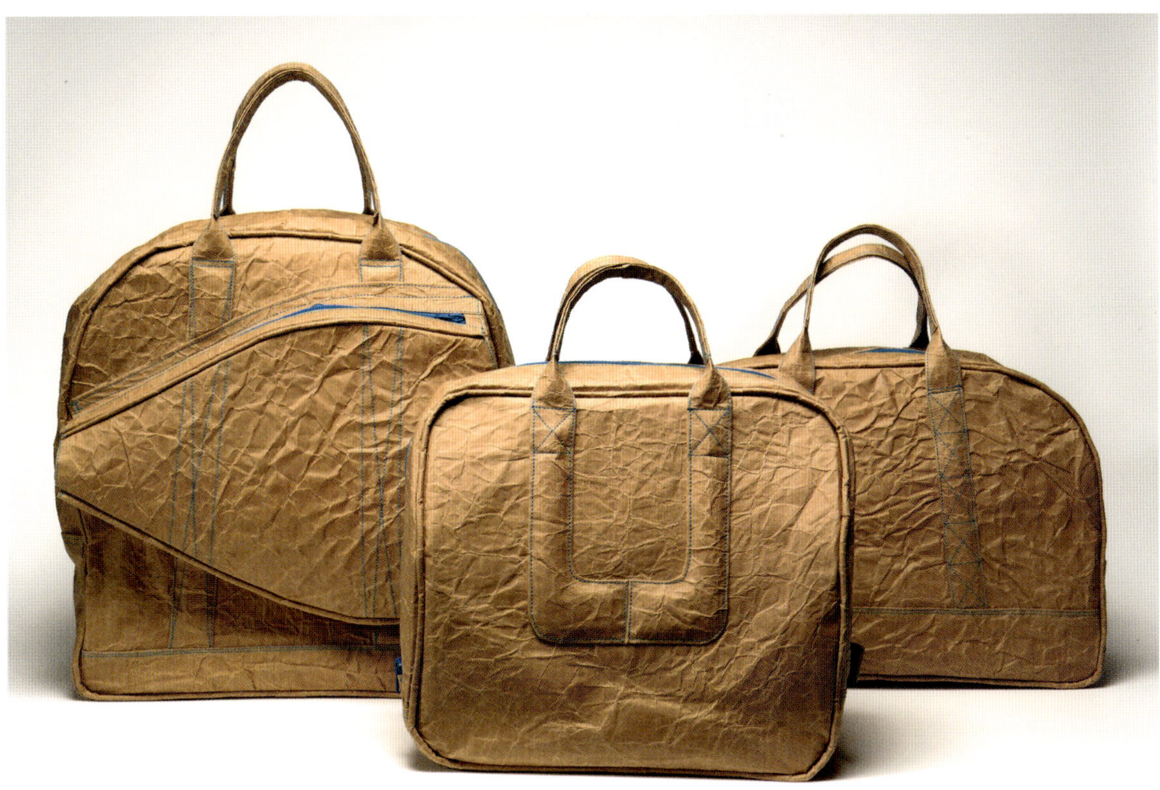

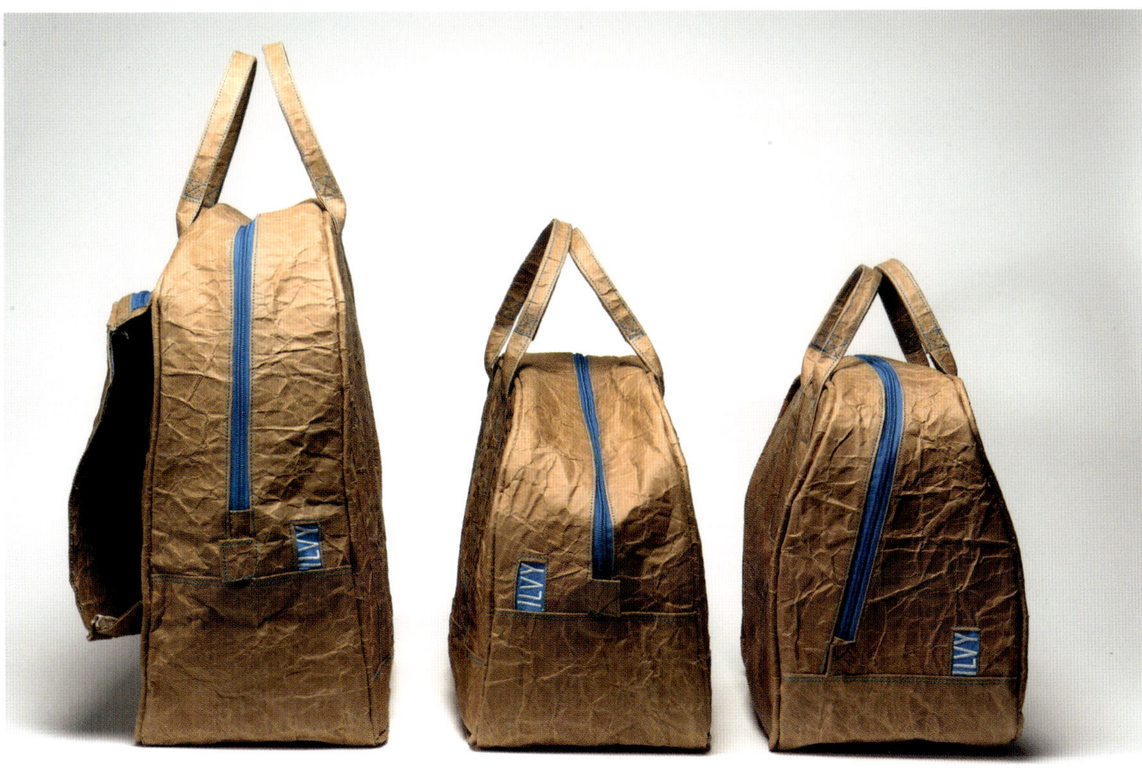

FOLD BAGS
DE: Ilvy Jacobs

These bags demonstrate a new view on everyday bag design and creates a new silhouette for paper bags.

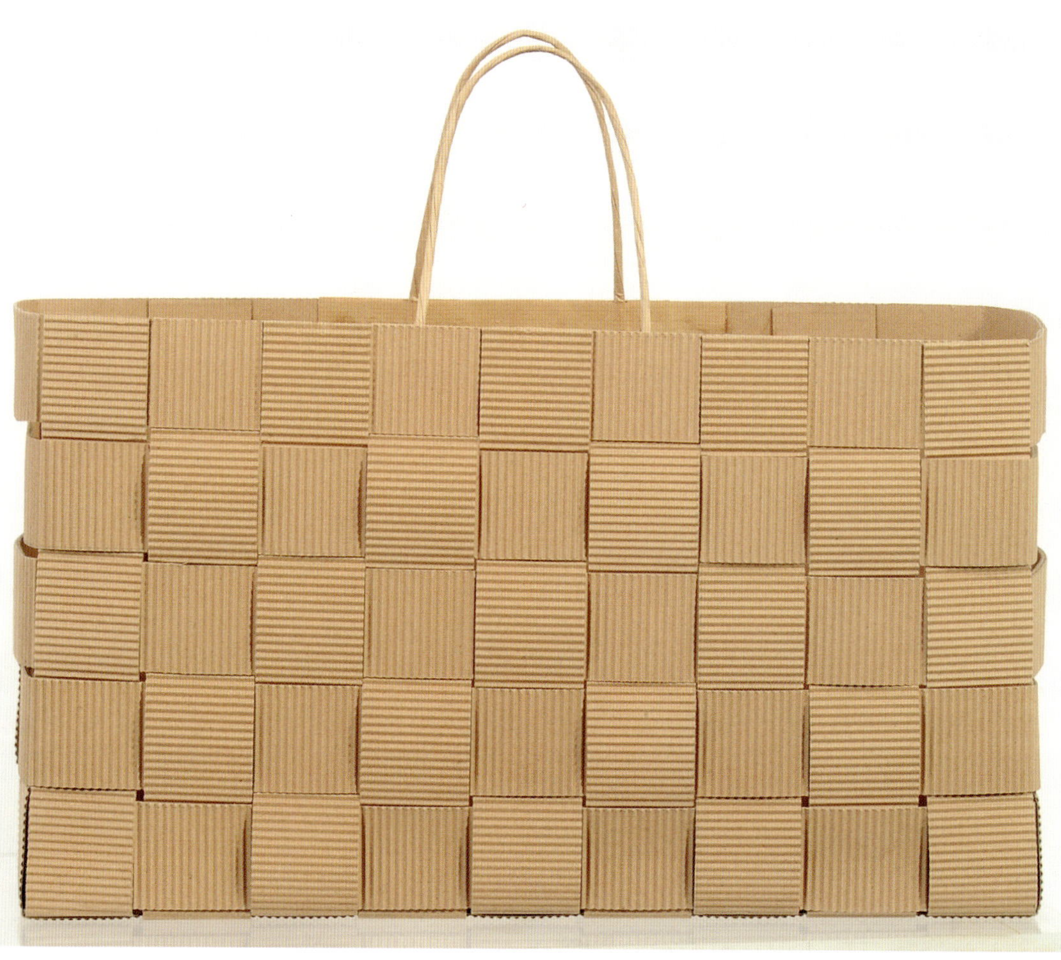

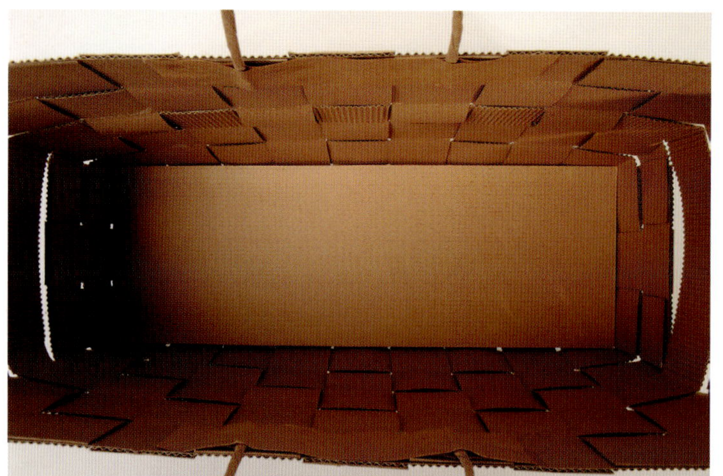

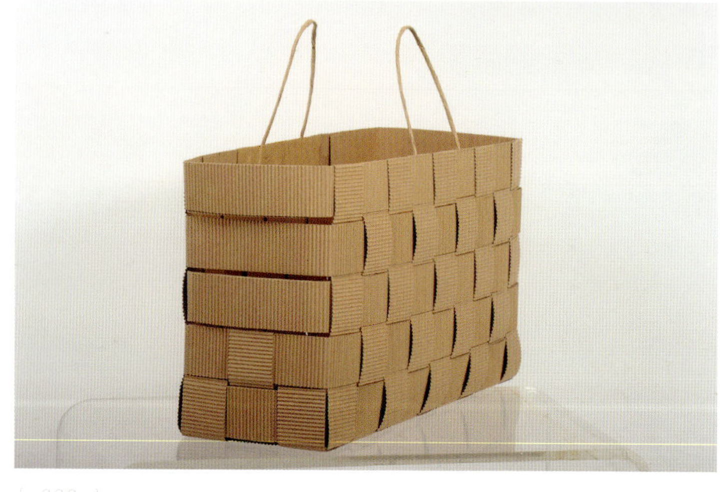

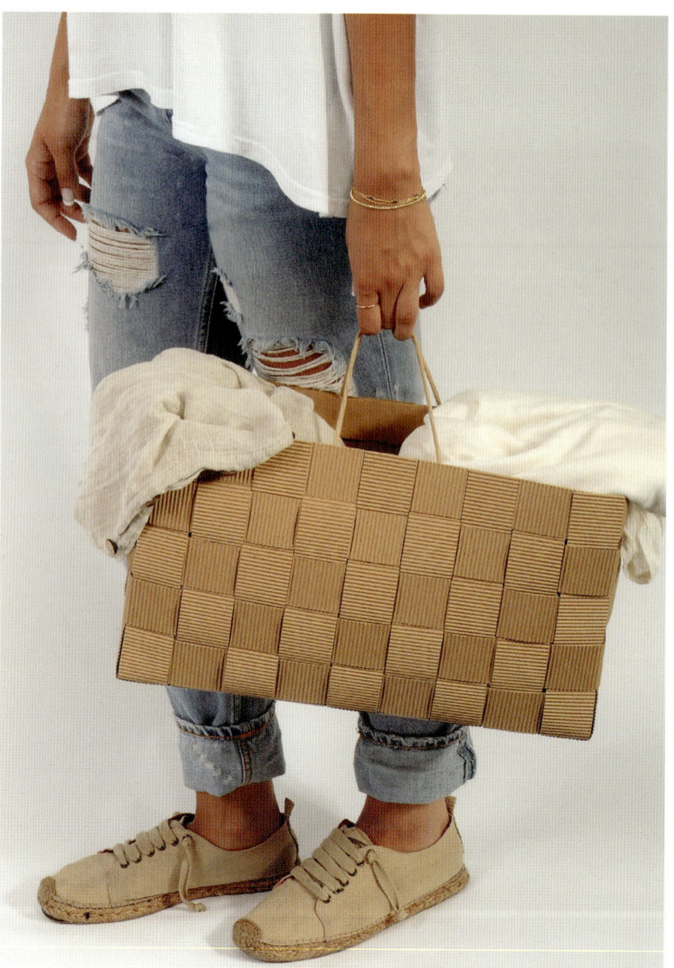

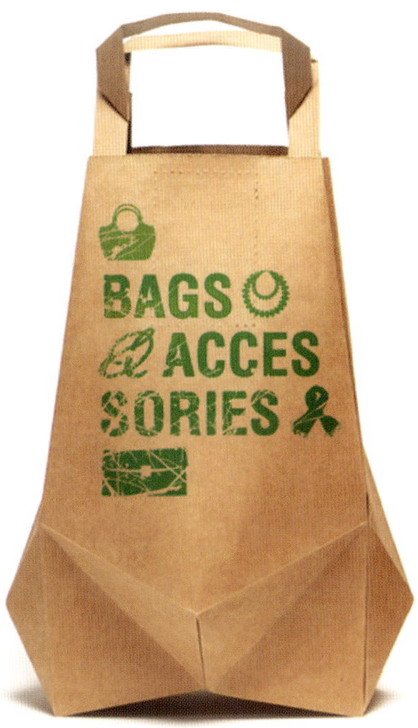

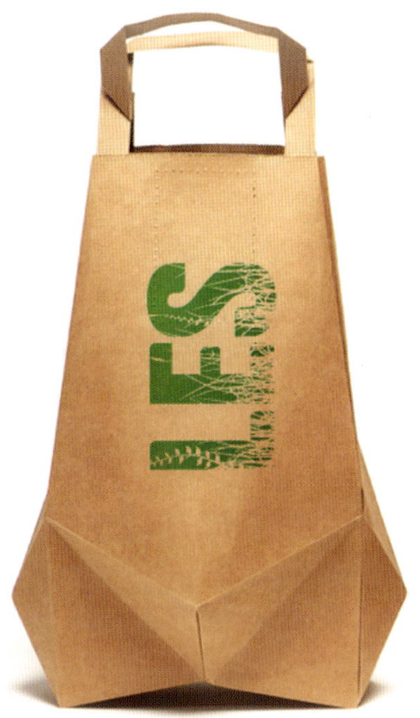

WOVEN SHOPPING BAG
DE: Despina Meimaroglou

Made of strips from single-face, corrugated boards, this bag was woven together at this particular angle to give the design strength and durability.

LES STORE
DA: Playoff

With calculated folding, this bag comes in a geometrical shape, while the brown color of kraft paper complements the green logo.

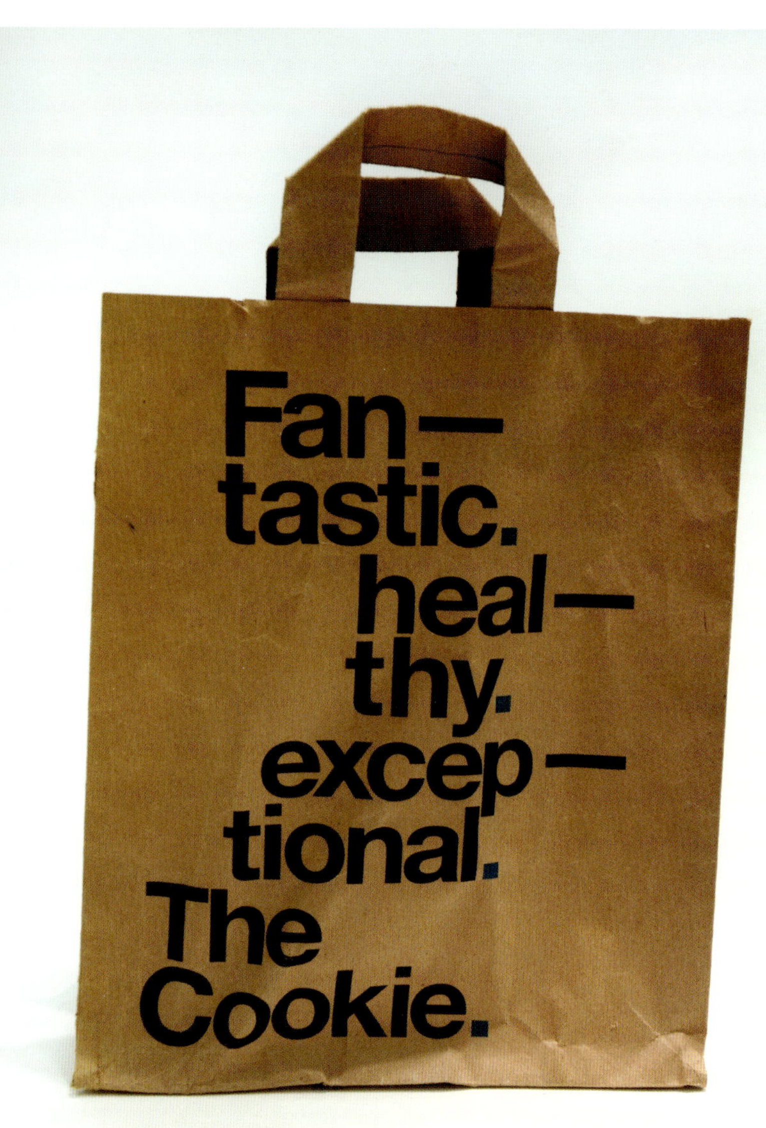

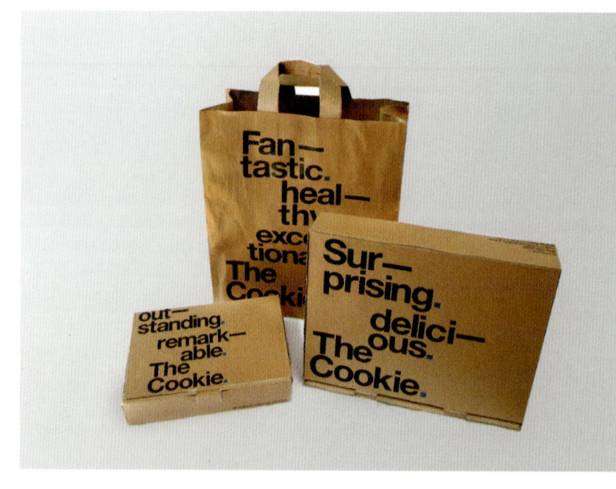

THE COOKIE
DE: Andrea Garza Escamilla

Designed for an oatmeal cookie shop, the designer wanted the designer
create special bags to communicate that this type of cookie is health and
delicious. She did that by creatively breaking the words breaking the words
into pieces like cookie crumbs.

LIANG DIAN DESIGN CENTER
DA: Ames Studio

Designed for the opening of the Liang Dian Design Center, this gift bag has
a hole to encourage recipients to discover beauty through a new perspective.
It resonates with the brand identity - a center devoted to promoting the
appreciation of Chine.

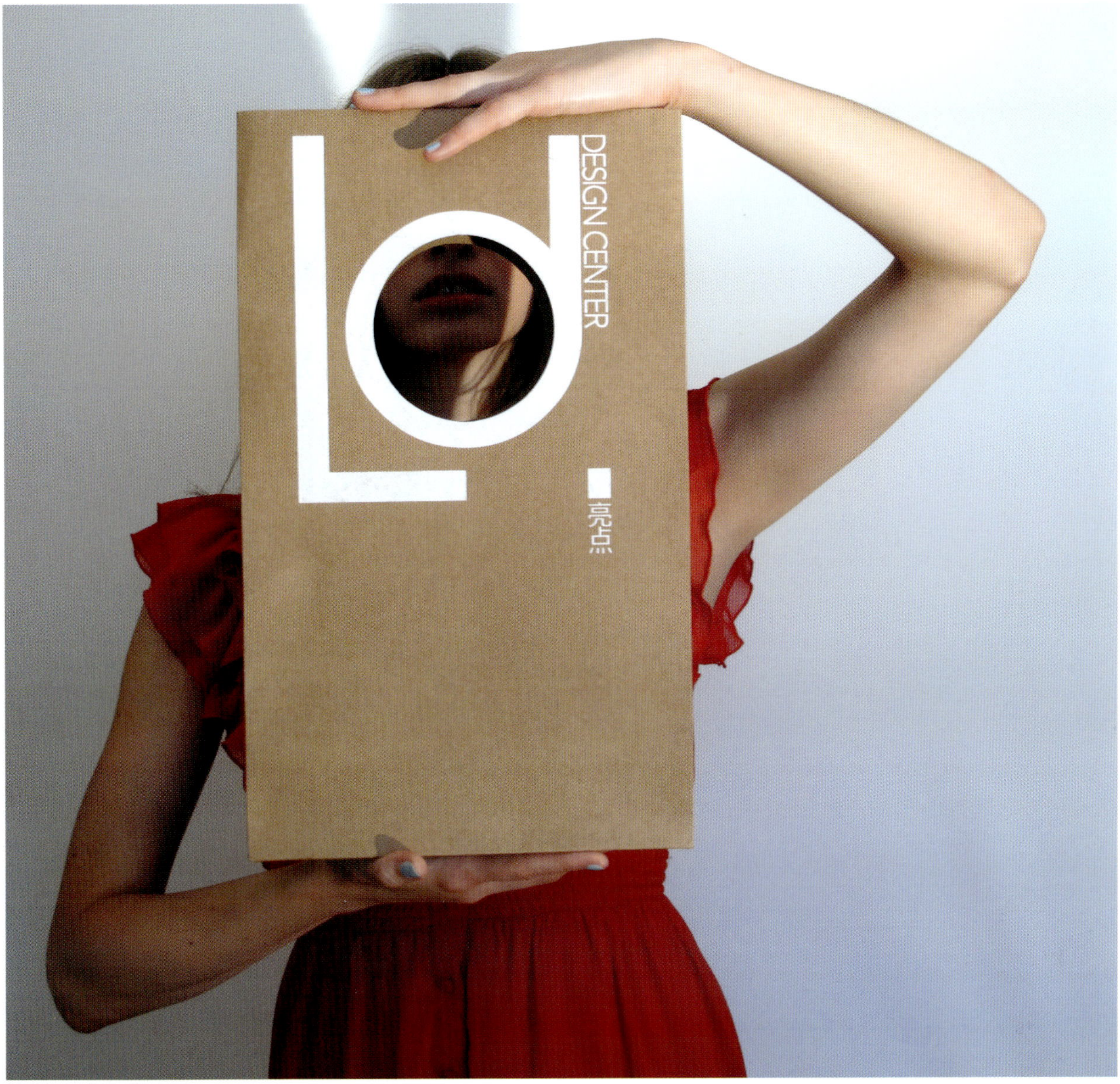

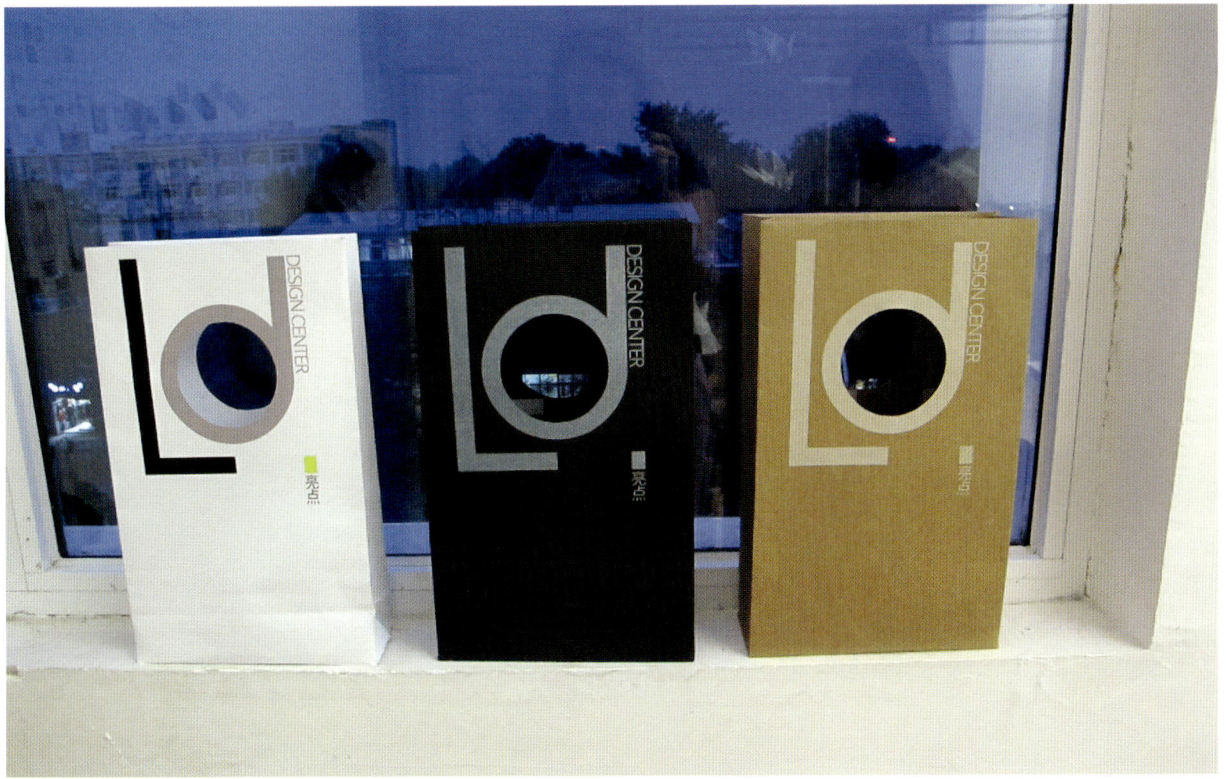

Ld
DESIGN CENTER
亮点

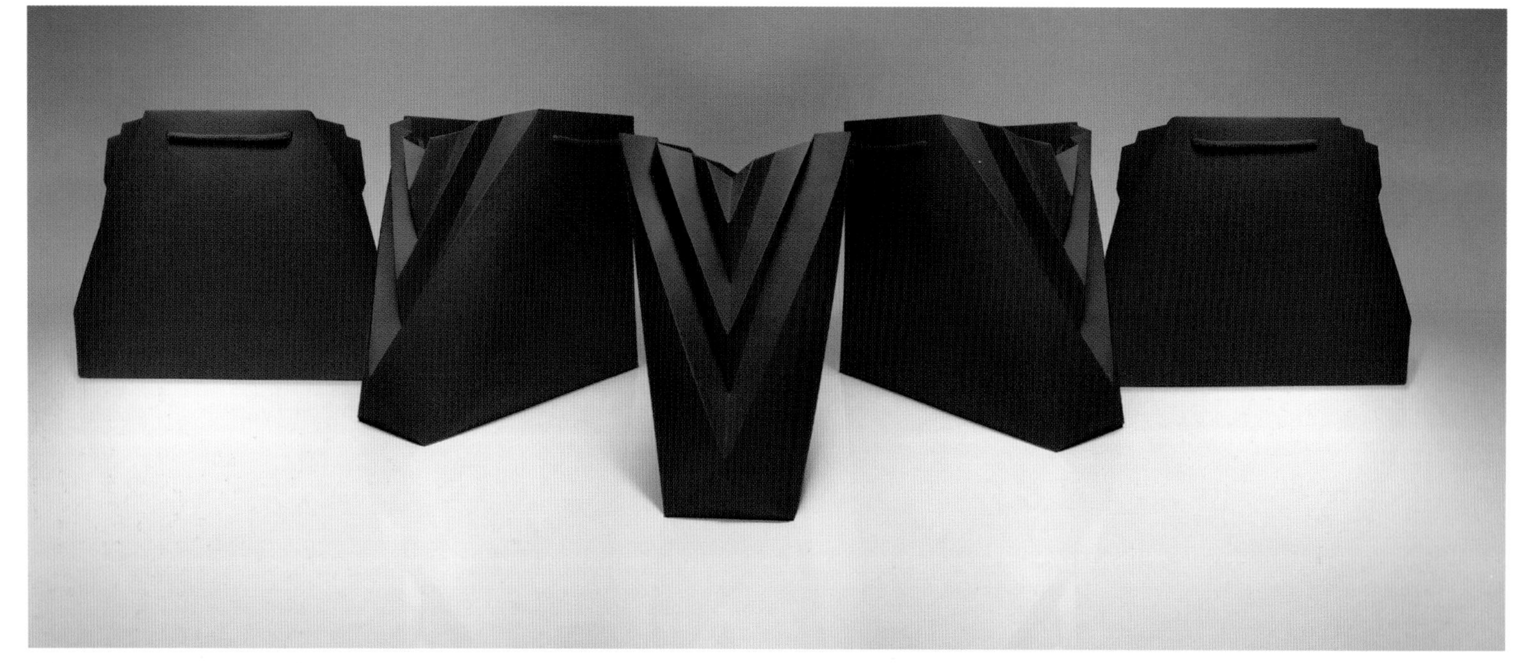

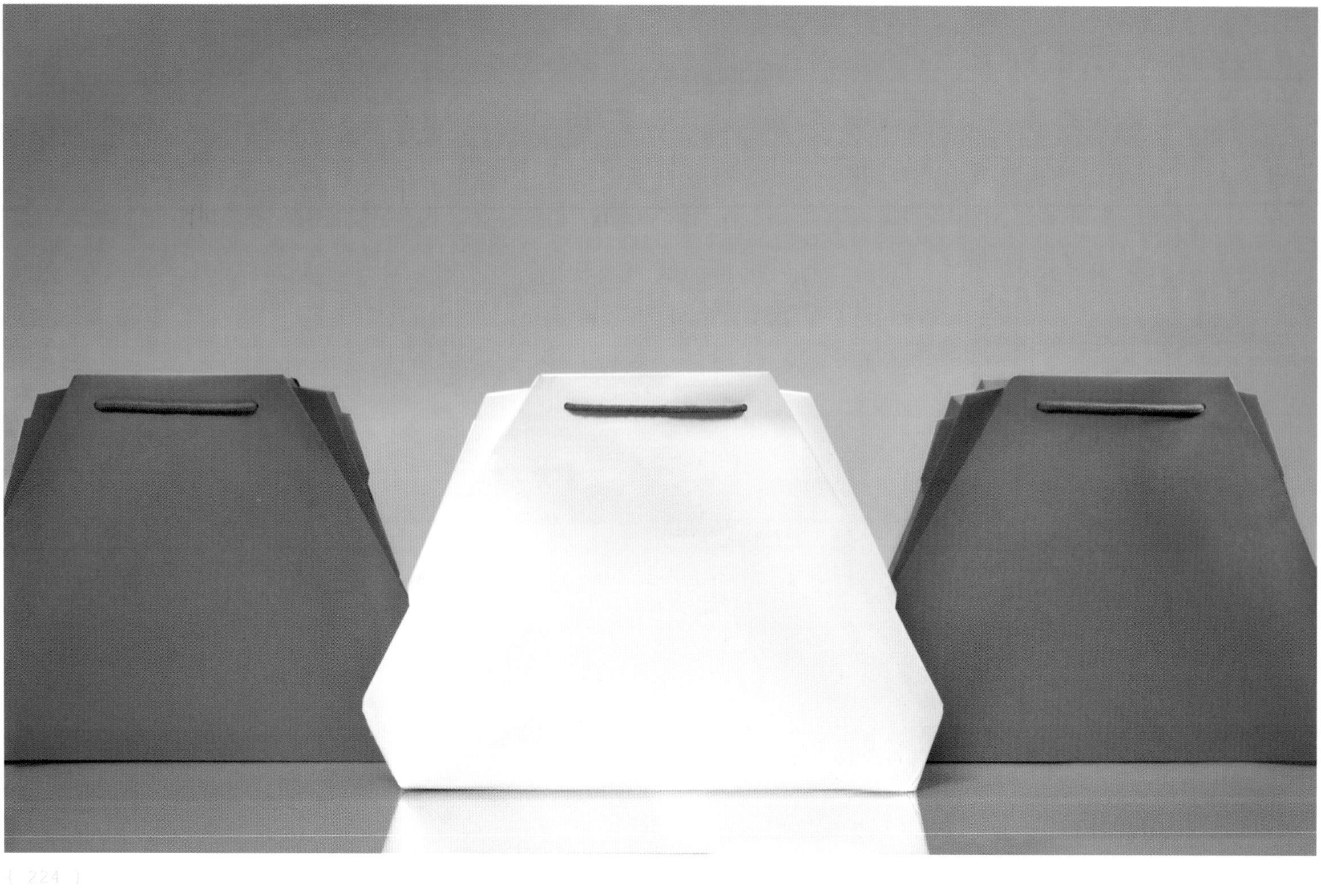

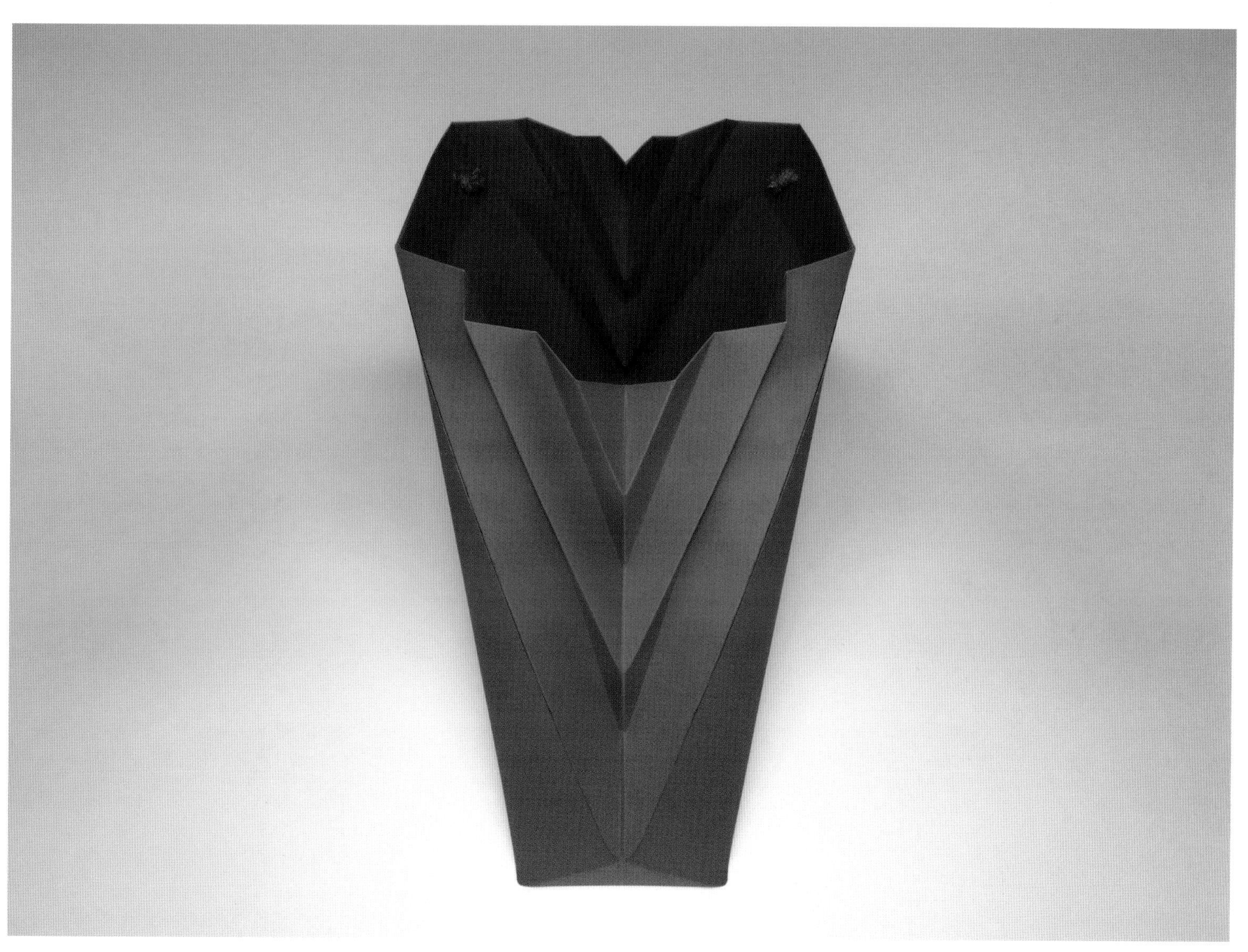

PLEATED SHOPPING BAG
DA: Design Packaging(Evelio Mattos, John Turner)

Exploring ways of applying origami patterns to shopping bags, this design is
characterized by the bold pleated ornament on the sides, while the inverted
bottom fold allows it to collapse like a regular bag.

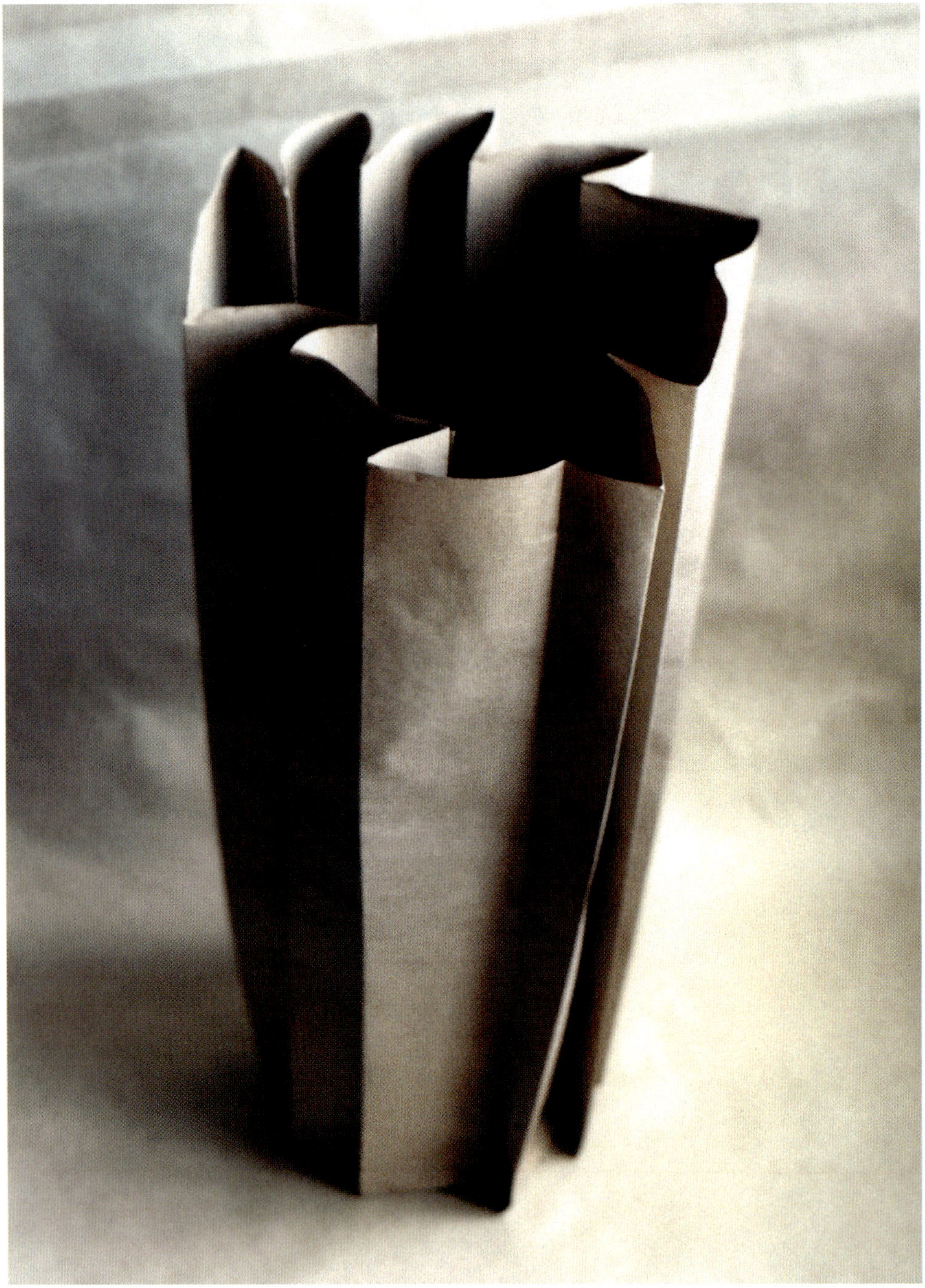

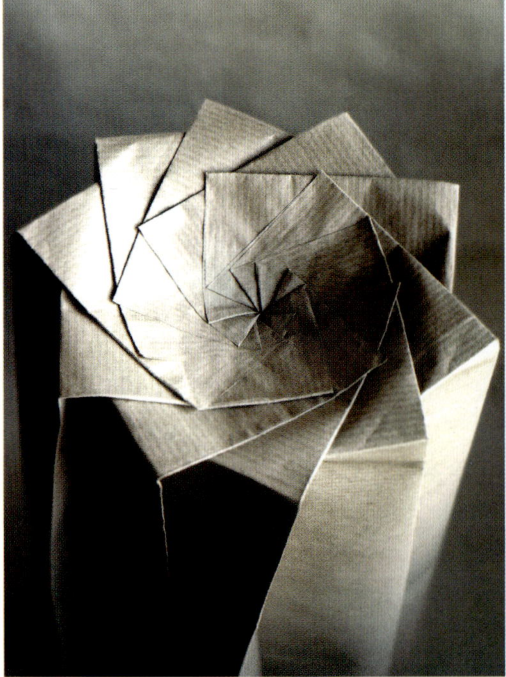

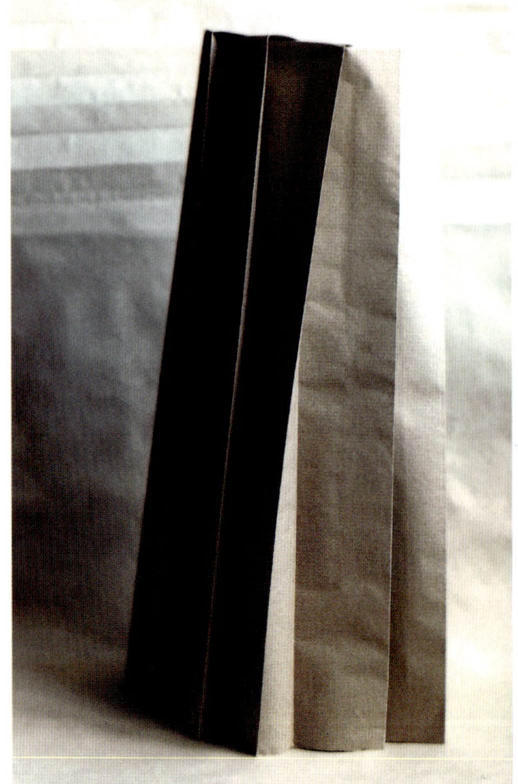

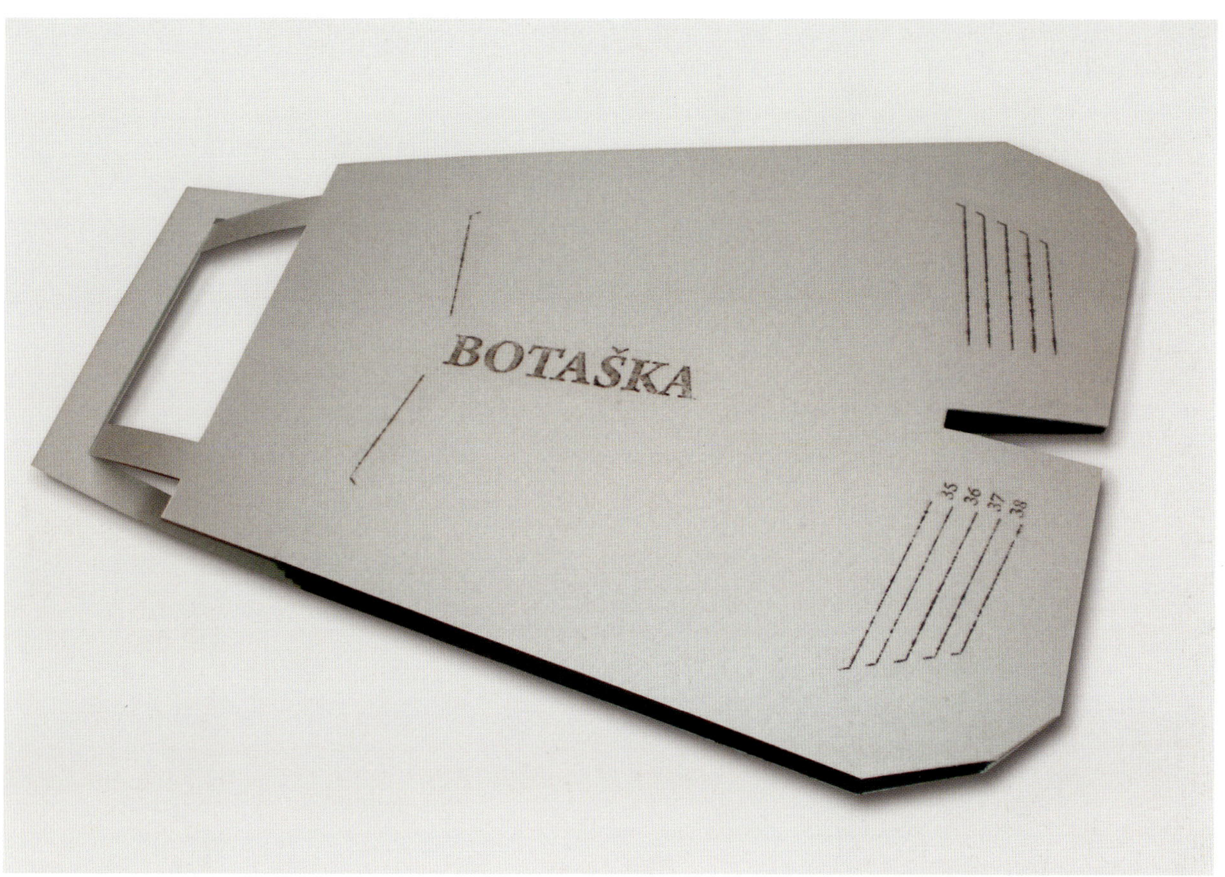

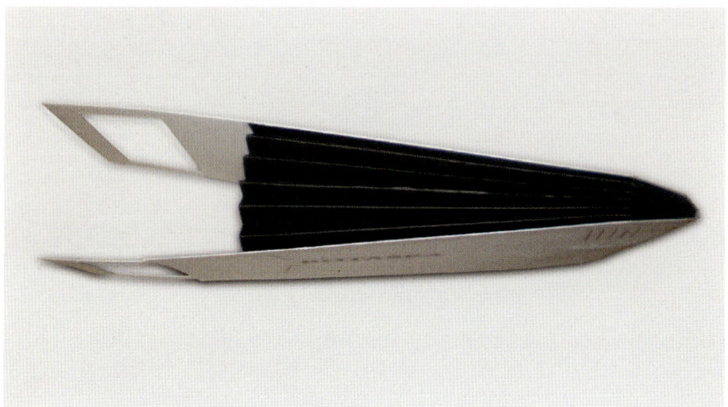

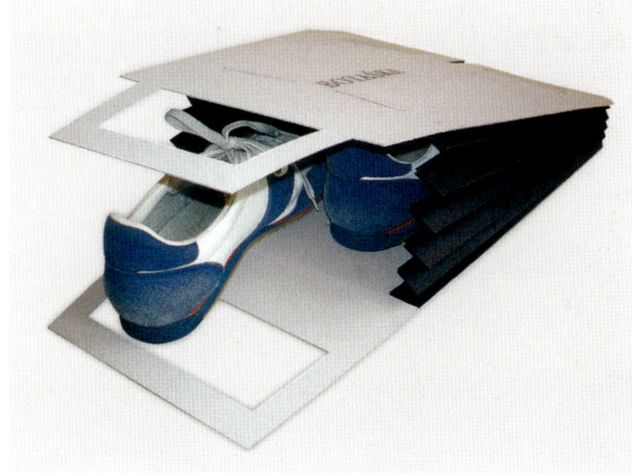

TWISTED SHOPPING BAG
DE: Izabela Adriana Wit

Inspired by the art of origami, this bag was the result of folding a rectangular piece of recycled brown paper. Users are allowed to change the volume according to their needs.

BOTASKA
DE: Iva Jancova, Zuzana Stiefova

To store shoes with less space, "Botaskawas" was developed using cardboard and paper, coming in three sizes to fit all types of footwear.

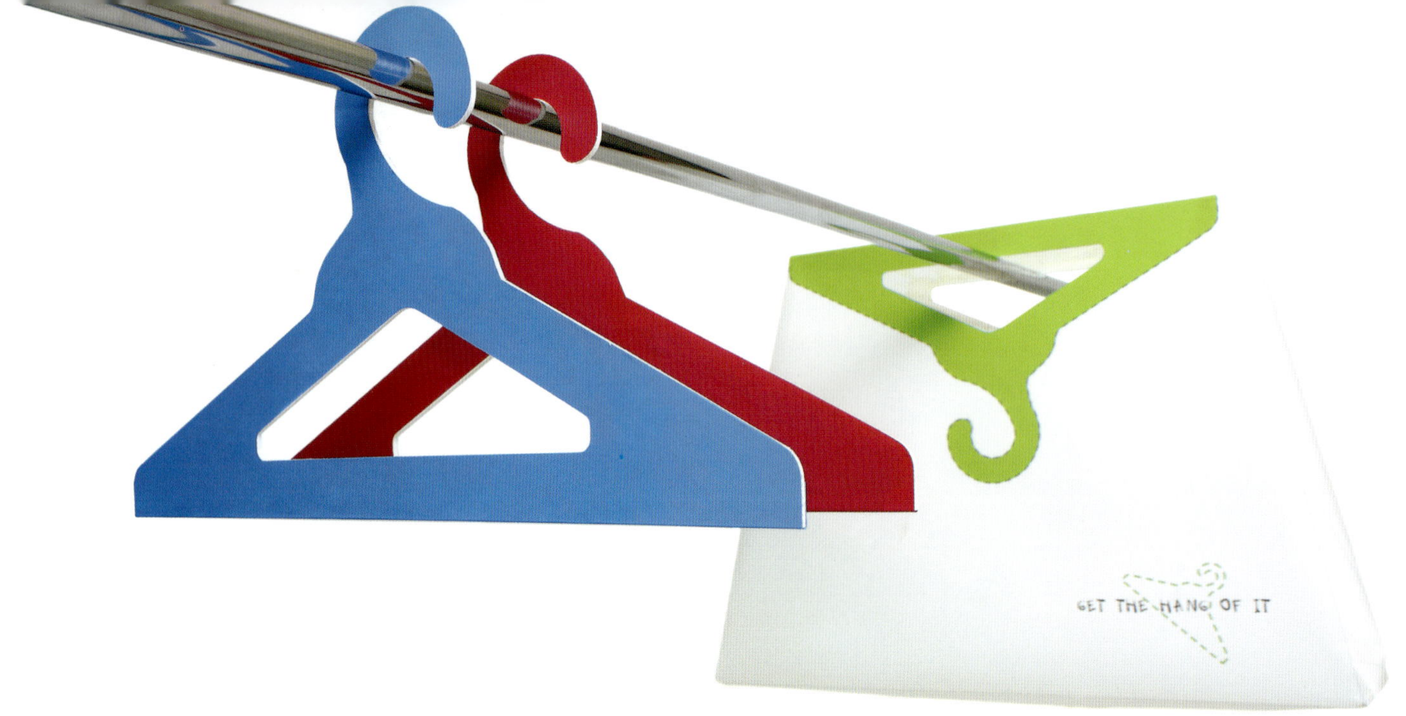

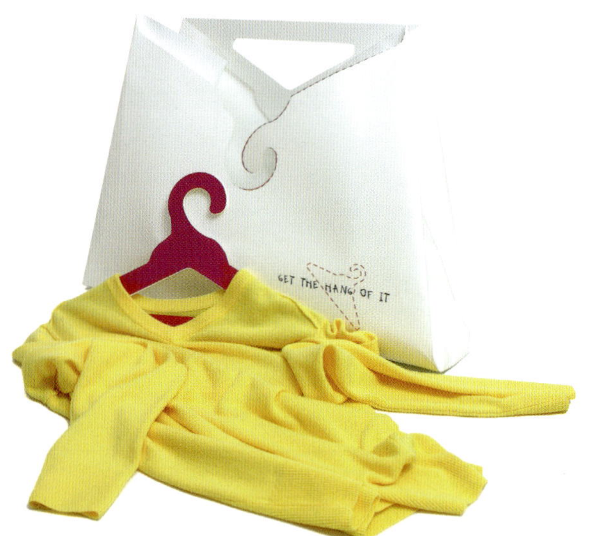

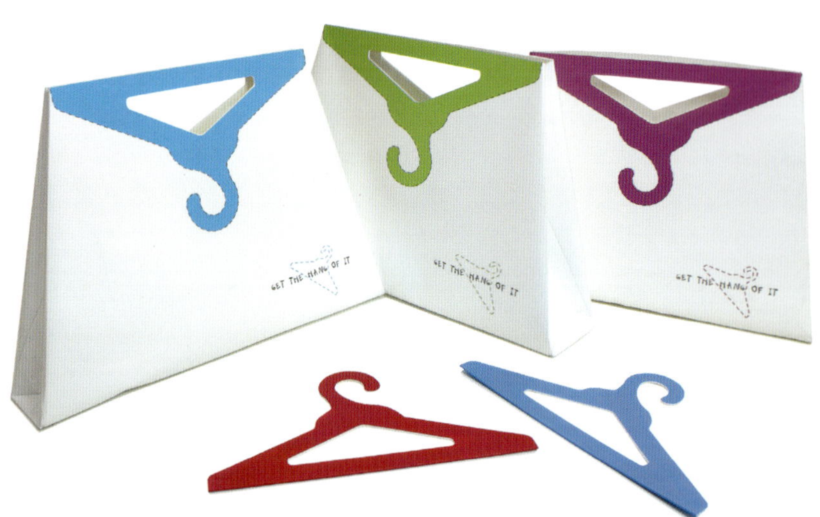

GET THE HANG OF IT BAG
DA: DEDE DextrousDesign

With two special handles (two cardboard hangers) users can hang up their newly purchased clothes at once with this shopping bag.

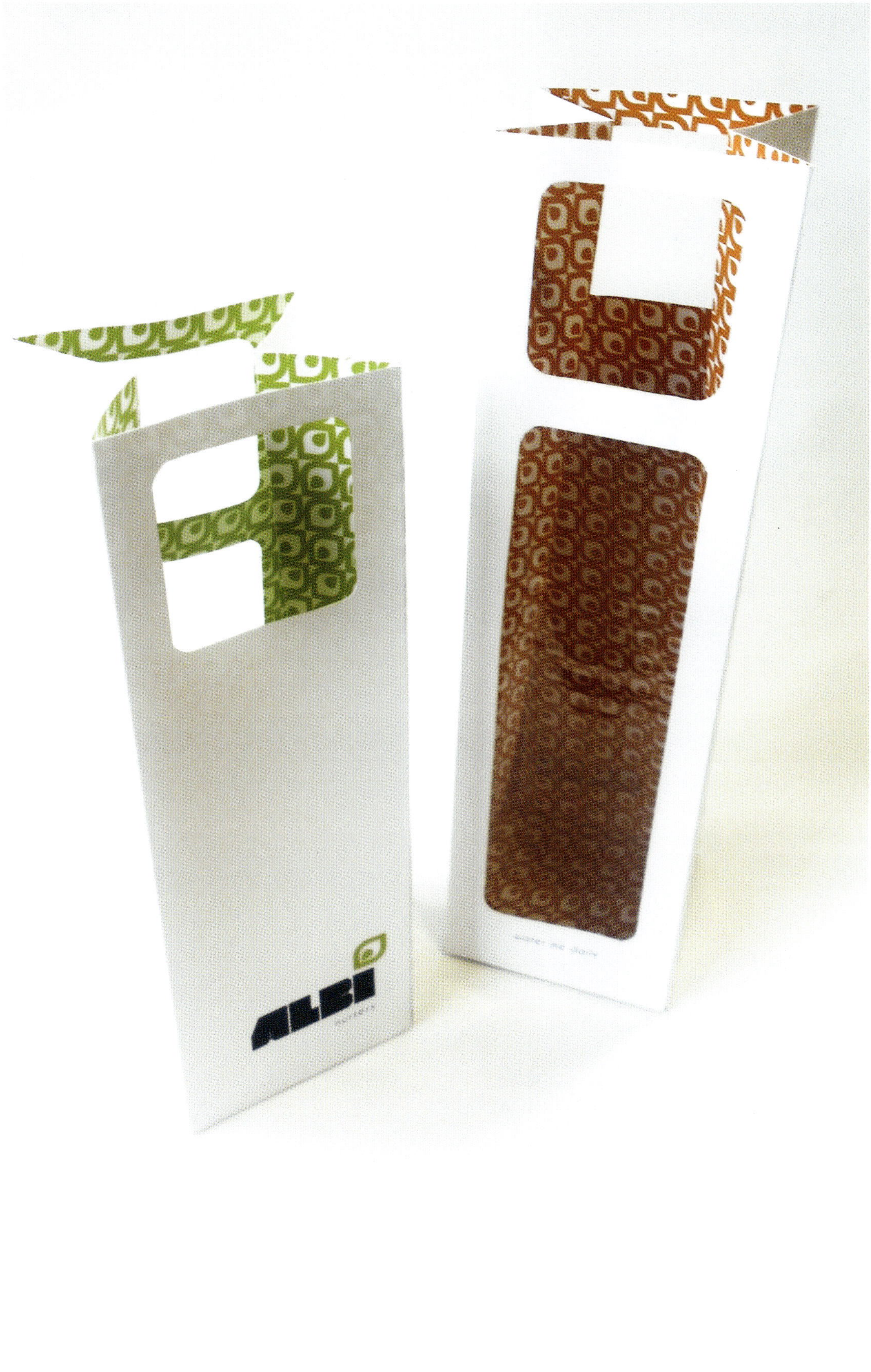

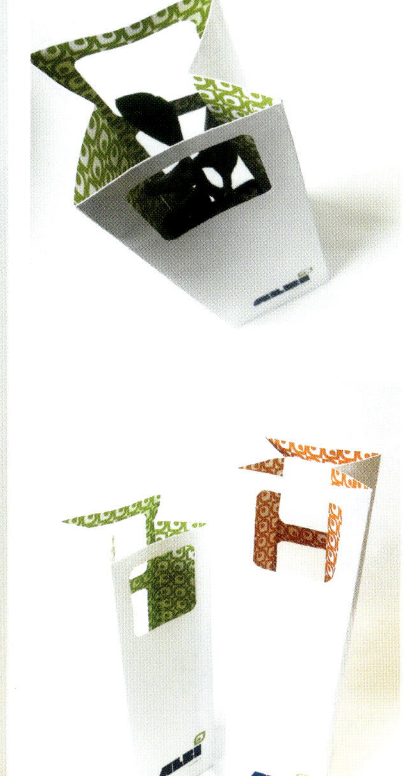

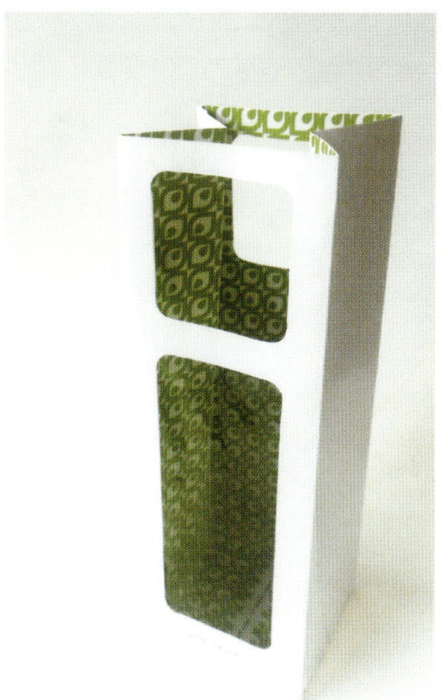

ALBI - BAGS FOR NURSERY
DE: Kelly Torres

Based on the concept "albi," which simply means white, designer kept the outside white and clean, and the interior, painted with colorful patterns that symbolize nature. The color is revealed through a big window on the back.

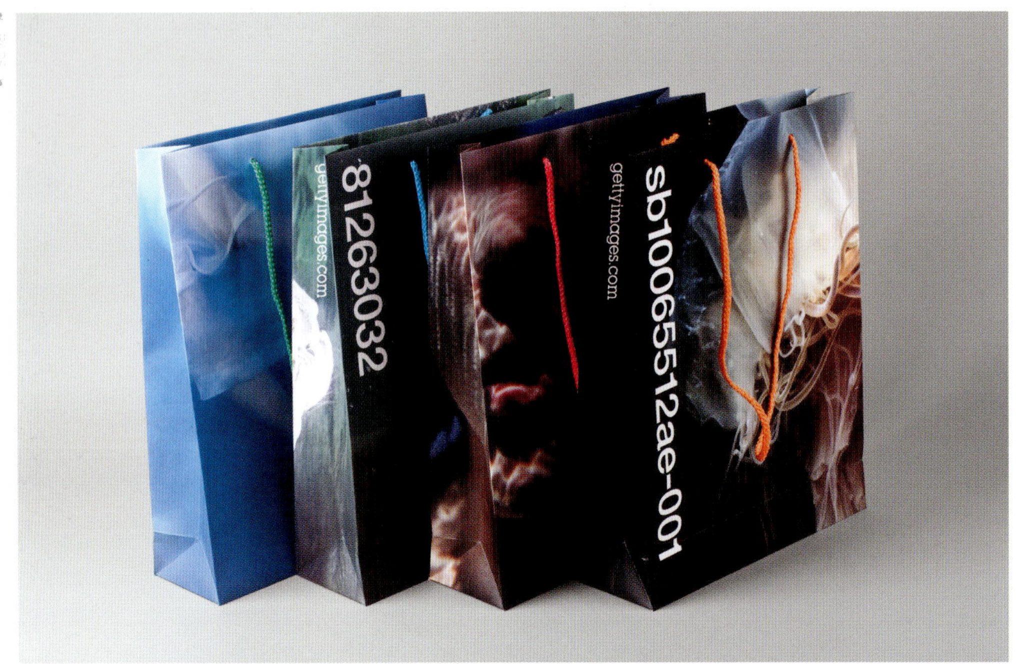
81263032
gettyimages.com
sb10065512ae-001
gettyimages.com

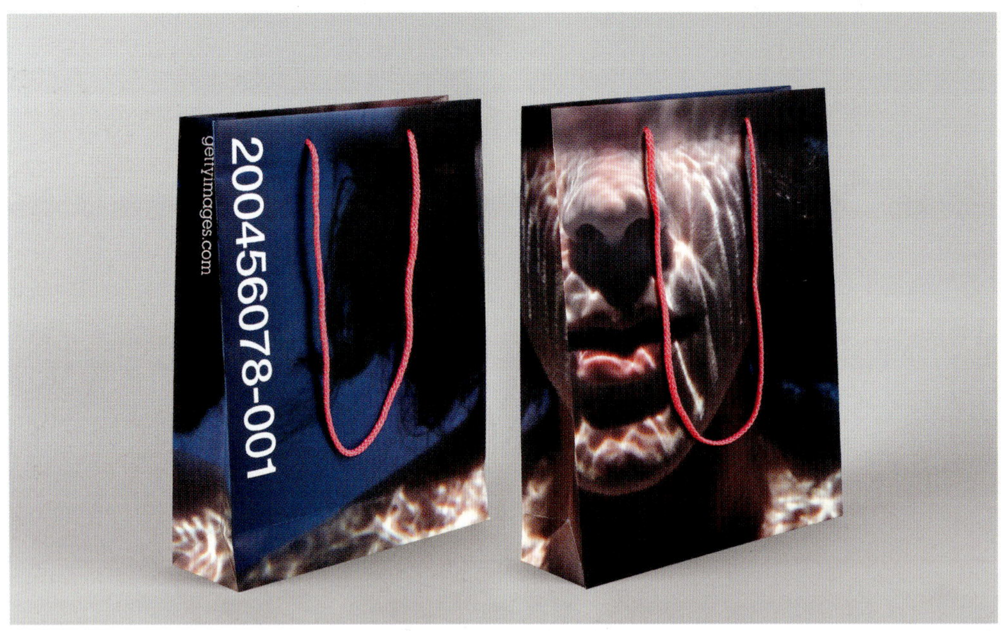
200456078-001
gettyimages.com

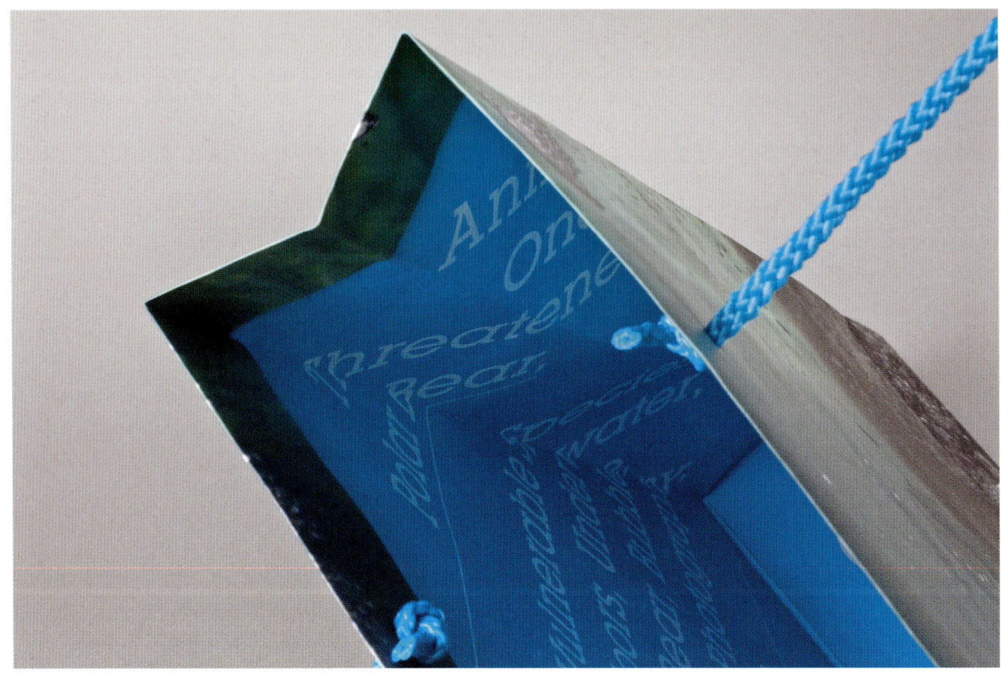
Animals On
Threatened
Bear

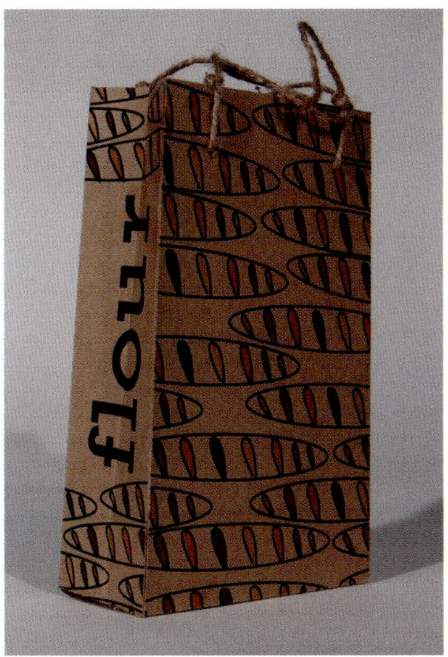 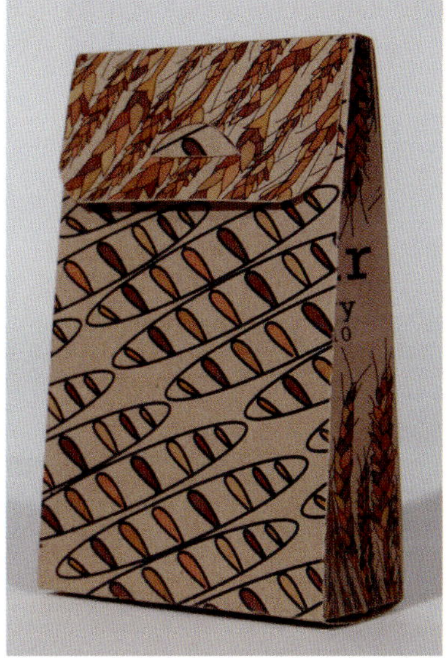 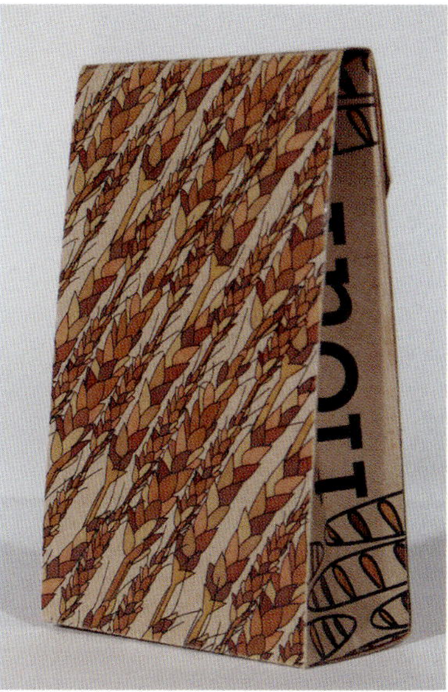

GETTY IMAGES- BAGS
DE: Michael C. Place(Build)

These bags were created with striking images printed boldly on the sides. The eye-catching look is strengthen by using fluorescent handles on the bags.

FLOUR BREAD CO. BAGS
DE: Becca Dunn

Becca Dunn decided to brand a bakery, using her own illustrations of wheat and bread in earthy tones, to create an inviting impression, while hinting at the healthy quality of the product itself.

CAREALE SHOPPING BAG
DE: Natalie Gwen Bradhurst

Designed for a boutique cheese shop called "Careale," (Latin for "cheese kitchen") this bag resembles a wax covered cheese wheel wrapped in twine. The negative space created by the cut out wedge allows for a handle.

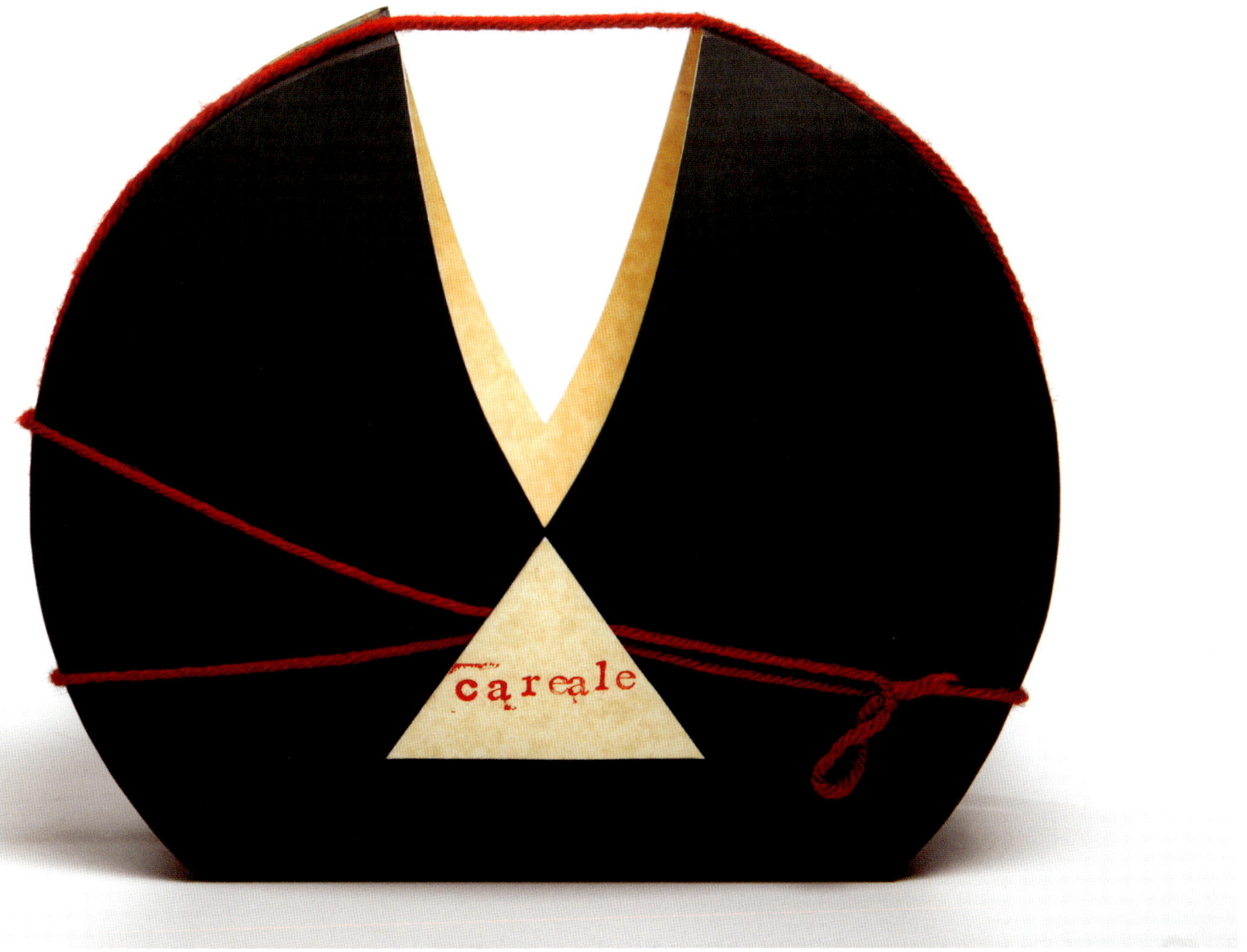

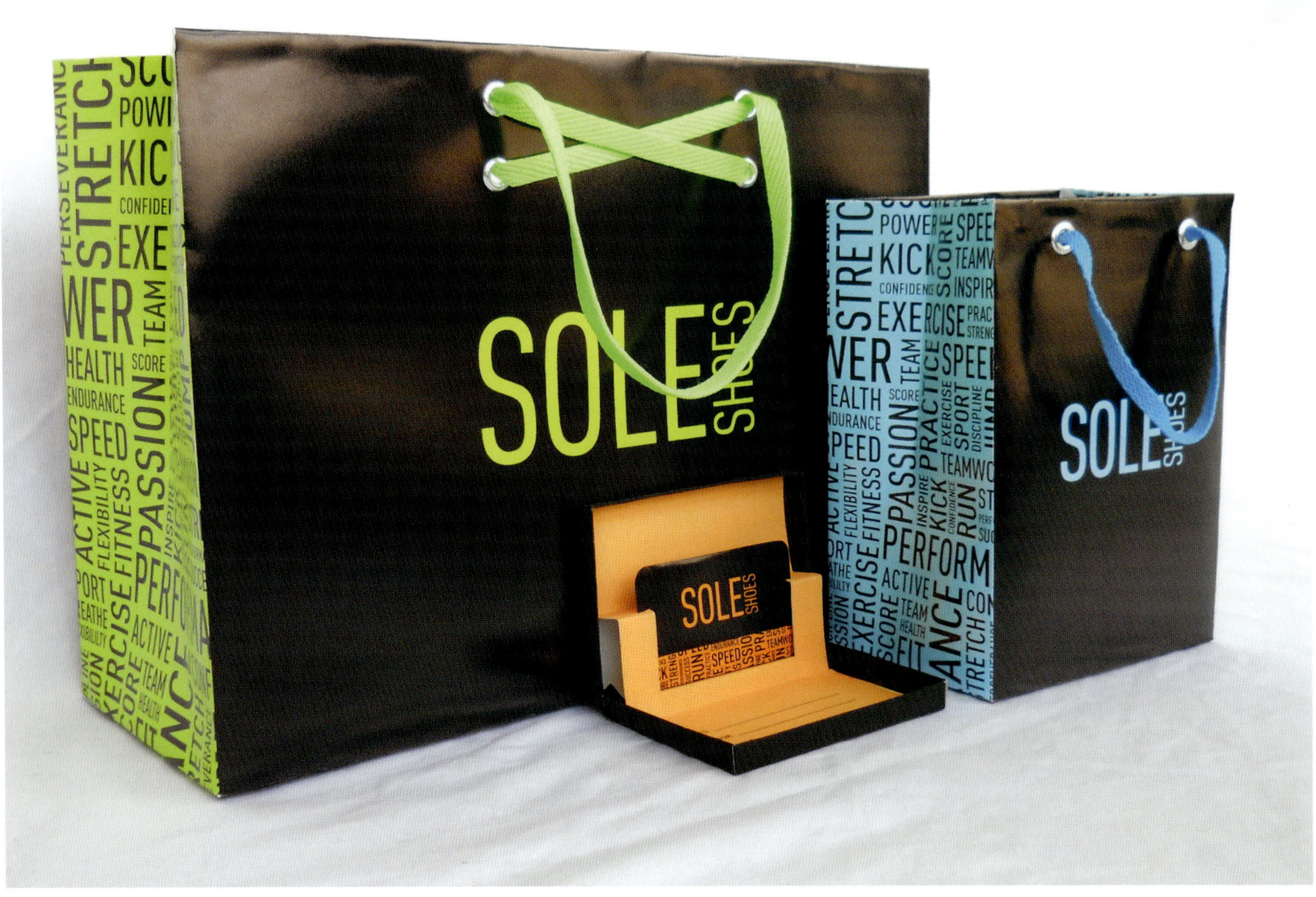

SOLE SHOES SHOPPING BAG

DE: Megan K. McKenry

Megan McKenry created an athletic appeal with neon colors and a word collage
that depicts the theme. This bags uses shoelaces as handles that consumers
can use for their new shoes.

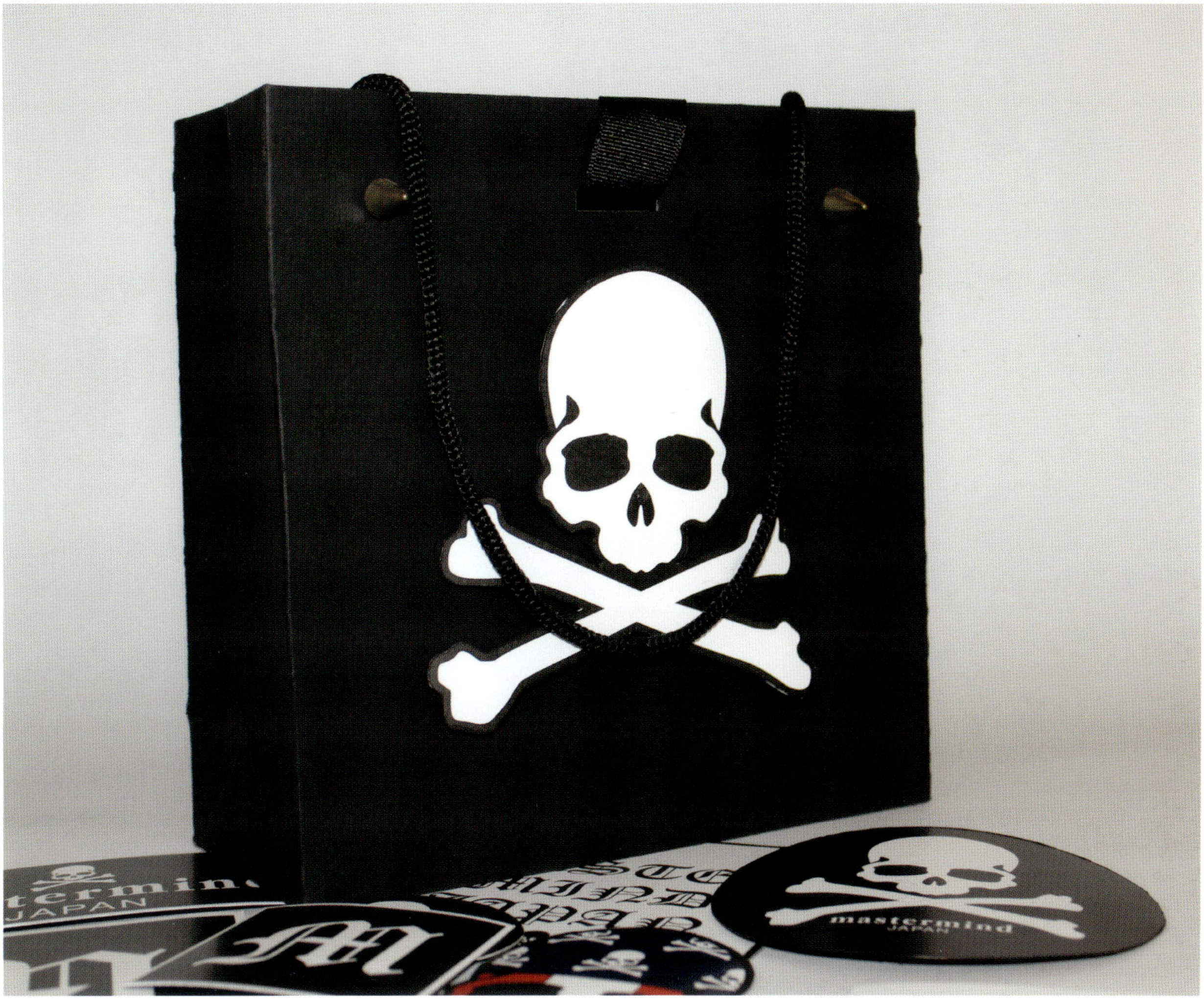

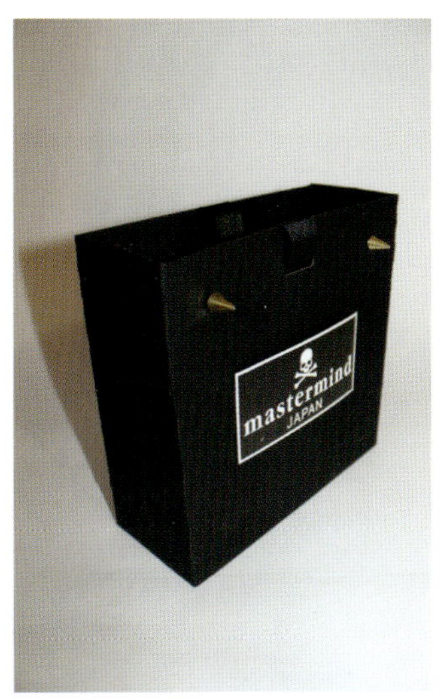

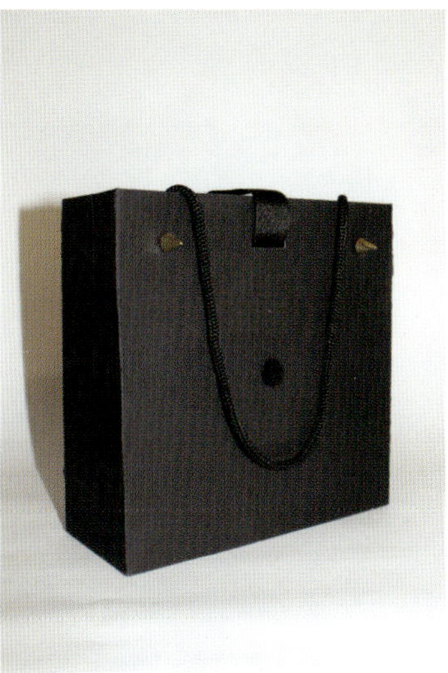

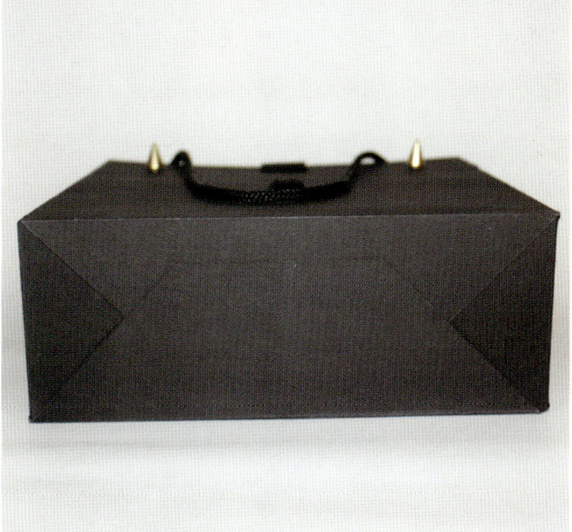

SHOPPING BAG CONCEPT
DE: Gabriel Castro

This bag appears to be simple, but recipients will be given some accessories like brass rivets, spike studs etc. to embellish the bag the way they want it.

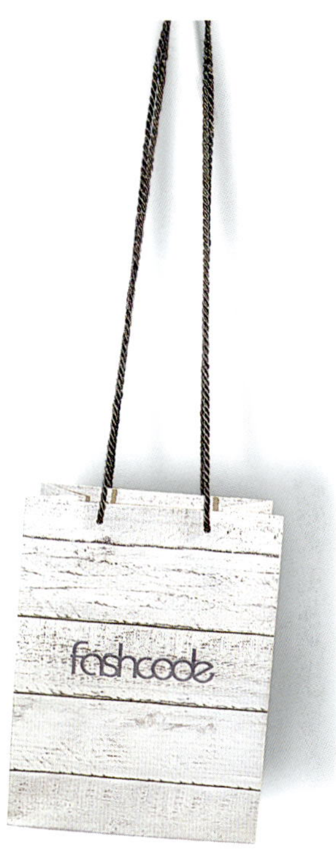

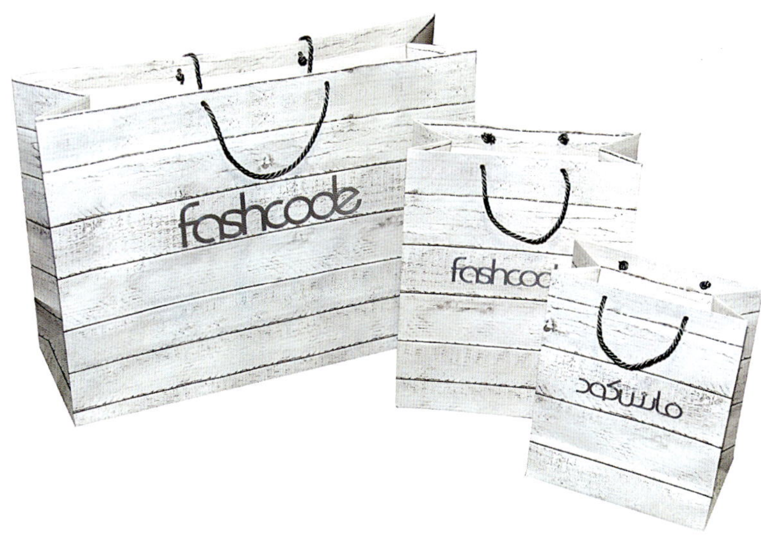

FASHCODE
DA: Paragon Marketing Communication

This shopping bag was printed with the texture
of a rough wooden surface, with the brand name
showing in a neon-sign-like typeface.

RAMADAN BAG
DA: Paragon Marketing Communication

Designed for the Ramadan celebration, this bag
was printed with the traditional Lantern symbol
for Ramadan, with an optical illusion that makes
it interactive.

LOVE ME, POSSESS ME
DE: Sidney Lim YX

Vibrate flowers were painted to represent the
lure of products in a consumer society. They
are delicate but strong, fighting to escape the
confines of the text frame to attract consumers'
attention.

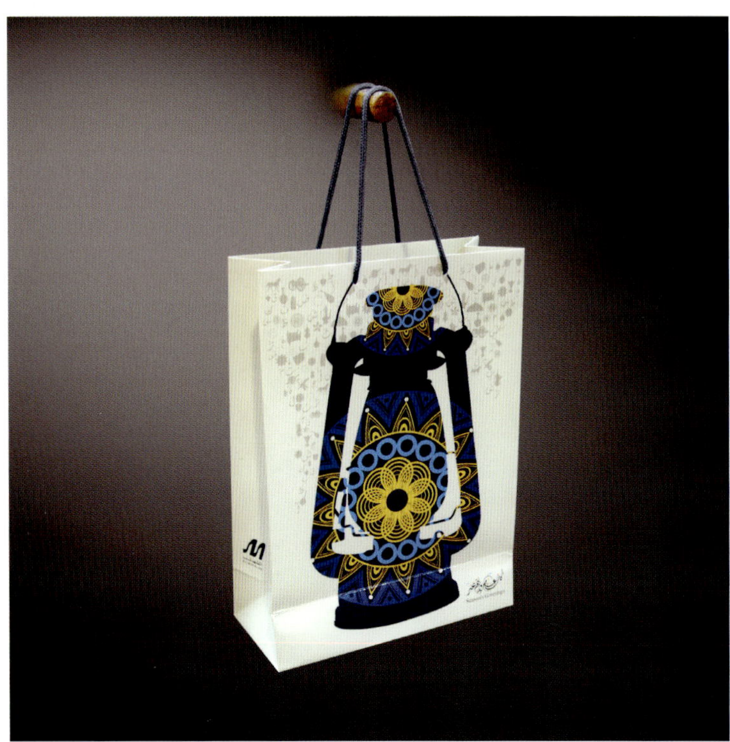

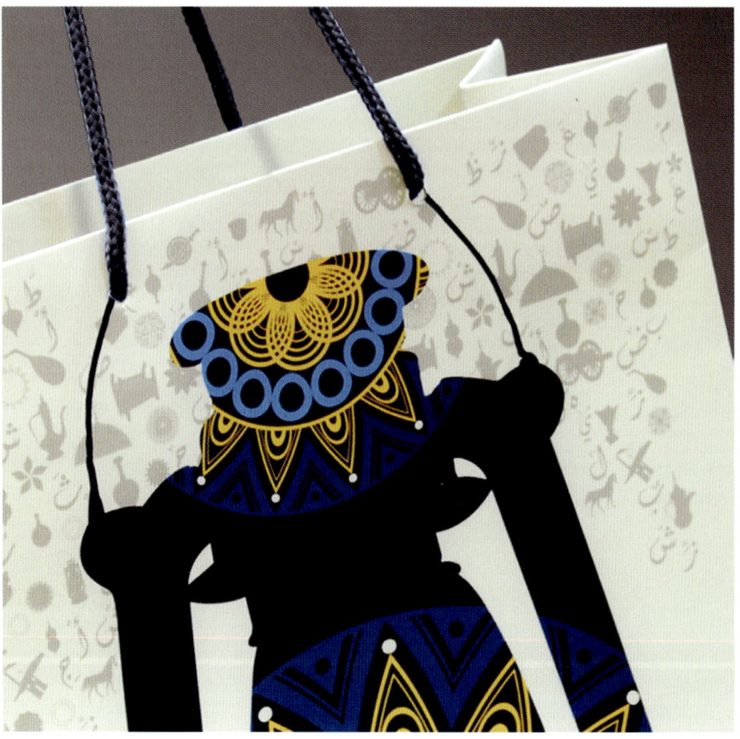

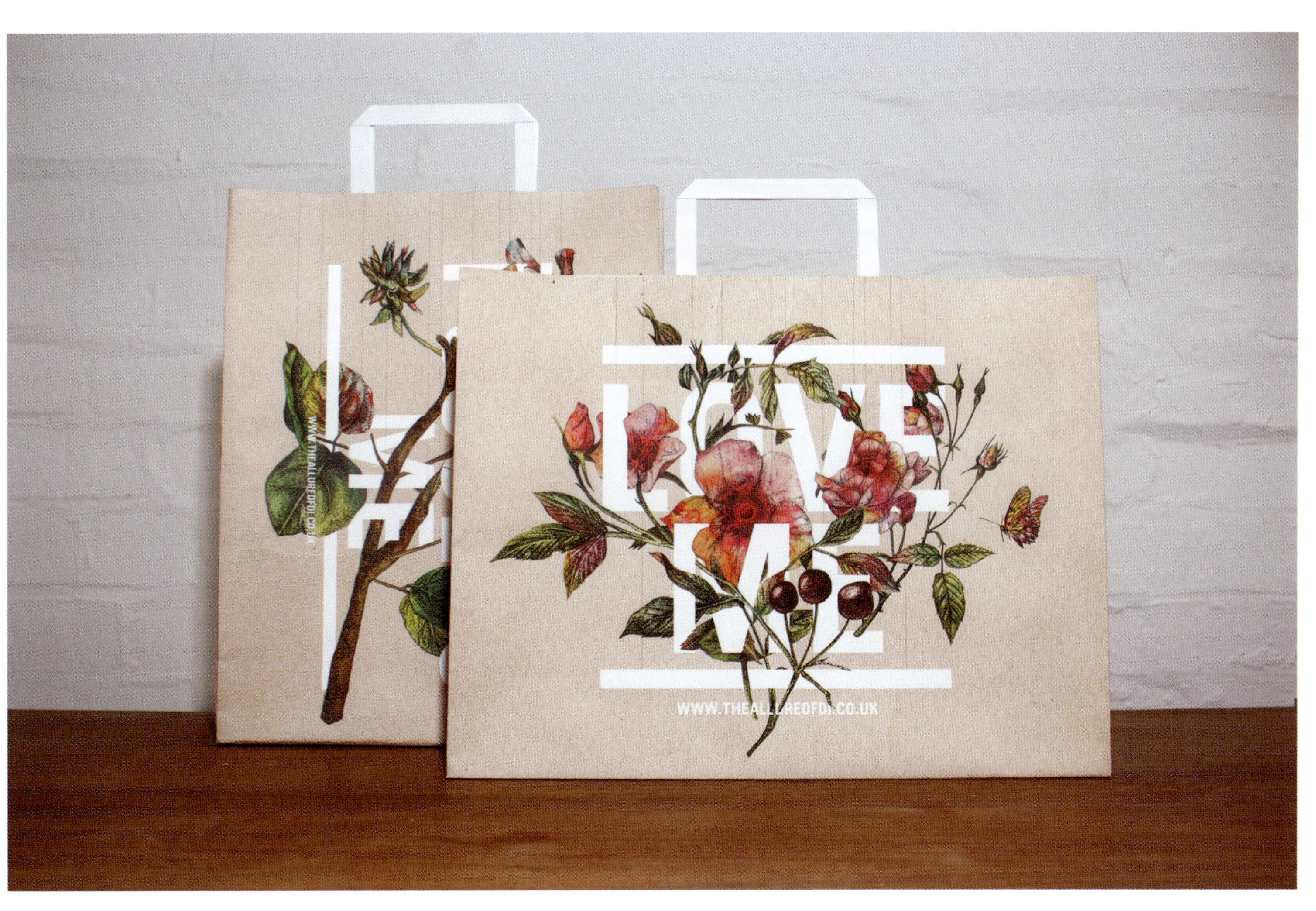

LOVE ME
WWW.THEALLUREOFDI.CO.UK

ACKNOWLEDGEMENTS

We would like to thank all the designers and contributers who have been involved in the production of this book. Their significant contribution is indispensable in the compilation of this book. We would also like to express our gratitude to all the producers for their invaluable opinions and assistance throughout this project. And to the many others whose names are not credited but have made specific input in this book, we thank you for your continuous support.

FUTURE COOPERATIONS: If you wish to participate in SendPoints' future projects and publications, please send your website or portfolio to editor01@sendpoints.cn